Reliability and Validity in Neuropsychological Assessment

Second Edition

CRITICAL ISSUES IN NEUROPSYCHOLOGY

Series Editors

Antonio E. Puente
University of North Carolina at Wilmington

Cecil R. Reynolds
*Texas A&M University
and Bastrop Mental Health Associates*

Reliability and Validity in Neuropsychological Assessment

Second Edition

Michael D. Franzen

Allegheny General Hospital
and Medical College of Pennsylvania/Hahnemann University
Pittsburgh, Pennsylvania

Kluwer Academic / Plenum Publishers
New York, Boston, Dordrecht, London, Moscow

Library of Congress Cataloging-in-Publication Data

Franzen, Michael D., 1954–
    Reliability and validity in neuropsychological assessment/Michael D. Franzen—2nd ed.
        p.   ; cm. — (Critical issues in neuropsychology)
    Includes bibliographical references and index.
    ISBN 0-306-46344-X
        1. Neuropsychological tests—Evaluation.   2. Neuropsychological tests—Validity.   I.
Title.   II. Series.
        [DNLM: 1. Neuropsychological Tests.   2. Neuropsychology—methods.   3.
Psychometrics—methods.   4. Reproducibility of Results.   5. Sensitivity and Specificity.
WL 141 F837r 2000]
    RC386.6.N48 F73 2000
    152—dc21

                                                                                    00-028725

ISBN 0-306-46344-X

 ©2000 Kluwer Academic/Plenum Publishers, New York
233 Spring Street, New York, New York 10013

http://www.wkap.nl/

10   9   8   7   6   5   4   3   2   1

A C.I.P. record for this book is available from the Library of Congress

Preface

Much has happened since the publication of the first edition of this book. Little of what has happened could have been predicted. The one accurate prediction was that clinical neuropsychology would continue to grow in terms of methods and knowledge as well as in importance in health care overall. The impact of managed care was not in the crystal ball. The rise in interest in the detection of response bias or in premorbid estimates was not seen in 1989. Both of those activities were viewed as being secondary and subsidiary to the "actual" testing. I did not foresee the rise in interest and sophistication in psychometric issues among clinical neuropsychologists, although certainly I am gratified by this development.

When I began my career, I had a great deal of difficulty trying to publish papers that were studies of reliability and validity, although certainly validity studies had a better shot at being accepted. Today, psychometrically based studies are routinely published in a newer journal, *The Clinical Neuropsychologist*, and to a somewhat lesser extent in other journals such as *Archives of Clinical Neuropsychology, Journal of Experimental and Clinical Neuropsychology*, and *Psychological Assessment*. Clinical neuropsychologists are more sophisticated in discussing issues of sensitivity, specificity, advanced concepts in reliability, and confirmatory factor analysis.

Writing the second edition of this book was a much more labor-intensive effort than the first edition. The names of certain of my colleagues would pop up time after time in my reviews of the journals. In fact, during some late nights I would silently curse the productivity of some of these colleagues whose output was slowing the completion of the book. Psychometric research is not sexy, but it has the potential to inform our clinical practice in an enormous way. Therefore, these researchers deserve our thanks, and in the morning light I would retract my nighttime curses. The first edition of this book did not initiate this wave of psychometric sophistication, but it did ride the crest. Other books (e.g., Mitrushina, Boone, & D'Elia, 1999; Spreen & Strauss, 1998) address the issues of normative information from a different perspective. The intent of this book is to review the extensive research and hopefully provide a direction for additional investigation.

To evaluate the degree to which the numbers produced by assessment possessed the characteristics of stability and meaningfulness, or of reliability and validity, experimental and mathematical methods were applied that had been developed in other areas of psychometrics (literally, the measurement of psychological functions). But because clinical neuropsychology still remained at least partly a medical endeavor, it was somewhat slower than some areas of psychological measurement to evaluate its instruments by psychometric methods. There were even some individuals who totally eschewed the use of assessment methods that produced numbers. That is not the case today. The practitioners who are most closely identified with psychometric methods are those clinical neuropsychologists who use a battery approach to assessment. But even those individuals who use a flexible approach, sometimes called a *process approach*, rely on smaller tests that produce numbers. It is difficult to find a contemporary clinical neuropsychologist who does not use at least a few standardized tests in evaluating a patient. The evaluation of the psychometric properties of clinical neuropsychological assessment instruments has assumed a more prominent position and a higher priority than it held previously.

The psychometric evaluation of assessment instruments is a continual activity. This is true, first of all, because psychometric theoreticians keep producing innovations. Second, the psychometric properties of the instruments depend on the characteristics of the subject populations. As individuals change or as different emphases develop for a population, the instruments need to be reevaluated. This book should be seen as a takeoff rather than as a summation point.

The purpose of this book is not to indict certain assessment instruments or to champion other instruments. Rather, the purpose is to identify areas of needed research. Recommendations regarding clinical use are made in certain cases; however, if we were to use only those instruments that have been completely evaluated and found to be completely satisfactory, our repertoire of assessment techniques would be very small indeed. This last statement is not meant to be a justification for the use of incompletely evaluated instruments or for the use of instruments that have been evaluated and found to lack reasonable reliability or to generate no valid interpretations. We have an obligation to choose the best instrument or to develop a better one. Some instruments may be useful in some situations and useless in others. We should use the results of research to guide our choice of assessment instruments.

It is hoped that this book will alert the clinical researcher to the need to conduct basic research into the psychometric properties of neuropsychological instruments. It is further hoped that clinicians will use the book to make decisions regarding the use of instruments for particular patients in particular situations. It is also hoped that students will be able to use this book to learn about instruments or to generate ideas for thesis or dissertation research.

Acknowledgments

I'd like to thank the coauthors of the first edition of this book, Robert Sawicki and Doug Robbins, who helped shape the initial manifestation. I'd like to acknowledge the enormous contributions of my colleagues in clinical neuropsychology, without whose work this book would not have been possible, or even necessary. I'd like to thank my editor, Mariclaire Cloutier, who showed great patience in awaiting the completion of the manuscript. Most of all I'd like to acknowledge Debbie, who showed great forbearance while I toiled, and Joe, Tim, and Rose who accepted Dad's preoccupation and who learned to write at their computers with professional journals propped open at the side.

Contents

Chapter 21

Preliminary Measurement Considerations in Clinical Neuropsychological Assessment

As the name implies, clinical neuropsychology draws from more than just one discipline. Looking at the name alone, however, gives a somewhat simplified view because more than just simply neurology and psychology comprise modern clinical neuropsychological practice. Current influences include behavioral therapy and assessment, internal medicine, rehabilitation, endocrinology, aphasiology, and public health, among others. Other sources of influence exist because clinical neuropsychology exists in a context of social and cultural variables. The development of clinical neuropsychological assessment techniques is influenced by referral, and to an increasing extent, reimbursement sources. The rise of managed care has affected the amount of time allowed for a neuropsychological evaluation as well as the procedures allowed. When the clinical neuropsychologist is given precertification for time periods less than he or she would like to use, the question faced is whether to truncate the evaluation using shorter procedures or to absorb the cost of nonreimbursed time. More focused instruments requiring less time become more heavily used. When the managed care reviewer denies certain tests as not being covered, the clinical neuropsychologist must either find an acceptable alternative or absorb the cost once again. There is a clear need to educate managed care professionals, and research regarding reliability and validity becomes even more important.

Partly because of the wide divergence of sources of clinical neuropsychology, a wide variety of assessment techniques and instruments have been used. The assessment methods involve everything from behavioral observation to timed pencil-and-paper tests. Many of the earlier assessment methods in clinical neuropsychology were derived from behavioral neurology and the medical model. These assessment instruments tend to be qualitative in nature and are scored largely on the basis of informal internal norms. Lately, there has been some activity aimed at standardizing these assessment procedures so that their use results in quantitative indices. In this way, many of the qualitative assessment procedures have become amenable to numerical analysis. Influences from managed care have increased the need for shorter, more accurate assessment techniques. Influences from forensic sources have increased the need to know about the diagnostic specificity of the instruments as well as brought into high focus the evaluation of effort.

During World War II, many experimental psychologists were pressed into service as part of the war effort. These psychologists formed one of the first substantial groups of what have come to be known as *clinical psychologists*. Clinical psychology had previously existed largely as a concept, but it was at this time that the expansion of clinical psychological activities accelerated. These wartime psychologists had been trained in laboratories and in the experimental method. Their conceptions of measurement had been formed largely by current psychometric theory. These psychologists brought their psychometric and experimental traditions to the clinical settings in which they found themselves or else adopted clinical techniques to their experimental methods. For example, A.L. Benton's early publications were on the use of the Rorschach test to detect malingering by experimentally manipulating the administration instructions (Benton, 1945). Many of the patients in these clinical settings were soldiers who had suffered some form of neurological impairment. It was this situation that was probably most responsible for the growth of psychometric and experimental influences on clinical neuropsychological assessment.

Today, clinical neuropsychological assessment has developed into a much broader and more sophisticated method than it had been in the past. There have also been developments in psychometric theory. Although classical test theory remains a primary influence on our conceptions of reliability and validity, psychometric theory is no longer associated only with classical test theory. There have been developments in measurement to include different forms of scaling, nonparametric as well as parametric statistics, and different theoretical conceptions of the process of measurement. As in any relationship between theory and practice, the movement from the theoretical to the practical side has been somewhat slow. However, as clinical neuropsychology becomes more aligned with the scientific field of psychology and psychological training, in contrast to its early background in the medical field, more clinical neuropsychologists will receive at least part of their training from psychometric and measurement theoreticians. This latter process will increase the quantitative sophistication of neuropsychological assessment.

We are not yet at the point where clinical neuropsychological assessment has become a field in which theory, science, and practice are successfully melded. Even where there are associations between theory and practice, the overlap may be minor. Many of the applications of psychometric theory to the evaluation of neuropsychological assessment instruments have occurred only in the area of classical test theory. However, we are seeing more applications of modern psychometric theory to the evaluation of neuropsychological assessment instruments. One example is the use of item response theory to evaluate the Knox Cube Test. More importantly, we are seeing a rational approach to evaluating neuropsychological assessment instruments. Not all "types" of reliability or validity need to be evaluated for each evaluation instrument. The choice of a design or paradigm within which to evaluate a neuropsychological assessment instrument should be as carefully pondered as the choice of an instrument for a particular clinical question.

There is not a hegemony of measurement theory in clinical neuropsychological assessment, and perhaps it is not necessary. There are several different types of assessment and measurement strategies. These types of assessment use standardized tests to differing degrees. Differences are also found in the extent to which parametric statistics have been used in analyses of the data resulting from the use of the assessment types. For example, many of the assessment strategies used by individuals who rely heavily on the clinical intuitive method associated with the behavioral neurology tradition result in qualitative information that is binary: The individual is either impaired or normal. The original intent of gathering this type of information was to uncover behavioral deficits that had a strict correspondence with localized lesions. Of course, not much in the way of statistical analyses is possible with this type of qualitative information. However, some assessment instruments sum the number of qualitative signs to produce a number that is amenable to statistical manipulation and analysis. The Benton Visual Retention Test is an example of such a test, and there is the additional possibility of performing a qualitative analysis on the type of error exhibited by the subject.

Other assessment instruments rely on the production of numbers related to summed errors over a set of homogeneous items. This approach is seen in the psychometric tradition represented most directly in neuropsychology by the work of Ralph Reitan. Here, the number is thought to represent the placement of an index along a continuum of skill. Higher numbers indicate that the person has a larger degree of skill (or, depending on the scaling direction, has committed a larger number of errors and therefore has a smaller degree of skill) than an individual who has produced a smaller score. The same rationale has been used in the development of many smaller tests of specific neuropsychological functions. The advantage of the battery approach is that it allows an analysis of the profile and multivariate relationships among the shorter tests that comprise the battery. In addition, because the tests in the battery have been normed on the same population, comparisons across subtest performances can be meaningfully interpreted.

A final approach is one that is unique and still somewhat controversial: the measurement strategy used in the Luria–Nebraska Neuropsychological Battery (LNNB). Although the LNNB was originally discussed as an attempt to use Luria's qualitative method in a standard psychometric framework, it became apparent that an even more different measurement strategy was possible. The scale scores of the LNNB are derived by summing qualitative errors and transformations of qualitatively different tasks into a set of single scores. The scales were originally headed by the names of the processes that were central to the various tasks, but the names were later removed in favor of numbering the scales. The scale scores do not represent homogeneous skills; instead, they can be used to make probabilistic statements about extratest behavior. The interpretation of the LNNB can be conducted by first examining scale elevations, then examining scale profiles, and then by conducting a qualitative analysis of individual item performance.

Perhaps some of these distinctions can be clarified by reference to a classification of measurement theories. Michell (1986) discussed three different theories of measurement with reference to acceptable statistics: representational theory, operational theory, and classical theory (not to be confused with classical test theory). At the risk of oversimplifying Michell's discussion, representational theory can be described as the use of numbers to represent the empirical relationships between the objects of measurement. Operational theory views measurement as an operation that produces numbers. Classical theory views measurement as the assessment of quantity. Here, numbers are not necessarily assigned; instead, numerical relationships are discovered.

In terms of these theories, the psychometric tradition can be seen to be embedded in the representational theory. The process of measurement results in numbers that reflect or represent a level of skill (or some other construct) that can be related to a level of some other skill when both skills are measured along the same scale. Or, alternately, the first number can be correlated with a number reflective of some other property, such as the degree of self-report anxiety. Representational theory applies only to single test scores. When the battery is interpreted on the basis of profiles, the applicable body of thought is classical theory. In profile interpretation, one goal is to uncover the numerical relationships among the subtests as well as between the subtest profiles and external indices such as the diagnostic group or indices of extratest behavior.

The measurement and production of numbers involved in summing qualitative signs are associated with operational theory. The operation of challenging the subject to perform certain behaviors and then summing the successes results in a number that does not necessarily reflect a skill, but that can be analyzed by means of statistical manipulations. The operational theory of measurement is also implicit in the use of the behavioral assessment techniques that have been applied mainly to the assessment of the functional levels of skill in neuropsychologically impaired individuals involved in a rehabilitation program. The score on a test of cooking behaviors is not interpreted as representing cooking skill per se. Rather, the score is thought to be related to overall success in performing chains of behaviors embedded in some aspect of independent functioning.

The measurement theory implicit in the LNNB appears to be a combination of operational theory and classical theory. The overlap with operational theory is apparent from the preceding discussion regarding the summing of qualitative signs. The relationship to classical theory results from the lack of reliance on a definite construct that homogeneously underlies the procedure and from the use of profile and multivariate strategies for interpretation. Elevations on certain scales in conjunction with lower scores on other scales are thought to be associated with certain diagnoses.

Despite the heterogeneity of underlying measurement theories, there is a common link across many neuropsychological assessment strategies: the production of numbers. The numbers open the possibility of mathematically analyzing the data and investigating the characteristics of the instruments in an empirical and systematic fashion. Not all neuropsychological assessment strategies can be evaluated in this manner. Notable exceptions are the interview and the history. However, for those assessment strategies for which numerical analysis is appropriate, it is important to conduct those analyses to better understand the instruments, and ultimately to better understand brain–behavior relationships and our patients. The utility and accuracy of information and interpretations derived from the interview and history need to be evaluated as well; however, the methods used to evaluate them are markedly different from those methods used to evaluate the quantitative assessment methods.

A few words may be said here about the intended purpose of this book. This book is not intended as a step-by-step manual by which a person can engage in investigations of the reliability and validity of neuropsychological assessment instruments. Instead, it is intended to highlight pertinent issues and to alert clinical researchers and clinicians to issues that need to be dealt with when they are researching or evaluating neuropsychological instruments.

The discussions rely to some extent on prior knowledge of psychometric theory and methods. It is assumed that the reader has some familiarity with factor analysis. Of course, it is also assumed that the reader has some familiarity with neuropsychological assessment. To that extent, the book reflects certain biases regarding what basic knowledge is required of the modern clinical neuropsychologist. It is true that the use of standardized psychometric instruments is not preferred over the use of instruments that require intuitive interpretation or instruments that are scored qualitatively. It is also true that not only psychometrically standardized instruments and interpretation systems have a place in clinical neuropsychological assessment. Qualitative methods are necessary and complementary to psychometric methods. However, the psychometric methods are essential components of neuropsychological assessment.

Some statements regarding the choice of instruments reviewed in the second part of the book are also necessary. The instruments were chosen on the basis of a few principles. First, the procedures must constitute part of contemporary clinical neuropsychological practice. Second, they must be amenable to empirical, quantitative investigation. Third, there must be published research evaluating their psychometric properties. In the library research for this book, it is possible that certain instruments favored by other clinical neuropsychologists have been overlooked. Undoubtedly, these omissions will be identified in the written reviews of the book; such is the nature of public scrutiny, and the final step in the scientific method is public scrutiny and debate. However, not all readers will be able to publish their opinions, and of these individuals, personal communication is requested.

Another limitation on the instruments chosen for this book involves the traditional conception of neuropsychological assessment. Many instruments used by clinical neuro-psychologists who are interested in ecological issues and in the treatment of neurologically impaired individuals are not represented here. Since the publication of the first edition of this book, there has been increased interest in ecological issues. As even more clinical neuropsychologists become interested in these areas, we may see a shift toward the use of other instruments and the development of new instruments to measure variables, such as aspects of interpersonal behavior, that are not typically and traditionally seen as being in the purview of clinical neuropsychologists. This shift would be welcomed as the role of the clinical neuropsychologist changes from that of a consultant to surgeon to that of a treating professional responsible for certain aspects of a patient's overall health care. Unfortunately, at the present time, there is not sufficient material to allow including those instruments in this book. Exceptions exist for those instruments that have a long history of use by clinical neuropsychologists, such as the Minnesota Multiphasic Personality Inventory (MMPI). Therefore, there are reviews of the use of the Rorschach and the MMPI in the second part of the book. However, reviews of other instruments will have to wait until their frequency of use in clinical neuropsychological practice increases sufficiently to justify their inclusion.

Since the time of the publication of the first edition of this book, there have been many developments, some of which could have been predicted, some of which were surprising. The impact of managed care could not have been predicted in 1989. Some of the influences of managed care may be unpredictable even yet. Managed care calls for shorter evaluations, but reviewers are also more likely to authorize the use of standard batteries such as the Halstead–Reitan or Luria–Nebraska. The increase of interest in cognitive neuroscience-based instruments and computerized testing was predictable. Computerized testing has increased at a steady rate. This rise then suggests new areas of research. What is the relationship between computerized and standard administration forms of tests? If tests are administered in mixed formats across time, how does that affect the psychometric proper-ties? At least one study suggests that test–retest reliabilities may be lower when mixed administration formats are used than when the same format is used on both occasions (Campbell et al., 1999). These are all part of the future of research and practice in clinical neuropsychology.

General and Theoretical Considerations in the Assessment of Reliability

The term *reliability* is often used to describe the temporal stability of a set of measurement procedures. Other frequent uses of the term are related to internal consistency and agreement among different users of the procedures. These different usages all relate to a single concept, namely, the estimation of the influence of error on the scores resulting from the use of the test or set of procedures. A perfectly reliable test is a test that measures without error. Error-free measurement is a practical impossibility. Instead, it is an ideal to which test authors and developers attempt approximations. As well as being an impossible ideal to attain in a practical sense, reliability is also an impossible concept to evaluate directly. All of the methods and designs discussed in Chapter 3 are able only to estimate the reliability of the test. As will be seen in the more complete discussion in Chapter 3, the methods and designs are attempts to estimate the degree of error that influences test scores by systematically varying the possible sources of error. The success of the endeavor is related to the quality of the methods and designs and to the ability of the researcher to comprehensively describe the possible sources of error.

The purpose of this chapter is to consider the concept of *reliability* itself. The most common form of reliability evaluation involves obtaining test scores on two occasions, under two conditions, or from two examiners, and correlating the two sets of scores. The correlation coefficients describe the extent of covariation between the two sets of scores, and the square of the coefficient describes the amount of shared variance. All of the usual methods and designs used to estimate reliability are based in classical test theory and depend on this theory for their assumptions. The major assumption is that the observed score is composed of a true score term and an error score term, and furthermore, that the error term values are independent of each other and normally distributed. More recent developments in test theory, such as Rasch model measurement and generalizability theory, have different assumptions and require a substantial rethinking of the notion of error-free measurement.

ITEM RESPONSE THEORY

Perhaps the earliest form of item response theory (IRT) was contained in Frederick Lord's dissertation that was later published in monograph form as *a theory of test scores*

(1952). In that book, Lord described his dissatisfaction with classical test theory, particularly in regard to its assumptions. Lord demonstrated that, when the assumptions are made to fit the test-taking situation, rather than the other way around, there are startling implications for the relationship of ability to the distribution of test scores and error terms. In particular, Lord felt that it could not be assumed that the relationship of ability to the distribution of scores was linear, nor could it be assumed that errors were independent of true score. There has been much controversy regarding whether IRT or classical test theory best fits the specifics of most test situations. We will not attempt to resolve this controversy. However, by surveying some of the advances in IRT, we find some implications for clinical neuropsychological assessment, particularly in the way in which we regard reliability.

One of the most important differences between classical test theory and IRT lies in their respective focus for analysis. Classical test theory uses test scores as the unit of analysis. Test scores are usually an arithmetic sum or average or some weighted sum of component items. The focus of IRT is the item itself. Clinical neuropsychological assessment is a mixed breed of psychological assessment traditions. The influential assessment methods have included the qualitative analysis of discrete performance on individual tasks, as exemplified by the behavioral neurology tradition, as well as the quantitative analysis of test scores, as exemplified by the psychometric traditions used by R.M. Reitan and others. However, most evaluations of the reliability of neuropsychological assessment procedures have been limited to applications of the classical test theory to summative test scores. This is true even of the qualitative assessment procedures, in which the subject's performances on various procedures are summed into a single score. Even where psychometric methods are used, IRT allows one to evaluate the single items that are the focus of the response pattern analysis that takes place following interpretation of the summative score.

Classical test theory is the ascendant form of psychometric theory taught in graduate psychology programs. Most clinical neuropsychologists are familiar with classical test theory. Item response theory is less well known among general psychologists (that is, among nonpsychometric specialists), and a brief overview is appropriate. Contrary to the usual assumption that ability has a linear relationship to test score, Lord (1952) gave a mathematical proof that the relationship was actually curvilinear. In subsequent publications, Lord refined his notions. An excellent discussion of current thought on the topic can be found in Lord (1980). Other relevant publications at a level appropriate for clinical neuropsychologists include Baker (1985), Hambleton (1983), and Andrich (1988).

Aside from the level of ability of the subject in performing the skill under consideration, IRT posits three influences on item score values: the guessing parameter (the probability that a subject completely lacking in the skill will answer correctly), the item difficulty parameter (the level of skill where the item has .5 discrimination), and the item discrimination parameter (the probability of a correct response at a given level of difficulty). In graphing the relationships among these variables, we obtain the item characteristic curve (ICC). The ICC is the cumulative or additive shape of the various logistic functions that describe the relationships among the variables for differing levels of ability.

Perhaps the most common model used in practical applications of IRT is the one-parameter logistic or Rasch model (Andrich, 1988). The multiple applications of the Rasch model are due, in part, to the work of Wright (e.g., Wright, 1977). It is also due to the model's relative simplicity. Only one parameter is allowed (or assumed) to vary, namely, item difficulty. The two-parameter normal-ogive model allows items to vary along two dimensions: difficulty and discrimination. Finally, the three-parameter model, which adds the dimension of variability in guessing, is perhaps a more complete model, but it is also more complex, and computer programs using it to analyze data are not readily available.

The advantage of IRT of focusing on the level of the item as the unit of analysis has already been mentioned. There are other advantages, depending on the appropriateness of IRT to a given data set. First, if a model is accurately specified for a population, the parameters estimated from various samples drawn from that population will be linearly related. This characteristic is known as *invariance of the item parameters*. A second advantage is known as *invariance of ability parameters*. Even if the estimation of the parameters has been based on two subjects' performance on two different items, the ability parameters can be compared across the two individuals, assuming that the two items measure the same dimension of ability. A third advantage is perhaps the most important for clinical neuropsychology. It is related to the fact that IRT allows estimates of the precision of measurement or the degree of error for different levels of ability.

In clinical neuropsychological assessment, the ability of the subjects varies greatly. There are some conditions, such as advanced dementia, in which there are generally uniform and severe decrements in performance. There are also conditions, such as those that may result from infiltrative tumor or cerebral vascular accidents, in which a decrement in a single skill may be present alongside normal or even superior performance in another skill. In addition, neuropsychological skills may be conceptualized as existing along a continuum of level of performance. An adequate test should contain items that differ in difficulty, so that it will detect the early signs of degenerative disorders or document the incremental improvements following injury and treatment. Historically, clinical neuropsychological assessment did not need to attend to these considerations. The main questions were related to the diagnosis of organicity or, in more sophisticated settings, to the localization of the lesion. Answering these questions required little in the way of reliability assessment. The items were usually scored as either correct or incorrect. If a given item was performed incorrectly, organicity was diagnosed. If a given item was failed and another item was passed, localization was suggested. Now clinical neuropsychologists are asked to measure the level of skill to help predict behavior in an open environment, or they are asked to measure changes in skill level over time, and clinical neuropsychological assessment instruments need to be evaluated for differing levels of accuracy at differing levels of skill.

Weiss (1985) discussed some of the implications of IRT for clinical assessment conducted by computer. An important current concern of clinical neuropsychological assessment is accurately determining the levels of ability across different skills. Doing so may require uneconomical uses of both the examiner's and the patient's time. In addition, increasing the time required for an assessment may decrease the motivation of a subject to comply with the test procedures. Adaptive testing—that is, testing that conforms in the order of the presentation of items—is one method of reducing the amount of time needed to assess an individual. Item response theory will allow the construction of computer programs that evaluate subjects, choosing the order of presentation on the basis of the accuracy of the subject's responses to past items.

GENERALIZABILITY THEORY

Generalizability theory is concerned with the systematic description of sources of variance that impact on the reliability and validity of measures. The original statement of this set of concepts can be found in Cronbach, Rajaratnam, and Gleser (1963). Generalizability theory was proposed to overcome objections to what were seen as shortcomings in classical test theory. As noted previously, classical test theory assumes that the act of measurement results in obtaining a true score combined with an error term, and that one of the goals of statistical analysis of the obtained scores is to estimate the amount of variance associated with error or uncontrolled factors. The methods involved in this estimation process required that observations be obtained under equivalent conditions (e.g., the same test administered twice or parallel forms administered to the same subjects). The shortcomings of classical theory were most apparent in direct behavioral observation, where exactly the same conditions were unlikely to be found in different measurement situations.

Cronbach et al. (1963) examined the reasons for reliability estimation to determine whether some alternate to classical theory existed for behavioral observations. They decided that the reason an investigator estimates the reliability of a measure is to facilitate generalization from the measure to some other set of conditions. Estimating test–retest reliability is a method of determining the extent to which one can generalize from the scores obtained in one temporal condition to the scores likely to be obtained in another temporal condition. Similarly, we are interested in interrater reliability because we wish to know the extent to which we can generalize from the scores obtained by one rater to the scores obtained by another rater. Because the apparent raison d'etre of reliability studies was to estimate the degree of generalizability possible, Cronbach et al. (1963) decided that a more useful form of analysis would focus on generalizability. The approach taken by these authors involves a systematic manipulation of the variables thought to impinge on generalizability and a measurement of the effects of such manipulations on values of the test scores.

The advances allowed by generalizability theory included the capacity to test the statistical significance of the effects of undesirable sources of variance. These advances can most clearly be seen in the later book by Cronbach, Gleser, Nanda, and Rajaratnam (1972). The overall idea was to systematically vary the sources of "error" and thus to allow the researcher to partial out the sources of variance in a factorial design. Cronbach et al. (1972) examined the forms of reliability and validity and subsequently relabeled the forms as universes of generalizability.

Here, the value of a score is determined by the conditions under which the score is obtained. There is no single set of conditions, known as *facets* in generalizability theory, that needs to be considered in the evaluation of every assessment instrument. Instead, the researcher is responsible for determining the sufficiency and appropriateness of each set of facets. Some examples of facets are observers, items, test forms, time, and contexts. The researcher also specifies the universe to which he or she wishes to generalize. The universe contains the various levels of the facets to which the assessment instrument will be applied. For example, a neuropsychological assessment instrument may not have alternate forms and may be used in psychiatric and neurological populations, may require active participation by the examiner so that the examiner's behavior is part of the eliciting stimuli for the test, and may be designed to be used to measure change across time. In this case, the relevant facets include observers, occasions, and the two populations, but not parallel forms.

The basic requirements of generalizability theory are that the universe be described unambiguously, that a person's score in one condition be independent of whether the person has been observed in another condition, and that the scores be on an interval level. Neither the content of the universe nor the statistical properties of the scores within conditions have any bearing on the use of generalizability theory. The analysis results in the computation of a generalizability coefficient, which is the squared coefficient of correlation between the observed score and the universe score. The universe score may be defined as the mean score over all relevant observations. Two types of error are possible under generalizability theory: the first type includes all components of variance; the second type includes only those components that are considered extraneous and whose influence is undesirable to the researcher in that situation.

Generalizability theory provides an experimental design for the evaluation of assessment procedures. When the analysis uncovers statistical significance associated with a certain dimension, it is possible that there will be inaccuracies in generalizing across that dimension. In a G (generalizability) study, the statistical significance of the interaction between two independent variables indicates that generalizability over one dimension in the interaction is variable for different levels of the second dimension. In a D (decision) study, the statistical significance of the interaction between two independent variables indicates that predictions made regarding the effects of manipulating the first variable are variables for different levels of the second variable. This conclusion may seem confusing at first, but it is actually consistent with the way in which statistically significant interaction terms are interpreted in normal factorial designs. The difference is that now there are implications either for the reliability of an instrument or for the validity of the inferences drawn from the use of the instrument. This discussion has concentrated on the evaluation of single scores; however, it should be pointed out that Cronbach et al. (1972) provided methods for applying their strategies to composite scores and multiscore tests.

Generalizability theory considers both reliability and validity and can be seen to provide a general model for the evaluation of both in a single conceptual scheme. Broadly speaking, a G study involves recording data that will allow estimates of the components of variance relevant to the use of a given measurement strategy. A D study involves recording data that will outline the limits of validity of certain conclusions or decisions based on the use of the instrument. The analog of a G study is a reliability investigation, and the analog of a D study is a validity investigation.

To use generalizability theory, we must consider which facets are important in clinical neuropsychological assessment. There is no easy answer to this question. The important facets vary for each instrument and for each use to which the instrument is put. Many clinical neuropsychological assessment instruments involve a considerable amount of interactive behavior between the examiner and the subject. For those instruments, the observer is an important facet. For neuropsychological assessment instruments for which it is important to measure change over time, the facet of occasion is important. For those instruments that are used to assess the level of skill along a continuum or in different diagnostic groups, the facet of population is important.

Although the formal characteristics of generalizability theory may seem to be imposing, the statistical methodology in applying generalizability theory is actually quite traditional. Shavelson and Webb (1991) provide an excellent small volume that describes the basic statistical methodology, namely analysis of variance (ANOVA) procedures, that underlie the application of generalizability theory. These authors make the point that dependability refers to the accuracy with which an observed score can be assumed to be representative of the average score obtained under all possible conditions for that subject. These conditions include event occasion, rater identity, and test form, among others.

CONCLUSIONS

Although the concept of *reliability* is taught to psychologists in training as if it were a clearly defined concept with standard measurement procedures, it is actually a somewhat slippery concept that needs to be carefully conceptualized. Furthermore, the empirical estimation of reliability requires planning and active decision-making. With the exception of the Knox Cube Test (Stone & Wright, 1980)—for IRT and the Memory Assessment Scales (Williams, 1991)—for generalizability theory, the estimation of the reliability of clinical neuropsychological assessment instruments has been based largely on classical test theory. This tendency is consistent with trends in general psychological assessment, but it may be insufficient to provide the information required to choose an instrument for a particular situation.

The degree of reliability is likely to vary at the different levels of skill of the individual. One way to deal with this variability is through the use of local norms (Elliott & Bretzing, 1980). However, this procedure is costly and time-consuming and does not allow an estimation of the amount of variability associated with different populations or different geographical locations. On the other hand, the use of IRT allows the estimation of reliability at different levels of skill with the use of a single experimental sample, and the use of generalizability theory allows an estimation of the amount of variance associated with attempts to generalize across different populations.

Another benefit of IRT is the ability to estimate reliability for a single item. This fact is very important for clinical neuropsychology because here interpretation is often based on a consideration of performance on individual items. This is true both of assessment instruments that have been designed by traditional psychometric construction methods of homogeneous content and varying difficulty level, such as the Wechsler intelligence scales, and of instruments that have been designed by less traditional construction methods, such as the Luria–Nebraska, in which items are grouped into scales on the basis of shared central skill areas. In the first case, interpretation might be based partly on the point at which the performance of the subject starts to fail. In the second case, interpretation might be more directly based on a comparison of failed and passed items.

The benefits of the use of generalizability theory are partly related to the fact that it allows the researcher to take measurement error out of the realm of the ineffable and imprecisely estimable and to place it squarely in the arena of manipulatable and observable phenomena. The use of generalizability theory also causes clinical neuropsychologists to be more conservative in their interpretation of instrument evaluation results and to be more cautious in their predictions to situations outside the research setting.

None of the preceding statements are intended to argue for the replacement of traditional reliability estimation methods by either IRT or generalizability theory. Instead, the argument is for the inclusion of both of these newer methods with the older methods. Because reliability is abstract, we can understand it better and more completely through the use of multiple estimation strategies. This book contains test reviews and critiques that focus mainly on the evaluation of reliability and validity as traditionally conceptualized.

These reviews offer one way of understanding the numbers that result from the use of the measurement strategies. The innovative strategies discussed in this chapter represent different approaches that provide complementary ways of understanding the numbers, and that will ultimately increase our understanding of our patients.

The previous edition of this book predicted greater acceptance and assimilation of the newer methods (IRT and generalizability theory) into psychometric research regarding clinical neuropsychological assessment. The reality has been slower. There is no need to discard the traditional methods; in fact, these methods provide us with essential information. But is it hoped that the application of the newer methodologies will result in greater sophistication and technical advancement.

3

Practical and Methodological Considerations Regarding Reliability

Reliability refers to the level of consistency or stability in the values of the scores that an instrument elicits. Reliability has different manifestations and methods of evaluation. It is possible to speak of split-half reliability, test–retest reliability, or alternate-forms reliability. Although these types of reliability require different methods of measurement, they are all ways of indexing the amount of variance in a test that is the result of error in measurement. Thus, reliability measurement is an attempt to estimate the percentage of error variance (Anastasi, 1982).

Another commonality of these forms of reliability is that they all involve the computation of a measure of association, agreement, or concordance. In split-half reliability, a computation relates the score from one half of the test to the score from the other half. In the test-retest method, the score obtained on one occasion is related to the score obtained on another occasion. This chapter considers the concept of reliability in the context of the statistical computations used to estimate a measure of reliability, as well as the forms of reliability and their related methodologies.

First, it is necessary to examine some of the broader issues that arise in the discussion of reliability. The present conceptualization of reliability as the estimate of error in measurement is formulated from classical test theory. There are more modern conceptualizations of reliability such as in item response theory or generalizability theory, but for now the discussion is confined to classical test theory. The methods of classical test theory are generally simple and are given an excellent exposition in Gulliksen (1987). The theory of classical test theory is, at its base, simple. A given score is thought to consist of two parts: the true score and the error. The true score is the actual value attained by a given individual on the construct if it were to be measured completely accurately by the test. The error is the value of the extraneous influences on the measurement process.

For example, an individual may receive a score of 96 on a test that measures mathematical ability. This individual's true score might actually be 97. However, because the individual had not had much sleep the night before, the score was lowered by 2 points. Because the individual guessed correctly on a couple of items, the score was raised by 4 points. Because the test did not assess all areas of mathematical ability equally and instead was loaded more highly on an ability (say, trigonometry) with which the individual was not very familiar, his or her score was lowered by another 3 points. The individual then ends up

15

with a measured score of 96. The error component of the observed score may be comprised of more than one influence. In addition, these influences may either lower or raise the observed score.

All of these fluctuations in score are subsumed under the rubric *error*. The error portion of the measured score contains all of those influences that cause the measured score to deviate from the true score. In general, reliability estimates are attempts to measure the proportion of variance that is due to these extraneous, usually unstable, influences. Reliability may therefore be thought of as the degree to which a measurement instrument is able to consistently elicit a stable score from an individual. An important consequence of this definition is that reliability is not binary; rather, it is continuous. A test itself is not reliable or unreliable, but it can possess a low or a high degree of reliability.

Two different forms of error can lower the reliability of a test (Carmines & Zeller, 1979). Random errors are those extraneous influences that fluctuate over different occasions. An example of random error in neuropsychological testing is the influence of the time of day. As another example, the performance of a child tested at school is likely to be different on a Monday morning than on a Friday afternoon.

Nonrandom error is the result of those influences that systematically affect the observed score. Nonrandom error always raises or lowers the observed score to the same extent. For example, an individual's scores on the Wechsler Adult Intelligence Scale-Revised (WAIS-R) may be consistently lower than her or his scores on the WAIS. Because of nonrandom error, one of these forms may be over- or underestimating this person's IQ.

The concept of reliability poses some special problems for neuropsychological assessment instruments. An individual's score on a neuropsychological examination would not always be expected to remain stable, as for example, in the case of serial testing of an individual who had recently suffered a blow to the head. On the contrary, one would expect that the scores would improve over time as, for example, the edema subsided and as the individual learned to compensate for impaired abilities. The important consideration is that, for reliable scores, one would not expect the values to change in the absence of outside influences.

Brown (1970) defined reliability as the ratio of true variance in test scores to the total variance. This definition has its roots in the psychometric tradition. It will help us determine an appropriate statistical format for the evaluation of reliability. In a behavioral sense, reliability can be defined as the ability of a test to elicit a stable performance from the subject in the absence of outside influences. This definition can help us to conceptualize the observable referents of reliability.

STATISTICAL METHODOLOGY IN RELIABILITY MEASUREMENT

Let us now turn to a discussion of the different statistical methods of measuring reliability. Generally speaking, reliability is measured by computing some form of a correlation coefficient, usually a Pearson product moment coefficient. Some readers will recognize that, given our definition of reliability as the consistency of scores, an appropriate statistical model might be some form of analysis of variance. After all, the analysis of variance is well suited to determining the differences in two sets of observations. However, it actually tests for the difference between the means of the two groups of observations. It is possible for the individual scores to change drastically without affecting the analysis of variance as long as the group means remained relatively unchanged.

Using the correlation coefficient as the index of reliability helps us to address some of these problems. The correlation coefficient examines the extent to which the two sets of observations vary together. That is, a correlation coefficient keeps intact the differences between two paired observations instead of combining them in some group statistic. But the correlation coefficient does not reflect the difference in the value level of the observations. For example, if we take a set of observations and add 20 points to each and then correlate the second (created) set with the original set, we obtain a perfect correlation coefficient of 1.0.

The use of a correlation coefficient, therefore, is not perfect either. However, it is preferable to the use of the analysis of variance. One reason for this preference is that the correlation coefficient provides an index of the stability of the position of the observation in the distribution of scores. Second, its focus is on the individual observation instead of on the group mean. If there is a question regarding changes in level from one set of observations to the second, an analysis of variance (or in some cases, the use of a chi-square or other nonparametric statistic) can be performed in addition to a calculation of the correlation coefficient, or else a simple examination of the group means may help to answer questions related to level. In fact, the optimum reliability evaluation may include both correlational procedures and analysis of variance procedures.

There is more than one correlation coefficient, and the choice of which to use must be made on the basis of the characteristics of the data (Carroll, 1961). The most popular coefficient is the well-known Pearson product–moment correlation coefficient. The Pearson product–moment coefficient is computed by first calculating standardized deviation scores for each of the observations and then summing the cross-products of the deviation scores and dividing by the number of observations. This algorithm results in a number that ranges from 1.0 to −1.0. A zero indicates that there is no linear relationship between the two sets of observations; 1.0 indicates that, as the values in one set increase, the values in the other set increase accordingly; and −1.0 indicates that, as the values in one set increase, the values in the other set decrease. The assumptions of the Pearson product–moment coefficient include:

1. The relationship between the two sets of observations is linear.
2. The error terms are uncorrelated.
3. The error terms are normally distributed with a mean of zero.
4. The independent variable is uncorrelated with the error term.

The Pearson product–moment coefficient is relatively robust to violations of some of its assumptions, such as normality and equal-interval measurement (Havlicek & Peterson, 1977). However, violations of the other assumptions sometimes result in an inflation of the value of the coefficient. Therefore, it is best to use the Pearson product–moment coefficient when one is relatively sure that the assumptions are met.

In addition, the Pearson product–moment coefficient is most accurate when the data it describes are continuous, are of interval level, and have reasonable variability. The use of the Pearson product–moment coefficient with categorical data results in an overestimation of the correlation between the two variables under consideration. The fewer the categories, the larger the overestimation. The use of the Pearson product–moment coefficient with data with restricted range presents the other side of the problem. Restriction of range (or lack of variability) results in attenuation of the value of the correlation coefficient.

When the data to be correlated are dichotomous, it is better to calculate the phi coefficient, which is computed on the basis of the information contained in a 2×2 contingency table constructed from the two levels of each of the variables. Phi can be computed from the entries in a 2×2 contingency table as follows:

$$\text{Phi} = (a + b)(c + d)(a + c)(b + d) \tag{1}$$

where a is the entry in the upper left cell of a 2×2 contingency table, b is the entry in the upper right cell, c is the entry in the lower left cell, and d is the entry in the lower right cell (Hays, 1973).

When the data to be correlated are dichotomous in one set of observations and are continuous in the other, then the point–biserial coefficient should be used. Both the phi coefficient and the point–biserial coefficient are versions of the product–moment coefficient, which can be used when the characteristics of the data do not match the assumptions of the Pearson product–moment, but for which it is necessary to obtain an estimate of the product–moment coefficient (Nunnally, 1978). An extension of the point–biserial coefficient is the tetrachoric correlation. This coefficient is computed when both variables are dichotomous but the researcher is interested in an estimate of what the product–moment correlation would be if the variables were continuous.

The next two indices to be discussed (Spearman's rank-order coefficient and Kendall's tau) are not, strictly speaking, correlation coefficients. They are actually descriptors of the extent to which the data tend toward monotonicity as well as of the direction of the relationship between the two sets of data (Hays, 1973). Monotonicity refers to the degree to which the observations on two variables are similarly ranked. A monotone-increasing relationship is one in which an increase in one variable is accompanied by an increase in the other. A monotone-decreasing relationship is one in which increases in one variable are accompanied by decreases in the other. Monotonic relationships are not necessarily linear. Therefore, these two statistics are also applied in those cases where the relationship between the two variables cannot be assumed to be linear.

The Spearman rank-order coefficient is calculated by treating the rank orderings as numbers and calculating the correlation between these two ranks, for example, between the rank of Subject A at time 1 and again at time 2. Under conditions of a bivariate normal distribution, the Spearman rank-order coefficient can be used as an estimate of the Pearson product–moment coefficient. However, in those cases, it is more convenient to calculate the product–moment coefficient.

The Kendall tau is calculated by first counting the number of times the pairs invert, that is, the number of times when that rank order of the two observations is not the same in the two sets of observations. This information is then used in the following formula:

$$\text{Tau} = \frac{2(C - D)}{n(n - 1)} \tag{2}$$

where C is the number of concordant pairs, D is the number of discordant pairs, and n is the sample size. The Kendall tau may be interpreted as a proportion of agreements to disagreements in the two rank orders. Neither Spearman's rank-order coefficient nor Kendall's tau

test when factor analysis is used. The first, called *coefficient theta*, is used in principal components analysis and can be interpreted as a form of Cronbach's coefficient alpha. Coefficient theta is an estimate of the maximum value of alpha (Greene & Carmines, 1980). The second statistic, called *coefficient omega*, is used in common factor analysis and can also be interpreted as a form of alpha. However, omega provides an estimate of the internal consistency reliability averaged across all of the common factors that arise in the analysis.

Clinical neuropsychological assessment instruments sometimes rely on a consideration of profiles in interpreting the results. For those multiscale instruments of which this is true, it may be important to have some estimate of the reliability of the profile. Conger and Lipshitz (1973) and Conger (1974) have provided some formulas for this purpose. Budescu (1980) offers four methods of calculating similarity among profiles, each of which could be used in a test–retest design to evaluate the stability of cognitive profiles. These formulas have not been used in evaluating clinical neuropsychological instruments with the exception of the Wechsler Intelligence Scale for Children—Revised. However, this is an important area that needs to be addressed.

Still another form of reliability refers to the stability of test scores obtained across examiners. There are two concepts involved in the determination of the stability of scores across raters. *Rater reliability* refers to the stability of the position of individuals in their respective distributions. Therefore, rater reliability is most appropriately measured by some form of a correlation coefficient. *Rater agreement* refers to the extent to which there is stability in the actual scores assigned to individuals. Both rater reliability and rater agreement are important in those cases in which the score of an individual is not arrived at totally objectively but is instead determined by some judgment on the part of the examiner. There are several measures of rater agreement, and the choice of one depends on the scaling characteristics of the ratings, the number of scoring categories possible, and the way in which agreement and disagreement are defined (Tinsley & Weiss, 1975). In addition, Zwick (1988) recommended assessing the marginal homogeneity of the raters. If the raters have similar marginals, the use of a coefficient derived by Scott (1955) is suggested instead.

INTERPRETATION OF RELIABILITY INFORMATION

When choosing a test, it is important to evaluate it on the basis of its psychometric properties, including its reliability. Therefore, it is important to consider the meaning of the reliability coefficient in relation to the test. The type and degree of reliability expected are based on a careful consideration of the purpose of the test as well as on a careful consideration of the construct that the test purports to measure. Most neuropsychological tests seek to measure basic intellectual and cognitive abilities. Therefore, most neuropsychological test procedures could be expected to exhibit a large degree of test–retest reliability. However, the degree of internal consistency reliability varies with the theoretical homogeneity of the construct measured by the test.

The magnitude of the reliability coefficient depends partly on the characteristics of the sample for which the coefficient is calculated. If the sample from which the coefficient is derived has limited variability, the coefficient will be attenuated because of the effects of the restriction of range. A sample that has a wide range of abilities associated with the construct will exhibit greater reliability than will a more homogeneous sample.

In addition, reliability is influenced by other characteristics of the group. The result of this influence is the existence of different reliability estimates for different groups. Therefore, it is important to examine the reliability estimate for the group relevant to the assessment at hand.

Adequate reliability is important if one is to interpret the score as reflecting an accurate measurement of the targeted construct. Another concept in the interpretation of reliability involves the standard error of measurement. *Reliability* refers to the stability of scores. *Standard error of measurement* refers to the significance of the differences between scores. Thus, it is affected by both the stability and the accuracy of the measurement. It can be used to interpret scores only from one individual, not across individuals. The standard error of measurement is calculated by means of the formula

$$SE_{meas} = SD_t(1 - r_{tt}) \tag{3}$$

where SD is the standard deviation of the test score and r_{tt} is the reliability of the test. By adding the standard error of measurement to the obtained score at one end and subtracting it at the other end, one can generate a confidence interval. The true score will be in this interval 68% of the time. As the standard deviation increases or the reliability decreases, the standard error of measurement increases.

The interpretation of score differences for the same individual is another important issue. One may wish to know whether the difference between an individual's score on the WAIS-R Performance scale is significantly different from that same individual's score on the WAIS-R Verbal scale. The statistic that can answer that question, the standard error of the difference, can be calculated by the use of either the standard error of measurement of the two scales or the reliability of the two scales. In the first formula, the standard error of differences between the two scales is expressed as the square root of the sum of the squared standard error of measurement for each of the two scales:

$$SE_{diff} = SE2_{meas} 1 + SE2_{meas} 2 \tag{4}$$

In the second formula, the standard error of differences is expressed as

$$SE_{diff} = SD(2 - r_{11} - r_{22}) \tag{5}$$

where SD is the standard deviation of the two scales (this formula applies only when the scales are made comparable by standardization) and r_{11} and r_{22} are the reliabilities for the respective scales.

By now the importance of reliability assessment has become apparent. Most generally speaking, the reliability coefficient associated with a given test provides an estimate of the precision with which measurement is conducted by means of that test. It allows one to estimate the value of the true score by partialing out the influence of error. There are different methods of assessing reliability, each of which attempts to partial out the influence of a different type of error. Test–retest reliability attempts to partial out the error associated with transient situational variables. Internal consistency reliability attempts to partial out the influence of error due to imperfect content sampling and content homogeneity. Alternate-form reliability attempts to partial out the influence of error due to imperfect content sampling. Scorer reliability attempts to partial out the influence of interscorer differences. In each of these cases, the estimation of the true score depends on the removal of the effect of an error source from the observed score. Because the estimation of the true score proceeds indirectly, it is important to make sure that all possible sources of error for a particular test have been identified. For example, if one wanted to assess an ability that was presumed to be relatively stable, one would choose a test that demonstrated adequate test–retest reliability. If the test could be scored completely objectively, one would not need to assess interscorer reliability. Reliability must be assessed and used with reference to the theoretical underpinnings of the test and the match of those underpinnings with the assumptions and information consequences of the methodology used.

Reliability refers to several different types of stability, such as temporal, equivalence, and internal stability. Each type of reliability estimation is an attempt to assess the accuracy of the measurement. As can be inferred from this discussion, reliability is never precisely measured; it can only be estimated. To give the most accurate estimate of the accuracy of the measurement, it is therefore necessary to obtain as many types of reliability estimation as are theoretically and practically possible with the particular instrument under question (Fiske, 1971).

ITEM RESPONSE THEORY

In the previous chapter, we discussed some of the theoretical implications of item response theory. We now consider some of its practical applications in clinical neuro-psychology.

In recent years, a new and exciting development has occurred in the psychometric evaluation of assessment procedures. This development is alternately referred to as the *Rasch model*, the *latent trait model*, or *item response*. Until now, most of the adherents of item response theory (IRT) have been mathematical psychometricians. This is true because of the complexity of the mathematics involved and the speed at which the area has developed, necessitating that interested persons keep abreast of a burgeoning body of highly complicated and sometimes contradictory mathematical material just to be conversant with the field, let alone to understand the material well enough to use it sensibly (Hambleton & Cook, 1977).

Recently, with the advent of programs that can be used to analyze data from tests using IRT, with the slowly growing consensus on the applicability of IRT to certain types of test data, and with the organizing of workshops and conferences dealing with the topic, IRT has started to trickle down into the armamentarium of methods used by psychologists to assess tests.

IRT assumes that the performance of a subject on a test can be partly predicted by the abilities or traits of the subject. These traits cannot be directly measured—hence the title *latent trait*. The emphasis of IRT is on the item. Rather than evaluating the summed score of the items that make up a test, each of the items is evaluated. Earlier, it was stated that classical test theory stipulates that the score on an item is composed of the true score and error. IRT stipulates that the latent response to an item is composed of two values: (1) the product of the latent trait times its correlation between the latent trait and the latent response and (2) the error component, which has a mean of zero and a distribution that is constant for all values of the latent trait (Bejar, 1983). IRT attempts to estimate the item's character-istic curve, which is determined by three parameters: the difficulty of the item, the ability of the subject, and the discrimination of the item. It is possible to hold constant any of those three parameters and to estimate the value of the third. It is this flexibility that gives IRT its wide applicability (Lord, 1980).

The first applications of IRT have been to achievement testing in the primary schools. However, it is easy to see that applications to ability and achievement testing in neuropsychological assessment are a logical extension. Item response theory does not require that all items be given to each subject, which is one of the requirements that limit classical theory. Therefore, IRT is well suited to the evaluation of an instrument in which the ceiling and floor specifications limit the number of items administered to each subject, such as the Stanford–Binet and the WAIS-R. In addition, with IRT, it is possible to perform an assessment of equivalent forms that is much more fine grained than that allowed by the current methods. It assesses not only the equivalence of test scores but also the equivalence of the difficulty and discrimination of items. Until now, there have been few published reports of the use of IRT to evaluate neuropsychological assessment techniques (for an exception, see Stone & Wright, 1980). However, it is only a matter of time before IRT will be further applied to neuropsychological data in an attempt to further understand the psychometric properties of neuropsychological instruments. For example, IRT can be useful in the detection of biased items, that is, items with differential functioning (Hambleton, Swaminathan, & Rogers, 1991).

Elemental Considerations in Validity

Validity is a term that is often invoked in decisions to use neuropsychological tests. Unfortunately, the context of this use is usually negative, as when a test is cited as invalid. The use of the term implies that a test can be determined to be either valid or invalid. Of course, most clinical neuropsychologists agree that a test that is "valid" for one population may be "invalid" for another. If this is true, can a test ever be evaluated as universally valid or invalid? A second question relates to how a test is evaluated as valid or invalid. This is a question of both method (How do we evaluate a test?) and of epistemology (How do we know what we know?). Although method may be discussed separately from epistemology, the obverse is not necessarily true. That is, how we know something is highly related to how we investigate that something. This chapter discusses general issues in the relationship between epistemology and method, and Chapter 5 discusses the methodological issues more directly.

Historically, validity in clinical neuropsychological research has involved either the demonstration that scores derived from a test can accurately separate neurologically impaired individuals from unimpaired individuals or the demonstration of a statistical relationship between scores on a neuropsychological test and the results of a medical neurodiagnostic procedure such as postmortem surgical investigations or CT scans. We say that we know the validity of a test by systematic, empirical investigation. Limiting neuropsychological validity studies to these variables was the result of the questions posed to the neuropsychologist in the clinical setting. Clinical neuropsychological assessment did not have its own canon of methods or its own set of mature scientific principles. To a large extent, clinical neuropsychology still does not have these. However, along with the development of clinical neuropsychology as a form of behavioral science with unique training requirements and professional identity has come a growth in methods that, although not unique in principle, are unique in application.

These developments have made necessary the examination of the concepts of both *reliability* and *validity* as applied to clinical neuropsychological assessment. The methods for investigating these concepts are formed partly by the nascent body of neuropsychological assumptions and principles and partly by the changing questions that are posed to the neuropsychologist in the clinical setting. Instead of being asked to localize the site of a lesion, clinical neuropsychologists are being asked to predict the limits of the behavior of a patient in the open environment or to determine whether a substantial change in skill level has occurred as the result of applications of a rehabilitation strategy.

Earlier, we stated that we know the validity of a test by empirical observations. However, there is a leap that needs to be made before statements can be made regarding the validity of a test. That leap is from the specific results of a particular procedure to statements regarding the test used as part of the procedure. The investigation is actually an evaluation of the conclusions drawn from the use of the test. These conclusions may relate to localization or to prediction issues, but they always depend on the procedure used and the context in which the procedures are used. These issues are usually discussed in terms of internal and external validity, and they are applied to the interpretations of the results of empirical investigations. Threats to internal validity are presented by those events or processes that cast doubt on the reasonableness of the conclusions drawn. Threats to external validity are presented by those events or processes that cast doubt on the generalizability of the results to other populations. These terms may be easily applied to the investigations of neuropsychological tests and may also be appropriate to discussions of the conclusions drawn from the use of these tests in a clinical situation. It may be misleading to speak of a test as valid or invalid when our research actually investigates specific hypotheses.

There is yet another consideration linking validity to method. In discussing personality constructs, Fiske (1971) argued that there was too much variance in the results when constructs are measured by different methods. Instead, Fiske proposed that the unit of analysis be the construct-operation unit. Huba and Hamilton (1976) replied that there was too much convergence among the data to support such a notion. Even though different instruments give slightly different results, they seem to share a central construct, as demonstrated by covariation among the instruments. Huba and Hamilton implicitly suggested that the best way to measure a construct is through multioperationalization; however, they did not suggest a way to concatenate the data into a single index. Fiske (1976) replied that the presence of even small variations in relationships among different methods of measuring constructs indicates the need to include the method as an integral part of the measuring unit.

Not all of these arguments may be applied to clinical neuropsychological assessment; however, parts of the arguments are very pertinent to the present discussion. Clinicians are familiar with the pattern of results when a patient performs well on a test of verbal memory but not on a test of visual memory. Alternately, the patient may perform well on a test of recognition memory, but not on a test of free recall. When these results occur, clinical neuropsychologists do not generally throw up their hands and conclude that the results are due to method variance but that the construct is singular. Instead, more than one construct is used to explain the pattern of results.

Clinical neuropsychologists often attempt to delineate the actual skill or ability that is deficient by presenting a task to a patient under different conditions. A useful method for conceptualizing this set of relationships is to consider aspects of the stimulus (e.g., the sensory modality used and the potency of the stimulus compared to other stimuli in the environment), aspects of the processing required to perform the task (mental arithmetic vs. the use of paper-and-pencil or verbal encoding vs. abstract visual encoding), and aspects of the response (motoric, verbal, and recognition). In this way, we arrive at an assessment of the ability of the individual to copy abstract line drawings and not an assessment of the construct of construction apraxia. The construct-operation unit may be specified by means of the three aspects of the behavior requested: stimulus, processing, and response. Validity investigations can then be aimed at the evaluation of the conclusions drawn from the results of a specific test procedure.

It is still important to consider the underlying central trait, that is, memory. The trait may help us to generate hypotheses that can then be tested with data. For example, knowing that spatial skills are related to certain types of mathematical skills allows us to generate some hypotheses regarding performance on mathematical tasks when a subject demonstrates spatial manipulation deficits. One of the tasks is to determine the conditions and subjects for which the relationships occur or do not occur. By focusing on the construct-operation unit, we do not as easily commit the error of assuming that the traits measured are singular. By focusing on the construct-operation unit, we can remain close to the behavioral data and can use a more parsimonious set of cognitive constructs.

THE NATURE OF VALIDITY

In the area of general psychological research, there is an unsettled debate about whether validation is tripartite or unitary. Cronbach and Meehl (1955) suggested that validity is composed of three varieties: criterion-related (comprising both predictive and concurrent validity), content validity, and construct validity. Other theorists, such as Landy (1986), have suggested that validity has a unitarian nature. In this view, validation is a multidimensional activity by which the type of validity is determined by the inference attempted. Landy suggested that validation be viewed as hypothesis testing. Taking this suggestion a step further, one concentrates on evaluating the validity of the inference rather that on the validity of the test.

Discussions of the validity of a test may be clarified by considering the conditions, populations, and types of generalization that form the parameters of the inference. Instead of stating that a given test is valid, we should state instead that it is valid (or invalid) for drawing certain conclusions when it is administered to a certain individual in a certain setting. Doing so helps to make it clear that validity has as its central concern the evaluation of hypotheses formed by attempts to generalize past the test situation.

Some people draw distinctions between constructs (such as reasoning ability) and observable facts (such as the accuracy of an individual's attempt to solve some problem). The construct helps one to make predictions beyond the individual, the setting, and the observed behavior by hypothesizing a central commonality. In this way, we reduce the uncertainty of each new clinical question by pointing out the similarities with other previously answered questions. Concentrating on the observable fact allows greater accuracy in predicting a specific outcome. There is an obvious tradeoff in this situation: the greater the extent to which constructs are used, the greater the generality of the predictions made. On the other hand, the obverse is true of the reliance on observable facts: the greater the extent to which the predictions are restricted to observable facts, the more accurately can predictions be made in a given situation. The distinction is not just semantic, for the clinician is faced with a decision that has implications for the eventual validity of inferences.

There is no single answer to the question of how extensive the level of abstraction should be in naming the skills evaluated by clinical neuropsychological methods. In one sense, the task is completed during the assessment when the clinician gathers data from extratest sources, that is, clinical and collateral interviews, behavioral observations, and reviews of previous test results. The limits of the inferences drawn regarding the visual–spatial skills of a subject as determined by a test score are partly determined by data regarding the performance of the subject on real-life tasks that require visual–spatial skills. Unfortunately, the strategy of allowing all of the limitations of generalizability to be described by extratest data removes the process from quantification and public observation. A preferable strategy is to limit the description of the construct being assessed to the most basic level of behavioral description that can still allow generalizability to other situations but not to other skills. As a result, the inferences remain in the public scrutiny of the community of clinicians and researchers. The inferences can then be quantified and empirically evaluated.

For example, a test of visual–spatial skills may require the subject to reproduce a simple abstract line drawing after having viewed the test stimulus for 10 seconds. Because the task requires memory, motor skills, and visual–spatial perception, it would be misleading to label the test as purely an index of visual–spatial constructional skills. Performance on the test may not generalize to situations in which memory is not required. Although it may seem more cumbersome to describe the test as assessing visual–spatial motor–reproduction skills for which short-term memory is required, it is less cumbersome than the theoretical excess baggage required to explain discrepancies in performance between a situation that requires memory and a situation that does not require memory. The clinician can identify which skill component of the construct-operation unit is actually deficient by comparing the results of the application of various construct-operation units (tests or procedures) that vary only slightly in the content of their components. This method is similar both to Luria's method of qualifying the symptom and to Teuber's concept of double discrimination. However, to show the similarity to double discrimination, the goal of assessment must be changed from physical localization to functional localization. For example, if a patient performs poorly on a test of visual-recognition memory but performs adequately on tests of verbal recognition and verbal free recall, we might hypothesize that some aspect of visual encoding is impaired.

Limiting construct descriptions to the lowest possible level of necessary abstraction has its roots in the concept of face validity and has implications for both construct and content validity. A prerequisite for naming a test as an index of a given neuropsychological skill is that the test appear to tap the construct of interest. A test of visual–spatial constructional skills should contain tasks that require the subject to perform using those skills or else that require the performance of skills highly related to the construct of interest, for example, drawing to command.

We return now to a consideration of the construct-operation unit. As an abstract entity, the construct is not actually measurable. When we specify the construct-operation unit, we provide both an abstract definition of the skill and a public observational system for assessing that skill. The validity of the inferences drawn from test scores is related to the similarity of the method to the demands of the environment in the performance of the behavioral products of the skill. Memory tests generally assess the skill of an individual in receiving, encoding, and retrieving discrete bits of information in a relatively distraction-free environment. Those particular conditions are rarely met in the free environment. As a result, predictions from test scores may be inaccurate (that is, may have limited validity) in describing the performance of the subject in everyday memory tasks. By concentrating on the construct-operation unit, we explicitly accept the theoretical considerations underlying the use of the test, namely, that memory performance differs under differing levels of distraction. We may wish to devise and use two tests, one with and one without distraction methods. When we desire to make predictions to extratest behavior, we would choose the test with the method that best approximates the conditions under which the subject is expected to perform. Or conversely, we may specify the environmental limitations and conditions under which performance of the central task is expected, for example, telling the subject to learn new material under minimal distraction.

VALIDITY AND NONNEUROLOGICAL VARIABLES

There is always a problem with omitting variables. When we omit relevant variables in our research, we consign to error variance those sources of variance that might otherwise be explained systematically. Clinical neuropsychological assessment tends to look at the score derived from a test and the possible membership in a certain class, such as a diagnostic subgroup. In doing so, it ignores the context of the evaluation, the demographic characteristics of the subject, the learning history of the subject, and the influence of conative variables such as level of motivation or affective state. This occurs even though theory states that these variables are important. The role of these variables is relegated to the domain of clinical inference, intuition, or decision. The price paid for this omission ranges from unfortunate (in the form of lowered validity coefficients) to inexcusable (in the form of misleading information resulting in disservice to the patient). These variables can be theoretically argued to have import in the decisions regarding the validity of inferences drawn from test scores; however, in reality, the import of these variables is an empirical question yet to be answered.

At this point in the development of clinical neuropsychological assessment as a scientific endeavor, it may not be possible to directly specify the effects of nonneurological variables on assessment results. It is still necessary to attempt to delineate these effects. We are evaluating the validity of inferences drawn from test results. Therefore, we need to rule out the extraneous effects of conative variables, or else we need to make some statements regarding the likely effects of these variables. Table 4.1 describes a model for determining the possible relevant variables. The variables are divided into three major classes: examiner variables, contextual variables, and subject variables.

The effects of these variables may be different for different levels of other variables in the model. That is, the variables may have moderating effects on each other. An obvious example would be the gender of the examiner, which may have different effects, depending on the gender and the learning history of the subject. Again, these are all empirical questions that need to be addressed if we are to increase the validity of the inferences drawn

TABLE 4.1. Variables Affecting Test Results

Situation	Subject	Examiner
Setting	Gender	Gender
Reason for assessment (perceived objective, rationale provided)	History	Voice inflection
	IQ	Level of skill and experience
Forensic	Occupation	
For child: school versus medical setting	Reaction to examiner	

from our test results. It is likely that there are other variables that need to be placed on the table. More conceptual as well as empirical work needs to be done.

Fiske (1978) observed that most psychologists recognize (or pay lip service to) the importance of the person–situation interaction. His comments were made in the context of discussing personality assessment, but some of the same considerations apply to clinical neuropsychological assessment. It is not sufficient to state that anxiety plays a role in the assessment of memory functions or that forensic settings affect test results. It would be better, instead, to make the person–situation interaction the focus of our investigations. By stating and experimentally controlling the situations in which assessment takes place, we bring the moderating influence of these situations into the arena of public scrutiny, and the result is greater agreement regarding the confirmation or disconfirmation of the inferences drawn.

Every person is different. Each of us has different levels of skills as the result of genetic heterogeneity, different learning histories, and differing current states. However, faced with these differences, we should not throw up our hands at the insurmountability of the task. As Fiske (1978) recommended, it would be more productive to attempt to determine whether any regularities exist in the phenomenon under study and to uncover the conditions in which these regularities exist.

CONCLUSIONS

Validity is a term that is better applied to inferences than to tests. We can know little about the validity of a test, but we can know the accuracy of the hypotheses and inferences associated with its use. It may be difficult to change the language of a profession, but doing so could have beneficial effects on our use of test instruments. When we focus on the validity of inferences, we draw attention to the construct-operation unit. In essence, we become more behavior-minded; our conclusions are limited by the characteristics of the observed data rather than by references to categorical abstracts. In addition, when we focus on the validity of inferences, we focus on the decision-making processes of the clinician. No test can be valid in the hands of an inadequately trained clinician. We also become more aware of the nonneurological variables impinging on test performance. Much work needs to be done, but we can be cheered and motivated by the fact that much work has already been done. We know some of the basics regarding the different performance by diagnostic groups on certain tests. We now need to determine the basics regarding performance that differs because of other variables.

Validity as Applied to Neuropsychological Assessment

The concept of test validity basically corresponds to the question of whether a test or an assessment procedure supplies the kind of information needed for a particular interpretation. This issue is very important because the test scores in and of themselves are meaningless unless they refer to a defined realm of observable phenomena. In clinical psychology, the consequence of interest may be a particular personality style or behavioral disorder. For clinical neuropsychology, the consequence of interest may range from whether brain impairment exists to the implications of the test results for adaptive behavior. Before particular issues that affect the validity of neuropsychological tests are described, general applicable concepts of validity and threats to validity are reviewed.

TYPES OF VALIDITY

Recent texts reinterpret validity as "validation"; that is, the issue of interest is not only what a test measures, but also what a test's strengths and weaknesses are in terms of particular subjects, interpretive questions, and settings. Answers to these questions may be found in various sources: the test manual, test reviews, general test standards, and published research. Throughout this book, the reviews of neuropsychological assessment instruments use the test manuals as sources as well as the publicly available research data from the literature and, in some cases, from conference presentations or directly from the researcher. Validity is not a unitary construct, nor is it a construct that can be readily and permanently decided by a single piece of research. In addition, there is sometimes disagreement among clinical neuropsychologists on the topic of test validity. We do not attempt to resolve the issues of disagreement, but attempt to enlarge the discussion of validity by including issues of contextual and comparative quality as discussed by Cronbach (1984). We also attempt to keep the discussion focused on a very important central point: tests themselves are not valid or invalid, but inferences drawn from test results can be described as either valid or invalid.

VALIDITY: BASIC DEFINITIONS

Validity may be defined in an empirical sense as a statistical relationship between the results of a particular procedure and a characteristic of interest, that is, between a contrived procedure and other independently observed events (Anastasi, 1982; Nunnally, 1978). These relationships may be defined in terms of the content of a test, related criteria, and underlying constructs. All of these can be qualified in terms of contextual and subject variables.

Content Validity

Content validity is the degree to which a test adequately samples from the domain of interest. For example, if a test is intended to be sensitive to the global aspects of memory dysfunction, there need to be sufficiently representative tasks that access the construct defining "global memory processes" as understood by the test developer. Therefore, it is important that the developer describe the definition of the construct fairly completely, so that discussions in the literature can focus on the theoretical adequacy of the definition, rather than on content validity. In our example of a test of memory, if the test designer subscribed to the Atkinson and Schiffrin (1968) model of memory, the content of the test would optimally include tasks that demonstrate the acquisition of information at the sensory level, decay from short-term storage, decay from long-term storage, and the effects of rehearsal and interference.

The process of content validation begins when the initial test items or procedures are selected during the design of an instrument. Careful selection and design in the initial stages will help to ease the task of later validation. Most arguments used to support content validation are theoretical and logical. Content validation may be most easily evaluated or demonstrated when the procedure is an operational version of a well-defined theory or a component of a theory. A "table of specifications" (Hopkins & Antes, 1978) that demonstrates the translation of theory into test items can further facilitate the demonstration of content validity.

A table of specifications can be described as a two-dimensional matrix in which one dimension represents the skills or traits of interest and the other dimension represents the behavior characteristic of the interest areas. This diagram can be used to determine the number of items that ought to be assigned to a given topic area as well as the type of item (e.g., timed vs. untimed or spoken vs. written) that need to be included. With the use of these guides, a neuropsychological battery can be expected to include diverse and apparently unrelated items, whereas a test of language comprehension should contain items that are more consistent with each other.

As an example, Table 5.1 demonstrates a table of specifications for the Visual Processes Scale of the Luria–Nebraska Neuropsychological Battery (LNNB). This table has been greatly simplified for descriptive purposes. The functions described here could also be further specified as visual recognition of objects, visual recognition of line drawings, visually mediated inferential reasoning, and so on, and topic areas could be weighted according to their perceived theoretical importance (2056 of the items could be selected to represent operations based on mental rotations).

Items are usually derived by a variety of methods, ranging from examples of behavior

TABLE 5.1. Specifications for the Luria–Nebraska
Neuropsychological Battery: Visual Processes Scale

Function	Simple	Complex
Visually mediated recognition	Items 86, 87	Items 88, 89
Figure–ground perception		Items 90, 91
Spatially mediated perception	Items 94, 95, 96	
Mental imagery		Items 97, 99

that are directly stated in the theoretical model (e.g., the expectation of increased skin conductance as anxiety increases) to the selection of items by expert judges. In terms of neuropsychological procedures, the sensory modality (visual, auditory, or tactile) through which a stimulus item is presented and the likely internal processes used to achieve a solution (rote vs. reasoned) are all important to content validity as well as to construct validity. The pertinent issue is the likely generalizability (Nunnally, 1978) of the information derived from an item and, consequently, the likely generalizability of the test as a whole. In dealing with content validity, the test designer must be aware of the tradeoff between lack of specificity or insufficient sampling of the domain and tedious redundancy that does not usefully articulate the characteristic of interest.

The success with which a test designer resolves this tradeoff balance is an issue for future validational research. Later investigators may propose a contrasting theory or may suggest a different set of items as better translating the initially proposed theory. When tests are shown to have limited content validity, the issue raised is insufficient to the purported domain of interest. The causes of limited content validity are usually incomplete understanding of the underlying theory, lack of a guiding theory, or a tendency to assume greater generalized interpretations of item performance at the time of construction. One's intent may be to design a widely applicable neuropsychological screening test, but the items may all require that the subject copy simple geometric designs. There is a large subset of brain-impaired subjects (e.g., subjects with specific impairments in language skills) for whom performance on such a test will not be diagnostically useful.

Face validity is often erroneously used as a synonym for *content validity*. However, a more accurate description of the relationship between content validity and face validity is that face validity is a category of content validity. Face validity refers primarily to the perceptions of the examinee. The subject forms some conclusions regarding what the test is measuring on the basis of the content or language of the test procedures. In more ambiguous test situations (e.g., personality evaluation), the examinee's assumptions about the nature of the test may be widely disparate from the examiner's intent. Face validity becomes an important concern to the extent that the perceptions of the examinee affect his or her performance on the test; the result may be confounded with the intended measurement purpose of the test. An examinee is more likely to participate in an assessment that uses procedures that appear to provide information that will answer his or her concerns.

Face validity can also affect the decision-making process of potential users of the test. The astute clinician will ultimately choose tests on the basis of the available empirical literature, but the original decision to investigate the utility of a test may be influenced by the "look" of a test. Face validity may also influence later empirical validation work by researchers other than the test designer. Subsequent investigators may assume different intents for the items or test scales based on their interpretation of the intent of an item or the meaning of a scale name. Some of these problems can be avoided by including in the manual a specific discussion of the theoretical background of a test as well as a discussion of particular item and scale intents. The manual can also describe the scale titles as somewhat arbitrary labels and give titles that have readily shared meanings in the community of test researchers and consumers. The latter is not always possible because there is no standard dictionary of neuropsychological terms. Even if such a dictionary existed, there would not be universal acceptance of the definitions, given the diverse theoretical, epistemological, and procedural backgrounds of the group of individuals who constitute the practitioners of clinical neuropsychology.

It is advisable to give titles that have a relatively large amount of acceptance and agreement among clinical neuropsychologists. It is further advisable to give names to the scales and to the skill areas purported to be measured that reflect behavioral descriptions rather than unobservable constructs. For example, a test might be described as a test of memory, but it would be more accurate to describe the scales and procedures as being measures of new learning, immediate recall, or delayed recall. From the preceding discussion, it can be seen that, although face validity does not play a direct role in the empirical definition of a test, it does play a mediating role in the understanding and evaluation of the test data.

Content validity plays a large role in the development of a test. Most of the evaluative processes involved in investigating content validity are based on logical considerations. Nunnally (1978) suggested a few ways in which content validity can be evaluated. For example, if a scale is thought to measure a single construct, the items can reasonably be expected to demonstrate a fair amount of internal consistency, a relationship that can be empirically evaluated. For those constructs thought to be affected by experience, content validity can be evaluated by demonstrating improved performance following a training procedure. Content validity can also be evaluated by comparing performance on the test in question with performance on other tests thought to tap the same or similar constructs. Anastasi (1982) suggested a qualitative method of checking content validity by having subjects think out loud during the testing. Of course, this suggestion has limited utility for assessing brain-impaired populations.

Still another method of assessing content validity is to conduct an error analysis. When persons with similar brain dysfunctions fail an item, a review of their error patterns for signs of consistency may suggest how the brain dysfunction translates into behavior. For example, failures during the block design subtest of the WAIS-R that are due to the individual's breaking the external configuration of the target design have been related to right cerebral dysfunction (Kaplan, 1983).

The demonstration of content validation is limited by the extent to which extraneous factors affect test performance. The relative contributions of motivation, academic experience, prior intellectual resources, socioeconomic status, sex, and psychological status must be understood before an accurate assessment of content relevance and generalizability can be conducted. Differences in timing procedures, administration instructions, or scoring procedures may cause relationships with external criteria to vary considerably. Clinical education optimally emphasizes the role of these variables in the process of measurement, but it is wise for both researchers and clinicians to be mindful of the need to minimize the effect of the variables on the derived score.

Criterion Validity

Anastasi (1982) described criterion-validating procedures as those that demonstrate a test's effectiveness in a given context. Criterion validity is commonly expressed as the correlation between a test score and some external variable, which may be another test that is assumed to measure the same characteristic of interest or future behavior that is assumed to demonstrate the characteristic of interest. In the former case, one usually speaks of concurrent validity, as allied behavior is measured at the same time. In the latter case, one usually speaks of predictive validity, as performance on the test being evaluated is used to temporally predict the criterion, whether it is diagnostic group membership or behavioral change.

Although the information is rarely offered in test manuals, a validity coefficient may be computed as the correlation between the score achieved on a particular test and some criterion variable. For example, one may correlate the relationship between a score on the Category Test (Reitan & Wolfson, 1993) and a dummy-coded variable indicating diagnostic group (i.e., 1 = normal, 2 = neurologically impaired). In this case, a significant positive relationship would indicate that a high score on the Category Test was associated with a subject's being part of the neurologically impaired diagnostic group. Assignment to the diagnostic group would have to be made on the basis of external, independent criteria, such as a neurological evaluation, the results of neuroradiological evaluation, or previous history.

The validity coefficient can be negatively affected by the degree of homogeneity of the sample. This can occur both numerically and conceptually. Numerically, the magnitude of the correlation coefficient decreases as the overall sample becomes more similar in test scores because of the restriction of range. Conceptually, a high validity coefficient might be associated with a particular type of neurological impairment, but not with others. Validity coefficients can also be affected by gender, level of education, age, and so on. This is important information for determining the utility of the instrument; however, it can be disheartening when it is not intended by the test author.

The relationship between a validity coefficient and decision theory is important in deciding the significance of the validity coefficient. Decision theory, as applied to tests, is a mathematical operationalization of the decision-making process. Early models of the theory were based on the net improvement in accuracy over the base rate (the natural frequency of occurrence of a given phenomenon) that one could gain at various levels of validity. Applications to psychological instruments were developed by Cronbach and Gleser (1965). We may see the application of the theory in the following example: If we were to identify all persons as neurologically impaired, even a test with a perfect validity coefficient ($r = 1.0$) would not contribute additional information to the decision. On the other hand, if we knew ahead of time that approximately 70% of the people referred for neuropsychological evaluation were neurologically impaired, that same test with the perfect validity coefficient would improve our accuracy by approximately 16%. If the prior base rate were 20%, the same test would improve our accuracy by 80%. As a rule of thumb, a base rate of 50% optimizes the utility of an instrument. As the likelihood of seeing a condition becomes more rare, the utility of an instrument in terms of improving on the base rate decreases. The cost–benefit ratio of developing and applying an instrument for rare conditions is low. It might be more useful to learn the qualitative and historical symptoms of the disorder and to assess for them rather than to develop a specific identification instrument. Tables for computing the relationship between base rate and validity coefficients for specific decision levels can be found in Taylor and Russell (1939).

An elaborate alternative to computing a validity coefficient is a research design sometimes referred to as the *method of contrasted groups* (Anastasi, 1982). Here, the researcher evaluates the results of testing two groups that are assumed to be different on the criterion that is of interest. For example, persons with no known neurological impairment and persons with known neurological impairment are both administered the Luria–Nebraska Neuropsychological Battery. The scores are then compared by some statistical method. A traditional method of comparing test performance has been to test for the significance of the difference between mean scores for the two groups. Unfortunately, the two groups may contain members whose scores lie in the region of overlapping distributions of the two groups. An alternate and preferable method begins with a use of the statistical technique known as *discriminant function analysis*. The results of such an analysis produce a linear composite that may be used to demonstrate maximal separation between the two diagnostic groups. The weightings derived from this analysis may then be used to assign the subjects statistically to "predicted" groups. Predicted group membership is then compared with actual group membership, and an accuracy rate, or "hit rate," is computed. The latter part of this analysis is referred to as *classification analysis*.

Although many examples of this set of procedures may be found in even a quick review of current journals, misapplications of the procedures are common. In applying such a design, two major points should be kept in mind. First, the discriminant function analysis and the classification analysis are separate procedures. The discriminant analysis identifies those variables that significantly contribute to the function that statistically separates the groups of interest, and the classification analysis applies an equation based on those significant variables in order to predict group membership. Optimally, applying the equation to the group on which it was derived should result in a relatively high hit rate. Second, demonstrating a significant hit rate in such a derivation sample is only the first step in determining predictive validity. It is not until the derived equation can significantly predict group membership in a second, or cross-validation, sample that predictive validity can be said to have been demonstrated for that set of test procedures.

The use of such a design is a sophisticated demonstration and is open to many sources of contamination. One of the major sources is sample representativeness. If the procedure being evaluated is intended to have broad applications rather than to demonstrate the presence of a particular type of neurological impairment, and if the effects of ancillary subject characteristics are to be ruled out, both the diagnostic subgroup characteristic of neurological impairment and the diagnostic subgroup characteristic of "normality" need to be as heterogeneous as possible. To the extent that they are not heterogeneous, the generalizability of the validating investigations needs to be clearly defined. In addition, the usual subject-matching procedures in the contrasting-groups methodology should be observed just as they would be in any clinical research.

The hit rate itself may be contaminated. Willis (1984) demonstrated that the meaning of a given rate of accuracy may be inflated if one does not take into account the prior probabilities of group membership (the base rate). Thus, when one is comparing two diagnostic groups, 50% accuracy is not the correct point for chance assignment if prior membership had been 70% and 307 for the two groups.

Concurrent validity of neuropsychological tests is more complex than is a similar analysis of general psychological measures. Although neuropsychological tests may be related to other tests that purport to measure similar brain functions, concurrent neuro-physiological measures (i.e., a CT scan, an EEG, an MRI, and an rCBF) can also provide a major source of validation. The cost of such a validational exercise may be prohibitive even if it is rewarding. In reviewing such demonstrations, several issues must be considered. First, what is being demonstrated? Although the CT scan may be accurate in detecting acute subdural hemorrhage, it is significantly less accurate in detecting subtle, residual subcorti-cal changes that may leave an individual profoundly perseverative or memory-impaired. The individual may appear impaired on the neuropsychological test but not on the CT scan. If one wishes to demonstrate the general utility of the neuropsychological measure, a series of both physiological and behavioral measures may be a more accurate set of criteria.

Second, what is the population to which the measures will be applied? Although severely impaired individuals may be more likely to present classically demonstrable physiological findings, unless such individuals are the intended population such criterion-validational exercises are likely to be inappropriate because of their limited general-izability. In those cases, it may be necessary to use some other forms of criteria.

Third, how will the instrument be used in clinical settings? Physiological criteria may be useful for instruments that will be used primarily for diagnostic or localization purposes. On the other hand, behavioral measures may be more appropriate for instruments that are intended to provide information for intervention programs or to document the course of recovery. Clinical neuropsychologists are often in the uncomfortable situation of having to make statements regarding the behavior of an individual in the free environment based on test data. The field is in need of instruments that have been validated against behavioral criteria.

Generally speaking, greater numbers of criteria and greater degrees of heterogeneity in the sample used in the validation of an instrument will enhance the clarity with which the utility of a test can be defined. In validating an instrument, it is important to remember that the identification of the populations, the context, and the questions for which a particular instrument is inappropriate are just as important as the identification of the populations, the context, and the questions for which an instrument is appropriate.

Construct Validity

Construct validity was conceptually introduced by Cronbach and Meehl (1955). Construct validity can be described as that aspect of the validation process that attempts to demonstrate the dimensions or traits that the test was designed to measure. Construct validation is an ongoing process. It runs through the demonstration of content and criterion validity and, in addition, is built from exploratory and confirmatory hypothesis-testing of the procedure of interest. The goal of construct validation is to build a nomothetic net or inferential definition of the characteristics that a test seeks to measure. In many ways, the process of construct validation returns the investigators to the beginning of the design of the instrument because the relationship between the test and its underlying theory is constantly at issue.

To return to a point made earlier (in the discussion of criterion validity), devising demonstrations of what a test does measure as well as what it does not measure is a crucial aspect of examining the validity of the inferences drawn regarding a particular test. The results of such demonstrations help us to understand how a particular pattern of behaviors occurred during a test as well as to define how a test may be improved. This latter point is often ignored during the construction of test procedures. No instrument or procedure should be assumed to be completely finished at the time that it is introduced. Instead, we should expect that, as investigations of the technique refine our understanding of that technique, and as knowledge in the area of brain–behavior relationships grows, the technique itself, if viable, will evolve. This is not to give permission to test authors to publish incompletely specified or incompletely investigated new tests. Test authors have ethical imperatives to publish only test materials that have met minimum guidelines as specified in the American Psychological Association standards (American Educational Research Association, American Psychological Association, & National Council on Measurement in Education, 1985).

There are several common ways to investigate the construct validity of a test. The most basic research method is theory testing. By using a theory or a set of alternative theories of brain–behavior relationships, one may test hypotheses regarding test performance following definable brain injuries. In this way, one would expect the items of a test that tap functions attributed to the damaged area to show the most frequent failures, and the items tapping functions not usually attributed to the damaged area to be relatively error-free. At a simpler level, performance on a test thought to be sensitive to brain dysfunction should be able to discriminate neurologically impaired individuals from individuals who are not neurologically impaired. The scores on such a test should vary with the degree of brain compromise or cognitive inefficiency. Psychiatrically impaired persons, especially those individuals with major psychiatric disorders, might also be expected to show varying degrees of impaired performance on the test.

Serial testing during recovery from brain injury can also provide a useful test of construct validity. For example, knowing that edema is more likely to cause general impairment during the first few weeks after brain injury, one may expect more impaired test performance early in the course of recovery, with improvement in test performance following expected recovery time lines. Similarly, as compensatory skills are taught in rehabilitation programs or as the individual learns to compensate for the deficits with feedback from the environment, one may see significant changes in some functional areas. Using the logic of Finger and Stein (1982), one might also expect that the most severely and directly damaged functions would show deficits more impervious to recovery. This latter point is especially true if very fine component skills are assessed with the instrument.

An alternate approach to construct validation focuses on predictions regarding performance on other tests that are postulated to measure the same traits as the original test or other tests that measure underlying traits. In this fashion, one might expect that a measure of a certain cognitive skill would show moderate correlations with measures of general intelligence, little or no relationship to a measure of trait anxiety, and a strong correlation with an instrument purported to measure the same cognitive skill. As noted earlier, an important aspect of these validational investigations is the degree to which the investigator accurately understands the intent of a test and the theory underlying the test.

Campbell and Fiske (1959) operationalized this design into a model that evaluates a measurement technique in terms of discriminant and convergent validity. Discriminant validity is defined by relationships with tests assumed to be unrelated to the test of interest.

One expects divergent coefficients to be nonsignificant or very low. Convergent validity is demonstrated by positive significant correlations with tests thought to measure the same or a similar construct. Furthermore, higher correlations are expected between two procedures that use the same methodology instead of different methodologies (e.g., behavioral observation vs. self-report). This method of analysis is usually identified as the *multitrait–multimethod matrix*.

With such an analysis, the postulated underlying trait dimension is measured by a variety of procedures, including the test under consideration, that use both the same and different methodologies. At the same time, those methodologies are used to measure a different trait. In this way, the traits are crossed with the methods. The intercorrelations among these measures constitute the multitrait–multimethod matrix. The results thought to support the instrument under evaluation include a pattern of positive correlations with other tests measuring the same trait and low to zero correlations with instruments measuring the unrelated traits.

Jackson (1969) criticized the multitrait–multimethod design and offered an alternative. The majority of Jackson's criticisms focus on the issue that Campbell and Fiske's method compares individual correlations without examining the overall structure of the relationships. This is an important point because the pattern of correlations may be affected by the way in which variance is distributed in measuring the traits under consideration.

To obviate these concerns, Jackson (1969) suggested that a factor analysis of the monomethod matrix be conducted. During such an analysis, the correlation matrix is first orthogonalized and submitted to a principal-components analysis, followed by a varimax rotation. The number of factors is set to equal the number of postulated underlying traits. Although Jackson's suggestion offers some advantages, it may be of limited use in cases in which relationships exist among the traits under consideration, as in the neuropsychological assessment of many interrelated cognitive skills. Secondarily, when the monomethod matrix is used, the influence of different measurement methods may not be examined. Cole, Howard, and Maxwell (1981) investigated the result of using a mono-operationalization of constructs and reported that the overall effect is to spuriously deflate validity coefficients. Therefore, the two methods (i.e., Campbell and Fiske's and Jackson's) may be seen as complementary. In a rigorous attempt at construct validation, it is useful to apply both.

Cole (1987) also criticized the multitrait–multimethod matrix in general and suggested an alternative. Some of Cole's criticisms parallel Jackson's. That is, Cole noted that there are no specific guidelines for the evaluation of the size of the resulting zero-order correlation coefficients. In addition, Cole stated that the collection of multiple measures of multiple constructs is an endeavor that is extremely expensive in clinical settings and that is therefore rarely done. Finally, Cole noted that the multitrait–multimethod matrix is sensitive to the presence of correlated errors. The errors may be correlated because of a similarity in the time of day at which certain aspects of the assessments are conducted or because of certain of the instruments being administered by the same person.

Cole suggested instead the use of confirmatory factor analysis to analyze the data and investigate discriminant and convergent validity. Confirmatory factor analysis allows for a statistical test of the hypothesis, unlike examination of the multitrait–multimethod matrix, which allows for only a description of the relationships among variables. Confirmatory factor analysis can also test for the presence of correlated errors and can control for their effects. Finally, the use of confirmatory factor analysis allows the clinical researcher to analyze less costly data sets by allowing the use of monotrait–monomethod data sets (for the evaluation of factorial validity), monotrait–multimethod data sets (for the evaluation of convergent validity), and multitrait–monomethod data sets (for the evaluation of discriminant validity), as well as the analysis of multitrait–multimethod data sets (for the evaluation of both discriminant and convergent validity).

The drawbacks of confirmatory factor analysis are related to its requirements. Usually, a very large data set is necessary for confirmatory factor analysis. In addition, complete data sets are required for each subject. Confirmatory factor analysis cannot handle missing data. The data set must also be multivariate normal; failure to meet this requirement will affect the results of the test of significance considerably. Finally, the covariance matrix must contain multiple measures of each construct. Another requirement of confirmatory factor analysis can be seen as a benefit; that is, the factor structure must be specified before analysis, and therefore the researcher must more fully consider the implications of the chosen data analysis before analyzing the data.

Exploratory factor analysis provides another way to examine construct validity. As before, the investigator starts from the theory underlying the test or from an alternative theory thought to explain test performance. This type of factoring can be seen to be a rudimentary version of confirmatory factor analysis, as opposed to exploratory factor analysis, which makes relatively few assumptions regarding the underlying structure of a set of data.

For example, in the validational work with the LNNB, predictions were made from Luria's theory regarding the likely number of dimensions that would underlie a given LNNB subscale. These predictions were based on operational definitions of conceptually similar tasks that represented a given component function. Oblique rotations were initially selected because factors were assumed to be interrelated. In many cases, the assumptions from the theory were confirmed (for a review see Golden et al., 1982d).

Exploratory factor analyses may also be used to develop support for conclusions regarding the construct validity of a test. A test composed of a variety of subscales may be reduced to factorially simple dimensions. Once the factors have been identified, a linear-weighted composite (a factor score) may be used to determine the relative contribution of a given factor to the specified test performance. The factorial validity coefficient of a test may then be computed by correlating test scores with the factor score (Anastasi, 1982). For example, if a motor speed factor were identified, the relative contribution of motor speed to test performance could be computed.

Marker variables can also be used in factor-analytic construct validation. A marker variable is usually a descriptive rather than a conceptual measure. Its meaning is relatively better understood than that of the test procedure being evaluated. Age, gender, education, and IQ are common marker variables; however, the scores generated by accepted neuropsychological measures may also be included as markers. When reviewing the results of such a factoring procedure, the researcher looks for factors on which the marker variables are significantly loaded. Consideration of the meaning of the marker variables contributes to an understanding of the construct meaning of the tests of interest that also load on that factor.

Serial factor analyses with the same sample or across independent samples demonstrate the stability of a test's underlying dimensions across time or across samples. Although temporally stable results may be less desirable for those measures thought to be sensitive to the current neuropsychological status of an individual, the latter method (independent samples) is highly desirable for those techniques that are not intended to be impairment specific. Examining the factor structure of a test across different populations is important for a further reason. We earlier had discussed the notion that reliability of a test may vary across different populations or across different levels of skill of the individual taking the test. This set of concepts is addressed by item response theory. Reliability and validity are related in various ways, and the validity analog to these reliability issues is that relationships among factors and scores of a test may vary across populations. To complete group comparisons or interpret data from patients in different populations (e.g., WMS-III scores in closed head injury and in epilepsy) three conditions must be met. First, the observed scores must represent the same theoretical construct. Second, the scores must index the constructs with equivalent scales of measurement. Third, these theoretical constructs must be measured with equivalent precision (Lord & Novick, 1968). The extent to which these conditions are met can be evaluated using confirmatory factor analytic methods as has been done for the Wechsler Memory Scale—Revised (Jurden, Franzen, Callahan, & Ledbetter, 1996).

A final method that may be used in construct validation is also useful for refining a measure. The method of examining the homogeneity of a scale was previously discussed in the context of evaluating the reliability of a test. On scales that are assumed to measure a general underlying dimension, especially scales that use a sum across items to derive the score, the correlation of individual item scores with the total scale score may be used to identify items that are less likely to be related to the underlying trait. As an example, let us consider a 15-item scale intended to measure perceptual constancy, for which the test's author intended to sum the individual item scores to produce a single score that would represent an individual's degree of perceptual constancy. Correlations between the items and the total scale score would indicate the degree to which each item is related to the trait as measured by the instrument. Items whose scores are low would be candidates for revision, which could improve the overall validity of the homogeneous scale. Yet another consideration is the application of this procedure to the contrasted-groups design to evaluate the extent to which the trait is homogeneous across the intended subject pools (Anastasi, 1982).

Diagnostic Validity

A common use of neuropsychological assessment is to provide a diagnostic impression. Unfortunately, this application of neuropsychology has not received wide attention in studies examining the validity of neuropsychological assessment instruments. There are two major aspects of diagnostic validity; the first is whether a single test can accurately identify individuals with a given diagnosis. The second is whether combinations of tests can accurately identify or classify individuals.

In examining the diagnostic validity of a single test, we go beyond the simple concepts of contrasted groups and attempt to apply that information to a single case. For contrasted groups designs, the relevant information is whether groups of subjects with different diagnoses have statistically different mean values. With large numbers of subjects in the groups being contrasted, small mean differences can be significant. The utility of this significant difference for interpreting results in the assessment of a single individual may be limited. In examining diagnostic validity, the relevant information involves the distribution of scores. Here, a greater amount of overlap in the distribution of scores for the two groups would enhance the accuracy of the test in diagnosing individuals.

In the simplest case an optimal cutoff score is chosen and the use of that cutoff in classifying subjects is evaluated with the use of a two-by-two contingency table. Classification of the subjects into the groups using the cutoff score is compared to classification by some external criterion. The cells of the contingency table can be labeled True Positives, False Positives, True Negatives, and False Negatives. True Positives are those subjects identified using the test as having the diagnosis who actually have the diagnosis using the external criterion. False Positives are those individuals incorrectly identified by the test as having the diagnosis when the external criterion classifies the subjects as not having the diagnosis. True Negatives are those subjects identified by the test as not having the diagnosis when the external criterion agrees that the diagnosis is not present. False Negatives are those subjects identified by the test as not having the diagnosis when the external criterion identifies the subjects as actually having the diagnosis.

Let us examine a hypothetical case in which a test to identify Alzheimer's dementia is used to classify 100 subjects, and in which 50 of the subjects actually carry the diagnosis on the basis of postmortem examinations. The test identifies 75 subjects as having the diagnosis with the following cell values.

A True Positives—50 (67%)	B False Negatives—0 (0%)
C False Positives—25 (33%)	D True Negatives—25 (100%)

Here the sensitivity (A/A + C) of the test, or the percentage of subjects with the diagnosis who are correctly identified as having the diagnosis, is 67%. The specificity of the test, or the percentage of subjects correctly identified as not having the diagnosis (D/B + D), is 100%. The diagnostic accuracy is the total percentage of subjects correctly identified as either having or not having the diagnosis. In this case the diagnostic accuracy is 50 + 25 divided by the total number of subjects, or 75%.

Finally, when diagnostic accuracy or classification is the focus of the test results, it is important to consider the positive and negative predictive values. Positive predictive value (PPV) is the probability that given a positive test finding, the diagnosis is present (A/A + B). Negative predictive value (NPV) is the probability that given a negative test finding, the diagnosis is not present (D/C + D). The higher the PPV, the more confidence we can place in interpretation of a positive finding. The higher the NPV, the more confidence we can have in a negative test finding. In this way they are related to sensitivity and specificity, which are conceptualized as being properties of the test (Blacker, 1992). PPV and NPV are somewhat different ways of looking at the relationship of test results to diagnostic validity and are conceptualized as being influenced by base rates of the diagnosis in the sample being studied.

Because diagnosis is frequently made on the basis of combining multiple bits of information, not many tests have been evaluated with these concepts in mind. A noteworthy exception is in the area of detection of malingering in which great attention has been paid to these issues. One recent exception is a study by Guilmette and Rasile (1995), who reported the capacity of the Rey Auditory Verbal Learning Test, the Logical Memory subtest of the WMS-R, and an Expanded Paired Associate Test to identify subjects with and without mild brain injury. They found that the Logical Memory subtest had the largest diagnostic accuracy (83%) and sensitivity (87%), but the Rey Auditory had the greatest specificity (100%). But even in this study, the validity of decisions made with multiple pieces of input was not a major focus of the study.

Meta-Analysis

Yet another recent development in research methodology promises to have great impact on validity research. This is the area of meta-analysis. Early conceptualizations (Glass, McGraw, & Smith, 1981; Hunter, Schmidt, & Jackson, 1982) focused on the methods of concatenating the results of multiple studies to come to some logical conclusions. The basic notions were that multiple studies sometimes provided what appeared to be contradictory results. Traditional literature review methods can result in varying conclusions depending upon the perspective of the reviewer. The meta-analytic approach attempted to provide an objective method of viewing the data from various studies in a single framework in order to reach reliable conclusions (Rosenthal, 1984).

To compare results of different studies, it is necessary to use a common metric. Most meta-analyses utilize some form of effect size, usually a ratio of mean differences to some index of variability. The effect sizes of different studies can then be compared or averaged. Another method is the confidence profile method in which evidence is synthesized to provide estimates of the effect of an independent variable or intervention (Eddy, Hasselblad, & Shachter, 1992). There are several advantages and limitations associated with meta-analytic techniques, and these opposing variables have received considerable attention as meta-analysis has developed (Cooper & Hedges, 1994; Wachter & Straf, 1990). For example, the selection and identification of relevant studies may have associated systematic error, and methods have been proposed to remediate this possibility (Hunter & Schmidt, 1990; Jacob, 1984). Applications of meta-analysis have required the development of new statistical methods (Hedges & Olkin, 1985). Indeed, the field of meta-analytic analysis has become a cottage industry.

Of course, there have also been criticisms of meta-analysis. These criticisms have sometimes involved the potential for bias in obtaining data for the analysis. The file drawer problem refers to the fact that only positive findings tend to get published and negative findings tend to occupy file drawers, biasing the data available for meta-analysis. One way of dealing with the problem of availability of studies is the fail-safe n. The fail-safe n is a way of estimating the number of additional studies with contradictory results that would be necessary to reduce an obtained effect to a specified lower level (Durlak, 1995; Wolf, 1986). Other critics see meta-analysis as a clumsy attempt to combine otherwise disparate studies with questionable results. Independent researchers frequently have independent conceptualizations and measurement systems. Averaging effect sizes across these studies may be misleading. It is important to realize that these same criticisms may also be applied to the qualitative literature review. However, meta-analysis allows quantitative methods of addressing these concerns, for example, coding the characteristics along which studies may differ (Wolf, 1986). Meta-analysis is not a magic panacea, but it is an improvement over qualitative, impressionistic methods of synthesizing research findings.

Meta-analysis can be used to summarize the findings in a field, but it can also be used to examine why or how different findings occur (Durlak, 1995). Meta-analysis can be partially understood as studies in which studies themselves are the observations or subjects. If the independent measures are characteristics of the studies (open-label vs. double-blind, random assignment vs. self-selection, direct observation vs. self-report) the comparison of effects sizes can help explain observed difference in study outcome.

The application of meta-analysis to clinical neuropsychological assessment research can be used to either provide estimates of average effects sizes in the relationship of diagnoses to test results or in the attempt to explain why different results may be reported in studies examining the same test in different populations or contexts. Hasselblad and Hedges (1995) have presented a method that can be used to evaluate the sensitivity and specificity of diagnostic tests. It appears that meta-analytic techniques have much to offer clinical neuropsychological assessment research, but this is still potential. Garb and Schramke (1996) provided an excellent example of meta-analysis to evaluate neuropsychological studies, particularly with regard to judgment research.

Ecological Validity

The concepts of ecological validity have received greater attention since the publication of the first edition of this book. However, with the exception of a book edited by Sbordone and Long (1996) there has been only a slight increase in actual published research using these concepts. It is hoped that the current chapter will help encourage further work, either conceptual and theoretical work or, more importantly, empirical work.

As noted earlier in this volume, the methodologies of clinical neuropsychological assessment have changed over time in response to influence from advances in psychometric theory, developments in neuropsychological theory, and changes in referral questions. As clinical neuropsychologists have been asked more frequently to predict factors such as return to work, need for supervision, or applicability of various educational interventions, the uses of assessment data have expanded. Therefore the concepts of validity for neuropsychological assessments have been expanded. In addition, there is greater emphasis on outcomes in the clinical arena. Part of this is the influence of managed care, but this influence builds on a substrate of prior interest in the practicality (outcome) of clinical assessments and interventions.

Williams (1996) discussed ecological validity in the context of everyday assessment— the assessment of skills necessary for practical (everyday) activities. These activities include simple employment, job-related skills, construct specific skills such as the language skills involved in conversation, following instructions, or discursive writing. He points out that consideration of these skills is essential in the rehabilitation field and that the increase of interest in ecological validity may be a result of increased participation of neuropsychologists in this clinical activity. However, yet another impetus may come from increased participation of neuropsychologists in the legal arena. Here it is not uncommon that a cross-examining lawyer may inquire as to the practical consequences of certain test scores. Finally, because neuropsychology is psychology, it involves the measurement and prediction of behavior, and it seems only natural that the validity concerns of neuropsychological assessment are expanded to include ecological considerations.

Although ecological validity is a term that is being increasingly used in discussions of the evaluations of neuropsychological tests and assessment techniques, there is a lack of definitional specificity in the definition. The term "ecological validity" has been used primarily to describe aspects of the assessment task and the perceived relation of that task to everyday tasks, that is, tasks that are found in the open environment. For example, Crook, Youngjohn, and Larrabee (1990) have devised a set of procedures that they describe as being more ecologically relevant and valid than previously devised techniques for the assessment of memory. Although their test, the Misplaced Objects Test, is a standardized procedure that is administered in the assessment clinic, the behaviors involved have a topographical similarity to behaviors in "real life." Implicit in the current usage of the term "ecological validity" is the idea that somehow the assessment procedure is similar to some aspect of free behavior in the open environment and that the results of the assessment procedures can somehow predict free behavior in the open environment.

In general, the validity of an assessment instrument is related to its ability to achieve the objectives of the assessment process, and ecological validity may not be an important consideration in all instances. When the objective of assessment is the prediction of behavior in the open environment or the prediction of functional capacity, the relationship of the assessment data to the environmental or ecological variables becomes pertinent.

Defining Components of Neuropsychological Ecological Validity

Franzen and Wilhelm described ecological validity as having two aspects. The first aspect, verisimilitude, is the topographical similarity of the data collection method to a task in the free environment, presumably the target prediction task. The second aspect, veridicality, is the extent to which test results reflect or can predict phenomena in the open environment. Verisimilitude may be more important in the design of neuropsychological assessment instruments. In designing the procedures of the instrument, one would need to carefully consider the intended use of the information. For example, in designing an instrument to evaluate the ability of a patient to remember instructions at work, one would want to assess verbal memory, memory for narrative, and memory for conceptually linked discrete behaviors because all of those types of memory are likely to be involved in the relevant task. Once the instrument is designed, aspects of veridicality become more important. Both aspects of ecological validity need to be evaluated, although the relative emphasis will vary with the test studied and the purposes for which the test may be applied.

Usually, ecological validity in neuropsychological assessment involves a description of skill deficits. The presence of a deficit is then related to the capacity of the subject to perform a certain behavior. A more complete conceptualization of ecological validity will involve the correlation of a neuropsychological assessment technique with a behavior and not just a correlation with a deficit (Chelune, 1982). This consideration is an expansion of the aims of neuropsychological assessment beyond the traditional aim of uncovering a deficit, which is the legacy of behavioral neurology. The consideration of behavior and not just deficit increases the relevant population of interest from impaired subjects to normal subjects; do the scores derived from the test correlate with performance on the criterion behavior in a sample of nonimpaired individuals?

The prediction of behavior can be evaluated in either the universe of specific, although complex behaviors, such as driving skills as well as in the prediction of molar outcomes, such as success in rehabilitation or return to work. In the first case, a single test may be useful in predicting the criterion, as in the preceding example of the use of a verbal memory test to predict capacity to remember work instructions. In the second case, because molar outcome is dependent upon a combination of behavioral skills, a group of tests may be necessary for accurate predictions. In addition, the capacity of the subject to link together molecular skills may need to be assessed.

Experimental Design

There are two basic classes of experimental design that can be utilized in evaluations of the ecological validity of neuropsychological assessment instruments: the concurrent and the longitudinal designs. In the concurrent designs, the results of neuropsychological assessment instruments are evaluated in terms of their ability to statistically predict performance on everyday tasks. For example, the relationship between score on a test of sequencing skills and the ability to follow a recipe in cooking may be investigated.

The longitudinal design involves prediction not only in the statistical sense, but also in the temporal sense. For example, scores on a test of abstract problem-solving may be examined in terms of their ability to predict success in rehabilitation or return to work. Application of the longitudinal design would also allow the neuropsychologist to investigate whether relevant predictors change over time. The scores on memory tests may be reasonable predictors of return to work when the memory assessment is conducted in an acute setting, but scores on a test of executive functioning may have greater predictive power in a reentry setting. Dodrill and Clemmons (1984) reported the results of a longitudinal design to investigate the ability of neuropsychological evaluations to predict adjustment in young adult epileptic patients between 3 and 11 years after the evaluations were conducted. The authors reported that the neuropsychological variables, especially the language variables, were more effective in prediction than were the emotional variables (MMPI scale scores).

Limits on the Determination of the Ecological Validity of Neuropsychological Assessment

There are at least three reasons why prediction of behavior in the open environment is not an easy task at the present time. First, there is little information regarding relationships between test results and actual behavior. Second, the evaluation of relationships between test results and behavior in the open environment will itself be difficult. The set of relationships between these two sets of phenomena is likely to be complex and moderated by other variables. These moderating variables may include the speed of information processing and the degree of distractibility. Third, the controlled aspect of the assessment situation may rule out the use of learned compensatory mechanisms that have proven to be successful for the subject. In the second case, test results may overpredict behavioral performance; in the third case, test results may underpredict performance.

Clinical neuropsychology has developed from the perspective of identifying behavioral patterns associated with lesion locations or etiological variables. As a result, certain tests such as the Halstead Category test, while useful in the determination of organic dysfunction, have little in the way of topographical similarities to real-world activities. This is not to say that these same tests may have correlates with behavior in the open environment. The component skills of the Category test may have real-world referents. For example, the Category test requires visual recognition skills, aspects of memory, nonverbal abstraction skills, and systematic problem-solving skills. However, it would be difficult to find an environmental situation in which a person was asked to perform the actual task involved in the Category test. In addition, for some neuropsychological constructs, there may be limited practical implications. As an example of this situation, Hart and Hayden (1986) discuss the lack of real-world examples of ideomotor apraxia.

Statistical Models of Interactive Predictor Variables

Contemporary neuropsychological theoretical models are multivariate, and the preceding evidence indicates that ecological validity models will, of necessity, be multivariate as well. The multivariate nature of neuropsychology should be no surprise to any student of psychology. Although the inferences drawn from the end product of assigning numbers to neuropsychological assessment procedures frequently may relate to physiological processes and structures, it is important to remember that neuropsychology predominantly involves the study of behavior. As such, the same issues that attend the study of behavior in general, i.e., psychological investigations, will impact upon the study of neuropsychological phenomena, albeit with the further complication of issues of physiology and anatomy. In explicating his notion of ecological validity, Brunswick (1955) stated his view that behavior is multiply determined and probabilistic in nature. If this position is true for the study of behavior in general psychology, it can be no less true for the study of behavior in neuropsychology.

Levels of Analysis

In evaluating the ecological validity of neuropsychological tests, there are multiple levels of analyzing the data obtained, but not all of these levels will be relevant to evaluating the twin aspects of verisimilitude and veridicality. Verisimilitude will require an analysis of information at a theoretical level or at a conceptual level. Veridicality involves a theoretical and an empirical level of analysis.

Relationship to Other Forms of Validity

Perhaps the best way to conceptualize ecological validity is to consider it in the context of general aspects of the validity of assessment techniques. Validity is best conceptualized not as a characteristic of tests, but rather as a characteristic of inferences. That is to say, we do not evaluate the validity of a test, but instead we evaluate the validity of an inference in using a test with a certain population. The different forms of validity become different methods of evaluating the utility and accuracy of the inferences drawn from the test results. The different forms of validity may be seen to overlap. For example, factorial validity may overlap with construct validity in an instrument that purports to evaluate both visual and verbal memory. In the same way, ecological validity is not an entirely independent concept.

Aspects of ecological validity, especially the degree of verisimilitude, tend to overlap with face validity. The relevant question here would be whether a test that is said to measure memory contains tasks that resemble everyday tasks that require memory processes. In the same way, aspects of ecological validity related to empirical relationships may overlap with predictive validity. The relevant question here would be whether an instrument said to measure memory can predict memory performance in the open environment.

Just as there can be no general answer to the question of which is more important, discriminant validity or concurrent validity, there can be no general answer to the question of which is more important, ecological validity or traditional validity. The related issues revolve around questions of understanding versus questions of application. Brooks and Baumeister (1977) have considered these issues in the context of research investigating mental retardation, but the points made are relevant here as well. Two themes become apparent. The first theme is the development of a theory of brain–behavior relationships and the second theme is an understanding of the condition of neurological impairment. The first theme, which relates to traditional validity, requires the researcher to consider issues of internal and external validity. The second theme, which relates to ecological validity, further requires the researcher to consider what Brooks and Baumeister (1977) term "metatheoretical constraints," namely the implications of motivation, the nature of the underlying condition, and the idiosyncratic manifestation of cause and effect in a specific real-life situation.

On the other hand, House (1977) points out the importance of traditional validity and research concerns because true causes may not be discernible from direct natural observation. Direct observation in the natural environment is constrained by interacting and confounding influences that complicate the process of drawing inferences regarding causation. Comparisons between traditional validity and ecological validity involve questions of understanding versus questions of application. The clinical researcher must consider both sets of questions.

Relationship of Clinical Assessment to Functional Assessment

As defined earlier, one of the considerations of ecological validity is the extent to which the neuropsychological instrument obtains ecologically relevant information (verisimilitude). One way to obtain ecologically relevant information is to design test procedures that elicit behaviors that are topographically related to the target behaviors. Another way to obtain ecologically relevant information is to evaluate the capacity of the subject to perform the behaviors in the environment. For reasons of economy, direct behavioral observations are rarely conducted. Instead, subjects may be given standard stimuli and asked to perform environmental behaviors. An example of this sort of functional assessment is the Loewenstein Direct Assessment of Functional Status (Loewenstein et al., 1989). Here, among other tasks, the subject is given a short list of grocery items and is then taken into a room where multiple grocery items are placed on a table. The task is to select correctly the items on the list. Another task on the Loewenstein involves writing a check and balancing a checkbook.

Alternately, other functional assessment instruments attempt to obtain ecologically relevant material in one of two other methods, either through questionnaires administered to collateral sources or through ratings obtained from professionals. Sometimes, ecologically relevant information is derived from the subject as in the case of the Cognitive Failures Questionnaire (Broadbent, Cooper, Fitzgerald, & Parkes, 1982). However, relying on the neuropsychologically impaired subject to provide information regarding level of skill or deficit is problematic because the subject may be unaware of the deficit or may report inaccurate data (McGlynn & Schacter, 1989; Godfrey, Partridge, Knight, & Bishara, 1993).

Ecological validity is a complex concept that can be conceptualized as involving both verisimilitude, or extent of similarity to relevant environmental behaviors, and veridicality, or degree of accuracy in predicting some environmental behavior or molar outcome. Because of the history of clinical neuropsychology, few clinical neuropsychological assessment instruments have been evaluated in terms of their ecological validity. However, this topic will acquire increased importance as clinical neuropsychologists become more active in applied treatment activities.

Social Validity

Just as the forms of neuropsychological assessment and its uses have been influenced by outside sources, the conceptualization of validity can be influenced by forces outside the specific field of neuropsychology. The realm of clinical interventions is undergoing a shift of emphasis brought about by the incorporation of outcomes research. Similarly, behavioral interventions are increasingly being evaluated by the impact of the intervention on the patient and on the patient's social environment. In both of these areas, an important consideration is the response and appraisal of the patient and other consumers of the intervention. As managed care makes greater inroads into the clinical arena, we will probably see a proliferation of outcomes research related to assessment. The questions raised here are not only whether the assessment was accurate in localization or diagnosis, but also whether the information was useful in impacting the choice of treatment or affecting the general clinical outcome in some demonstrable way. As part of that question, the concept of consumer satisfaction will need to be addressed.

Another consideration in the examination of ecological validity is the extent to which the target behavior is important to the functional capacity of the subject. This is a term that has been called social validity by some behaviorists (Hawkins, 1988). The issue is the extent to which the chosen unit of observation, or target behavior, is related to an issue of concern to the subject or to others in the social environment. For example, an assessment instrument used in the clinic may be found to be a good predictor of memory for shopping lists, but the task of remembering shopping lists may be irrelevant to a certain subject's life. The information relevant to this decision would involve self-report by the subject, the report of others in the subject's environment such as family members or caregivers, or expert opinion derived from neuropsychologists, nursing staff, or occupational therapists.

Social validity will have greater relevance to the process of neuropsychological assessment than to the evaluation of a single instrument. As a result it may share methods and concepts with decision analysis and research in clinical neuropsychological assessment. Because social validity concerns extend beyond the interpretation of results to the consequences of that interpretation, it enlarges the evaluation of the neuropsychological assessment results into a consideration of the system in which that assessment occurs. Therefore, we may witness in the future an even greater change in neuropsychological assessment methods and instruments as influences apart from the traditional influences of basic neurosciences, neuropsychological theory, psychometric theory, and referral source begin to have their effect.

An implication of including social relevance in the evaluation of ecological validity is that the values of the information source become an important part of the evaluation process. The question cannot be simply answered by examining whether a subject can perform a behavior; we must additionally ask, "Is the behavior important, and if so, to whom is it important?" There might be instances in which there are differences of opinion as to whether the target behavior or the assessment index is important. For example, an elderly resident of a nursing facility may not feel that it is important for her to be able to remember the names of staff or connect the names with the correct faces because the staff will provide care regardless of how she addresses them. On the other hand the care facility staff may feel that learning and using the staff's names will help the staff behave positively toward the subject, and the clinical neuropsychologist may possess the value that it is always better to improve a subject's functional memory. Another example might involve a severely head-injured patient's opinion that it is important for him to be able to plan and execute a cooked meal when the professional staff feel that his severe motor deficits significantly reduce the likelihood of such a behavior occurring.

The inclusion of values in the consideration of ecological validity is not meant to cloud the issues, but instead is meant to make explicit processes that already occur in the clinical setting. Clinical work does not exist in a social vacuum. Instead, all clinical activity occurs in the context of social contingencies partly under the control of the funding agent whether it is the government, the insurance company, a family member, or the patient herself. In addition, the social contingencies are under partial control of spouse and family members, care provider staff members, and other members of the clinical assessment team. By including social considerations, we allow ourselves a chance to examine the relevance, fairness, and utility of the values underlying some of our clinical decisions.

Including the issue of social validity complicates the evaluation of assessment instruments. One problem is that the demands of each person's open environment are different. The tasks and skills required in one job setting or in one cultural setting may not be applicable to another setting. The problem of individual environments does not obviate the need for basic assessment instruments. For one thing, basic assessment instruments, or instruments that have been designed to answer questions of organic integrity, localization, or diagnosis, maintain an important place in the overall assessment process. Most of these instruments are nomothetic with available comparisons to normative information. The normative comparisons can help provide information related to the level of skill demonstrated by the individual subject. The diagnostic information presented by the instruments can help in indicating treatments that may be helpful. Or alternately, the diagnostic information may help particularize the treatment approach most likely to be successful. For example, a memory assessment instrument may indicate that Alzheimer's disease is a probable diagnosis, indicating that serial assessments may be necessary or that arrangements for family members to help take responsibility should be made. Alternately, a memory assessment instrument may indicate that the manifest memory failure is due to difficulty in encoding, pointing to treatments that facilitate encoding. Although the problem of individual environments may seem to discourage the assessment of social validity, this challenge actually underlines the need for developing a more full armamentarium of assessment techniques. In that way, the clinician can obtain a more full view of the functioning of the subject.

Test Bias

Test and item bias can be seen as the validity analogs of item response theory in reliability. As a brief review, one of the central concepts of item response theory is that error terms may be correlated with true scores such that the reliability of a test may systematically vary as a function of skill level of the individual being assessed or as a function of the difficulty of the item regardless of the skill level of the individual being assessed. Although test or item bias appears to have pejorative connotations, at its essence bias refers to the notion of differential validity. The question that the methods of item bias attempts to answer is, "Does this item have different relations with the criterion depending upon characteristics of the individual being assessed?"

An important point needs to be raised here. Because tests can be used to permit or deny access to services or benefits or used to define classes, the application of test results can be used in a discriminatory fashion. That is, if the test results of males and females are used to allow admission to a certain college, more males than females may be admitted if males tend to score higher than females on the test. Whether or not this is a discriminatory practice is a sociolegal question. If the test equally predicts success at that college for males and females, then the test is not biased. However, if the test predicts accurately for males, but over- or underpredicts for females, then the test, or certain items, can be said to be biased. Bias is a property of the test, while validity is a property of the application of test results (Shepard, 1982).

There are several excellent introductions to test bias including Berk (1982a), Camilli and Shepard (1994), Osterlind (1983), and Holland and Thayer (1988). A basic method of examination for test bias is to examine the accuracy of prediction to criterion for different groups for which there might be hypothesized different relations. If classification is the issue one might first see if application of a cut rule results in different proportions of different groups of subjects classified to the criterion. For example, if the application of an optimal population cut rule for the Boston Naming Test results in different proportions of African-Americans and Caucasians classified as demented and there is no reason to expect different prevalence of the disorder in the two groups, the test might be biased. In that case, different cut scores may be developed (Lichtenberg, Ross, & Christensen, 1994).

The relationship of item bias to unfairness and its correctives is fraught with political overtones. In this context of conflicting values, decisions regarding the application of test results if not the actual interpretation of test results would be made on an unstable basis. Although there is currently no major ethical or professional conflict or dilemma related to test bias, one can see how these might arise by examination of the industrial/organizational psychology literature and the literature related to selection (Brown, 1994; Cascio, Zedeck, Goldstein, & Outtz, 1995; Gottfredson, 1994; Sackett & Wilk, 1994). Despite these difficulties, it is important that the psychometric evaluation of neuropsychological tests in the future take into consideration the possibility of test bias and evaluate for its presence. This is essential if clinical neuropsychology is to develop as an international endeavor and not just a collection of national efforts. Even in a single national group, the increasingly multicultural nature of society requires that cognitive and emotional evaluations be sensitive to potential sources of variability in test scores.

The evaluation for test bias is important for both new tests and established tests. At an earlier level of test construction, it would be important to evaluate for the presence of item bias. Camilli and Shepard (1994) separate bias assessment methods into internal and external. In external methods, if the criterion can be assumed to be error free, the potential for either overprediction or underprediction is evaluated. In internal methods, the examination is for different item difficulty indices for different groups. It may be difficult to identify item bias when it is present in a large proportion of items for a test. Bias can be conceptualized as the measurement of intended content being contaminated by the effects of demographic variables (Suen, 1990). There are several methods available for evaluating item bias.

The first method is called the delta plot. Here, the inverse normal transformation of item difficulty indices (p) for items for one group is plotted against those for another group. Outliers from the regression line may represent biased items. In the chi-square approach, groups are divided into ability levels and the difference in p is calculated by level. In the Mantel–Haenszel approach, two groups are matched on ability level (e.g., total score). Then an odds ratio of the two difficulties for individual items is calculated. If the items are not biased, the odds ratio should equal 1. Finally, item response theory (IRT, as first presented in Chapter 3) can be used. The item characteristic curve can be compared across groups. Alternately, individual item parameters can be compared. Third, the fit of the two groups to the IRT can be examined (Ironson, 1983).

CONCLUSIONS

From the preceding information, one may conclude that Cronbach's (1984) redefinition of test validation as test evaluation is a sensible approach that neatly captures the meaning of validity. As a result of many studies in a variety of conditions, a procedure can be defined in terms of the populations about whom it is maximally informative, the conditions under which it is maximally applicable and the decisions to which it is maximally applicable, and the decisions to which it is maximally contributory. Although it may be easy to become lost in the excitement of investigating a new instrument or new uses for an old instrument, it is important to remember that the ultimate purpose of validating a test is to inform the clinician or the consumer about the kinds of decisions that may be made, based on the results of the procedure in question.

The ultimate evaluative-validational demonstration of a test is its clinical utility. Tests survive to the extent that they provide information that is useful in the individual case as well as on the average. The various forms of validation are markers that indicate to a clinician the relative importance of a pattern of performance and the likelihood that a given pattern of performance is diagnostically or predictively contributory to the overall understanding of the patient.

The Wechsler Adult Intelligence Scale-Revised and Wechsler Adult Intelligence Scale-III

The Wechsler Intelligence Scales are the most popular method of estimating IQ in clinical settings. There have been Spanish (Escala Inteligencia de Wechsler or EIWA) and Japanese translations (Hattori & Lynn, 1997) as well as adaptations for British and for Canadian subjects (Pugh & Boer, 1991). The Wechsler Adult Intelligence Scale-Revised (WAIS-R; Wechsler, 1981) is, as its name implies, a revised form of the Wechsler Adult Intelligence Scale, which was first published in 1955. There were two main reasons the original version was revised. First, some of the items on the WAIS had become dated and were replaced with more contemporary items. An attempt was also made to make the test more culture-fair by including items related to black people and black history. Whether these attempts succeeded is an empirical question. Second, with the passage of three decades, the norms for the WAIS were unlikely to describe deviation intelligence. Scores could be interpreted as deviation IQs from the original sample, not from the general contemporary population.

The structure of the WAIS was maintained in the WAIS-R. There are 11 subtests, each of which is purported to measure components of intelligence. These 11 subtests are grouped under two general headings: the Information, Digit Span, Vocabulary, Arithmetic, Comprehension, and Similarities subtests are included in Verbal IQ (VIQ), and the Picture Completion, Picture Arrangement, Block Design, Object Assembly, and Digit Symbol subtests are included in Performance IQ (PIQ). All of the subtests are included in Full Scale IQ (FSIQ). Interpretation can take place at the level of the subtest scores, the PIQ and VIQ scores, or the FSIQ scores. Although the WAIS and the WAIS-R appear similar in content, structure, and procedure, there are important differences in the scores obtained from the two tests (Ryan, Nowak, & Geisser, 1987). Wechsler (1981), Lippold and Claiborn (1983), Smith (1983), Simon and Clopton (1984), Wagner and Gianakos (1985), and Whitworth and Gibbons (1986) have all reported that use of the WAIS-R results in significantly lower estimates of IQ than does use of the WAIS in multiple populations.

The lower estimates of IQ resulting when more contemporary assessment methods are used is a very common phenomenon that is seen in almost all revisions of intelligence tests. The lower estimates are necessary to counteract another phenomenon that has been labeled the Flynn effect. The Flynn effect is a consistent observation that regardless of the choice of standardized method used to evaluate intelligence and regardless of the population studies, IQ scores tend to increase between 2 and 3 points per decade. This is not likely to be due to general increases in average human intelligence, as any observer of politics or even of daily human behavior can easily ascertain. Instead, this increase may be due to shifts in the typical knowledge and skills of the average individual. If the deviation IQ is to have a consistent meaning as an index of difference from the average, then the normative transformation must change as well.

Although it is not as clear whether this gain is true for other neuropsychological skill areas, it certainly seems to be the case for general intelligence. The gain has occurred for standardized tests of intelligence in American (Flynn, 1984) and in Scottish subjects (Flynn, 1990), as well as for tests of intelligence in other countries even when those tests are relatively less dependent on culture (Flynn, 1987). The reasons for this gain have been debated without complete resolution, but regardless of the reason, the effect poses problems for clinical assessment unless tests are renormed consistently. Flynn (1998) provided suggestions for compensating for obsolete norms prior to the publication of revised intelligence tests.

NORMATIVE INFORMATION

The WAIS-R was normed on a sample of 1880 individuals in the United States who were between 16 and 74 years of age. By the use of information contained in the 1970 U.S. Census, the sample was stratified into groups on the basis of sex, age, race, geographic location, occupation, education, and urban versus rural residence. Raw scores on the WAIS-R are converted to scale scores by comparing the performance of the subject with the performance of the normative sample. The subtest scale scores have a mean of 10 and a standard deviation of 3. By examining the conversion tables for the age groups, one can see that it is mainly decrements in Performance subtests that make the age norms necessary. Although scale scores are available for the different age groups, the determination of IQ is made by obtaining scale scores based on the performance of the normative sample as a whole. It is when the subtest scale scores are summed that the age norms are used in the determination of IQ. IQ scores have a mean of 100 and a standard deviation of 15. Although the standardization sample did not demonstrate differences in performance due to race, Marcopulos, McLain, and Guiliano (1997) offer evidence that at least for elderly subjects race (Caucasian vs. African-American) was an important predictor of performance.

RELIABILITY

The scoring reliability of the WAIS-R was evaluated in a study reported by Ryan, Prifitera, and Powers (1983). In this study, 19 Ph.D. psychologists and 20 psychology graduate students scored two WAIS-R protocols that had been obtained from vocational counseling clients. The consequent IQ scores varied as much as 8 points across scorers. The variability in the scores of the two groups (Ph.D.s vs. students) was approximately equal, except in the case of the PIQ, where the Ph.D.s had a larger variance in scores that was statistically significant for both of the protocols. The results of this study underline the necessity of strict adherence to the standardized scoring system when using the WAIS-R.

The manual for the WAIS-R (Wechsler, 1981) gives split-half reliability information for each of the subtests except for the speeded subtest of Digit Symbol and the power subtest of Digit Span. In both of these cases, the test–retest reliability is reported. Reliability information is given for each of the nine age groups and is then averaged, by means of Fisher's r-to-z transformation, to yield a reliability coefficient averaged across the age groups. The reliability coefficients for the IQ scores were obtained by a methodology for computing the reliability of a composite group of tests. The split-half reliability coefficients are corrected for the length of the tests by use of the Spearman–Brown formula, but no information is given regarding the nature of the split. The reliability coefficients range from .68 for Object Assembly to .96 for Vocabulary. The reliability coefficients for the IQ scores are .97 for VIQ, .93 for PIQ, and .97 for FSIQ. It is important to remember that the IQ reliability coefficients are estimates based on composite scores. Equivalent internal consistency reliability coefficients have been reported in two separate samples of psychiatric inpatients (Boone, 1992a; Piedmont, Sokolove, & Fleming, 1989).

Test–retest reliability is presented for each of subtests as well as for IQ scores. The test–retest values were computed from the results of two administrations to a group of 71 subjects between the ages of 25 and 34 years and a sample of 48 subjects between the ages of 45 and 54 years. The intertest intervals ranged from 2 to 7 weeks. The test–retest reliability coefficients ranged from .69 for Digit Symbol in the 25- to 34-year-old group to .94 for Information in the 45- to 54-year-old group. The IQ test–retest coefficients were substantially high, the lowest being .89 for the PIQ in the 35- to 44 year-old group and the highest being .97 for verbal IQ in the 45- to 54-year-old group. There was no test for the difference in level across the two test sessions. This is a potentially important issue, as studies have indicated that, at least for the WAIS, there are substantial gains in IQ scores across time even in the presence of significant correlation coefficients (Catron & Thompson, 1979; Matarazzo, Carmody, & Jacobs, 1980). Carvajal, Schrader, and Holmes (1996) reported test–retest data similar to that in the manual but with 18- to 19-year-old subjects.

Hopp, Dixon, Grut, and Bacekman (1997) administered the WAIS-R to elderly normal subjects (aged 77 to 87 years) at 6-month intervals over a 2-year period. The WAIS-R demonstrated highly stable internal consistency estimates across periods as well as stable score values. When healthy elderly individuals were administered the WAIS-R twice across a 1-year period, there was a high correlation but also an average increase of 3 points in FSIQ (Raguet, Campbell, Berry, Schmitt, and Smith, 1996). Snow, Tierney, Zorzitto, Fisher, and Reid (1989) found good reliability for IQ scores but not for subtest scores or VIQ–PIQ discrepancy scores in a sample of healthy elderly individuals. This lack of reliability for the VIQ–PIQ split was also found in the standardization sample (Matarazzo & Herman, 1984). The temporal reliability of WAIS-R IQs in 16-year-old subjects tested twice across either a 3-month or an 18-month interval was equivalent to the values reported in the manual (Thompson & Molly, 1993).

The temporal stability of the WAIS-R in populations that would be administered the test for clinical reasons is also pertinent. Ryan, Georgemiller, Geisser, and Randall (1985) report a wide range of gains or losses on retest in a heterogeneous sample, and this change was correlated with years of education. Watkins and Campbell (1992) found that the WAIS-R had good reliability in a sample of mentally retarded adults who were tested over an average interval of 2 years and 8 months. Boone (1992a) reported good temporal reliability in psychiatric inpatients tested twice across a 2- to 8-week interval. Hawkins and Sayward (1994) found that the test–retest reliability in psychiatric inpatients tested again after discharge (mean interval was 15 months) was comparable to the values reported in the manual.

The presence of significant practice effects is as important as knowledge about reliable practice effects. Axelrod, Brines, and Rapaport (1997) found that subtracting 6 points from the FSIQ resulted in the best approximation of original FSIQ when a group of normal individuals was administered the WAIS-R twice across a 14-date interval. There may be differences in stability when the subjects are initially impaired. Therefore, it is vital that information be gathered regarding the test–retest reliability of the WAIS-R in those populations that are likely to be administered the instrument more than once. Rawlings and Crewe (1992) presented information regarding the average gains in IQ scores when individuals with traumatic brain injury (TBI) were tested at 2, 4, 8, and 1 months post-injury as compared to individuals with TBI who were tested twice at 2 and 12 months post-injury. Over the 12-month period, FSIQ increased nearly 14 points, VIQ increased nearly 9 points, and PIQ increased nearly 20 points. These researchers concluded that the practice effects were secondary to the improvement via recovery of skill in these subjects. In another look at this issue but with a different sample of head-injured patients as subjects, mean improvement scores were less than half those reported in the other study (Moore et al., 1990). Here, improvement correlated negatively with months post-injury, which may also account for the differences between the two studies.

McSweeny, Naugle, Chelune, and Lueders (1993) presented a method for evaluating individual change based on regression analysis of test–retest values in subjects known to be stable that may be helpful when comparison subjects with similar clinical characteristics are available.

The stability of test scores is important, as is the stability of other indices such as VIQ–PIQ splits and indices of scatter. Paolo and Ryan (1996) reported that when 61 normal elderly subjects were tested twice over an average period of 65 days, although the VIQ–PIQ split showed good reliability, there was great variability in both intersubtest and intrasubtest scatter with 52% disagreement of relative strengths and weaknesses.

The manual also presents information regarding the standard error of measurement for each of the subtest scores and the IQ scores for the nine age groups. These values are then averaged to provide an estimate of the overall standard error of measurement. The values are presented as scaled score units. These values range from .61 for Vocabulary to 1.54 for Object Assembly. The standard error of measurement values for the IQ scores are 2.74 for the VIQ, 4.14 for the PIQ, and 2.53 for the FSIQ. Naglieri (1982) presented values for confidence limits for the IQ scores. However, there is a problem with the values reported in the manual and by Naglieri. There are three formulas for the computation of the standard error of measurement. The formula used in the manual provides an estimate of the amount of error variance in the score and does not provide confidence boundaries for the scores, as the manual incorrectly states. Knight (1983) presented the values computed from the formula, which allow an interpretation of the confidence boundaries. Ryan, Paolo, and Brungardt (1990) present data regarding the reliability of the WAIS-R in elderly people and recommend its use in that population.

The manual provides a table of the minimum value required for the reliability of differences between pairs of scale scores and between the IQ scores. Atkinson (1991a) examined the reliability of intersubtest comparisons in mentally retarded subjects and found somewhat lower reliability than was reported in the manual for the normative sample; however, this difference did not seem to be of sufficient magnitude to invalidate interpretations based on these differences. D.E. Boone (1998) examined the specificity of variances for the subtests in psychiatric inpatients and found evidence in support of ipsative comparisons and interpretation only for the Information, Arithmetic, Vocabulary, Comprehension, Similarities, Picture Arrangement, and Digit Symbol subtests. Whether this finding applies to other populations and the relationship of the specific variance estimates to the size of the observed comparisons needs further explication, but hypotheses regarding ipsative comparisons with the remaining subtests should be interpreted cautiously when the observed differences are close to the standard errors. Atkinson (1992a) presents values for ipsative comparisons in individuals with mental retardation. This set of data is perhaps more relevant to neuropsychological practice than similar data gained from studies of individuals with no impairment.

Many people erroneously interpret a statistically reliable difference between PIQ and VIQ as a clinically significant one. This is an especially important issue when the VIQ–PIQ split is used to generate hypotheses about the presence of organicity. For example, according to the manual, a VIQ–PIQ split of 12.04 is statistically reliable at the .05 level for the 16- to 17-year-old group. However, Knight (1983) reported that more than 25% of the normative sample in that age group exceeded that difference. Clearly, a difference of that magnitude cannot be clinically significant. Grossman (1983) also examined the prevalence of different magnitudes of VIQ–PIQ splits in the normative sample for the WAIS-R. He reported that 10% of the normative sample, averaged across age groups, had a VIQ–PIQ split of at least 18 points. The normative sample was chosen partly on the basis of a negative history of neurological impairment. The fact that a large percentage of subjects manifested reliably large VIQ–PIQ splits argues against the use of the split to diagnose organicity. Piedmont, Sokolove, and Fleming (1989) had earlier cautioned against strict interpretation of the split when the minimum values reported in the manual are met. Atkinson (1991b) presented values for VIQ–PIQ differences based on confidence intervals placed around an estimate of the true score regressed against the mean rather than observed scores. [But see also Atkinson (1992b) for corrections].

An important distinction must be made among the reliability, the abnormality, and the validity of the VIQ–PIQ split (Berk, 1982b). Reliability of the split refers to a computation that denotes the probability that a split of a certain magnitude will occur as the result of error of measurement. Abnormality of the split refers to the observed percentage of subjects manifesting a split of a certain magnitude. Validity of the split refers to the clinical meaning of a split of a certain magnitude. Ryan (1984) calculated values for the abnormality of VIQ–PIQ differences in the normative sample. Associated with each difference value is a probability level that can be interpreted as the proportion of subjects who exhibit that magnitude of difference. Ryan reported that a difference of 28 points could be found in 156 individuals of the normative sample. The fact that a split of that magnitude could occur in normal subjects emphasizes the need for an empirical evaluation of the validity of the VIQ–PIQ split.

To assess the validity of the VIQ–PIQ split in neuropsychological diagnosis, Bornstein (1983b) examined the VIQ–PIQ split in patients with unilateral and bilateral cerebral dysfunction using a sample of 89 patients. Of these patients, 20 had left-hemisphere dysfunction, 24 had right-hemisphere dysfunction, and 45 had bilateral dysfunction as determined by neurodiagnostic techniques. It was found that the left-hemisphere patients had significantly lower VIQ than PIQ; however, the mean difference was only 4.9 points. Similarly, the right-hemisphere patients had significantly lower PIQ than VIQ, but the mean difference was 10.7 points. Most tellingly, the bilaterally dysfunctional patients had significantly lower PIQ than VIQ, and the mean difference was 7.8 points. It appears that cerebral dysfunction may have effects on the VIQ–PIQ split, but the absence of a control group in this study lessens our confidence in such a conclusion. However, the results of this study in conjunction with the examination of the VIQ–PIQ data in the WAIS-R normative sample emphasize the tenuous nature of performing a neuropsychological diagnosis using WAIS-R data only.

Some authors have suggested that the VIQ–PIQ split in unilateral lesions is differential by sex. McGlone (1977, 1978) presented data and Inglis and Lawson (1981) provided a literature review that seem to support this idea. However, a report by Bornstein (1984) concludes that sex does not make a difference in the validity of this split. Snow, Freedman, and Ford (1986) reviewed published studies that evaluated the possibility of differential laterality results in WAIS and Wechsler–Bellevue scores for males and females. They concluded that the effect of sex was nonrobust and might therefore be a reflection of a relationship between sex and other variables, such as education level. Sundet (1986) examined VIQ–PIQ differences in 83 subjects with unilateral brain impairment. When the magnitude of the split was used, only 70% of the subjects were correctly classified as left- or right-hemisphere-impaired. Female subjects were not found to be any more or less lateralized than male subjects. The argument is far from settled, and researchers will need to take sex into account when planning the design and executing the statistical analysis of a future study to examine this idea.

The WAIS-R may be valuable in providing collateral evidence of the existence of lateralized deficits once the existence of cerebral dysfunction has been determined. The differences in VIQ–PIQ splits for the unilaterally damaged subjects in the above study conform to the expectations derived from the widely held assumption that verbal abilities are largely mediated by the dominant hemisphere, whereas spatial tasks are largely mediated by the nondominant hemisphere. To investigate the possibility that a more empirically derived indicator of lateralized deficits may result in more useful neuropsychological information, Lawson, Inglis, and Stroud (1983) performed a principal-components factor analysis of the WAIS-R normative data. They derived a solution with two factors, the first of which they interpreted as general intelligence, and the second of which they interpreted as laterality. These authors then derived a weighted-sum method of combining subtest scale scores into a single laterality index. They then used a formula for computing the reliability of a composite score from the reliabilities of the constituent scale scores and reported an average split-half reliability of .78 for their laterality index. A test–retest coefficient was similarly derived from the data contained in the WAIS-R manual and an average value of .79 was reported. A very important point needs to be made here. The values for reliability reported by Lawson et al. (1983) were derived from a sample of normal subjects. These authors contended that their index is valid only for unilaterally damaged males, although no data are presented to substantiate that claim. The laterality index appears to be a good idea, but much more work, including an investigation of the reliability and validity of the index in the population for which it is intended, is needed before it can be recommended for clinical use.

Pattern analysis, or an examination of the scatter of scores among the subtests of the WAIS-R, is often recommended as an interpretive strategy. The rationale is based on the discovery of statistically significant differences among the subtest scale scores by use of the confidence boundaries published in the manual. Silverstein (1982a) pointed out that the published confidence boundaries are based on differences that compare only two subtests at a time. However, interpretation is based on a comparison of all of the subtests. The experiment-wide error in this case is likely to increase the probability of a type 1 error. Instead, Silverstein recommended that the Bonferroni approximate correction for experiment-wide error be made. Unfortunately, even with this correction, the problem of the clinical interpretation of statistically significant differences remains, as discussed earlier in the case of the VIQ–PIQ split. Silverstein (1991) provides information regarding the reliability of the score differences. Crawford and Allan (1994) describe the use of the Mahalanobis Distance statistic as an index of scatter among subtests and concludes that it is appropriate for use with subjects from the United Kingdom. The utility of the Mahalanobis Distance statistic for United States subjects needs to be investigated. Schinka, Vanderploeg, and Greblo (1998) present a table that details the frequency of observed differences in pairwise comparisons among subtests of the WAIS-R. What is needed is an investigation of the meaning of these differences. Although clinical lore has held that the amount of scatter increases in the presence of brain damage, Ryan, Paolo, and Smith (1992) found no differences in the degree of scatter in a comparison of brain-injured subjects with the standardization sample.

VALIDITY

The factor structure of the WAIS-R is an important issue in the evaluation of the construct validity of the instrument as well as an important issue in the interpretation of the test results. Silverstein (1982b) conducted a principal-factor analysis on the standardization data from the normative sample as reported in the manual. The number of factors was determined by Kaiser's rule of latent roots > 1.0 and the parallel analysis method (Franzen & Golden, 1984a). Silverstein then compared the similarity of the factor solutions for the nine age groups and for the WAIS and WAIS-R standardization data by using the coefficient of congruence. Unfortunately, this descriptive statistic is highly influenced by the number of variables that have the same algebraic sign in their factor loadings. Because of the characteristics of the data, the resulting coefficient of congruence is highly inflated and is misleading to interpret. However, by visual inspection of the averaged factor loadings, it is apparent that there is some similarity between the solutions for the WAIS and for the WAIS-R. Allen and Thorndike (1995a) examined the stability of the Verbal Comprehension, Perceptual Organization, and Freedom from Distractibility factors across each age group in the standardization sample using cross-validation of covariance structure models and found that those factors were stable. Atkinson (1991c) presented tables and a method for constructing confidence boundaries around the factor scores to examine for reliable change over time as well for interfactor comparisons. Rossini, Kowalski, Dudish, and Telcher (1991) reported a low correlation of .49 for the Freedom from Distractibility factor when undergraduate students were measured twice across a 2-week period. The results of this study are suggestive but inconclusive, as the restriction of range from using normal subjects as well as the unresolved question as to whether this factor reflects state or trait characteristics lend to its uncertainty.

Parker (1983) performed factor analysis on the standardization data from the manual. The method used was a principal-factor analysis with varimax rotation. The number of factors extracted was stopped after two, three, and four factors to afford comparison with earlier studies that had reported those numbers of factors when analyzing WAIS data. Except for the method of determining the number of factors, this study is identical to that of Silverstein (1982b), even using the same subjects. However, because Parker reported the results separately for the age groups, the study is of interest to us. The analyses were conducted separately for each of the nine age groups in the normative sample. Parker concluded that the three-factor solution reported for the WAIS is also tenable for the WAIS-R, and that this solution is stable across the age groups. This solution consists of verbal comprehension, perceptual organization, and freedom from distraction. There was no test performed to compare the appropriateness of one solution to another. Instead, the factor solutions were visually inspected. Using a similar methodology, Atkinson and Cyr (1984) reached a similar conclusion from a sample of 114 psychiatric inpatients as did Atkinson, Cyr, Doxey, and Vigna (1989) using a sample of head-injured male subjects, and Zillmer, Waechtler, Harris, Khan, and Fowler (1992) in a sample of patients with a diagnosis of cerebral vascular accidents.

Ryan, Rosenberg, and DeWolfe (1984a) reported an attempt to replicate the results of the factor analysis performed by Silverstein (1982b) in a sample of 85 VA vocational-counseling clients. The authors used a principal-factor analysis with varimax rotation. They did not report what criterion they used to terminate the extraction of factors. They interpreted the two resulting factors as verbal concentration and perceptual organization similar to the earlier solution. They then used the coefficient to congruence to determine the similarity of the factor structures. Unfortunately, the use of the coefficient of congruence was inappropriate. The coefficient of congruence is inflated when many of the factor loadings of the variables have the same algebraic sign (Levine, 1977). In examining the table of factor loadings reported by Ryan et al. (1984a), we see that they all have the same algebraic sign, so that the results of this comparison are highly suspect. Gorsuch (1974) warned against the use of the coefficient of congruence when comparing the results of factor analyses unless only the factor loadings are known. In this case, the authors would have been better advised to use the salient variable similarity index (Cattell, 1949; Cattell, Balcar, Horn, & Nesselroade, 1969). The distribution of the coefficient of congruence is unknown, so it is difficult to agree with the conclusion of these researchers that the factor loadings agree at more than a chance level.

A methodological improvement over the Parker (1983) study would involve a rigorous statistical comparison of the various solutions. O'Grady (1983) performed a maximum-likelihood-confirmatory-factor analysis on the nine age groups in the normative sample. Oblique and orthogonal one-, two-, and three-factor solutions were compared with the null model of no common factors by the use of an index of fit expressed as a chi square. In each case, there were no significant differences between the fit afforded by the null model and the fit afforded by the model being tested. The important implication is that none of the solved factor models account for the relationships among the subtests better than the other models examined. O'Grady (1983) suggested that the single model be adopted for the sake of parsimony. However, the possibility that a five- or six-factor model may account for the data better cannot be ruled out by this study. Allen et al. (1998) performed a confirmatory factor analysis in a sample of 169 males with schizophrenia. These researchers report that the three-factor model as derived from the standardization sample provided a good fit to the data from the experimental sample although the factor on which the Digit Symbol subtests loaded was different across the two samples.

It seems safe to say that the precise factor structure of the WAIS-R remains an empirical question. Fraboni and Saltstone (1992) attempted to resolve the number of factors question through the use of cluster analysis and concluded that the one-, two-, and three-factor solutions were each feasible. Although this study may seem inconclusive, it does help explain why there are disparate results across the factor analytic studies. The clinical utility of the factor models also needs to be addressed. Atkinson et al. (1990) concluded that the three factors (Verbal Comprehension, Perceptual Organization, Freedom from Distractibility) possess adequate temporal stability, indicating the possibility that they reflect stable intellectual traits. Kowalski and Rossini (1990) had also reported excellent reliability for the three factors in each of the age levels in the standardization sample.

Parker and Atkinson (1995) suggested that the three factors of the WAIS-R might be more accurately calculated using multiple regression techniques with the loadings of all of the subtests and not just the most highly contributing subtests to each factor. However, the three factors calculated in the originally suggested manner appear to have reasonable relationships to neuropsychological variables. The three factors of the WAIS-R were cross-validated in a sample of patients with suspected head injury, and those factors were also found to significantly correlate with relevant neuropsychological measures. The WAIS-R factors again correlated with hypothesized neuropsychological variables in a sample of head injury patients (Sherman, Strauss, Spellacy, and Hunter, 1995). Berger (1998) correlated the factor scores from the WAIS-R to data from the Halstead–Reitan in a sample of 112 patients. A complex set of relationships was uncovered, indicating that although the factors have a relationship to conceptually similar variables from the Halstead–Reitan Neuropsychological Battery (HRNB), those factors should not be interpreted in isolation in neuropsychological populations.

Blaha and Wallbrown (1982) reported the results of a hierarchical factor analysis of the standardization data reported in the WAIS-R manual. They concluded that the structure of the WAIS-R is composed of a general intelligence factor that includes two factors. The two secondary factors appeared to be similar to the verbal comprehension and the perceptual organization factors found in previous research.

The construct validity of the WAIS-R IQ scores is so widely accepted that the test is frequently used as a criterion for the examination of the validity of other tests of intellectual functioning (e.g., Raggio, 1993). The assumption is based on convention and frequency of usage. But the studies relating the WAIS-R to other intelligence tests can also be seen as evidence for the validity of the WAIS-R in a bootstrapping manner. There does not seem to be a single theoretical methodology for conceptualizing intelligence evaluation that has achieved hegemony over the field. The best test of the construct validity is the extent to which the test results conform to the theory of intelligence on which the test is based, regardless of whether a distinction between simultaneous and sequential processing or between verbal and nonverbal processing underlies intelligence. It is that concern that the factor analytic studies address. Another important consideration is what the subtests themselves measure. There have been few studies investigating this issue. Larrabee and Curtiss (1995) report that the Digit Span subtest loads on an attention/information processing factor in a study of various neuropsychological measures. Zillmer et al. (1992) report that the Comprehension and Picture Arrangement subtests were the most highly related to lesion site in patients with cerebral vascular accidents, but the predictive power of scores on these subtests needs to be explored.

As noted previously, in the factor analytic studies the structure of the WAIS-R appears to be similar in clinical populations to its structure in the standardization sample. Another piece of evidence in favor of interpreting WAIS-R data from neuropsychiatric patients comes from Crockett (1993), who found that all but 10% of his sample of 697 patients could be classified into the prototypical patterns found in the standardization sample.

SHORT FORMS

As with any test with multiple subtests, there have been several suggested short forms of the WAIS-R. In fact, research reports describing short forms of the WAIS-R have constituted the largest single group of publications regarding the WAIS-R. The suggested short forms range from administering only the even or odd items, a practice that is not recommended, to the various short forms in which only selected subtests are administered. The number of subtests used in these short forms range from only two subtests to seven subtests. Kaufman, Ishikuma, and Kaufman-Packer (1991) have suggested dyad, triad, and tetrad short forms. Boone (1992b) evaluated these forms as well as other dyad short forms in a sample of 100 psychiatric inpatients and concluded that based on administration time, ease of scoring, reliability, and validity in predicting long form IQ, the Kaufman triad of Information, Picture Completion, and Digit Span was superior to the others. When the dyad short forms were compared to the Satz–Mogel (item reduction) short form, the two methods were found to be equivalent (Boone, 1991). However, McCusker (1994) found that the four-subtest form was the best predictor across inpatient versus outpatient status, age, gender, and race. Mattis, Hannay, and Meyers (1992) found the Satz-Mogel short form to be misleading in tumor patients. Robiner, Dossa, and O'Dowd (1988) found that the Satz–Mogel short form was superior to the dyad and tetrad forms in patients with head injury. Watkins, Edinger, and Shipley (1986) concluded that although not optimal, the Satz–Mogel short form was acceptable for use in medical patients.

Thompson (1995) found that a four-subtest short form overestimated IQ scores in a sample of young individuals living in criminal justice institutions, and Ryan (1985) reported similar results in a sample of neurological patients. Silverstein (1990a) had reviewed one of the forms (Information, Arithmetic, Picture Completion, and Block Design) and found it to be more reliable than in the original reports, but the real test is in the comparison to other short forms. In general, short forms that reduce the number of items within subtests rather than reducing the number of subtests possess less reliability (Cella, Jacobsen, & Hymowitz, 1985; Silverstein, 1990b). Nagle and Bell (1995a) found no differences in accuracy of prediction of IQ by a dyad, a triad, and tetrad short form in a sample of young educable mentally retarded subjects, but this result may have been partially due to the floor effects seen in this population.

Callahan, Schopp, and Johnstone (1997) investigated the seven-subtest form of the

WAIS-R suggested by Ward (1990) and found that the three index scores were not significantly different from the values obtained from the long version in a sample of 459 patients with closed head injury. In fact, 95% of the subjects had predicted/observed Verbal IQ differences of 6 or fewer points. These researchers suggest that the short form, which takes only half the administration time, be administered when an estimate of intellectual or academic potential is desired in this population, leaving more time for more specific neuropsychological measures.

Abraham, Axelrod, and Paolo (1997) compared seven different short forms in a sample of 306 clinical patients and found that Ward's (1990) seven-subtest form was most accurate in predicting Full Scale IQ. In yet another examination of the seven-subtest short form, subjects from the standardization sample were grouped by education level and by age. In general, the highest correlation between short form and long version scores were for FSIQ, followed by VIQ and by PIQ. No differences by age level were found, but the two groups with higher levels of education (13 to 15 years and > 15 years) had somewhat lower reliabilities than the group with the least amount of education (< 8 years). Satterfield, Martin, and Leiker (1994) found the seven-subtest short form to be superior to three other short forms in a sample of 130 patients who had been referred for psychological or neuropsychological evaluation. Cyr and Atkinson (1992) found that the use of age-related scores in the calculation of short form scores did not make a difference in short form values in psychiatric inpatients. Silverstein (1987) reported that the use of multiple regression weights does not differ much from the use of equal weights in the calculation of IQ from short forms. Brooker and Cyr (1986) provided tables for the conversion of short form results to IQ estimates. This table was cross-validated by Ryan, Utley, and Worthen (1988). Silverstein (1985) presented data related to the reliability and validity of a two- and a four-subtest short form. Cyr and Brooker (1984) recommended that both reliability and validity be considered in the choice of a short form and provided a diagram to aid in decision-making.

The accuracy of prediction of the seven-subtest short form was impressive in a sample of head-injured patients where the average difference was 1 point (Iverson, Myers, Bengston, & Adams, 1996). In the same study the average difference for subjects with dementia was 3.5 points. Ryan, Weilage, Paolo, Miller, and Morris (1998) found that the seven-subtest short form predicted IQ scores generally within 5 points of actual IQ in their sample of females with documented brain damage. There was a larger range of differences in a sample of 54 African-Americans with brain damage, but the seven-subtest short form provided estimates generally within 1 standard error (Ryan et al., 1997). Although they did not report individual difference scores, Iverson, Guirguis, and Green (1998) found that the seven-subtest short form correlated highly with IQ in schizophrenic patients. Two different computational formulae have been suggested to predict IQ from the seven-subtest short form, but there may not be practical differences in the applications of these two formulae (Iverson, Myers, & Adams, 1997). A separate computational formula has been suggested for British subjects (Crawford, Allan, & Jack, 1992), and a comparison of the seven most frequently used short forms indicated that the seven-subtest short form did not consistently under- or overestimate actual IQs (Crawford, Mychalkiw, Johnson, & Moore, 1996). Because of inaccuracies in prediction, Drudge, Cyr, and Eccles (1989) recommended against the use of dyad and tetrad short forms in psychiatric patients. Randolph, Mohr, and Chase (1993) found that short forms either over- or underpredicted IQs in samples of patients with Alzheimer's, Parkinson's, and Huntington's diseases; however, because the correlations were high these researchers recommended the use of correction factors to improve accuracy.

The psychometric characteristics of the short forms are just as important in their interpretation as the psychometric characteristics of the long form are in its interpretation. Schretlen, Benedict, and Bobholz (1994) reported estimates of short form reliability and standard error of measurement for the seven-subtest short form. However, these estimates used the theoretical standard deviation of 15 points rather than the observed values. Axelrod, Woodard, Schretlen, and Benedict (1996) subsequently recalculated the reliabilities and standard errors of measurement using the observed standard deviations from the standardization sample, and these values should probably be used. Ward and Ryan (1996) calculated the times savings and reliabilities values for 565 possible short forms of the WAIS-R and found that the optimal forms were ones that had already been considered in the research. Thompson and LoBello (1994) calculated the reliable and deviant values for range of subtest scores for the short forms and suggested these values might be used as a guide to decide when to administer the whole test. Although an intriguing notion, the relationship of the range to external criteria needs to be addressed.

The estimation of IQ scores in aged subjects may present unique challenges owing to somewhat limited representation of the very aged in the original standardization sample for the WAIS-R. Ryan, Paolo, and Van Fleet (1994) investigated the test–retest reliabilities in 61 normal subjects aged 75 to 87 years when they were tested twice an average of 65 days apart. These investigators stated that the stabilities for the three tetrad short forms and for the seven-subtest form are basically comparable to the long form values. The Kaufman tetrad short form may be superior in the elderly to other short forms with two, three, or four subtests (Paolo & Ryan, 1991). Although initial reports indicated that the Satz–Mogel short form may be accurate in the elderly (Osato, Van Gorp, Kern, Satz, & Steinman, 1989), later investigations questioned this conclusion. Paolo and Ryan (1993) reported that the temporal reliability of the Satz–Mogel short form in elderly subjects was adequate for the FSIQ and VIQ, but not for the PIQ. However, when decisions regarding loss or gain were made using the short and the full forms, there was only 67% agreement for the FSIQ, and these researchers recommended against using the Satz–Mogel short form in this population.

Ryan, Georgemiller, and McKinney (1984) found differences between a four-subtest short form and the long form, but these researchers felt the correlations were high enough to allow screening for abnormality. Hoffman and Nelson (1988) cautioned against the use of short form to classify elderly subjects even though the correlations with long form scores may be high (Margolis, Taylor, & Greenlief, 1986). This suggestion was echoed for subjects with mental retardation (Watkins, Himmell, Polk, & Reinberg, 1988), for subjects in a general psychiatric setting (Thompson, Howard, & Anderson, 1986), and for subjects in a vocational rehabilitation setting (Banken & Banken, 1987; Clayton, Sapp, O'Sullivan, & Hall, 1986). Schretlen and Ivnik (1996) reported that the Mayo's Older American Normative Studies (MOANS) IQ scores could be reasonably predicting using MOANS scores from the seven subtests used in the normative short form. In most populations, the seven-subtest form may be the best choice, although the full form is generally preferable to any short form. Watkins, McKay, Parra, and Polk (1987) warned against the use of short forms because of the limitations in prediction in their own sample of outpatients. Clearly the use of a short form must be balanced between time demands and accuracy standards.

Another important population is that of subjects with head injury. Roth, Hughes, Monkowski, and Crosson (1984) warned of overestimation in patients with suspected neurological impairment, suggesting the need for a correction factor. Ward and Ryan (1997) compared various short forms of the WAIS-R in a brain-injured sample and did not indicate a significant advantage for any one form when both accuracy and time savings were considered. Other short methods of estimating IQ include the Kaufman Brief Intelligence Test (K-BIT). Because the K-BIT does not require a motor response, it might seem preferable in a neuropsychological setting. However, the short forms are generally more accurate than the K-BIT (Eisenstein & Engelhart, 1997). Slater and Van Wagoner (1988) reported that neither the item-reduction nor the subtest-reduction method is superior in adolescents with closed head injury.

Because there is a Spanish translation available for the WAIS, the Escala de Inteligencia Wechsler (EIWA), it is important to investigate the properties of short forms in that version. Demsky, Gass, and Golden (1997) reported that based on the standardization data, the two-subtest and the four-subtest versions offer similar results to the English version, lending support to their use.

CONCLUSIONS

The WAIS-R is a nearly ubiquitous instrument in clinical evaluation settings. Its reliability has been relatively well investigated, although its reliability still needs to be examined in special populations such as epileptic subjects, the learning disabled, and elderly individuals with dementia. But it is the validity of the instrument that is most in need of evaluation. The WAIS-R and its predecessors, the WAIS and the Wechsler–Bellevue, have become the standard criteria against which other tests of intelligence are evaluated on their concurrent validity, for example, the Stanford–Binet (Carvajal, Gerber, Hewes, & Weaver, 1987). This information alone does not allow conclusions regarding the construct validity of the WAIS-R. There have been many studies investigating the various short forms of the WAIS-R, and although not all of these studies have provided consistent results, it appears the seven-subtest form is superior in most populations.

The utility of the WAIS-R in neuropsychological evaluation is not completely explicated. The best approach may be to use the WAIS-R as an index of academically related intellectual skills without invoking diagnostic interpretation strategies. For example, Nagle (1993) found that the WAIS-R could be used to predict academic achievement (WRAT-R) in educable mentally retarded adolescents. On the other hand, Leonard (1994) found that the WAIS-R could not predict academic success in learning disabled students attending college. Part of this negative result may be due to the restriction of range since the definition of learning disability requires an average IQ at minimum. In adults, there may be disagreement between the results of the WAIS-R and the WRAT-R (Spruill & Beck, 1986).

Attempts to use the WAIS-R may have results similar to the attempts to use the WAIS, such as that of Strauss and Brandt (1986), who found that the WAIS was unable to identify subjects with Huntington's disease, although it did possess descriptive power in terms of the level of impairment. A more sophisticated analysis was conducted of the WAIS-R by Moses, Pritchard, and Adams (1997), who examined WAIS-R profile configurations in relation to Luria–Nebraska Neuropsychological Battery (LNNB) and HRNB profiles.

These researchers found that only the elevations of the WAIS-R profiles and not the configurations were related to LNNB profile information and to a lesser extent to HRNB profiles. Moses, Pritchard, and Adams conclude that the WAIS-R may be useful as an index of neuropsychological impairment, but not as an indicator of diagnostic information.

Patterns of performance on the WAIS, such as the use of hold–don't hold scales, have also been suggested, most notably by Fuld (1983), who suggested that a certain pattern of subscale scores could help identify the central cholinergic deficiency thought to be responsible for the memory deficits found in Alzheimer's disease. Tuokko and Crockett (1987) did not find this pattern in healthy elderly people. However, both Filley, Kobayashi, and Heaton (1987) and Heinrichs and Celinski (1987) have reported results that suggest that this pattern is not specific to an etiology of cholinergic deficiency; it may also be found in patients with closed-head injury or other brain impairments. Goldman, Axelrod, Giordani, Foster, and Berent (1992) reported that the Fuld profile has low temporal stability as well as low sensitivity. Massman and Bigler (1993) reviewed 18 studies that used the Fuld profile and concluded that there was insufficient sensitivity (24%), although specificity was high (93% for normal controls and 88% for patients with vascular dementia).

Russell (1987) suggested strategies for interpreting the WAIS in a neuropsychological setting. However, many of these suggestions are in need of rigorous experimental evaluation and, further, may not apply to WAIS-R results. Chelune, Eversole, Kane, and Talbott (1987) found that the WAIS and the WAIS-R generated different subtest profiles in the same subjects. The WAIS-R continues to be extremely popular in clinical neuropsychological practice. The accumulated empirical evidence supports its continued use, but it is essential to separate the clinical lore from the empirically supported uses.

The manual for the WAIS-R mentions correlational studies that have related the WAIS and the Wechsler–Bellevue to other psychometric measures of intelligence; it then goes on to state that similar conclusions can be drawn regarding the WAIS-R. This is a dangerous suggestion. For example, the WAIS-R results in higher IQ scores than does the WISC-R when individuals with below average scores are tested twice when their ages are appropriate to the respective instrument (Rubin, Goldman, & Rosenfeld, 1990). The opposite order of scores is seen in normal 16-year-old subjects (Quereshi, Treis, & Riebe, 1989). Fortunately, since the publication of the manual a number of studies have investigated many different aspects of the test. Knight (1997) reviewed some of the relevant studies for use of the WAIS-R in a clinical neuropsychological context and encouraged practitioners to interpret test results in the light of base rate information as well as the patient's history. There is evidence to suggest the neuropsychological relevance of the factor index scores (Berger, 1998; Parker & Atkinson, 1995; Sherman et al., 1995). In addition, Atkinson (1991d) has provided tables to use in comparing the results of evaluations with both the WAIS-R and the WMS-R, an idea that has been incorporated into the third editions of these tests, with a subsample of the standardization group being used to co-norm the two tests. The process of evaluating the validity of the WAIS-R is not complete, although it is likely to become overshadowed by the WAIS-III. What has been helpful and what is further needed is direct empirical evidence regarding the Wechsler intelligence scales that impinges directly on the issue of validity. This evidence could come from discriminant convergent validity methodologies, predictive validity methodologies, or concurrent validity correlational methodologies.

THE WECHSLER ADULT INTELLIGENCE SCALE-THIRD EDITION (WAIS-III)

The Wechsler Adult Intelligence Scale is now available in a third edition (Wechsler, 1997a), which along with a reorganization of subtests, an updated normative base, and an expanded age range to 89 years old, has the benefit of being co-normed with the Wechsler Individual Achievement Test in the 16- to 19-year-old range and co-normed with the Wechsler Memory Scale-Third Edition (Wechsler, 1997b) in 1250 subjects of the 2450 subjects in the total WAIS-III standardization sample. This co-norming allows psychometrically sophisticated comparisons of scores obtained from the administration of the tests in conjunction with each other.

As with previous editions of the WAIS, the standardization sample was stratified for sex, race, and geographic region consistent with the proportions of those variables in the 1995 U.S. census. In addition, subjects were sampled from education levels of <9 years, 9 to 11 years, 12 years, 13 to 15 years, and >15 years. An additional 437 subjects were tested so that each of the education levels at each age group would contain at least 30 subjects. The data from these additional subjects were not included in the calculation of norms, but were used for research studies.

There was some reorganization of the component subtests of the various IQ indexes. The Vocabulary, Similarities, Arithmetic, Digit Span, Information, and Comprehension subtests comprise the Verbal IQ Index. The Picture Completion, Digit Symbol-Coding, Block Design, Matrix Reasoning (a new subtest), and Picture Arrangement subtests comprise the Performance IQ Index. The Full Scale IQ Index contains all of those 12 subtests. The additional Index scores are Verbal Comprehension, Perceptual Organization, Working Memory, and Perceptual Speed.

There are three additional subtests. Letter–Number Sequencing is included in the Working Memory Index, Symbol Search is contained in the Perceptual Speed Index, and Object Assembly is an entirely optional subtest. It is possible to translate each of the subscale raw scores to an age-corrected standardized score as well as a percentile value and a reference group score. The manual provides statistical information to allow comparison of Index scores, pairwise comparisons of subtest scores, as well as comparison of a single subtest to the mean of the subtests for that Index. The reliability of the observed difference as well as the frequency of occurrence in the standardization sample (abnormality) is provided in the manual. It is also possible to evaluate the difference between the Digit Span forward and the Digit Span backward performance. Internal consistency (split-half) reliability estimates as well as temporal (mean retest interval 34.6 days) reliability estimates are given in the manual. Interscorer reliability estimates are also given in the manual.

The manual presents a plethora of statistical and psychometric information, but subsequent publications have expanded on this information. For example, LoBello, Thompson, and Evani (1998) presented tables to allow analysis of subtest scatter when six Performance subtests are administered (facilitating the calculation of the Processing Speed factor index score) or when optional subtests are substituted for standard subtests that have been spoiled.

The validity of the WAIS-III was evaluated via comparison with other tests. The WAIS-R correlates with the WAIS-III .94–VIQ, .86–PIQ, and .93–FSIQ. FSIQ declined 2.9 points from the WAIS-III to the WAIS-R, VIQ declined 1.2 points, and PIQ declined 4.8

points. The WAIS-III was correlated with the WISC-III in a sample of 184 subjects 16 years of age. The correlations were .88–VIQ, .78–PIQ, and .88–FSIQ. Correlations for the factor index scores were similar. The Raven's Progressive Matrices correlated .64 with the WAIS-III FSIQ, .79 with the PIQ, and .49 with the VIQ in a sample of 26 subjects. The correlation between WAIS-III FSIQ and the Stanford–Binet IV Global Component score was .88 in a sample of 26 subjects. The mean scores were very similar for the two tests. Correlations of the WAIS-III with the WIAT ranged from low (.18 between Working Memory and Oral Expression) to moderate (.82 between Full Scale IQ and Math Reasoning).

The construct validity of the WAIS-III was examined through exploratory factor analyses which generally resulted in a four-factor solution, corresponding to the four Factor Index scores. Confirmatory factor analysis indicated that the four-factor solution provided the best fit to the data for the entire standardization sample as well as for each of the age groups with the exception of the 75- to 89-year-old group, in which case the five-factor solution provided an incrementally better fit. The fifth factor consisted entirely of the Arithmetic subtest.

Correlations between WAIS-III index score and tests measuring similar constructs tended to provide support for the validity of the WAIS-III. In each case the sample sizes were somewhat limited and replication in independent and larger samples would be helpful. The WAIS-III was also administered to groups of individuals with various neurological disorders, alcohol related disorders, schizophrenia, mental retardation, Attention Deficit Hyperactivity Disorder (ADHD), learning disabilities, and hearing impairment. The results are meant as examples and not as rigorous studies.

CONCLUSIONS

In terms of standardization and psychometric sophistication, the WAIS-III is a vast improvement over the WAIS-R. It remains to be seen if these improvements result in greater clinical utility, validity, and precision. The age extension and the downward extension of ability are among the most needed changes. The WAIS-III will be the focus of extensive studies that will describe the limits and power of the instrument in a neuropsychological context. In the absence of those studies, the only characteristic to recommend the WAIS-III over the WAIS-R is the updated and improved normative base. Certainly, it is only a matter of time before even more becomes known about the WAIS-II than is currently known about the WAIS-R.

The Wechsler Intelligence Scales for Children—the WISC-R, WISC-III, and WPPSI-R

WECHSLER INTELLIGENCE SCALE FOR CHILDREN-REVISED (WISC-R)

The Wechsler Intelligence Scale for Children-Revised (WISC-R, Wechsler, 1974) is, as its name suggests, a revised and updated version of the WISC, which was first published in 1949. It attempts to measure intelligence by assessing 10 abilities. (Actually, there are 12 with the supplementary Digit Span and Mazes subtests.) Its scoring procedure results in a scaled score for each of the subtests. These scores have a mean of 10 and a standard deviation of 3. The scaled scores are combined to produce scores for Verbal IQ (VIQ), Performance IQ (PIQ), and Full Scale IQ (FSIQ). The IQ scores have a mean of 100 and a standard deviation of 15. The WISC-R is an extremely popular instrument that has been translated into different languages including Saudi (Qataee, 1993). The WISC-R has since been revised and updated as the Wechsler Intelligence Scale for Children-Third Edition (WISC-III). However, owing to similarities between the two instruments, critique of the WISC-R will help inform use of the WISC-III.

In revising the WISC, some items that were thought to be ambiguous or culturally biased were eliminated, new items were devised to replace them, and a few more items were added to increase the reliability of the test. The WISC-R was normed on a stratified sample that was designed to be representative of the U.S. population with regard to age, sex, race, geographic location, occupation of household head, and urban versus rural residence (Wechsler, 1974). There were 2200 children in the normative sample ranging in age from 6.5 to 16.5 years old. These children were divided into 11 age groups for the purpose of deriving the scaled scores.

Reliability

The scorer reliability of the WISC-R was assessed by Bradley, Hanna, and Lucas (1980). These authors constructed two WISC-R protocols for two hypothetical 10-year-old females whose intended IQ was 110. One of the protocols was constructed without ambiguous responses or administration errors. The other protocol was constructed with ambiguous responses, errors with regard to starting and stopping points, and a few highly unusual responses. These protocols were given to 63 members of the National Association of School Psychologists, who were then asked to score the protocols. Although the manner in which the data are presented does not allow us to estimate the amount of variance that was due to scorer error, the standard deviation of the IQ scores for each of the protocols is presented. The standard deviation can be used as an estimate of the variability among the scorers. The standard deviation for FSIQ for the difficult protocol is 4.3; that for the easy protocol is 2.9. These values indicate that, even with unambiguous responses rated by trained test administrators, there will still be some variability in test scores that is attributable to the scorer.

Split-half reliability coefficients were computed for all of the subtests except the power test of Digit Span and the speeded test of Coding. The manual reports that an odd–even split was used for most of the subtests, but it does not identify these subtests, nor does it say what method was used in the other cases. The Digit Span and Coding reliability estimates were based on test–retest values for 50 children in each of the age groups. The reliability coefficients were computed separately for each of the 11 age groups. The reliability coefficients for the IQ scores were computed by means of a formula for composite scores. Overall reliability coefficients were computed by averaging the values for each of the age groups by means of an r-to-z transformation. The reliability coefficients ranged from .73 for Picture Arrangement to .86 for Vocabulary. The reliability coefficient for VIQ was .94, for PIQ it was .90, and for FSIQ it was .96. Dean (1977) reported split-half reliability coefficients for a sample of behavior-disordered male children that are very similar to the values reported in the manual, indicating that these coefficients have some degree of stability in a sample of "nonnormal" children.

The reliability of the WISC-R with special populations needs to be addressed because the original reliability estimates were derived on normal populations. Hirshoren, Kavale, Harley, and Hunt (1977) investigated the internal consistency reliability of the performance IQ of the WISC-R for a sample of children who had been deaf before language acquisition. This is an interesting study because it not only provides information on the WISC-R in a special population, but it also allows us to examine the reliability of the part of the WISC-R that supposedly measures intelligence without the influence of language in a sample that has less language ability than the normative sample. Reliability estimates for the sample of deaf children were computed by the use of Cronbach's coefficient alpha. The reliability coefficients for the Performance subtests were not significantly different from the values reported in the manual, with the exception of the Picture Arrangement, for which the reliability estimates for the deaf sample were significantly higher than the value reported in the manual. The overall reliability of the Performance IQ score was equal to that reported in the manual.

The test–retest reliability for the scores was also computed and reported in the manual. A total of 303 children spread across three age groups were retested after an interval of approximately 1 month. Once again, the subtest scores were combined, so that composite reliability estimates were computed for the IQ scores. The reliability coefficients were corrected for the variability of the norm groups. All of the corrected scores for the age groups were averaged by use of the r-to-z transformation. These values ranged from .65 for Mazes to .88 for Information. The average corrected reliability estimates for the IQ scores were .93 for the VIQ, .90 for the PIQ, and .95 for the FSIQ. There were no tests for the difference in absolute level over time.

Vance, Blixt, Ellis, and Bebell (1981) investigated the test–retest stability on a sample of 75 learning disabled and retarded children. The intertest interval was 2 years. Because reliability deteriorates over time, these values were likely to be lower than those reported in the manual, which had an intertest interval of 1 month. Correlation coefficients were computed for each of the subtest scores as well as for the IQ scores. In addition, t-tests were performed to assess the change in the absolute value of the scores. The correlation coefficients for the Verbal subtests ranged from .63 for Similarities to .80 for Digit Span. The correlation coefficients for the Performance subtests ranged from .59 for Picture Completion to .80 for Object Assembly. The correlation coefficients for the IQ scores were higher; .80 for the VIQ, .91 for the PIQ, and .88 for the FSIQ. Anderson, Cronin, and Kazmierski (1989) examined the stability of WISC-R scores in a sample of 113 learning disabled students evaluated twice within an interval of 3 years. They found that reliability was somewhat low, and in particular the Verbal IQ decreased in this sample. It may be that special populations develop more slowly than nonclinical individuals, but the low stability over an extended period is problematic for an instrument that is supposed to measure relatively stable traits in the absence of adverse events. It is interesting to note that a similar decline in Verbal IQ was reported in a sample of gifted children tested twice over a period of 1 to 4 years. The classification of gifted remained fairly consistent (Cahan & Gejman, 1994). Spangler and Sabatino (1995) examined gifted American children and found that the WISC-R IQ scores were stable over a 3-year and a 6-year period; however, there were significant changes in subtest performance. Neyens and Aldenkemp (1997) found that WISC-R IQ scores showed a significant change in 58% of Dutch children tested three times within an interval of 6 months.

Despite the significant positive correlations between time 1 and time 2, there were significant differences in absolute level for five of the subtests: there were significant decreases for Similarities, Vocabulary, Digit Span, and Block Design, and there was a significant increase in the scores for Picture Arrangement. There was also a significant decrease in Verbal IQ. An important caveat needs to be issued before these results can be interpreted. All of the subjects in this study were students who had abnormal conditions that might impede their development. IQ scores are deviation scores for certain age groups. Therefore, decreases in IQ for these groups may reflect the fact that, while their cohorts are developing normally, these subjects are developing more slowly or are remaining static in their ability levels. The plausibility of this explanation is heightened by the pattern of significant changes. Three of the four significant decreases were in Verbal subtests, and the only IQ score to change was Verbal IQ. It is in the verbal abilities that we would not expect the subjects to keep pace with their cohorts. Although this hypothesis may help to explain these differences, the results of the study imply that changes in level may occur in WISC-R scores over time. Evidence to support this hypothesis must come from empirical studies of other populations.

The standard error of measurement values was computed for each of the subtests. However, as discussed in the chapter on the WAIS-R, the formula used by the manual results in an estimate of the variance attributable to error rather than in confidence boundaries for the test scores. The magnitude of the determination of the significance-of-difference scores between subtest scores and between IQ scores is also given. The danger of interpreting these statistically significant differences as clinically significant parallels the danger in the same kind of interpretation of scores on the WAIS-R. The reader is referred to that section for a more thorough discussion of the issue.

There are actually three levels on which to evaluate the split between the VIQ and the PIQ. The manual deals with the reliability of the split, or the probability that the magnitude of the split did not occur by chance. The second level involves the abnormality of the magnitude of the split, or the proportion of the subjects tested who exhibited that magnitude of split. In reviewing the relevant research, Berk (1982b) stated that abnormal splits are about twice the size of reliable splits at the same probability levels. That is, if a split of 10 points is reliable at the .05 level, a split of 20 points is probably abnormal at the .05 level. The last level is the validity of the split. This consideration can be restated as a question: What is the clinical significance of a 10-point split? Kaufman (1979) stated that there may be many reasons for a VIQ–PIQ split, and it is up to the clinician to determine the reason in each case. In reviewing the research, Berk (1982b) concluded that the validity of the VIQ–PIQ split in the WISC-R is yet to be determined and recommended against its use in a clinical setting.

Often, interpretation of the WISC-R depends on an examination of the pattern among the scale scores or among the IQ scores. This is especially true of the use of the WISC-R in neuropsychological assessment. As a result, the reliability of the pattern of scores needs to be assessed if one is to be confident of such interpretations. Assessing the reliability of the univariate scales is insufficient for this purpose because it fails to take the multivariate structure of patterns into account.

Conger, Conger, Farrell, and Ward (1979) examined the profile reliability of the WISC-R across the age groups of the normative sample. They found that, although the factor structure of the WISC-R appeared to be relatively invariant across age, the salience of those factors changed across age. By assessing the reliability of various types of profile analysis, they were able to recommend the following strategies for profile analysis: comparison of IQ scores, comparison of the VIQ with the PIQ, and comparison of individual scale scores with the average of all scale scores. These profile strategies possess sufficient reliability to recommend their use. The next step would be to assess the validity of these strategies and to discover the clinical meaning of differences in these profiles.

Dean (1977) examined the relationship of various suggested interpretive pattern strategies by using a sample of 41 Caucasian male children who had been referred for psychological evaluation because of their manifestation of behavior disorders. With the exception of the rule that emotionally disturbed children demonstrate Picture Arrangement scores that are greater than their Picture Completion scores, and Object Assembly Scores that are greater than their Coding scores, each by 3 scaled score points, the examined rules demonstrated reasonable accuracy in classifying the children as emotionally disturbed. The interpretation of this study is hampered by its design. No normal children were included in the study; therefore, we do not know how accurate these rules are in classifying children in general. However, this is the type of study that needs to be done to assess the clinical utility of profile analysis.

Intercorrelations among the subtests were computed separately for each of the age groups and are reported in the manual. These values were then averaged by means of an r-to-z transformation. In addition, the manual presents information regarding the correlation of each subtest with the relevant IQ scores, which are corrected for membership in the composite that comprises the IQ score. The subtests are moderately correlated with each other.

Validity

The manual reports that concurrent validity of the WISC-R was assessed by correlation with three other tests of intelligence: the Wechsler Preschool and Primary Scale of Intelligence (WPPSI), the Stanford–Binet Intelligence Scale (using the 1972 norms), and the Wechsler Adult Intelligence Scale (WAIS). The WISC-R-WPPSI correlation study evaluated 50 children who were 6 years old. The two tests were administered in counterbalanced order with an intertest interval of between 1 and 3 weeks. The VIQ and the PIQ both correlated .8O, and the FSIQ correlated .82.

For the study that examined the relationship between the WISC-R and the WAIS, 40 children aged 16 years, 11 months were evaluated. Once again, the tests were administered in counterbalanced fashion with an intertest interval of 1 to 3 weeks. The VIQ correlated .96, the PIQ .83, and the FSIQ .95.

The study reported in the manual that examined the relationship of the WISC-R to the Stanford–Binet evaluated a sample of children divided into four age groups. Thirty-three children from the WISC-R-WPPSI study were also administered the Stanford–Binet. In addition, 29 children aged 9.5 years, 27 children aged 12.5 years, and 29 children aged 16.5 years were administered the WISC-R and the Stanford–Binet in counterbalanced fashion. These age-related correlations were averaged by means of the r-to-z transformation. The WISC-R VIQ correlated .71 with the Stanford–Binet IQ. The corresponding correlation for the PIQ was .60, and for the FSIQ, the value was .73.

White (1979) reported a study in which the WISC-R, the Wide Range Achievement Test (WRAT), and the Goodenough–Harris Draw-a-Man test were intercorrelated in a sample of 30 children, 20 of whom had been referred for diagnosis of learning problems, and 10 of whom were the children of friends of the researcher. Moderately high correlations between the WISC-R IQ scores and the WRAT and Draw-a-Man scores were obtained, whereas only moderate correlations were obtained between the WISC-R subscales and the WRAT and Draw-a-Man scores. These findings indicate moderate support of the WISC-R IQ scores as a predictor of academic achievement, as well as support of the WISC-R IQ scores as agreeing with the Draw-a-Man IQ estimates.

Other studies offer moderate support for the concurrent validity of the WISC-R. Wickoff (1979) reported that the IQ scores of the WISC-R correlated moderately with the Peabody Individual Achievement Test (PIAT) in a sample of children referred for an evaluation of learning problems. The VIQ was correlated best with the PIAT scores, followed by the FSIQ and the PIQ. The correlation values ranged from .40 to .78. Brooks (1977) examined the relationship between the WISC-R and the WRAT and Stanford–Binet in a sample of 30 children. The WISC-R correlated .95 with the Stanford–Binet. The correlations between the WISC-R and WRAT scores were more modest: .76 for the Arithmetic scale, .65 for the Spelling scale, and .06 for the Reading scale. Kaufman and Van Hagen (1977) examined the relationship between WISC-R and Stanford–Binet IQ scores in a sample of 45 retarded children. They reported correlations of .73 for the VIQ, .65 for the PIQ, and .82 for the FSIQ.

One method of assessing the validity of the WISC-R is to evaluate how well scores from the WISC-R can predict academic performance. Schwarting and Schwarting (1977) assessed the relationship between the WISC-R and the WRAT in a sample of 282 children who had been referred for evaluation because of suspected learning problems. The subjects were divided into two age groups of 6 to 11 and 12 to 16 years. Particularly for the older group, the WISC-R PIQ did not correlate well with the WRAT scores. However, for the VIQ and the FSIQ, the correlations were moderate, ranging from .56 to .75. Hartlage and Steele (1977) reported moderate correlations between WISC-R IQ scores and WRAT scores in a sample of 36 children. All of the correlations were significant; they were as low as .36. Hale (1978) reported the results of an investigation into the ability of the WISC-R to predict WRAT scores in a group of 155 schoolchildren. When all three of the WISC-R subscores were entered into a multiple-regression formula to predict each of the three WRAT scale scores, only the VIQ was found to significantly, independently predict the Reading and Arithmetic scores of the WRAT.

The information gathered from the studies discussed in the foregoing points out the significant relationship between the WISC-R and measures of academic achievement. The important point to remember is that, although significant, the relationships are moderate; often, only 10% of the variance is shared by the tests. This result may be construed as acceptable, as there are other variables that impinge on academic achievement; however, it is important to determine what makes up the variance in the IQ tests that is not shared by tests of academic achievement. The much higher correlations with the Stanford–Binet argue for the validity of the WISC-R, but we are faced with correlating a test said to measure IQ with a test that is also said to measure IQ. What is really needed is a study that correlates WISC-R IQ with real IQ, whatever that may be. Because IQ is traditionally measured by the use of the tests, such a study is not foreseeable until some basic work has been done on the theoretical definition of IQ.

Construct Validity

Kaufman (1975a) investigated the factor structure of the WISC-R by performing several factor analyses on the normative data published in the manual. For each of the 11 age groups, a principal-components factor analysis with varimax rotation was performed, as well as principal-factors factor analysis with varimax, oblimin, and biquartimin rotations of two-, three-, four-, and five-factor solutions. No statistical analysis of the different solutions was performed. However, the appearance of the WISC three (interpretable)-factor solution was fairly consistent across age groups. These three factors are usually interpreted as Verbal Comprehension, Perceptual Organization, and Freedom from Distractibility.

A corollary question involves the factor structure of the WISC-R in a sample of children who are not free from neurological impairment. This is especially appropriate because an instrument such as the WISC-R is more likely to be used to evaluate a child for whom there is suspicion of impairment than it is to be used to provide an assessment of a child for whom there is no suspicion of impairment. Richards, Fowler, Berent, and Boll (1980) examined the factor structure of the WISC-R by using a sample of 113 epileptic children aged 6 to 12 years old and a sample of 124 epileptic children aged 12 to 16 years old. These authors used maximum-likelihood factor analysis with oblimin rotation. For both groups, the solved-factor structure consisted of a Verbal Comprehension factor and a Perceptual Organization factor. For the older group, the third factor was interpreted as Freedom from Distractibility.

Groff and Hubble (1982) examined the factor structure of low-IQ children in two age groups. The first group consisted of 107 children between the ages of 9 and 11 years with an average FSIQ of 70.4. The second group consisted of 78 children between the ages of 14 and 16 years with an average FSIQ of 66.5. Principal-factor analysis was performed on the data. The method of rotation was not reported. Three, four, and five factors were examined, and the three-factor solution was chosen as the clearest explanation of the data, although the criterion for deciding this point was not given. The three factors for both of the groups were interpreted as Verbal Comprehension, Perceptual Organization, and Freedom from Distractibility. Although the factors were consistent across the two groups, the Distractibility factor accounted for 14% of the shared variance in the older sample and for 20% of the shared variance in the younger sample. Apparently, the importance of the factors is sensitive to age.

Another study investigated the factor structure of the WISC-R in low-IQ children, this time in 80 mentally retarded children between the ages of 6 and 16 who had an average IQ of 58.1. Van Hagen and Kaufman (1975) conducted principal-components factor analysis with varimax rotation of factors with a minimum eigenvalue of 1.0; principal-factor analysis with varimax rotation of two-, three-, four-, and five-factor solutions; and principal-factor analysis with oblimax and biquartimin rotations of two-, three-, four-, and five-factor solutions. They reported that the three-factor solution, as determined in the factor analysis of the standardization sample, was fairly stable across factor analytic methods in this sample of mentally retarded children with a few exceptions: the Verbal Comprehension factor for the standardization sample had greater agreement with the retarded children's Freedom-from-Distractibility factor and the Freedom-from-Distractibility factor had greater agreement with the standardization sample's factor of the same name than did either of the other factors with their namesakes. This finding indicates that there are differences in the factor structure of the WISC-R for retarded subjects in spite of the seeming similarities to each other. An important clinical consequence is a more cautious interpretation of the WISC-R for retarded subjects.

Silverstein (1982b) performed correlated multiple-group-components factor analysis on the standardization data for 7.5-, 10.5-, and 13.5-year-old age groups and compared the two- and three-factor solutions. He found that the two-factor solution was at least as accurate as the three-factor solution in describing the data. Tingstrom and Pfeiffer (1988) found that the two-factor model was obtained in a sample of 155 learning disabled children and in a sample of 272 non-learning disabled children who had been referred for neuropsychological evaluation.

Wallbrown, Blaha, Wallbrown, and Engin (1975) performed a hierarchical factor analysis of the normative data from the WISC-R manual. They interpreted a general intelligence factor that was composed of a verbal–educational factor and a spatial–perceptual factor. This solution was stable across age groups, as determined by a visual inspection of the factor loadings. The differences between the solution in this study and the solution in the Kaufman (1975a) study can be attributed to the different factor-analytic techniques. Hierarchical factor analysis assumes a general factor with component factors. Principal-components factor analysis assumes that a few factors will explain the variance in the data. It is interesting to note the similarities in the solutions. Both of the studies conclude that a verbal and a spatial factor are involved in the WISC-R.

Interpretation of the factors is necessary to the clinical utility of the scores. Kaufman (1975a) recommended that the scale scores of the subtests that comprise the factor scores for a given subject be changed to percentile scores and then be translated into IQ scores through the use of a table found in the WISC-R manual that gives percentile equivalents of IQ scores. Noting that the table gives IQ equivalents only in 5-point increments, Sobotka and Black (1978) presented tables that allow a quick transformation of the scale scores of the three factors into IQ scores for use in clinical interpretation. These authors stated that interpretation then follows the usual procedure for IQ scores. However, these resultant factor "IQ" scores have unknown psychometric properties. Nothing is known of their internal consistency or stability. Gutkin (1978) presented a method for a linear combination of subtest scale scores into IQ scores for the factor scales, as well as a table of reliable differences between the scores. Gutkin (1979) then extended these tables to provide separate estimates of the values for each of the age groups. However, aside from their computed composite reliabilities, little is known about the psychometric properties of these scores. Little is known of the validity or meaning of either the Sobotka and Black (1978) or the Gutkin (1978) factor "IQ" scores.

Grossman and Johnson (1982) reported that the Verbal Comprehension and the Freedom-from-Distractibility factors significantly predicted Wide Range Achievement Test (WRAT) scores in a multiple-regression formula, but that the Perceptual–Organization factor did not. Squared multiple-correlation coefficients indicated that, although the relationships were significant, they accounted for only 25% to 36% of the variance in the WRAT scores. More needs to be known about these factor scales before they can be recommended for clinical use. After reviewing the literature, Wielkiewicz (1990) concluded that scores on the Freedom from Distractibility factor may be low for reasons other than distractibility, including learning disability, low motivation, and poor short-term memory. He hypothesizes that this factor may actually be a reflection of executive functioning in children.

The factor analysis studies have produced results that are similar to the rational structure of the WISC-R. This similarity can be construed as support for the construct validity of the WISC-R. It is necessary also to provide external evidence of the construct validity of the WISC-R. The correlational studies of the WISC-R with the WPPSI, the WAIS, and the Stanford–Binet are only preliminary steps in this direction. What is needed is evidence that IQ scores as determined by the WISC-R are indeed related to intelligence.

There is evidence to suggest that performance on the WISC-R is related to other factors in addition to intelligence. Brannigan and Ash (1977) classified 73 children (out of a sample of 100) as either extremely impulsive or extremely reflective and then compared the WISC-R scores of the two groups. The reflective subjects were found to have significantly superior performance on the VIQ, the PIQ, and the FSIQ.

Another variable that is often thought to have an effect on performance on the WISC-R is race. One of the purposes behind revising the WISC was the minimization of racial bias in the test. Race is a heated issue in our society, and the arguments regarding it are often more emotional than rational. Sometimes, although rarely, the proponents are able to agree on basic facts. One of those facts is that black children perform more poorly on the WISC-R than do Caucasian children. The divergence of opinion and the genesis of irrationality occur when the reason for this difference in performance is proposed. Some people declare that the WISC-R is a culture-fair instrument and that the difference in performance reflects a genetic difference in ability. Other people declare that the difference in performance reflects the bias of the test, that is, that the WISC-R measures abilities and information to which Caucasian children are more likely to be exposed.

According to an extensive review by Sattler and Gwynne (1982b), there is no evidence that the race of the examiner influences performance on the WISC-R. The more pressing question is whether the test itself is sensitive to race. As might be expected in a case such as this, there are studies that purport to present evidence for both of the competing viewpoints. Vance and Engin (1978) administered the WISC-R to 154 black children. Because there were significant differences between the scale scores, the authors concluded that the WISC-R is a valid instrument for the assessment of black children. It is difficult, if not impossible, to agree with the conclusions of these authors. There is no evaluation of the validity of the WISC-R, nor is there even a comparison of the performance of the black children to the performance of Caucasian children.

Mishra (1983) examined the predictive validity of the WISC-R IQ and factor scores in relation to Wide Range Achievement Test scores of 64 Mexican-American children. There were small and insignificant correlations between the WISC-R factor scores and the WRAT scores, indicating a limited predictive validity of the WISC-R factor scores for this sample of Mexican-American children. There were significant but moderate correlations between the IQ scores and the WRAT scores, indicating some predictive validity of these measures for the achievement of these children.

Munford, Meyerowitz, and Munford (1980) looked at the difference between WISC and WISC-R scores of Caucasian children and then compared these results to those of an earlier study that had examined the same differences in black children. They reported that, whereas there were no differences between WISC and WISC-R scores for the Caucasian children, the black children performed significantly worse on the WISC-R than they did on the WISC. Although this evidence is suggestive, two obstacles block the interpretation of this study. First, the study that examined Caucasian children evaluated only 20 subjects, as did the study that examined black children. The Caucasian children also performed more poorly on the WISC-R, but their differences did not reach significance. Second, the conclusions would be stronger if the data had been analyzed as part of the same design. Poteat, Wuensch, and Gregg (1988) examined the relationship between WISC-R and California Achievement Test scores and found no differences between Caucasian and African-American children.

Mishra (1982) examined the performance on three of the WISC-R subtests (Information, Similarities, and Vocabulary) by 40 Caucasian and 40 Navaho children. Differences in performance across individual items were assessed by the use of a log-linear transformation of the data and the maximum-likelihood-ratio chi square. Mishra concluded that 15 of the items evoked performance differences attributable to race. There was no evaluation of performance differences on scale scores, which is another pertinent method of examining this question. However, it is likely that such a difference may exist.

In what is probably methodologically the best of the studies investigating this question, Oakland and Feigenbaum (1979) evaluated the internal consistency, the item difficulty, the item-total correlations, correlation with the California Achievement Test (CAT), and the factor structure of the WISC-R in subjects who were stratified by race (Caucasian, black, and Mexican-American), family size, family structure, socioeconomic status, urban versus rural residence, age, health, and birth order. The analysis for internal consistency, item-total correlations, and concurrent validity (CAT scores prediction) was performed by correlating the values for the subtests for one group with the values for another group. The analysis for item difficulty involved an analysis of variance in which the groups were the independent variables and the item difficulty indices were the dependent measures. The factor analyses were evaluated by correlating varimax loadings on the first principal component and by similarly correlating both of the solved factors after rerotation of one solution to maximize the contiguity between the two vectors. The results indicated that the internal consistency values, the item-total correlations, and the factor structures were relatively unaffected by the independent variables. However, there were differences in item difficulty indices and concurrent validity that were due to the independent variables, indicating differential sensitivity of the WISC-R to race.

Humphries and Bone (1993) found that WISC-R differences with the WRAT- R did not differentiate between students with a specific learning disability and students who were slow learners. However, this lack of effect may have been due as much to the lack of specificity in the WRAT-R as to an insufficiency of the WISC-R. Of greater impact is the lack of significant differences in factor scores including Freedom from Distractibility scores when students with ADHD were compared with students with internalizing disorders (Semrud-Clikeman, Hynd, Lorys, & Lahey, 1993).

The WISC-R shows good agreement with rank ordering of performance on the Stanford Achievement Test-Hearing Impaired Version in a sample of 83 deaf children (Kelly & Braden, 1990). The WISC-R PIQ has been proposed as an adequate measure of intellectual functioning in hearing impaired children. Braden (1989) reported that the WISC-R PIQ has differential relationships with different criteria as measures of achievement in deaf children and, further, that this relationship does not change much with age.

The use of the WISC-R to determine the presence of brain impairment is a speculative endeavor. Warschausky, Kewman, and Selim (1996) reported that qualitative analysis of the errors on the Digit Span subtests of the WISC-R discriminated children with traumatic brain injury from normal control children, but this is a rare study to examine the relationship of WISC-R to the diagnosis of acquired brain damage. In addition, the specificity of the qualitative pattern of inconsistency on the Digit Span subtest to traumatic brain injury needs to be evaluated by examining the performance of children with other forms of cerebral dysfunction.

Once brain damage is diagnosed, the WISC-R can be used to delineate profiles of skills and deficits. Certainly, because of the WISC-R's omnipresence in child clinical settings, any validated use would be extremely welcome. Tramontana and Boyd (1986) evaluated the concurrent validity of the WISC-R in screening for neuropsychological abnormalities in a sample of 90 psychiatric patients with a mean age of 92.8 months. All of the patients were administered the WISC-R, the Aphasia Screening Test, and the age-appropriate form of the Halstead–Reitan or the Luria–Nebraska Neuropsychological batteries. When the results of the neuropsychological batteries were used to classify the subjects as 41 impaired and 49 nonimpaired individuals, there were significant differences on all WISC-R subscale scores except Objects Assembly. When the WISC-R and the Aphasia Screening Test scores were used as predictors in a discriminant function analysis, 91.1% of the subjects were correctly classified. However, the ratio of predictors to subjects was extremely low, limiting the potential generality of the results. In cross-validating the discriminant function with a sample of 84 psychiatric subjects, Boyd and Tramontana (1987) obtained a correct classification rate of 79.3%.

Because the results of the above investigations may suggest that the relationship between performances on the WISC-R and on the Halstead–Reitan and Luria–Nebraska batteries may be influenced by shared variance in the skills tapped, it is important to delineate the amount of overlap between the WISC-R and the neuropsychological measures. Sweet, Carr, Rosini, and Kaspar (1986) administered the WISC-R and the revision of the LNNB for children (LNNB-C) to a sample of 32 psychiatric patients, 28 neurologically impaired patients, and 32 normal subjects between the ages of 8 and 12. There were significant correlations between the WISC-R and the LNNB-C measures only in the neurologically impaired sample, a finding indicating that the information derived from the WISC-R may not be redundant with the LNNB-C, but that both may be influenced by neurological impairment.

A short form of the WISC-R involving a split-half administration of items has been suggested. Bawden and Byrne (1991) found that although the short form correlated well with the long form, the short form tended to overestimate IQ.

Conclusions

The WISC-R is an instrument for which reliability has been fairly well assessed. The reliability still needs to be assessed in certain populations, such as epileptic children or psychiatric inpatients, but these are minor points in comparison to the reliability assessment already performed. The major issue in the evaluation of the WISC-R is the determination of its validity. There have been no attempts to evaluate the discriminant and convergent validity of the instrument, such as might be done with the Fiske–Campbell methodology, nor have there been sufficient studies of the predictive validity of the WISC-R. Despite the lack of content validity studies, the WISC-R has become the criterion against which the validity of other tests of intelligence are being measured. This fact should not signal unconditional acceptance of the WISC-R; instead, it should alert us to the paucity of other instruments available to measure intelligence. A particularly important issue for neuropsychologists is the validity of the WISC-R in making diagnoses regarding organic impairment in children. The WISC-R is most appropriately used as a measure of the child's current IQ. Published reports of the use of the WISC-R continue to appear, but these decrease over time as the WISC-III replaces the WISC-R. It is likely that many of the criticisms of the WISC-R will not be sufficiently addressed, but it is hoped that studies of the WISC-III will ameliorate this lack. In fact, review of the WISC-III manual indicates that the studies and criticisms related to the WISC-R have influenced the development and initial evaluation of the WISC-III.

WECHSLER INTELLIGENCE SCALE FOR CHILDREN-THIRD EDITION (WISC-III)

Consistent with the observation that IQ scores on the basis of a given test tend to increase over time and with the need to provide accurate estimates of relative performance (deviation scores), the WISC has been revised yet again in a third edition—the WISC-III.

As well as changing some items to be more relevant to contemporary children and providing a more current normative base, the WISC-III accommodates the presence of different observed indices of age-associated variability about the mean scores by calculating asymmetric standard errors of estimate for the IQ scores and factor scores at different age levels. A potential further psychometric advantage was demonstrated by McGrew and Wrightson (1997), who used data smoothing procedures to generate more accurate estimates of scale scores, but as yet, there has been no application of these "improved" reliability and factor score estimates. Some of the subtests are optional (e.g., Symbol Search), and Reynolds, Sanchez, and Willson (1996) present tables for calculating Performance IQ when Symbol Search is substituted for Coding.

Reliability

Split-half reliability estimates for the subtests (except Coding and Symbol Search) were calculated on the standardization sample. These coefficients range from .87 for Block Design and Vocabulary to .69 for Object Assembly. Standard errors of measurement and confidence intervals were calculated on the basis of these reliability values. For precision, these confidence intervals are not averaged across index scores and are based on the standard error of estimation rather than the standard error of measurement. The standard error of estimation is distributed around the estimated true score. As a result, these confidence intervals are sometimes asymmetric around the obtained scores. The manual also presents information regarding the test–retest reliability in a subsample of 353 subjects from the standardization sample. The median intertest interval was 23 days. Full Scale IQ scores increased around 7 points across the two test occasions, with Performance IQs increasing 12 points and Verbal IQs increasing less than 2 points.

Interscorer reliability was reported for the Similarities, Vocabulary, Comprehension, and Mazes subtests. Four raters scored 60 protocols. Using the intraclass correlation, and averaging across age groups, the reliability values were .94 for Similarities, .92 for Vocabulary, .90 for Comprehension, and .92 for Mazes. The manual provides information regarding the statistical reliability (and not the statistical significance as stated in the manual) of the differences between index scores. In addition, the WISC-III manual reports the percentage of subjects in the standardization sample who obtained similar index score differences, so that the abnormality of the difference can be evaluated. The interpretative significance of these differences still needs to be delineated. The same information is available for differences between individual subscale scores and the mean of subtest scores for that index (Verbal or Performance) and differences among pairs of individual subtests. The manual also presents data regarding the frequency of different levels of subtest scatter. Finally, information is presented regarding the discrepancies between Digits Forward and Digits Backward. All of this information is desirable and beneficial. It is now up to the research community to provide interpretative validation of the various reliabilities and differences.

Other investigators have examined the temporal stability of the WISC-III in different populations. Bolen (1998) reported that temporal stability is lower for the IQ scores in low-IQ children based on a study of 70 children with a classification of educable mentally handicapped (EMH) who were tested twice over an interval of 3 years. The overall trend was for IQ scores to decline over that period; however, given the characteristics of the subjects, this decline may have been due as much to a failure on the part of the subjects to progress developmentally on a par with their age peers as it might have been due to instability of the test itself. When a larger sample (667 students) more representative of average was used over the same approximate time period, the reliability coefficients ranged from .87 (PIQ and VIQ) to .91 (FSIQ) with no significant differences across the two occasions.

Siegel and Piotrowski (1994) investigated the subtest composites suggested by Kaufman (1979) as a way of enhancing the interpretation of the WISC-III. The reliability estimates of these composites appear to be adequate, but the evidence for their application is based on theoretical and conceptual arguments. Actual empirical evidence is needed.

One of the most interesting characteristics of the WISC-III, at least for clinical neuropsychological applications, is information in the manual that allows the examiner to evaluate subtest differences and scatter. Aside from the reliability of magnitudes of those differences, it is useful to know the abnormality of those differences. Schinka, Vanderploeg, & Greblo (1998) presented a table of differences at various levels of frequency in the standardization sample.

The role of the examiner and the behavior of the examiner in determining performance of subjects can be an important factor interpreting scores. As a beginning point, Plante, Plante, Rahm, Bentar, an Couchman (1997) reported that eye contact during administration of the Digit Span procedure was nonconsequential in affecting performance of either clinical or nonclinical subjects.

Validity

The manual for the WISC-III reviews validity information for the WISC-R. Although this information is suggestive, it is not definitive, and explicit information regarding the validity of the WISC-III is in the formative stages. Schultz (1997) found that correlations between the WISC-III and Woodcock–Johnson Tests of Achievement-Revised were similar to the correlation found with the WISC-R in children evaluated serially. However, changes in level of IQ resulted in fewer children being identified as learning disabled. The manual reports intercorrelations among subtests as a way of examining the construct validity of the subscales. As predicted, the Verbal subtests generally correlate more highly with each other than with the Performance subtests and vice versa. Factor analyses indicate that a four-factor solution generally describes the relationships among subtests well. These four factors are interpreted as two factors found in the WISC-R, namely, Verbal Comprehension and Perceptual Organization, as well as two slightly different factors, Freedom from Distractibility and Processing Speed. These factor structures were developed using exploratory factor analysis methods and tested using confirmatory factor analysis methods. Only in the younger age groups did a five-factor solution seem to provide a greater fit to the data, but the fifth factor consisted only of the Picture Arrangement subtest. The four-factor solution was the best fit for a sample of clinical subjects and a sample of gifted subjects. Tupa, Wright, and Fristad (1997) found that using confirmatory factor analyses, the four-factor model provided the best fit to the data in a sample of 177 psychiatric inpatients. The factor structure may be very different in certain clinical populations. Sullivan and Montoya (1997) found a two-factor solution (Language Comprehension and Visual–Spatial Organization) in a sample of children with hearing impairments.

The four-factor structure of the WISC-III appears to be robust across age groups

(Allen & Thorndike, 1995a,b; Reynolds & Ford, 1994) and in the Canadian normative sample (Roid & Worrall, 1997). Kush and Watkins (1997) reported that the factor structure of the WISC-III in a sample of 161 African-American students enrolled in special education services approximated the factor structure reported in the manual. Using the original WISC-III, and not the Canadian version, Roid and Worrall (1997) replicated the four-factor solution in a nationally stratified sample of 1100 Canadian children. Maller and Ferron (1997) found that although the four-factor solution could be replicated using confirmatory factor analysis in a sample of deaf children, the error variances and factor covariances were not similar, indicating that different constructs may actually underlie the four factors in this special population. Even when only the 12 clinical subtests were used in the analysis, Konold, Kush, and Canivez (1997) replicated the four factor solution in children receiving special education services. Using maximum likelihood confirmatory factor analysis, Donders and Warschausky (1996a) found that the four-factor solution from the manual best fit the data on 171 children with traumatic brain injury.

In an examination of the construct validity of the factor scores of the WISC-III, Donders and Warschausky (1996b) performed a cluster analysis of the factors in a sample of 153 children who had experienced traumatic brain injury. They found four subtypes, and although three of these clusters appeared to reflect differences in level of performance, one cluster reflected selective impairment on the Perceptual Organization and the Processing Speed factors. Further external validation of this cluster may enhance the utility of the WISC-III in evaluating children with neuropsychological impairment. Glutting, Youngstrom, Ward, and Hale (1997) investigated the utility of the WISC-III factor scores in predicting achievement measured by Wechsler Individual Achievement Test scores, but found that the FSIQ provided adequate estimates with only small increments afforded by use of the factor scores. Donders (1997a) found that the Perceptual Organization and Processing Speed factor indexes of the WISC-III were sensitive to injury severity as measured by length of coma in children with closed head injury. There were group differences in PIQ, Perceptual Organization, and Processing Speed among mild, moderate, and severe closed head injury, but not for VIQ, Verbal Comprehension, or Freedom from Distractibility. The performance subtests may be more sensitive to acquired brain damage. The Freedom from Distractibility and the Processing Speed factors do not correlate well with other measures of attention, nor do these factors differ significantly as a function of diagnosis of ADHD versus learning disability (Riccio, Cohen, Hall, & Ross, 1997). Kush (1996) has similarly questioned the validity of these two factors based on his factor analysis of WISC-III data from 327 children with learning disabilities. The Freedom from Distractibility factor did not correlate with behavioral ratings of attention difficulties and hyperactivity (Lowman, Schwanz, & Kamphaus, 1996), nor does it seem to be lower than the Perceptual Organization or Verbal Comprehension factor scores in students with ADHD (Anastopolous, Spisto, & Maher, 1994). Although the Freedom from Distractibility factor has been suggested for clinical use, its construct validity is in need of further explication.

Glutting et al. (1997) report that the four factors provided a statistically incremental advantage to predicting performance on the Wechsler Individual Achievement Test (WIAT) in a nationally stratified sample of normal children involved in the norming of another test and in a sample of children referred for neuropsychological evaluation. However, the magnitude of this advantage was not clinically significant and the authors recommend the FSIQ as the best practical predictor of the WIAT.

Concurrent validity was examined by correlating the WSIC-III with the WISC-R with high correlations in the presence of score differences which involved lower scores for the WISC-III, as is expected when tests are renormed. The difference between WISC-R and WISC-III scores was reported by other investigators (Sapp, Abbott, Hinckley, & Rowell, 1997) who used a test–retest methodology rather than a concurrent validity design, and by Slate and Jones (1995) in a sample of 31 African-American students who received both tests across an interval of 3 years for the purposes of being evaluated for special education services. In general the WISC-III IQ scores are about 6 points lower than WISC-R IQ scores (Zimmerman & Woo-Sam, 1997). The WISC-III correlates well with the Stanford-Binet-Fourth Edition with only small differences between obtained IQ scores across the two tests in a sample of unselected volunteer subjects (Rust & Lindstrom, 1996). However, Lukens and Hurrell (1996) reported that Stanford–Binet, Fourth Edition IQ scores tend to be higher than WISC-III IQ scores in children with mild mental retardation. When children who had been evaluated using the WISC-III were evaluated 3 years later using the Differential Abilities Scale, there were high correlations between similar constructs and a 96% agreement in classification (Dumont, Cruse, Price, & Whelley, 1996).

The WISC-III was correlated with the WAIS-R in 16-year-old subjects, with higher values for the index scores than for subtest scores. In addition, the WAIS-R index scores were somewhat higher than the WISC-III index scores. The WISC-III was correlated with the WPPSI-R in 6-year-old subjects. Acceptable correlation coefficients were obtained with mildly higher index scores for the WISC-III. The manual suggests that the difference may be due to ceiling effects on the WPPSI-R and states that the WISC-III may be a more accurate measure in this age group.

The WISC-III and Otis–Lennon School Ability Test were administered to a small sample of 65 children aged 6 to 16 years. These correlation coefficients were moderate, ranging from .59 for nonverbal indexes to .73 for the full scale indexes. The WISC-III correlated more highly with the Differential Abilities Scales in a sample of 27 children. The WISC-III was correlated with the Tactual Performance Test, Trail-Making A and B, and the Finger Tapping Test in a sample of 30 children with either learning disability or attention deficit disorder. Here the correlation coefficients were low to moderate, with greater values for the Performance and Verbal IQs than for Full Scale IQ, probably due to a lack of specificity in the Full Scale IQ. The WISC-III correlated moderately to unsubstantially with the WRAT-R in a sample of 23 children with learning disability or attention deficit disorder. Correlations with group administered tests of academic achievement were moderate. There is a low correlation of the WISC-II with school grades, probably due to the large amount of error involved in measuring school grades.

The manual also reports the results of examining the WISC-III in different clinical groups, such as gifted children, mentally retarded children, children with learning disabilities, children with severe conduct disorders, children with attention deficit disorder, children with epilepsy, children with speech and language delays, and children with hearing impairment. The information is presented in the form of summary scores and examination of patterns. Of note is the fact that only 5.1% of the learning disability sample exhibited the ACID profile and only 20% of the sample exhibited a loosened criterion of only the ACID subtest being equal to or lower than the lowest score of the remaining subtests. Although these proportions were higher than in the standardization sample as a whole, they are still too modest to suggest interpretation for diagnostic purposes. As further caution against the use of this interpretative strategy, Watkins, Marley, Kush, and Glutting (1997) found that the ACID profile did not identify children with learning disabilities.

The WISC-R has been adapted for different nations and cultures, and the WISC-III is sure to follow suit. One such version, for Australian children, was evaluated by Rodriguez, Treacy, Sowerby, and Murphy (1998), who reported mean scores comparable to the American normative sample.

There has been some work developing interpretative strategies for qualitative analysis of the subtests WISC-III. One such strategy is to investigate 30-second intervals on the Coding subtest under the hypothesis that normal children should show increasing numbers of symbol pairs completed as time passes. Dumont, Farr, Willis, and Whelley (1998) found that declines in this number did not identify either diagnostic categories or levels of overall IQ. The lack of significant findings provides a caution against using these interpretative strategies in the absence of empirical support. Neither should these strategies be dismissed in the absence of data.

Short Forms

To a somewhat lesser extent than for the adult WAIS-R, there has been interest in the development of short forms of the WISC-R and WISC-III. Slater and Van Wagoner (1988) administered the WISC-R to a group of adolescents with closed head injury and then rescored the protocols based on either reduced subtest short forms or reduced item short form proposals. There were no significant differences between IQ scores obtained from the short forms as compared to the long forms; however, in the reduced item forms, there were significant differences between subtest scores obtained. The lack of significant differences may have been due to the limited sample size (61 subjects between the ages of 12 and 20 years and some subjects were administered the WAIS-R). Examination of the scores indicated frequent discrepancies. Thompson, Browne, Schmidt, and Boer (1997) found that the validity of a four-subtest short form of the WISC-III exceeded that of the Kaufman Brief Intelligence Test (K-BIT) in 42 adolescent offenders. The short form correlated .91 with the long form. Donders (1997b) developed a six-subtest short form of the WISC-III and provided information regarding internal consistency and factor structure of this short form. The next step will be to examine the external validity indices of this short form. The extreme of the short forms involves the use of the Vocabulary and Block Design subtests as the sole estimates of IQ (Herrera-Graf, Dipert, & Hinton, 1996). Not surprisingly, 50% of the research sample was misclassified using this short form. Kaufman, Kaufman, Balgopal, and McClean (1996) compared three short forms of the WISC-III using the standardization data and found that although all three forms possessed adequate reliability properties, the validity estimates were attenuated.

Dumont and Faro (1993) suggested a short form that was then evaluated by Mark, Beal, and Dumont (1998) in terms of its ability to identify Canadian students with regard to gifted status. Of 158 children, 29 were identified as gifted using the full form WISC-III, and of these 20 were identified as gifted using the short form. The remaining nine students were identified as potentially gifted. Of the 129 nongifted students, only five were misidentified as gifted using the short form. When the Dumont and Faro (1993) short form was evaluated in 44 Canadian students with learning disabilities, only insignificant differences with long form IQ were detected. Campbell (1998) examined the characteristics of seven different short forms of the WISC-III including those proposed by Kaufman and colleagues; by

Herrera-Graf, Dipert, and Hinton (1996); by Dumont and Faro (1993); and by Donders (1997b). The method of inquiry included calculating internal consistency, correlating the short form IQs with the long form IQs, and by correlating the short form IQ scores with the Kaufman Test of Educational Achievement Composite score. The Kaufman Information–Picture Completion short form and the Information–Arithmetic–Picture Completion–Coding short forms tended to overestimate IQ by at least 4 points. Using the entire set of criteria, the Vocabulary–Block Design and the Vocabulary–Similarities–Picture Completion–Block Design–Arithmetic–Coding short forms performed the best. Donders and Warschausky (1996c) reported that the Donders (1997b) short form IQ correlated with length of coma in children with closed head injury.

Conclusions

The WISC-III is psychometrically superior to the WISC-R. More data are needed regarding the validity of the test in relationship to identification of diagnostic groups. In addition, the use of the test would be greatly enhanced by validation of profile analysis schemes. Despite its shortcomings, the WISC-III is the preeminent means of evaluating IQ in children. Its use can safely be applied in the determination of cognitive performance in relationship to average performance and in the delineation of individual strengths and weaknesses based on interpretations of the subscales. However, the construct validity of the subscales could be more definitively explicated.

THE WECHSLER PRESCHOOL AND PRIMARY SCALE OF INTELLIGENCE-REVISED (WPPSI-R)

The Wechsler scale appropriate for younger children is the Wechsler Preschool and Primary Scale of Intelligence-Revised (WPPSI-R) which has a normative standardization base ranging from 3 years old to 7 years old. The structure is similar to the other Wechsler scales, with summary IQ scores (Verbal and Performance) available based on sums of individual subtests. The subtests are somewhat different from the WISC-III, and greatly different from the WAIS-III which is only to be expected given the developmental differences between the populations intended to be assessed by the different instruments. Similar to criticisms of the WAIS-R, the WPPSI-R may have ceiling effects as the IQ exceeds 135, resulting in conservative estimates of high IQs as well as inaccurate estimates of intersubtest scatter and VIQ–PIQ differences (Kaplan, 1993). The WPPSI-R, the WPPSI, and the WISC-R do not provide equivalent scores, with the highest IQ being provided by the WPPSI, the next lowest by the WISC-R, and the lowest scores being provided by the WPPSI-R (Quereshi & Seitz, 1994a). Urbina and Clayton (1991) had also reported higher scores for the WISC-R than for the WPPSI-R, a pattern also seen by Kaplan, Fox, and Paxton (1991) in children from high socioeconomic status groups and by Milrod and Rescorla (1991) in high-IQ children. The fact that the WPPSI-R provides lower IQ scores than the WPPSI should not be a surprise, given that this is a trend seen in the revision of all intelligence tests. However, the discrepancy between the WPPSI-R and the WISC-R gives pause for thought when those instruments would be used sequentially as a child develops. It remains to be seen if there are discrepancies between the WPPSI-R and the WISC-III.

The WPPSI-R has aroused some of the same interest as the other Wechsler scales, motivating examinations of the psychometric properties and dissemination of information related to the reliability of the scores themselves as well as the reliability of different interscale comparisons. Unfortunately, the examination of the reliability and abnormality of difference scores has not always been followed by examinations of the validity of inferences drawn from those comparisons or explications of the clinical implications of the differences. But the first essential step of calculation of reliability and examination of the frequency of the differences in the standardization sample (abnormality) has been accomplished. It is up to the clinical researcher to examine the implications of those differences and up to the responsible clinician to make reasonable interpretations.

LoBello (1991a) calculated the reliability of Verbal–Performance discrepancies at different age levels. Gyurke, Prifitera, and Sharp (1991) reported that the Verbal–Performance discrepancy varies as a function of level of Full Scale composite score, where higher levels of ability were associated with greater likelihood of larger discrepancies. Therefore, both the ability-related tables and the age-related tables should probably be used in the interpretation of an individual's test scores. LoBello (1991b) also provided age-related tables to determine reliable differences between mean subtest scores and individual subtest scores, which will help in the investigation of individual strengths and weaknesses. Thompson and LoBello (1994) calculated the reliability and abnormality of subtest range in short forms of the WPPSI-R as a guide to decisions to administer the entire test. By examining item overlap between the WPPSI-R and the WISC-III, Sattler and Atkinson (1993) calculated test age equivalents for different items and found that they correlated well across the two tests, lending support to the interpretation of individual items.

Individual interpretation of the Performance and Verbal scales is supported by the findings of Moore, O'Keefe, and Laehorn (1998), who reported that a test of nonverbal intelligence correlates highly with the Performance IQ of the WPPIS-R, to a lesser extent with the Full Scale IQ, and nonsignificantly with the Verbal IQ. The Verbal IQ and to a lesser extent the Full Scale IQ measured prior to kindergarten predicted academic achievement at the end of grades 1, 2, and 3. The Performance IQ did not predict academic achievement. A similar pattern of prediction was reported by Kaplan (1993) using a sample of 50 children tested prior to entry to kindergarten. The Full Scale IQ correlates with the Bracken Basic Concept Scale School Readiness Composite (Laughlin, 1995). Quereshi and Seitz (1994b) reported that in their sample of 72 children there were significant differences between boys and girls on the Verbal IQ scores as well as on the Comprehension and Vocabulary subtests. This advantage to boys was not found in the standardization sample or in a different study (Karr et al., 1993), and further investigation is necessary before the full implications can be understood.

Information regarding concurrent validity of the WPPSI-R is provided by the finding that the WPPSI-R tends to agree with the scores obtained from the Kaufman Brief Intelligence Scale and the Achievement scale of the Kaufman Assessment Battery for Children (Lassiter & Bardos, 1995). In addition, the WPPSI-R tends to provide similar scores as the Stanford–Binet-IV in samples of preschool children (Gerken & Hodapp, 1992; McCrowell & Nagle, 1994). The WPPIS-R and the McCarthy Scales of Children's Abilities give similar scores in preschool and kindergarten children (Karr et al., 1993). The WPPSI-R correlates well with the Woodcock–Johnson Tests of Cognitive Ability, although the Basic Cognitive Ability index scores tended to be about 4.5 points lower than the WPPSI-R FS IQ scores (Harrington, Kimbrell, & Dai, 1992). Faust and Hollingsworth

(1991) reported good agreement of the WPPSI-R with the McCarthy Scales of Children's Abilities but not with the Peabody Picture Vocabulary Test-Revised. In terms of predictive validity, Lowe, Anderson, Williams, and Currie (1987) reported that in a sample of 169 African-American children in a Head Start program, the WPPSI correlates .78 with the WISC-R and .73 with the WAIS-R when those tests are separated by 4 years and 12 years, respectively.

Various forms of factor analysis have been used to examine the construct validity of the WPPSI-R. A hierarchical factor analysis of the WPPIS-R indicated that a central factor (general intelligence) accounted for 33% of the total variance with a verbal factor and a spatial–perceptual factor accounting for the majority of the remainder of variance (Blaha & Wallbrown, 1991). Using principal-axis factor analysis, LoBello and Guelgoez (1991) found that a general intelligence factor could be further discriminated into Verbal and Performance scales that approximated the clinical groupings suggested in the manual. When the standardization sample data are subjected to maximum likelihood confirmatory factor analysis, the two-factor solution (Verbal and Performance scales) best fit the interrelationships among the subtests. The Verbal Comprehension and Perceptual Organization factors of the WPPSI-R tend to be stable across age groups when the covariance structures are examined (Allen & Thorndike, 1995b). In a confirmatory factor analysis of data obtained from the youngest children and the oldest children able to be assessed using the WPPSI-R, the two-factor solution was again found to be superior to either a one-factor or a three-factor solution (Stone, Gridley, & Gyurke, 1991).

Short Forms

A four-subtest short form of the WPPSI-R has been suggested (LoBello, 1991c). This investigator investigated the four-subtest short form in the standardization sample and found that the Comprehension and Arithmetic subtests (Verbal IQ) and the Picture Completion and Block Design subtests (Performance IQ) produced reasonable estimates of the full version score. Using the same four subtests but in a comparison of the WPPSI and the WPPSI-R, Tsushima (1994) reported IQ estimates that were very similar to each other, but no comparison to full version IQ scores were available to evaluate the accuracy of the estimates. Although there may not be a relationship between scatter among subtests in a four-subtest short form and the agreement with full version IQ, other short forms may result in inaccurate estimates as scatter increases (LoBello, 1991d). Thompson and Lobello (1994) presented a guide for determining when to administer the entire WPPSI-R when various short forms are used and different magnitudes of scatter among subtests are obtained.

Conclusions

The WPPSI-R has received some of the most careful scrutiny of the many measures used to evaluate cognitive functioning in very young children. Most of this scrutiny has occurred in the context of examining normal children or in academic settings. The information may be transferable to neuropsychological populations when the questions involve academic performance. However, research specifically investigating the relationship of WPPSI-R performance to neuropsychological impairment would enhance the utility of this instrument.

Tests of General Intelligence

GOODENOUGH–HARRIS DRAWING TEST

The Goodenough–Harris Drawing Test has its origins in the Goodenough Draw-a-Man Test, which was developed in 1926 and revised by Harris in 1963. It requires the subject to draw a man; alternate forms include instructions for the subject to draw a woman or to draw himself or herself. It is scored on the basis of 73 items related to the detail, the proportion, and the position of the drawing. The result of this scoring procedure is known as the Point Scale. There is also a set of quality scores, which are determined by comparison with a set of 12 drawings said to represent different levels of conceptual maturation. The Quality Scale can be transformed into IQ estimates. The Goodenough–Harris can be administered to either a group or an individual. Age-related norms are available for individuals between the ages of 5 and 15. The score values are normally distributed and increase with age (Scott, 1981).

Harris (1963) found that girls and boys performed differently on the woman and the man forms of the test and consequently provided separate tables for transforming the raw scores into standardized scores. He reported that correlations between the standardized woman and man forms were .76 for boys, .77 for girls, and .75 for both sexes combined. These findings were replicated by McGilligan, Yater, and Hulsing (1971). Harris (1963) further reported that the Point Scale correlates about .80 with the Quality Scale, a finding indicating that time may be saved by scoring only the procedurally easier Quality Scale. However, research investigating the respective accuracy of each scale in estimating IQ has not provided such positive results.

On the basis of a review of 19 studies, Scott (1981) reported that interscorer reliability coefficients range from .80 to .96, with values for the Point Scale being somewhat higher than for the Quality Scale. However, the absolute level of scores was significantly different for the scorers, a finding indicating that mean scores should be computed from the use of multiple scorers or that a study should use only a single scorer to measure change. Naglieri and Maxwell (1981) reported an interscorer reliability coefficient of .94 for a sample of 60 children between the ages of 6 and 8 years. The rescoring of the same protocols by a single scorer resulted in coefficients of .75 to .99 (Dunn, 1967; Levy, 1971; Yater, Barclay, & McGilligan, 1969); however, the differences in mean levels were not significant.

In the original study, the test–retest reliability values ranged from .68 for a 3-month interval to .91 for a 1-week interval (Harris, 1963). In later studies, the test–retest reliability coefficients ranged from .53 to .87 for the Point Scale for intervals of either 2 or 3 weeks in samples of 4- to 8-year-old children. A single study investigated the test-retest reliability of the Quality Scale and reported a coefficient of .73 for a sample of 10- to 13-year-old subjects, with a 4-month interval (Struempfer, 1971).

Harris (1963) reviewed several studies that investigated the criterion-related validity of the Harris–Goodenough by correlating its results with those of the Stanford–Binet, the Porteus Maze, Raven's Progressive Matrices, and the Primary Mental Abilities Test. The results were disappointing: the correlation coefficients ranged from .17 to .72, and most coefficients lay in the lower ranges. Joesting and Joesting (1972) found a correlation of .45 between the Goodenough–Harris and the Quick Test in a sample of 44 children ranging in age from 6 to 13 years. Naglieri and Maxwell (1981) reported that use of the Goodenough–Harris results in significantly lower IQ scores than does use of the WISC-R. The results of the Goodenough–Harris have correlated approximately .29 with measures of academic achievement (Dudek, Goldeberg, Lester, & Harris, 1969; Pihl & Nimrod, 1976). Scott (1981) reviewed 10 studies that used a multiple-regression methodology to determine the incremental validity of the Goodenough–Harris in predicting academic achievement in conjunction with other variables that are commonly used for that purpose. In each case, the Goodenough–Harris scores did not contribute enough independent variance to remain in the final equation.

One study attempted to validate the diagnostic validity of the Goodenough–Harris in classifying 48 subjects into four groups: paranoid schizophrenic, schizophrenic but non-paranoid, neurological, and normal controls (Watson, Felling, & Maceachern, 1967). These authors used seven different scoring systems but did not find acceptable accuracy for any of them. Aikman, Belter, and Finch (1992) reported poor prediction of either intelligence or academic achievement in child and adolescent psychiatric inpatients. Short-DeGraff, Slansky, and Diamond (1989) reported low correlations of the Goodenough–Harris with scores on the WPPSI General Information subtest.

Abell, Horkheimer, and Nguyen (1998) reported adequate interscorer reliability in a sample of 200 adolescent boys in residential treatment. The same study found that although the Goodenough–Harris correlated significantly with the WISC-R, predicted IQ scores were fairly consistently higher than actual WISC-R IQ scores. Conversely, Abell, Heiberger, and Johnson (1994) found that the Goodenough–Harris underestimated WAIS-R IQ scores in a sample of undergraduates. Abell, Von Briesen, and Watz (1996) reported that the Goodenough–Harris correlated with both the WISC-R and the Stanford–Binet, and that these correlations did not differ by level of IQ or by age. Based on a comparison to the WPPSI and measures of visual perception and construction, Short-DeGraff and Holan (1992) suggested that the Goodenough–Harris may be more appropriate as a screen for visual–motor integration and construction skills than as a screen for intelligence.

The Goodenough–Harris does not seem to be affected by ethnicity and culture, at least not in comparison of Native Alaskan undergraduates and white undergraduates (Skillman et al., 1992). Mehryar, Tashakkori, Yousefi, and Khajavi (1987) found that the Goodenough–Harris was related to socioeconomic class as well as academic achievement in Iranian children.

In conclusion, although the Goodenough–Harris appears to demonstrate adequate reliability, it has not demonstrated adequate validity even for the population for which it was intended. It is possible that it demonstrates validity in neuropsychological populations, but that is an empirical question that has not yet been adequately addressed. Further information regarding the equivalence of the group and individual form is needed.

THE LEITER INTERNATIONAL PERFORMANCE SCALE

The Leiter International Performance Scale (LIPS) is a nonverbal instrument that seeks to provide an estimate of the intelligence of an individual. As such, it has the potential of providing an assessment not only of congenitally impaired individuals but also of individuals with acquired receptive aphasia. It has two sections, which have split-half reliabilities of .89 and .75 (Arthur, 1949). In a sample of mentally retarded children, it had a test–retest reliability of .91 (Sharp, 1958). In a sample of language-impaired children, it had a test–retest reliability of .86. Black (1973a) administered the LIPS to a group of 100 children who had either acquired or developmental aphasia. With a 6-month interval, there was a .92 correlation between the scores obtained on the two occasions. The scores increased an average of 1 point, which was not statistically significant.

In evaluating the concurrent validity of the LIPS, Birch, Stuckless, and Birch (1963) reported correlations of .75 with the Stanford–Binet and .74 with the WISC in a sample of deaf children. Beverly and Bensberg (1952) reported a correlation of .62 between the LIPS and the Stanford–Binet in a sample of retarded children. Bensberg and Sloan (1951) reported a correlation of .75 with the Stanford-Binet in a sample of neurologically impaired children. Atkinson, Beve, Dickens, and Blackwell reported a correlation of .78 with the Stanford–Binet IV in their sample of developmentally delayed children. Black (1973a) reported a correlation of .55 with the Peabody Picture Vocabulary Test (PPVT) in a sample of 100 aphasic children. There was a statistically significant difference between the IQ scores provided by the PPVT and the IQ scores provided by the LIPS: the LIPS provided higher IQ scores. Similarly, Lewis and Lorentz (1994) reported that although the LIPS correlates significantly with the WISC-R and the WPPSI-R in a group of children of different ethnicities the LIPS provided significantly higher IQ scores than did the WISC-R for the Latino children. The LIPS was related to consanguinity, abnormal milestones for language and motor development, and the presence of abnormalities in the EEGs of Saudi Arabian children (Nester, Sakati, & Greer, 1992).

Because it is a nonverbal measure, it is important to study the LIPS in the hearing-impaired individual. In a 4-year longitudinal study, the LIPS was found to predict vocabulary development in hearing impaired children (Lindsay, Shapiro, Musselman, & Wilson, 1988). When the LIPS and the Stanford–Binet disagree at least one standard deviation in language-impaired children, the LIPS tends to overestimate IQ measured by the WPPSI and the Stanford–Binet tends to underestimate the WPPSI (Field, 1987). The LIPS overestimated WISC-R IQ in a sample of autistic children (Shah & Holmes, 1985). The LIPS showed greater agreement with the WISC-R than with the K-ABC Nonverbal scale, which also underestimated the WISC-R scores in a sample of hearing-impaired children in special educational programs.

White, Lynch, and Hayden (1978) administered the LIPS to six aphasic and six matched-control adult subjects. The scores obtained were comparable across the two groups. There was no attempt to investigate the validity of the IQ scores. Ratcliffe and Ratcliffe (1979) reviewed more than 15 studies that had investigated the validity of the LIPS.

They reported a median correlation with other tests of intelligence of .70 and concluded that the LIPS was an accurate measure except in cases of average intelligence. Indirect evidence for the construct validity of the LIPS can be found in Lynn, Mylotte, Ford, and McHugh (1997), who reported that scores on the LIPS twins followed the expected pattern of correlations among aspects of intellectual skill sensitive to genetics and environment.

Reeve, French, and Hunter (1983) administered the LIPS, the Stanford–Binet, and the Metropolitan Achievement Test (MAT) to 25 male and 35 female Caucasian kindergarten students. The LIPS and the Stanford–Binet were administered in counterbalance order with a 10-day interval. The MAT was administered 6 months later. The authors reported Kuder–Richardson 20 values of .81 for the LIPS and .89 for the Stanford–Binet. The Spearman–Brown prophecy formula resulted in values of .89 for the LIPS and .94 for the Stanford–Binet. The correlation between the two tests of intelligence was .70; the LIPS produced a nonsignificantly lower IQ by 1 point. The Stanford–Binet correlated .77 with the MAT, and the LIPS correlated .61 with the MAT. More work needs to be done in the evaluation of this instrument in adult language-impaired or non-English-speaking populations.

There is currently a new version of the Leiter, the LIPS-Revised, which has also been shown to be relatively free of ethnic differences (Flemmer & Roid, 1997).

THE MILL HILL VOCABULARY TEST

The Mill Hill Vocabulary Test is a paper-and-pencil measure of the ability of an individual to provide definitions for words. The original scoring of the test provides grade equivalents and percentile scores. These were converted into deviation IQ scores by Peck (1970). Impaired performance on this test has been associated with left-hemisphere lesions (Costa & Vaughan, 1962). Farley (1969) reported that the two subtests of the Mill Hill may result in different estimates of intelligence. There are no reports on the reliability of this instrument. Clare, McKenna, Mortimer, and Baddeley (1993) reported that schizophrenic patients scored lower than age-, sex-, and premorbid IQ-matched control patients.

The Mill Hill is sometimes used as an estimate of premorbid IQ, especially among patients with progressive dementia. O'Carroll and Gilleard (1986) reported that the Mill Hill is not related to any of four cognitive and behavioral measures that are indices of the severity of dementia. Furthermore, there were no differences noted between patients with Alzheimer's disease and patients with multiinfarct dementia. The Mill Hill is more popular in Great Britain than it is in the United States, where the National Adult Reading Test, revised as the North American Adult Reading Test, has become a more frequently used index of premorbid intellectual functioning.

THE PICTORIAL TEST OF INTELLIGENCE

The Pictorial Test of Intelligence (PTI; French, 1964) is a test that assesses intelligence in children without requiring a verbal response. It was standardized for children between the ages of 3 and 8 years. The manual reports test–retest reliability coefficients of .69 with an average interval of 55 months. Bonfield (1972) evaluated the stability of the PTI in a sample of 46 subjects who were residents of a state facility for retarded individuals. With approximately an 18-month interval, the overall correlation was .80; there was a nonsignificant 14-point increase in scores across time. When the subjects were divided into high-IQ (between 55 and 83) and low-IQ (between 40 and 55) groups, the high-IQ group had a correlation of .92, and the low-IQ group had a correlation of .50, indicating differences in stability across the range of ability. Because it does not require a verbal response, the PTI seems well suited for use with children who are language delayed or hearing impaired. Kennedey and Hiltonsmith (1988) report that the PTI correlates well with the K-ABC in preschool children with those types of problems.

Elliott (1969) investigated the concurrent validity of the PTI in a group of 12 female and 18 male 7- to 14-year-olds. The mental age scores of the PTI correlated .79 with the Wide Range Achievement Test (WRAT) Reading Scale and .73 with the WRAT Arithmetic Scale. The PTI subtests correlated with the WRAT in the range of .09 to .04. Coop, Eckel, and Stuck (1975) investigated the concurrent validity of the PTI in a sample of 46 children with cerebral palsy. All of the subjects were between the ages of 4 and 7. The PTI correlated .83 with the PPVT, .88 with the Columbia Mental Maturity Scale, and .76 with the Achievement Rating Scale.

Sawyer, Stanley, and Watson (1979) examined the construct validity of the PTI by factor-analyzing the subtest scores of 52 kindergarten and 38 second-grade children. Using principal-factors factor analysis, these authors found significant overlap among the subtests and a single-factor solution. They suggested that the overall score and not the subtests be interpreted. Dilworth and French (1990) reported on a downward extension of the PIT which they administered to 53 children aged 2 years. Their revision of the PIT correlated with the Bayley Scales of Infant development, suggesting that the instrument does assess aspects of intellectual functioning, but further validational research is warranted.

PEABODY PICTURE VOCABULARY TEST-REVISED

The Peabody Picture Vocabulary Test-Revised (PPVT-R; Dunn & Dunn, 1981) is an updated version of the original PPVT, which was published in 1959. It provides an estimate of intelligence by assessing the size of an individual's vocabulary. It can be quite a useful test in a neuropsychological setting because no verbal response is required of the subject. All that is needed is a yes or no signal, which can be arranged to allow for the deficits of the individuals. In addition, an eye-gaze response mode is available for individuals with motor impairment (Spillane, Ross, & Vasa, 1996). The current version is administered in two alternate forms, which were constructed with the use of the Rasch–Wright Latent Trait Item Analysis model. With the use of this statistical model, a growth curve for hearing vocabulary was estimated, and items for the two forms were chosen to fit similar locations on the curve, in this way maximizing the degree of item equivalence before the final test was fully constructed.

The PPVT-R was normed on a sample of 4200 subjects, who were stratified to conform to the demographic characteristics of the 1970 U.S. Census. There were 100 females and 100 males in each of the children's age groups. The age groups were formed every 6 months from age 2 to age 8, and every 12 months from age 8 to age 18. In addition, there were 828 adult subjects between the ages of 19 and 4.

The manual reports split-half reliability values for the various age groups. These values were calculated with the use of the Wright–Rasch model to correct for the fact that not all items were administered to all subjects. Correct responses between the basal and the ceiling items for each subject were divided into odd- and even-numbered items, and W-ability scores were calculated for each split and then correlated with each other. These values were then corrected for length by use of the Spearman–Brown formula. For the child sample, the median values were .80 for Form L and .81 for Form M. For the adult sample, split-half reliabilities were calculated only for Form L and only for the adults as a group, rather than by age. The split-half reliability coefficient for the adult sample was .82.

A subsample of the children's normative group ($n = 962$) was given both forms of the PPVT-R, and alternate-form reliability was assessed. For raw scores, the coefficient was .82. For standard scores, the value was .79. Test–retest reliability was assessed in a sample of 962 children, who were tested with intervals that ranged from 9 to 31 days. For raw scores, the coefficient had a value of .78. For standard scores, the coefficient had a value of .77.

Alternate-form reliability was assessed by Stoner (1981), who examined the reliability in a sample of 39 male and 40 female Head Start children. The children ranged in age from 3 years, 9 months to 6 years, 3 months. The correlation coefficient was .79. However, the standard score equivalents were significantly higher for Form M (93) than they were for Form L (89). The difference between the levels of scores was not examined in the manual, and these results therefore represent important findings. Tillinghast, Morrow, and Uhlig (1983) administered both forms of the PPVT-R to 120 children in Grades 4, 5, and 6. They reported an alternate-form reliability coefficient of .76. Eight days later, they administered both forms to the same children, but in reversed order, and found a reliability coefficient of .87. McCallum and Bracken (1981) reported alternate-form reliability coefficients ranging from .74 to .86 for black and Caucasian preschool children. In mentally retarded subjects, alternate-form reliability values ranged from .66 to .70 (Bracken & Prassee, 1981). Obviously, the value of the reliability coefficients varies with the characteristics of the sample. Worthing, Phye, and Nunn (1984) reported that Forms L and M appear to be equivalent for younger children, but there may be limitations with older students. Stevenson (1986) reported good alternate forms reliability of the PPVT-R in a sample of 60 adults referred to a state rehabilitation department.

Test–retest reliability has also been evaluated, mainly in samples of children. Scruggs, Mastropieri, and Argulewicz (1983) examined the stability of PPVT-R scores in extremely small samples of Anglo children ($n = 7$), Mexican-American children ($n = 22$), and Native American children ($n = 27$) on Form L over a 9-month interval. The rank value correlation was used because of the sample size. The values were .71 for the Anglos, .90 for the Mexican-Americans, and .74 for the Native Americans. The total sample coefficient was .90. When the PPVT-R was administered twice to a sample of 29 primary school students across an interval of 11 months, the correlation was .89, and there were no significant differences between the scores obtained on the two occasions (Bracken & Murray, 1984). Bracken and Murray (1984) report an 11-month reliability coefficient of .84 in first- to fifth-grade students. The PPVT-R is also reported to have adequate stability on a sample of hospitalized adolescents and young adults with a diagnosis of psychosis (Atlas, Fortunato, & Lavin, 1990). Based on a small sample of emotionally handicapped children, there may be differences in temporal reliability between Forms L, $r = .90$ and M, $r = .69$ (Levenson & Lasher-Adelman, 1988).

Evidence for validity in the manual is only theoretical according to Dunn and Dunn (1981), who stated that vocabulary is usually a good estimate of intelligence and cited a few validity studies that had been conducted with the original PPVT. Subsequent studies have helped flesh out our understanding of the validity of the PPVT-R. The PPVT-R correlates with the WRAT-R, and the WISC-R , especially the VIQ (Smith, Smith, & Dobbs, 1991).

An attempt at validation of the PPVT-R was reported by Quattrochi and Golden (1983), who correlated the PPVT-R with the scales of the children's form of the Luria–Nebraska Neuropsychological Battery. They found only a small correlation with the Receptive Speech Scale, although they had predicted a large value. The PPVT-R also had small correlations with the Visual, Arithmetic, Memory, and Intellectual Processes scales, indicating a confused picture regarding the construct validity of the PPVT-R. Construct validity was examined by Miller and Lee (1993) using structural equation modeling to examine the relationship of word length, date of entry into the English language, polysemy, and frequency of usage to the order of words as contained in the PPVT-R. The results indicated that these variables contributed a significant amount of variance (R-square = .62) to the word order, supporting the construct validity of the test. When subjected to a principal-components factor analysis along with the WISC-R and WRAT-R subtests, the PPVT-R tends to load on a factor interpreted as being verbal comprehension (Altepeter & Handal, 1986). Regression analysis indicated that PPVT-R may be related to perceptual organization as well as verbal comprehension (Hollinger & Sarvis, 1984). The PPVT loads on the verbal comprehension factor in a principal-components factor analysis with the children's HRNB (D'Amato, Gray, & Dean, 1988).

The PPVT-R does not predict school grades in a sample of fourth- to sixth-grade students (Tillinghast, Morrow, & Uhlig, 1984). The PPVT-R did correlate with PIAT scores obtained 10 months later (Naglieri, 1984). The PPVT-R showed the expected normal distribution of scores when administered to a group of 74 Canadian kindergarten children. The number of children found to be below cutoff for screening failure conformed to a normal distribution; unfortunately, there was no external criterion used in this study (Flipsen, 1998). It would be important to examine the extent to which the PPVT-R could accurately predict other measures of intelligence. One study suggested that the PPVT-R can be used as an estimate of WPPSI-R IQ (Vance, West, & Kutsick, 1989), although in another study, the PPVT-R did not correlate as well with the WPPSI-R in a sample of 4- and 5-year-old children (Faust & Hollingsworth, 1991). Carvajal et al. (1993) reported that the PPVT-R correlates well with the WISC-III with values of .75 (Vocabulary subtest score), .76 (Verbal IQ), and .60 (Full Scale IQ) in a sample of 33 third- to fifth-grade students. In another study, the PPVT correlated significantly with the WISC-R (VIQ–.87, PIQ–.78, FSIQ–.80) but tended to underestimate the IQ scores in a sample of incarcerated male delinquents (Rosso, Falasco, & Koller, 1984). A similar result was found in children in special education (Candler, Maddux, & Johnson, 1986), in children classified as hand-icapped (Beck & Black, 1986), in second-grade students not referred for evaluation (Davis & Kramer, 1985), and in children referred for educational evaluation (Altepeter & Handal, 1987). Slate (1995) reported that the PPVT-R correlated with the WISC-III in a sample of 32 young students with diagnoses of mental retardation, but the extent to which scores differed across the two tests was not reported.

As well as having correlation relationships with measures of intelligence the PPVT-R appears to be related to measures of achievement. The PPVT-R correlates significantly with the Reading subtest of the Wide Range Achievement Test-Revised in school-age children (Vance, Kitson, & Singer, 1985). The PPVT-R also correlates significantly with the Comprehensive Tests of Basic Skills (Beck, Black, & Doles, 1985).

In a study discussed previously (Stevenson, 1986) , both forms of the PPVT-R had significant correlations with the WAIS-R, although the PPVT-R underestimated the WAIS-R IQ scores. The PPVT-R appears to be related to the Kaufman Assessment Battery for Children or K-ABC (Zucker & Riordan, 1988). The PPVT-R correlates more highly with the Achievement scale of the Kaufman Assessment Battery for Children (K-ABC) than with the Simultaneous or the Sequential Processing scales of the K-ABC (D'Amato, Gray, & Dean, 1987); however, here again the PPVT-R tends to underestimate scale scores (Bing & Bing, 1985).

In looking at the classification of children as average or above average, the PPVT-R had an 83% agreement with the K-BIT (Childers, Durham, & Wilson, 1994). The PPVT-R agreed with the Stanford–Binet IV in a group of verbally advanced young children at 30 months of age but not at 24 months of age (Robinson, Dale, & Landesman, 1990). The PPVT-R correlated .69 with the Composite score of the Stanford–Binet IV in a sample of college students (Carvajal, Gerber, & Smith, 1987). In another study the Stanford–Binet IV and the PPVT-R correlated significantly and there was no significant difference between scores obtained; however, the classification differed for 50% of the sample of the 217 subjects aged 2 to 25 years (Tarnowski & Kelly, 1988), and in 55% of a sample of children aged 2 to 6 years old (Altepeter, 1985).

In what is a very relevant study for neuropsychology, the PPVT-R tended to underestimate WAIS-R IQS in a sample of 61 brain-injured patients in post-acute rehabilitation (Ingram et al., 1998). This result was also reported for a sample of rehabilitation department referred adults (Stevenson, 1986). The PPVT-R overestimated WAIS-R IQ in the lower ability ranges and underestimated it in the upper ability ranges in a sample of 60 normal adults (Altepeter & Johnson, 1989). This result was also reported in a sample of 40 adults who were inpatients in a psychiatric hospital (Mangiaracina & Simon, 1986). However, the PPVT-R consistently underestimated WAIS-R IQ in a sample of 21 mildly retarded adults (Prout & Schwartz, 1984).

An important aspect of validity is the extent to which bias may be present in the scores. By comparing Anglo and Mexican-American children, it was determined that although bias did exist in the form of significant item X group interactions in an ANOVA, there was not a greater number of items that were more difficult for one group than the other, suggesting that test scores were not biased (Argulewicz & Abel, 1984). Although there is no specific index for evaluating the presence of malingered performance on the PPVT-R, Morrison (1994) suggests that the PPVT-R can be used to estimate the probability that an individual is malingering intellectual impairment.

The PPVT-R appear to possess adequate reliability, although it is important to realize that it varies by sample characteristics, as most neuropsychological assessment instruments probably do. Just as the PPVT-R has consistent strong correlational relations with IQ measures, the PPVT-R consistently underestimates IQ scores. The clinician should be careful to avoid the temptation of using the PPVT-R scores as actual IQ estimates. Instead the regression formulae from the various studies could be used to develop equations to predict IQ scores more accurately, or else a correction factor could be added to the PPVT-R score to bring it more in line with IQ values. Yet another use of the PPVT-R may be to identify forms of learning disability by examining discrepancies with the Boston Naming Test (Halperin, Healey, Zeitchik, Ludman, & Weinstein, 1989) although this suggestion is in need of further empirical evidence.

THE QUEENSLAND TEST

The Queensland Test (McElwain, Kearney, & Ord, n.d.) is a combination of five subtests that require no verbal interaction for their administration. Three of the tasks (the Knox Cube Test, the bead-threading task from the Stanford–Binet, and Koh's Block Design Test) are borrowed from other tests. Thus, this test holds at least as much promise as its component tests; however, research regarding the tests collected as a battery is sparse, to say the least. Cartan (1971) administered the Queensland Test, the Stanford–Binet, and the WISC to a group of 10 boys with a mean IQ of 57. She found rank difference correlations of .85 between the Queensland Test and the FSIQ of the WISC. The rank difference correlation between the Stanford-Binet and the Queensland Test was not significant. In the same study, a group (an unspecified number) of adult males (mean age = 24 years) was administered the Queensland and the WAIS. The rank difference correlation was .87.

Because of its lack of reliance on language for its administration, the Queensland has potential for use with neuropsychologically impaired subjects. However, much more information regarding its reliability and its validity is needed before it can be recommended for clinical use.

THE QUICK TEST

The Quick Test is meant to be a rapid-estimation procedure for intelligence. In it, an individual is shown a series of cards on which four pictures are printed. The examiner says a word, and the subject is asked to point to the picture that best illustrates the word. There are three alternate forms, and the test's authors recommend combining the three forms in order to increase the accuracy and reliability of the test when sufficient time is available.

Normative data (circa 1960) is available on 458 nonimpaired subjects. The subjects were stratified according to demographic information from the 1950 U.S. Census. There were 23 subjects in each of the age groups from ages 2, 3, and 4 years, and then for every academic year from kindergarten to the senior year in high school. Unfortunately, the ages of about one half of these subjects were not recorded. Normative data are also available for 90 adult subjects between the ages of 24 and 45, and for 20 superior subjects at the 12th-grade level (top 10% of their class) and 20 subjects in their first and second years of college who scored in the 90th percentile on the Ohio State Psychological Examination. The normative data are published in the provisional manual (Ammons & Ammons, 1962). A list of published and unpublished research using the Quick Test is available in Ammons and Ammons (1979a,b). Sinnett, Holen, and Davie (1988) reported that the Quick Test requires a correction factor in the estimate of IQ scores in people over the age of 69 years. Vance, Hankins, and Brown (1988) reported no differences due to sex or race in normal subjects.

The provisional manual also provides alternate-forms reliability information based on a subsample of 40 of the preschool subjects. The mean correlation of the three forms was

.61. Other mean correlations among the three forms ranged from .96 for subjects between Grades 2 and 12 to .60 in a sample of seventh-graders. Rotatori (1978) evaluated the test–retest reliability in a sample of 50 retarded children between the ages of 6 and 16. With a 1-week interval, the reliability coefficients were .98 for the female subjects and .87 for the male subjects. The overall reliability coefficient was .92. Vance, Blixt, and Ellis (1980) reported that Forms 1 and 3 correlated .97 in a sample of 44 children who were receiving special-education services. There was a slight nonsignificant increase in scores across the interval. Abidin and Byrne (1967) administered all three forms to 32 adult organic subjects and 32 psychiatric inpatient subjects and reported overall correlations of .81 for Forms 1 and 2, .77 for Forms 1 and 3, and .84 for Forms 2 and 3. The correlations were slightly higher for the organic subjects than for the psychiatric subjects. There were significant differences between Forms 1 and 3 and Forms 1 and 2 for the organic subjects and between Forms 1 and 2 and Forms 1 and 3 for the psychiatric subjects. Joesting (1975) administered all three forms to 26 male and 31 female college students. There was no attempt to counterbalance or to investigate order effects. The correlations ranged from .55 to .80.

Ammons and Ammons (1962) attempted to investigate the concurrent validity by correlating the Quick Test with the Full Range Picture Vocabulary Test. In the various subsamples of the normative subjects, the correlations ranged from .13 to .97. Vance, Hankins, and Reynolds (1988) reported that the Quick test and the TONI are equivalently able to predict IQ scores on the WISC-R, but the difference between IQ scores obtained from the different instruments was not reported. In a different report Vance (1988) reported that nonsignificant differences existed between the WISC-R and the Quick Test. Other investigations have reported that the Quick Test correlated .68 with the Shipley Institute of Living Scale (Martin, Blair, & Vickers, 1979), .70 with the WISC-R FSIQ in Caucasian adolescents referred for court-ordered evaluation (Paramesh, 1982), and .50 with the WISC FSIQ in a sample of 40 retarded children (Lamp & Barclay, 1967). In each of these cases, there were significant differences in IQ values between the two tests used, calling into question the accuracy of using the Quick Test to estimate IQ. These results were supported by Abidin and Byrne (1967), who found significant differences between the two tests, and by Ciula and Cody (1978) and Law, Price, and Herbert (1981), who found systematic, but not significant, differences. Traub and Spruill (1982) concluded that the Quick Test was most inaccurate in the superior range of intelligence. DeFilippis and Fulmer (1980) reported that the relation between the Quick Test and the WISC-R varies both with level of IQ and with age. In their study of 99 students, the Quick Test tended to underestimate the WISC-R IQS of the high-IQ first- and fourth-grade students and to overestimate the WISC-R IQS of the lower-IQ fourth-graders and all of the seventh-graders. Marini (1990) investigated the relationship of the Quick Test to WISC-R scores in gifted Canadian students and found that although the Verbal IQ correlated highly with the Quick Test, the Performance IQ did not.

Husband and DeCato (1982) reported a correlation of .89 between WAIS IQS and Quick Test IQS in a sample of 40 subjects in a prison hospital; the differences between the two tests were not significant. DeCato and Husband (1984) subsequently reported moderately high correlations of the Quick Test with the Verbal IQ and Full Scale IQ of the WAIS-R but not with the Performance IQ in prisoners housed in a psychiatric ward. The Quick Test appears to be popular among prison psychologists because Simon (1995) also investigated the relationship between the Quick Test and the WAIS-R in criminal defendants and reported moderate correlations and no significant differences between IQ scores obtained on the basis of the two tests. Doss, Head, Blackburn, and Robertson (1986) concluded that the Quick Test was appropriate in estimating the IQ of adult offenders in the legal system, but this was largely on the basis of a tradeoff between time available and the accuracy of results obtained. Nash and Schwaller (1985) had developed a multiple-choice group administration form specifically for use in the prison setting.

Nicholson (1977) reported correlations ranging from .39 to .79 between subtests of the WISC-R and the Quick Test in a sample of 62 children between the ages of 6 years and 13 years, 11 months. These subjects had been referred for evaluation because of low achievement in school. All of the forms of the Quick Test were administered, and the result was the generation of 182 correlation coefficients; many of these correlations might have been due to chance relations. Levine (1971) tested 50 subjects, aged 60 to 100 years, and found a correlation of .91 between the Quick Test and the WAIS FSIQ, but the Quick Test resulted in significantly higher IQ values. A subsequent study by Price, Hebert, Walsh, and Law (1990) also found higher IQ estimates based on the Quick Test in comparison to the WAIS-R, especially with regard to Performance IQ. Craig and Olson (1988) reported that the Quick tended to underestimate WISC-R IQ scores by about 5 points but not WAIS-R IQ scores.

Predictive validity was investigated by O'Malley and Bachman (1976), who used the test records of 2213 students in Michigan. The Quick Test correlated .37 with grades achieved in the same year as the testing, .33 with grades achieved 3 years following testing, and −.03 with hourly wages earned 8 years after testing. To investigate the incremental validity of the Quick Test, the ability to predict WAIS IQ scores in 31 psychiatric inpatients was compared to psychiatrists' estimates of IQ. The Quick Test was found to be a more accurate predictor, although still inaccurate (Templer & Tarter, 1973). The use of psychiatrists' estimates is a questionable comparison procedure, as almost any test procedure is likely to be more accurate than the estimate of a group of professionals who do not have experience in standardized testing.

Orpen (1974) reported that the Quick Test is susceptible to instructional set. In this study the Quick Test was administered to 126 "Coloured" male pupils from South Africa who were in their last year of high school and 135 "Coloured" male pupils in their second year of high school. The subjects were randomly assigned to one of three groups: a group that was told that the Quick Test was a measure of achievement, a group that was told that the Quick Test was a measure of intelligence, and a final group that received the standard instructions. The subjects in the two special-instruction groups scored significantly higher than the subjects who received standard instructions, a finding underlining the need for carefully adhering to standardized administration.

The Quick Test appears to tap some construct of neuropsychological interest, as the score is correlated with late social outcome in head-injured patients (Acker & Davis, 1989). The data suggest that the alternate forms of the Quick Test may, in fact, provide estimates of IQ differently for different populations, and this possibility needs to be better documented. More information is needed regarding the test–retest reliability of the test. In addition, the Quick Test does not appear to be an entirely accurate estimator of WAIS and WISC IQ scores. Because the Quick test tends to consistently overestimate IQ, some form of a correction factor may increase the accuracy. For these reasons, the Quick Test probably should not be used to evaluate IQ except when time is extremely limited and only a rough estimate is needed. Dalton and Pederson (1987) developed optimal prediction regression formulae for the WAIS-R, but still suggested that the Quick Test only be used to estimate IQ scores under 100. The provisional manual is now 40 years old and is in need of replacement.

RAVEN'S PROGRESSIVE MATRICES

Raven's Progressive Matrices is intended to be a test of nonverbal intelligence. It consists of a series of increasingly difficult patterns with a piece missing. At the bottom of the stimuli is a set of six alternative pieces, one of which correctly completes the design. The test exists in three forms, Standard, Colored (intended mainly for children), and Advanced. Because it requires accurate perception of spatial relationships, it can also be seen to be a test of visual–spatial integrity. The manual (Raven, Court, & Raven, 1977) states that the test measures a person's ability to think clearly, irrespective of past experiences or present ability for verbal communication. It is stated to be standardized for subjects between the ages of 6 and 65.

The manual presents information regarding the reliability of the instrument in a wide range of subjects. In keeping with the multicultural applications of a test of nonverbal intelligence, the reliability of the instrument has been assessed in non-English-speaking populations. Internal-consistency reliability was assessed in a sample of 727 Greek school-aged children. The correlation coefficient had a value of .60 for the 6-year-old subjects and .98 for the 12-year-old subjects. The modal value was .90. The split-half reliability in a sample of Yugoslavian teenagers (unspecified age range and sample size) was .96. An assessment of the 1-year test–retest reliability in Congolese schoolchildren resulted in a correlation coefficient of .55. Information regarding the differences in absolute level was not reported.

The Colored Matrices have been recommended for young children, mental defectives, and older people. A group of 291 children was tested on the Colored Matrices in 1948 to provide normative information presented in the form of percentiles. Fifty-eight of those children were retested after an unspecified interval; the result was a correlation coefficient of .60 for the 6.5-year-old subjects and .80 for the 9.5-year-old subjects. A sample of 25 normal children and 29 emotionally disturbed children was tested three times with an interval of 3 months. For the normal subjects, the correlation between times 1 and 2 was .89; between times 1 and 3, .86; and between times 2 and 3, .90. For the disturbed subjects, the correlations between times 1 and 2 was .92; between times 2 and 3, .85; and between times 2 and 3, .92.

The manual also presents limited information regarding the validity of the instrument. Its criterion validity was assessed by correlating the matrices with intelligence test scores (the name of the intelligence test is not stated). For children, the correlation coefficients ranged from .54 to .86. For adults, the correlation coefficients ranged from .75 to .85. In children, the matrices correlated with scores from the California Achievement Tests in the range of .26 to .61, and with school grades in the range of .20 to .60. The manual states that the matrices correlate .70 with later school grades, but it does not specify the sample composition, the time interval, or the measure of achievement. Content validity was assessed by calculating the biserial item-total correlation; the result was a mean value of .52. A factor analysis extracted a single factor that the test's authors interpreted as g-factor intelligence. Although the report does not give enough information to allow an evaluation of the appropriateness of this conclusion, later studies have resulted in data that indicate that the initial conclusions were drawn from faulty methodology.

For example, Dolke (1976) performed a principal-components factor analysis with varimax rotation on the data from 521 Indian subjects. Extracting factors until the residual was not significantly different from zero resulted in a solution of five factors, none of which were interpreted as g. Dillon, Pohlmann, and Lohman (1981) hypothesized that the single-factor solution was an artifact of the dichotomous scoring method, and that the factor therefore actually represented a level of difficulty rather than a common construct. They therefore performed a factor analysis on the phi/phi coefficients derived from the item data. Using a principal-components factor analysis with varimax rotation, they derived two factors, one of which they interpreted as pattern addition–pattern subtraction and the other as pattern progression.

Dolke (1976) reported the results of an investigation into the psychometric properties of the Raven's Progressive Matrices in a sample of Indian subjects. The total sample for all of the data analyses involved 521 normal male subjects with a mean age of 42 years. To reveal the discriminability of the individual items, a random sample of 370 subjects was drawn from the larger sample. The highest and lowest scoring 27% of this subsample were formed into two groups. Then, a discrimination index was calculated based on the biserial correlation between group membership and score on the item. Conventional methodology labels a value of .35 as acceptable. Only 47 of the total 60 items demonstrated values greater than .35. Next, Dolke examined the sequence of items to see if their level of difficulty increased with their serial position in the test. Calculating the percentage of subjects passing each item, he found generally increasing difficulty, but with reversals in the sequence. A probit analysis conducted on the scores of all 521 subjects indicated that the level of difficulty did not proceed uniformly; instead, there was a discontinuous pattern with reversals, as well as a tendency for difficult items to be bunched in the middle of the sequence. In addition, the distance (measured in increments of difficulty) between the items was not well spaced.

Hall (1957) also reported an uneven progression of level of difficulty in his sample of 82 U.S. subjects, as did Bromley (1953) in his sample of 35 British subjects. Johnson and Oziel (1970) examined the item difficulty in a sample of 100 male nonparanoid chronic schizophrenics and 100 paranoid chronic schizophrenics and found no differences between the two samples, although as a whole there was an uneven series of item difficulties. These results indicate that a different sequence of the items may result in a more precise instrument.

An unspecified subsample of the subjects was retested after a 6-week interval; the result was a correlation of .80. An odd–even split of the items produced a Kuder–Richardson (K–R) 20 value of .67 and a Spearman–Brown value of .73. Hall (1957) found a higher K–R 20 value of .86. Finally, Dolke administered the General Aptitude Test Battery (GATB) to another unspecified subsample to obtain a correlation of .55 between the GATB IQ score and the score from Raven's Progressive Matrices. Hall found that Raven's Progressive Matrices correlated .72 with the WAIS FSIQ, .58 with the VIQ, and .71 with the PIQ.

The construct validity of Raven's Progressive Matrices has been examined. The result has been data that call into question whether the test actually is a measure of nonverbal

104

intelligence. Bock (1973) argued that because Raven's stimuli have the a priori easily verbalized descriptors of shading, shape, and size, the test is actually one of verbal abilities. He performed a factor analysis on the Raven's and the Tests of Primary Mental Abilities and found that the Raven's loaded heavily on the extracted verbal factor. Burke and Gingham (1969) administered the Raven's, the WAIS, and the Army General Classification Test to 91 male VA inpatient subjects. When principal-components factor analysis with varimax rotation was used, the Raven's loaded highly on the verbal factor. Urmer, Morris, and Wendland (1960) compared 20 nonneurological patients with 20 cerebrovascular-accident (CVA) patients and found significant differences in Raven's scores even when WAIS IQ was partialed out in an analysis of covariance. However, these results are difficult to interpret precisely because the CVA patients had a wide variety of location of lesions. After reviewing four studies investigating the Colored Matrices, Sigmon (1983) concluded that there were inadequate normative data, and additionally, that boys tend to perform better than girls.

A possible problem of Raven's Progressive Matrices is that the alternate answers are arranged in a horizontal line, which may influence the performance of individuals with unilateral neglect or visual hemifield deficits. Gainotti, D'Erme, Villa, and Caltagirone (1986) produced a form of the Raven's in which the alternatives are arranged in a vertical line; there were no differences in performance between the left-hemisphere- and right-hemisphere-lesioned subjects. However, the aphasic subjects performed significantly more poorly than the nonaphasic left-hemisphere-lesioned subjects, a finding indicating again that verbal skills may play a role in successful performance on Raven's Progressive Matrices.

Other studies have tried to investigate whether Raven's Progressive Matrices can be used to lateralize neurological impairment. Archibald, Wepman, and Jones (1967) tested 39 left-hemisphere and 29 right-hemisphere subjects using the Colored Matrices. They reported that the left-hemisphere subjects performed more poorly, but only at the $p < .06$ level of significance. Campbell and Oxbury (1976) tested stroke patients at 3 weeks and 6 months following stroke. Of all of the comparisons performed, only the right-hemisphere patients with unilateral neglect were significantly worse than the right-hemisphere patients without neglect. All of the patients improved over time. Colonna and Faglioni (1966); Costa and Vaughan (1962); DeRenzi and Faglioni (1965); and Zaidel, Zaidel, and Sperry (1981) concluded that performance on Raven's Progressive Matrices cannot be used to lateralize brain impairment. In a rigorous examination of the laterality question, Denes, Semenza, Stoppa, and Gradenigo (1978) evaluated 42 subjects with unilateral damage. To rule out the effects of contracoup, they used only subjects with ischemic cerebrovascular pathology. They also matched their subjects on the degree of their sensorimotor and visual field defects. The subjects were tested at admission and again 2 months later. All of the subjects improved over time, but there were no differences between the left- and the right-lateralized subjects.

In studies that concluded that lateralization is possible, Arrigoni and DeRenzi (1964) concluded that left-hemisphere subjects performed more poorly, but Piercy and Smith (1962) and Miceli, Caltagirone, Gainotti, Masullo, and Silvero (1981) concluded that right-hemisphere subjects performed more poorly. Basso, DeRenzi, Faglioni, Scotti, and Spinnler (1973) investigated Raven's Progressive Matrices performance in 159 subjects with unilateral brain impairment and 55 control subjects. The brain-impaired subjects were subdivided on the basis of the presence or absence of visual field defects, and the left-hemisphere-impaired subjects were further subdivided into aphasics and nonaphasics. As a whole, the brain-impaired subjects performed significantly more poorly than the control subjects. Out of all of the possible pairwise comparisons of the subgroups with the control subjects, only the right-hemisphere subjects with visual field defects and the aphasic subjects performed significantly more poorly than the control subjects. The right-lateralized subjects performed more poorly, although not significantly so, than did the left-lateralized subjects. The role of unilateral visual neglect was examined by Colombo, DeRenzi, and Faglioni (1976), who reported that these patients tended to choose alternatives from the side of the response sheet homolateral to their injured hemisphere, regardless of the correctness of the response chosen.

Zaidel and Sperry (1973) reported the results of an innovative technique to examine the laterality of Raven's Progressive Matrices. They examined seven commissurotomy patients between 2.5 and 7 years postsurgery. They reduced the number of responses possible from six to three. Although they allowed the subjects to view the stimuli, the possible responses were behind a screen and could be felt by only one hand at a time. The use of the left hand always resulted in a better performance, a finding indicating that Raven's may be a right-hemisphere task. However, the results are clouded by the presence of additional damage in the subjects secondary to epilepsy, the extremely small sample size, and the presence of a ventricular jugular shunt in one subject.

Given the studies described, it is safer to conclude that the Raven's cannot be easily lateralized. The results of Zaidel and Sperry indicate that this is an area that may bear fruit with the application of more creative methodology.

Costa (1976) argued that the reason that a clear consensus on laterality has not been reached is that the laterality and the locus of the lesion affect performance on the three subsets of the Ravens differently. This approach makes sense, as the summing of item scores often results in loss of information. Whether this approach will bear experimental fruit remains to be seen, but it does offer promise for future research.

In an examination of the concurrent validity of Raven's Progressive Matrices, Bolin (1955) administered the test to 76 college juniors and found a .65 correlation with the Otis Gamma Mental Ability Test, a .48 correlation with the American Council on Education Psychological Qualifying Exam total score, .29 with the linguistic portion of the same test, and .59 with the quantitative portion of the same test.

Raven's Progressive Matrices have readily recognizable advantages in testing language-impaired individuals. Brown and McMullen (1982) modified the administration of the test to allow movement-impaired subjects to indicate their responses by simple eye movements, further increasing the test's applicability.

STANFORD–BINET INTELLIGENCE SCALE

The Stanford–Binet Intelligence Scale has one of the oldest histories of any standardized test in current use in the United States. It is based on A. Binet's pioneering work in measuring the aptitude of French children for school and on Louis Terman's adaptation of that work for children in the United States. Because of the test's venerable history, it is surprising that the reliability of the current form of the Stanford–Binet has not been evaluated and that the validity of the Stanford–Binet has been meagerly evaluated. The manual (Terman & Merrill, 1972) reports that internal consistency has been evaluated only for the 1960 revision of the Stanford–Binet, and not for the 1972 renorming. The mean biserial correlation for each subtest is .67 for subjects between the ages of 6 and 14 years and .61 for subjects between the ages of 2.5 and 5 years. The new norms were generated from an administration of the Stanford–Binet to approximately 150 subjects in each of 21 age groups. The manual states that attempts were made to stratify the sample in terms of the demographic composition of the United States, but these attempts are not described. The safest conclusion to be drawn is that the reliability of the Stanford–Binet needs to be more fully evaluated.

There are three abbreviated forms that serve as approximations of alternate forms. Bloom, Klee, and Raskin (1977) administered the Stanford–Binet to 50 children with developmental disabilities. These authors found fairly high correlations between the full form and the abbreviated form (.99, .98, and .92). However, all of the abbreviated forms tended to underestimate the IQ derived from the full-length form. As many as 34% of the subjects had discrepancies of 5 points or more between their full-length Stanford–Binet IQ and their abbreviated-form IQS. The results of this study indicate that the short forms should not be considered alternate forms. Further, when an IQ score is desired, it would be better to administer the entire test.

Most studies of the Stanford–Binet have been mainly of the concurrent validity of the instrument; these studies have used a correlational design. For example, Harper and Tanners (1972) correlated the Stanford–Binet with the French Pictorial Test of Intelligence in a sample of 40 physically handicapped children, reporting a value of .79. Sewell (1977) administered the Stanford–Binet and the WPPSI to 35 black children from a lower-socioeconomic status background. He found correlations of .75 with the Verbal IQ score of the WPPSI, .70 with the Performance IQ, and .71 with the Full Scale IQ. In a test of the difference in absolute level, the WPPSI provided significantly greater IQ scores than did the Stanford–Binet. Davis (1973) found a correlation of .91 between the Stanford–Binet and the General Cognitive Index of the McCarthy scales in a sample of low-IQ kindergarten children. On the other hand, Harrison and Wiebe (1977) reported a correlation of only .45 between the same two tests in a sample of average-IQ preschool children. Apparently, the accuracy of the Stanford–Binet is different at different levels of ability.

An examination of the predictive validity of the Stanford–Binet found that it was more accurate in predicting WISC scores after a period of 3 years than was the WPPSI (Crockett, Rardin, & Pasework, 1975).

Brossard, Reynolds, and Gutkin (1980) investigated the question of whether the Stanford–Binet had differential validity as a function of race. They administered the Stanford–Binet and the Wide Range Achievement Test (WRAT) to 60 white children and 60 black children. They used the Stanford–Binet IQ scores to predict scores on the three WRAT subtests, separately by sex, and then tested for the significance of differences between the two races. There were no significant differences due to race.

Although the Stanford–Binet L–M is an often-used instrument for both clinical and research purposes, there is much that can be done to evaluate the instrument. In particular, studies of the reliability of the test are much needed. The test appears to have reasonable concurrent validity, but the construct and predictive validity of the test can be further evaluated. Some of these concerns have been addressed in the development of the fourth edition of the Stanford–Binet (Thorndike, Hagen, & Sattler, 1986).

Stanford–Binet Fourth Edition

The fourth edition of the Stanford–Binet is different from the earlier editions in important ways. There are a total of 15 subtests, but depending upon the age of the subject, between eight and thirteen subtests are administered to a single person. A composite score related to IQ is obtained just as with the earlier editions; however, no mental age score is given. (It is possible to calculate age equivalents.) Rather than a ratio IQ, the composite score is a deviation IQ with a mean of 100 and an average standard deviation of 16 points. In addition, four area scores are possible; Verbal Reasoning, Quantitative Reasoning, Abstract/Visual Reasoning, and Short-Term Memory. Each of the area scores has a mean of 50 and a standard deviation of 8 points. There is an Australian version of the Stanford–Binet IV and initial data indicate that it is comparable to its American version in terms of mean scores obtained in random samples (Rodriguez, Treacy, Sowerby, & Murphy, 1998).

The technical manual contains much useful information, but Atkinson (1989) has criticized the choice of standard error of measurement and presents a method of calculating true scores and constructing confidence intervals for these estimated true scores. Generally, the reliability of the Stanford–Binet IV is adequate except for its use in the preschool child. Schuerger and Witt (1989) investigated the temporal reliability of the Stanford–Binet IV and provide a table detailing the standardized error and percentages of subjects who evidenced changes greater than 15 points. One source of error is in the somewhat low interrater reliability of the Copying subtest (Mason, 1992). Because four area scores are now possible, it may be useful to examine scatter among these areas as well as among the individual subtests. Rosenthal and Kamphaus (1988) present tables of values for reliability of the scatter as well as the abnormality of the scatter. The validity of interpretations of scatter needs to be better explicated, especially since Kline, Snyder, Guilmette, and Castellanos (1992) reported marginal incremental validity of an index of scatter over Area SAS scores in predicting academic achievement. In reviewing the available validity data Laurent, Swerdlik, and Ryburn (1992) concluded that the Stanford–Binet IV is a two-factor (Verbal, Nonverbal) test in younger children and a three-factor (Verbal, Nonverbal Memory) test in children over the age of seven years. However, these authors also found that the Composite SAS was a valid measure of general intelligence. The factor structure of the Stanford–Binet IV may also differ as a function of skill level as McCallum, Karnes, and Crowell (1988) reported that the four-factor model as posited in the manual was a good descriptor of the data obtained in evaluating gifted children.

The Stanford–Binet IV correlates well with the WISC-R (Rothlisberg, 1987). The concurrent validity of the Stanford–Binet IV was also investigated by Rust and Lindstrom (1996), who administered it along with the WISC-III to 57 normal control subjects between the ages of 6 and 17 years. The correlation between FSIQ and Composite Standard score was .81, with an average difference between the two scores of less than 2 points. It should be pointed out that for some subjects the difference between IQ scores was substantial. It would be worthwhile to examine whether there is any regularity in terms of characteristics of subjects for whom the two tests tend to agree or disagree. For example, Lukens and Hurrell (1996) reported that the Stanford–Binet IV IQ scores were higher than WISC-III IQ scores in mildly retarded children even with significant correlations. Lavin (1996) reported similar correlations between the WISC-III and Stanford–Binet IV but did not find differences in mean IQ when the two tests were administered 24 days apart. The difference between IQ scores in individual subjects was not reported. Therefore, we cannot be sure if this set of results is actually different from those of Rust and Lindstrom (1996). Saklofske, Schwean, Yakulic, and Quinn (1994) reported high correlations but differences in scale scores between the Stanford–Binet IV and WISC-III in Canadian children with ADHD. Although the Stanford–Binet IV and WISC-R may provide congruent information when IQ scores are compared, the pattern of subscale performances may differ, at least for children with learning disabilities (Brown & Morgan, 1991).

McCrowell and Nagle (1994) found that the Stanford–Binet IV and WPPSI-R nonverbal scale scores differed although the verbal scales did not. Atkinson, Buec, Dickens, and Blackwell (1992) reported significant correlations but with large individual discrepancies between the Stanford–Binet IV and Leiter International Performance Scale in 24 children with developmental delays. The Stanford–Binet IV tends to result in higher IQ scores than does the Kaufman Assessment Battery even in the presence of moderately high correlations between the two instruments (Hayden, Furlong, & Linnemeyer, 1988). Carvajal, Gerber, Hewes, and Weaver (1987) reported substantial correlations between the Stanford–Binet IV and the WAIS-R, but individual differences in IQ scores were not reported.

The relationship between Composite Standard Age Score (SAS) and Area SAS (subscales) is not necessarily an average, at least not in subjects with mental retardation. Spruill (1996) reported that for these subjects, the Composite was closest to the lowest Area SAS, rather than being in the arithmetic middle.

Short Forms of the Stanford–Binet IV

Lawson and Evans (1996) reported on the relation of two-, four-, and six-subtest short forms to the full form with relatively high correlations. In evaluating these three short forms, Prewett (1992c) found roughly equivalent results for the four- and six-subtest forms with lesser confidence in the results of the two-subtest form. Glaub and Kamphaus (1991) developed a short form of the Stanford–Binet IV for hearing-impaired subjects. This short form uses only the Bead Memory, Pattern Analysis, Copying, Memory for Objects, and Matrices subtests. Nagle and Bell (1995b) found that an item reduction short form was closer to the long form Composite SAS than was a subtest reduction short form. Nagle and Bell (1993) also found differences between the long form and four different subtest reduction short forms in college students, and these differences became larger as the Composite SAS increased. Prewett (1992c) reported that the six-subtest short form recommended in the manual was superior to two-subtest short forms, but did not find differences in comparison to the four-subtest short form in students with low academic achievement. The four-subtest (Vocabulary, Quantitative, Pattern Analyses, and Memory for Sentences) short form was recommended when the long form cannot be administered.

Conclusions

The Stanford–Binet L–M had a seeming advantage over the WISC-R and WAIS-R in that measurement in the low and high extremes of IQ was more reliable. The WISC-III, and now the WAIS-III, has greater sampling in these ranges, lessening this advantage. The Stanford–Binet IV has the potential for advantage over the L–M form in that area scores as well as the composite score is possible. More empirical evidence regarding the characteristics of the Stanford–Binet IV in neuropsychological populations, especially with regard to subtest and area scatter, is needed to enhance its utility for the purposes of clinical neuropsychological assessment. Although there is general agreement in rank orderings of IQ scores between the Stanford–Binet IV and the WISC-III, the actual scale scores may differ in certain populations, indicating caution in considering these two tests to be comparable.

SLOSSON INTELLIGENCE TEST

The Slosson Intelligence Test is a short, easily administered test of intellectual ability that is derived from the Stanford–Binet. It is stated to be appropriate for individuals 1 month and older. It can be administered by people with average intelligence with a minimal amount of training. Its items appear to tap verbal comprehension and production, arithmetic reasoning, verbal–auditory memory, and general fund of knowledge. The reliability of the Slosson has not been evaluated.

There has been some research investigating the concurrent validity of the Slosson. The manual for the Slosson (Slosson, 1963) reports two studies that compare it to the WAIS and the WISC. However, these two studies used only 10 subjects (WAIS) and 15 subjects (WISC). More research is obviously needed. Johnson and Johnson (1971) compared the PIAT, the Draw-a-Man Test, and the Slosson to the Stanford–Binet and found the greatest correlation with the Slosson (.79) as well as no difference in mean IQ scores. Unfortunately, the individual differences were not reported. Stewart and Jones (1976) reviewed research correlating the Slosson with the Stanford-Binet and reported that most correlation coefficient values were in the .90s. This is not surprising, as the Slosson is based on the Stanford–Binet. A more relevant research design would be to relate the Slosson to other tests of intelligence. Covin (1977) reviewed four studies that compared the Slosson with the WISC and the WAIS; the samples were larger than those used in the manual. Covin found a range of correlation coefficients from .49 to .6. She then reported the results of her own study, which investigated the relationship between the Slosson and the WISC in 50 children who had been referred for psychoeducational assessment. She found moderate correlations between the Slosson and the WISC IQS for black students and somewhat higher correlation values for Caucasian students. The overall trend was for the Slosson to be more highly related to the VIQ than to the PIQ or the FSIQ. This trend is present in gifted students as well (Clarke & Scagliotti, 1989). Unfortunately, the Slosson may overestimate Full Scale IQ of the WISC-R and the Stanford–Binet in gifted children (Clark, McCallum, Edwards, & Hildman, 1987). Despite this overestimation, Karnes and Oehler (1986) reported that using a cutoff of 130 still results in accurate classification. Still more serious overestimation occurs when the Slosson is compared with the McCarthy (Bondy, Constantino, Norcross, & Sheslow, 1984).

The Slosson may have limitations when used to evaluate individuals with significantly low IQS. Kunen, Overstreet, and Salles (1996) reported that the Slosson correlated well with the Stanford–Binet, but tended to disagree with regard to category of mental retardation for subjects in that range. The Slosson may also have limitations when used with students with auditory processing problems as scores on the Slosson were lower than scores from the Test of Nonverbal Intelligence and lower than scores from the Clinical Evaluation of Language-Revised (Perez et al., 1995). However, the Slosson was superior to teacher ratings in predicting academic achievement for students in a remedial reading program (Eaves, Williams, Winshester, & Darch, 1994) and correlates well with all three subtests of the WRAT-R (Prewett & Fowler, 1992). When the revised Slosson was given to a group of children whose IQ (based on the abbreviated Stanford–Binet IV) ranged from 36 to 110, there was little consistency of assignment to intellectual category. However, there was good agreement with the overall classification of mentally retarded or not (Kunen, Overstreet, & Salles, 1996).

Lowrance and Anderson (1979) also compared the Slosson with the WISC-R in school-aged children. The subjects were 34 females and 35 males between the ages of 6 and 13. The authors reported a correlation of .79 with the PIQ and of .92 with the VIQ. The Slosson tended to provide higher estimates of IQ than did the WISC-R at the upper ranges of this distribution and lower estimates of IQ at the lower end of the distribution. Martin et al. (1979) correlated the Slosson with the California Short Form Test of Mental Maturity ($r = .73$) and with the Shipley Institute of Living Scale ($r = .69$) in a sample of 50 college students. The Slosson correlates fairly well with the WAIS-R, but as with the WISC-R, the Slosson results in higher IQ scores (Klett, Watson, & Hoffman, 1986).

The Slosson predicts oral reading skills fairly well and does so equally across genders (Flynt, Warren, Morton, & Smith, 1997). The Slosson exhibited a fair amount of agreement with the Woodcock Reading Mastery Test-Revised and the Reading subtest of the Wide Range Achievement Test-Revised in a sample of adult substance abuse patients (Johnson & Fisher, 1996).

As a short screening instrument, the Slosson appears to be attractive for clinical practice. However, there are little data regarding its characteristics in neuropsychological populations, especially in adults. Furthermore, scores from the Slosson tend to be higher than scores from other instruments even when those instruments correlate highly with the Slosson.

THE SHIPLEY–HARTFORD SCALE

The Shipley–Hartford Scale (also known as the Shipley Institute of Living Scale) was originally designed as a measure of mental deterioration in psychiatric patients (Pollock, 1942). It is a brief instrument that can be administered individually or in groups. It consists of two parts. The first part is a measure of vocabulary, and the second a measure of abstraction skills. The comparison between the two scores is said to demonstrate the amount of deterioration that has occurred. The Shipley–Hartford has recently generated interest as a screening instrument in the determination of general intellectual level. There are no reports of evaluations of any form of reliability.

The Shipley–Hartford has been evaluated only in terms of its concurrent validity. Prado and Taub (1966) investigated its accuracy in estimating IQ scores derived from either an abbreviated form of the WAIS or the Stanford–Binet in a sample of 59 psychiatric patients in a VA hospital and a second group of 55 employees of a state hospital. These authors reported that the Shipley–Hartford showed better agreement in individuals with above-average IQ. Black (1974b) reported similar findings in a sample of 40 subjects with penetrating head wounds. Again, the Shipley–Hartford predicted WAIS scores more accurately in above-average IQ subjects. Interestingly, the IQ scores derived from the two instruments agreed within 3 points in only 33% of the subjects. The two instruments agreed within 12 points in 80% of the subjects. Bartz (1968) reported that the Shipley–Hartford was a better predictor of WAIS IQ scores than was the Army Beta Test, although the overall correlation between Full Scale IQ values was only .73.

The Shipley did not correlate with grade point average in a sample of college students, but then again neither did the WAIS-R in the same sample (Wong, 1993). The Shipley has a smaller correlation with WAIS-R IQ scores than does the Henmon– Nelson Tests of Mental Ability, but the Henmon–Nelson tended to overestimate WAIS-R scores while the Shipley did not (Watson et al., 1992). It should be noted that one study has indicated that the Shipley may underestimate IQ in the above average range and overestimate IQ in the below average range (Heinemann, Harper, Friedman, & Whitney, 1985). The Shipley has moderate correlations with the Test of Nonverbal Intelligence, with the expected pattern of higher correlations between the Shipley Total and Abstraction scores than for the Vocabulary scores (Martin, Blair, & Bledsoe, 1990). Other studies indicated that the Shipley is useful in estimating WAIS-R IQ scores in psychiatric inpatients (Frisch & Jessop, 1989) regardless of level of education (Schear, Harrison, & Sherman, 1987). There is less accuracy in estimating WAIS-R IQ in normal control adults (Retzlaff, Slicner, & Gibertini, 1986). Because of age-related difficulties in abstraction skills, the Shipley may not be effective in the elderly (Heinemann et al., 1985; Morgan & Hatsukami, 1987).

THE KAUFMAN ADOLESCENT AND ADULT INTELLIGENCE TEST

The Kaufman Adolescent and Adult Intelligence Test (KAIT) is a standardized assessment procedure designed to measure aspects of crystallized and fluid intelligence (Kaufman & Kaufman, 1993). There are three subtests and one alternate subtest for each aspect of intelligence. For fluid intelligence the subtests are Rebus Learning, Logical Steps, and Mystery Codes; the alternate subtest is Memory for Block Designs. For crystallized intelligence the subtests are Definitions, Auditory Comprehension, and Double meanings; the alternate subtest is Famous Faces. The KAIT was normed and standardized on a nationally stratified sample of 2000 individuals between the ages of 11 and 94 years. The mean split-half reliability for the subtests is .96, and the mean test–retest reliability is .90 for a 1-month interval. Factor analyses generally support the composition of the crystallized and fluid intelligence indices. Examination of the adult data indicates that fluid intelligence scores tend to decrease with age, and indices of crystallized intelligence increased in young adulthood, remained stable in middle-age adulthood, and decreased after age 60 (Kaufman & Horn, 1996). These results were taken as evidence in support of the construct validity of the KAIT.

THE KAUFMAN BRIEF INTELLIGENCE TEST

The Kaufman Brief Intelligence Test (K-BIT) is a two subtest procedure that was designed to allow a short estimate of intellectual functioning (Kaufman & Kaufman, 1990). The two subtests, Vocabulary and Matrices, are combined to provide a Composite that can be interpreted as an estimate of Full Scale IQ. The K-BIT was standardized on a nationally stratified sample of 2022 people between the ages of 4 and 90 years. The K-BIT scores were related to race and education in the standardization sample (Kaufman & Wang, 1992).

Reliability Data

The manual presents data related to the reliability of the K-BIT. Split-half reliability coefficients are presented by age group and are generally between .74 for the Matrices subtest in the 5-year-old group and .98 for Vocabulary in the 55- to 90-year-old group. Test–retest reliability was evaluated by administering the K-BIT twice to 232 subjects between the ages of 5 and 89 years and values ranged from .80 for the Matrices subtest in the 13- to 19-year-old group to .97 for the Vocabulary subtest in the 20- to 54-year-old group. There was a gain of about 2 points associated with retesting.

It is important to also determine the reliability of the K-BIT in clinical samples because it is there that the use is more likely for clinical neuropsychologists. Eisenstein and Engelhart (1997) reported an internal consistency coefficient of .97 (Composite Score) using the intraclass correlation coefficient in a sample of 64 adult patients referred for neuropsychological assessment. In a sample of 24 adolescent offenders, using an average retest interval of 18 days, the K-BIT exhibited test–retest coefficients of .92 (Vocabulary) with a mean increase of 4 points, .79 (Matrices) with a mean increase of 3 points, and .92 (Composite) with a mean increase of 4 points (Thompson et al., 1997). Although these correlations are higher than those reported in the manual, the gains associated with retesting are also higher, and it may be that clinical subjects show more of a practice effect than the standardization subjects.

The manual also provides descriptions of initial validity studies. The descriptions of these studies are briefer than would be found in journal report. The K-BIT was correlated with other tests of intelligence including the Kaufman Assessment Battery for Children, the WISC-R, and the WAIS-R. The resulting values were moderate in degree and followed a trend in which the Vocabulary subtest correlated more highly than the Matrices subtest with other measures of aspects of intelligence, even when those other aspects were not necessarily verbal in nature. The Matrices subtest may be tapping some dimension of nonverbal intelligence not well accessed by other standard tests. When the K-BIT was compared with other short tests of intelligence (Test of Nonverbal Intelligence, Slosson), the Matrices subtest correlated more highly with the nonverbal tests, as would be expected. Correlations of the K-BIT with tests of educational achievement (Wide Range Achievement Test-Revised, Kaufman Test of Educational Achievement) were moderate to low.

Concurrent validity of the K-BIT has been examined by correlations with other tests of intelligence, both other screening tests and other full-length intelligence tests. The K-BIT exhibited adequate correlations with the Slosson Intelligence Test in both a small sample of college students and in a somewhat larger sample of incarcerated females (Bowers & Pantle, 1998).

Concurrent validity can be evaluated by comparing performance on the K-BIT to performance on the WAIS-R. Axelrod and Naugle (1998) found reasonable relationships of the K-BIT to the WAIS-R, although there was more accurate estimates of Full Scale IQ using the seven-subtest short form of the WAIS-R. Naugle, Chelune, and Tucker (1993) reported reasonable correlations of the K-BIT and WAIS-R, but the K-BIT provided IQ scores that were 5 points higher on the average. Eisenstein and Engelhart (1997) compared the K-BIT to seven different short forms of the WAIS-R in a clinical sample, and reported reasonable correlations, ranging from .82 for a two-subtest form to .88 for a four-subtest form.

Although no other tests were administered, Donovick, Burright, Burg, and Gronen-dyke (1996) administered the K-BIT to different groups of patients and found that average scores declined from the college students to the adults with closed head injury (CHI), children with learning disabilities, psychiatric inpatients, and neurosurgical patients in the acute stages of recovery. Donders (1995) examined the K-BIT in a sample of 47 children with traumatic brain injury (TBI) and found that although the K-BIT Vocabulary subtest correlated well with the WISC-III IQ indexes, the Matrices subtest did not. In addition, the K-BIT did not correlate with the length of coma. K-BIT Vocabulary may reflect crystallized intelligence and may therefore be useful as an estimate of premorbid functioning following TBI in children. However, the construct underlying the Matrices subtest is in need of further explication.

Together, these two studies indicate that although the K-BIT may be sensitive to some aspects of organic functioning, it may tap constructs different from those tapped by the WISC-III. On the other hand, Canivez (1995) and Prewett (1995) found that the K-BIT did correlate well with the WISC-III, although use of the K-BIT may result in somewhat higher IQ estimates than the WISC-III. The difference between IQ scores obtained on the WISC-R and IQ scores obtained on the WISC-II may also account for the fact that K-BIT scores generally show greater agreement with WISC-R scores (Prewett, 1992a) at least among incarcerated juveniles; however, the K-BIT may provide higher IQ estimates than does the WISC-III in school children referred for evaluation (Prewett, 1992b) . When the subjects are students with above average IQ scores, the K-BIT does correlate well with the WISC-III (Levinson & Folino, 1995).

The K-BIT agreed with the Peabody Picture Vocabulary Test-Revised in classifying preschool children as being average or above average (Childers, Durham, & Wilson, 1994). When the K-BIT was compared to the Stanford–Binet, correlations were respectable, but use of the K-BIT resulted in somewhat lower IQ estimates (Prewett & MacCaffrey, 1993).

Slate, Graham, and Bower (1996) used a somewhat unusual design in that the WISC-R was first administered to a sample of 44 adolescents with clinical diagnoses and then 3 years later, the K-BIT was administered with resulting high correlations. When the K-BIT was compared to a four-subtest short form of the WISC-III in predicting full-length WISC-III scores, the Vocabulary scale correlated .79 with the VIQ as did the Composite scale with the FSIQ , but the Matrices scale correlated only .45 with PIQ. Furthermore, corresponding scores differed by two standard errors or less in fewer than 50% of the individuals in the sample (Thompson et al., 1997). The K-BIT along with the WISC-III and Woodcock–Johnson-Revised Tests of Achievement was administered to a sample of 75 students with learning disabilities (Canivez, 1996). The identification of learning disability based on comparison with the Woodcock–Johnson was similar for the K-BIT and the WISC-III. Furthermore, the K-BIT correlated well with the WISC-III, but there were not the expected differences between Vocabulary and Matrices.

Factor analyses are also useful in the evaluation of construct validity. Confirmatory factor analysis of the K-BIT in relation to the WAIS-R evaluated six possible models and resulted in a four factor solution best fitting the data. The K-BIT Verbal Intelligence and

WAIS-R Verbal factors were separate factors with the K-BIT Verbal Intelligence factor having significant loadings from visuospatial variables. Therefore the K-BIT and WAIS-R verbal subtests probably measure somewhat different constructs (Burton, Naugle, & Schuster, 1995).

Reaction time has been suggested as an index of general intelligence. Buckhalt, Whang, & Fischman (1998) found reasonable correlations between reaction time and K-BIT scores with a stronger relationship involving the Matrices scores.

The K-BIT may be a reasonable method to estimate IQ in situations where time is limited and where direct IQ values are not sought, but the K-BIT may be inferior to the WISC-III, WAIS-R, or Stanford–Binet (Parker, 1993). Eisenstein and Engelhart (1997) reported that the K-BIT is inferior to short forms of the WAIS-R in predicting Full Scale IQ.

TEST OF NONVERBAL INTELLIGENCE (TONI)

The TONI was developed as a means to estimate intellectual functioning that was significantly impacted by verbal skill and that would therefore be less culturally sensitive. There are two forms, A and B. Both Form A and Form B have reasonable temporal reliability when measured over a 3-week interval. In addition, interform reliability was comparable to temporal reliability (McGhee & Lieberman, 1991). There is a second edition (TONI-2) as well as a version with multiple subtests related to either representational (pictorial) or abstract (geometric) items. Norms are provided in the manual for children of various ages, but the sample is limited to individuals aged 18 years or younger. A normative sample of adult aged subjects would be very helpful. Although female children tend to score higher than males, no significant differences were found in a sample of 311 children and adolescents receiving inpatient mental health services (Frey, 1996). Correlations between the TONI and the VIQ and PIQ from the WISC-R do not indicate a greater relation to nonverbal measures (D'Amato, Lidiak, & Lassiter, 1994). The TONI provided lower estimates of intelligence than did either the Kaufman Assessment Battery for Children or the WISC-R (Lassiter & Bardos, 1993). However, in comparing suburban Canadian children with native Canadian children, the relationship with the WISC-R performance IQ was higher in the native Canadian sample (Kowall, Watson, & Madak, 1990). The TONI does correlate with the WISC-R in a sample of Native American and Caucasian rural children (Whorton & Morgan, 1990). As expected, the TONI had a greater relationship to the Shipley Institute of Living Scale Total and Abstraction scores than to the Vocabulary score in a sample of undergraduate students (Martin, Blair, & Bledsoe, 1990). Despite its theoretical culture-fair assumptions, there may be bias in the TONI at least in evaluating eastern Indian children (Parmar, 1989). Vance, Hankins, and Reynolds (1988) concluded that the TONI is as adequate and accurate a predictor of WISC-R as is the Quick Test. In learning disabled students, the TONI was not able to reasonably predict WISC-R scores (Haddad, 1987). The TONI is promising, but the existing data provide conflicting and sometimes confusing information that can be resolved only with additional research.

The Halstead–Reitan and Luria–Nebraska Neuropsychological Batteries

North American neuropsychology is largely based on the psychometric tradition of measurement. Many neuropsychologists practicing in North America were trained in the context of graduate psychology departments. Because they received their training from psychologists, rather than from neurologists who may have provided ancillary training experiences, clinical neuropsychologists largely have chosen assessment instruments that involve standardized assessment. Many clinical neuropsychologists utilized a fixed battery approach in the past. In the early 1980s, the Battle of the Batteries consisted of adherents of either the Halstead–Reitan (HRNB) or of the Luria–Nebraska (LNNB) conducting studies, publishing results, and trading comments. It seemed as if neither battery would achieve hegemony. Surveys such as that described by Guilmette and Faust (1991) indicated that although the HRNB had greater frequency of usage, both batteries were commonly used. Since that time, changes in some of the influences on clinical neuropsychology have resulted in a lesser emphasis on comprehensive evaluations using instruments that have been normed and standardized on a single sample. Whether this is a positive trend is subject to review.

These influences include the development of sophisticated, highly focused assessment instruments such as the California Verbal Memory Test and the Warrington Recognition Memory Test in the realm of memory assessment. Yet another influence of change has been restrictions brought about by the carriers of reimbursement. Managed care organizations (MCOs) have severely limited the amount of time they will pay for in a neuropsychological evaluation. As a result, it is likely that fewer comprehensive evaluations are being conducted using full fixed batteries. A recent survey indicates that the use of the flexible battery approach has increased in frequency while the fixed battery approach has decreased (Sweet, Moberg, & Westergaard, 1996). Even with this decrease, the fixed battery will remain with us for a long time. If publications are any indication, there is not a strong decline in interest in these batteries as dependent measures (e.g., Haltiner, Temkin, Winn, & Dikmen, 1996; Hom, Haley, & Kurt, 1997). Nonetheless the battery approach may undergo some modification in the future. One likely scenario would be for components of batteries to be normed on the same sample but for those components also to be applicable in their single manifestations. An example of this approach can be seen in the Wechsler scales in which the same subset of subjects was used to norm the intelligence scales (WISC-III and WAIS-III), the achievement scales (Wechsler Individual Achievement Test or WIAT), and the memory scales (WMS-III).

Rather than the battle of the batteries as described earlier, the recent controversy regarding the HRNB has been criticisms from a leading proponent of the flexible approach (Lezak, 1995). Lezak has been very vocal regarding criticisms of the fixed battery approach. Earlier editions of her textbook had dismissed the LNNB, and the third edition contains a spirited and opinionated critique of the HRNB. Russell (1998) provided an ample response to the criticisms and suggested that Lezak had little understanding of the HRNB and of standardized testing. Some of Lezak's (1995) comments regarding the HRNB do seem to be misinformed, but some of Russell's (1998) responses assume a specific and particular use of the HRNB. It is true that there is an underlying assumption of pattern recognition being an important model of interpretation of the HRNB, but this assumption has not been well articulated by Reitan. It was Russell himself who in a series of writings (Russell, 1984, 1986, 1994, 1997) has provided the most cogent exegesis of this set of concepts. It is also true that other authors have provided different models of interpretation of the HRNB. For example, Jarvis and Barth (1994) presented a model, based on Reitan (1967), in which level of performance and the presence of pathognomonic signs also figure in the interpretation. Bradford (1992) also discussed process relationships in the interpretation of data from the HRNB. Regardless of the method of interpretation favored by an individual, the accuracy of that interpretation is evaluable empirically, and that, not opinion, is the main issue in critiquing an instrument.

THE HALSTEAD–REITAN NEUROPSYCHOLOGICAL BATTERY

The HRNB is the forerunner of comprehensive neuropsychological batteries. Ward Halstead collected the procedures from the psychological literature after an extensive review. Later Ralph Reitan extended and modified the battery. The intent of the battery was to identify the psychological aspects of impaired brain function. Although there is general agreement that the HRNB is highly reliable and valid (Hevern, 1980), there is much more empirical information regarding its validity than there is regarding its reliability. Perhaps because of its longevity, the HRNB or its subtests are sometimes used as criterion measures in evaluating new tests (e.g., Coleman, Moberg, Raglund, & Gur, 1997). The original HRNB consisted of the following seven tests which were selected for their ability to discriminate between subjects with frontal lobe lesions and patients with other lesions or normal subjects (Halstead, 1947; Reitan & Davison, 1974): (1) the Category Test; (2) the Tactual Performance Test (a modification of the Seguin–Goddard Form Board); (3) the Rhythm Test (which originally appeared in the Seashore Measures of Musical Talent); (4) the Speech Sounds Perception Test; (5) the Finger Oscillation Test (Finger Tapping Test); (6) the Critical Flicker Fusion Test; and (7) the Time Sense Test. The Flicker Fusion Test and the Time Sense Test are not typically included in current modifications of the HRNB, as they have not been shown to reliably differentiate neurologically impaired subjects from unimpaired subjects (Boll, 1981; Russell, Neuringer, & Goldstein, 1970). The five remaining tests produce seven individual scores, three scores (total time, memory, and location) being derived from the Tactual Performance Test (TPT). These scores are used to calculate an Impairment Index, which represents the proportion of the patient's scores that fall within the impaired range. An Impairment Index of .5 is considered the cutoff for overall performance within the impaired range.

Although the Impairment Index has proved to be a clinically useful measure, it is important to note that diagnostic conclusions regarding the simple presence or absence of brain damage that are based on this measure have been found to be less accurate than those obtained by clinical judgment based on tests, interviews, and medical history (Tsushima & Wedding, 1979). Because of the amount of time required to obtain the HII, an alternative index (Alternate Impairment Index or AII; Horton, 1995a,b) using some of the same tests was proposed. Further research indicated that the AII may not be as accurate as the HII in describing the degree of severity of brain damage (Horton, 1997). [Additionally, there is another summary index score available from the HRNB, namely, the General Neuro-psychological Deficit Scale (GND). This score sums information from the results of the individual subtests and appears to be sensitive to both localized and diffuse damage. The GND is discussed further in the section on validity.]

In addition to the tests listed in the preceding, many clinicians augment this core battery with tests of verbal and visuospatial memory (e.g., Dodrill, 1978, 1979; Matarazzo, Wiens, Matarazzo, & Goldstein, 1974; Russell, 1980), perceptual integrity (e.g., Reitan, 1966; Russell et al., 1970), and motor performance (e.g., Harley, Leuthold, Matthews, & Bergs, 1980; Matthews & Haaland, 1979). In addition to the original tests comprising the Halstead battery, Reitan has included several additional procedures: the Wechsler Adult Intelligence Scale, an aphasia and sensory-perceptual battery, the Trail Making Test, and a measure of grip strength. It should be noted that the titles "Halstead–Reitan Neuropsycho-logical Battery" and "Halstead–Reitan Battery and Allied Procedures" refer to three separate test batteries (adult, intermediate, and young children). The adult battery, the Halstead Neuropsychological Test Battery and Allied Procedures, is used for persons 15 years old and older. The procedures for children aged 9 to 15 years is the Halstead Neuropsychological Test Battery for Children and Allied Procedures. The battery for children aged 6 to 9 years is the Reitan Indiana Neuropsychological Test Battery for Children. Each of these batteries includes a minimum of 14 separate tests and 26 variables, as well as an aphasia and constructional praxis test of 31 separate items (Boll, 1981).

Normative Data

Table 9.1 provides a listing of cutoff scores for the adult HRNB and many of its commonly used additional procedures. The norms for this table were adopted from Halstead (1947), Reitan (n.d.), Russell et al. (1970), and Golden (1977, 1978a).

Although the research literature in general is supportive of the HRNB, it is important to note that the original norms for this battery (see Boll, 1981) were not well founded. It is questionable whether the 29 subjects that were used as normals in this research were appropriate. For example, ten of the subjects were diagnosed as having "minor" psychiatric problems, one subject was awaiting criminal sentencing (either life imprisonment or execution) at the time of testing, and four subjects were awaiting lobotomies because of aberrant behavior. In spite of these criticisms, the HRNB has proved to be quite robust in its ability to assess neurological impairment.

For those reasons, recent publications have sought to provide more comprehensive normative information. Bornstein (1986c) presented normative information on the differ-

TABLE 9.1 Ranges for Brain-Injured Performance on
the Halstead–Reitan Battery

Test	Impaired range
Aphasia exam	>6 points or 72 errors
Category test	>50 errors
Finger Agnosia	>2 errors
Finger Tapping Test (dominant)	<51 taps
Finger Tapping Test (nondominant)	<46 taps
Fingertip Number Writing	>3 errors
Grip Strength (dominant)	<40 kg
Grip Strength (nondominant)	<35 kg
Impairment Index	>.4
Rhythm Test	>4 errors
Speech Sounds Perception Test	>7 errors
Suppressions (all modalities)	>0
Tactile Form Recognition	>0 errors
Tactual Performance Test	
Total time	>942 seconds
Memory	<6 correct
Location	<5 correct
Trail Making Test (Part A)	>39 seconds
Trail Making Test (Part B)	>91 seconds

ences between left- and right-sided performance on the Grooved Pegboard, the Smedley dynamometer, and the Finger Tapping Test. Bornstein (1986a) examined the cutoff scores in relation to performance by 365 normal subjects and found that between 15% and 80% of the subjects would have been misclassified as impaired. Fromm–Auch and Yeudall (1983) presented normative data based on a sample of 193 normal adult subjects. Steinmeyer (1986) reviewed the available normative data and calculated metanorms for the HRNB. Alekoumbides, Charter, Adkins, and Seacat (1987) provided age and education corrections based on a limited sample of 235 patients.

Subsequently, Heaton, Grant, and Matthews (1991) published a set of normative information regarding the HRNB in which scores could be translated to standardized T-scores, stratified by gender, age, and education. The publication of this information started a controversy in which Reitan questioned the wisdom of using age or education corrections (Reitan & Wolfson, 1995a). The basic argument is that the demographically based corrections may be unnecessary because the effects of brain damage are stronger than any effects of age or education. Shuttleworth–Jordan (1997) and Vanderploeg, Axelrod, Shere, Scott, and Adams (1997) reexamined the data presented by Reitan and Wolfson (1995a) and instead concluded that the demographic corrections are necessary, especially when the effects of subtle neurological impairment may actually be masked by or mimicked by age or education, similar to earlier reports that age and education have consistent effects on test performance whether or not the subject is neurologically impaired (Sherer & Adams, 1993). The presence of age and education effects is consistent with current theory and empirical knowledge regarding neuropsychological test data, and it is probably wise to consider these factors when interpreting the results of the HRNB. However, there is another cautionary consideration here. The cell sizes for the various stratifications of age, education, and gender are not given in the Heaton et al. (1991) manual. However, using simple arithmetic and the total number of subjects, we can see that the normative bases may be quite limited in size, especially for the lower education and upper age ranges. As a result, even these norms should be interpreted with caution. Fastenau and Adams (1996) presented these and other criticisms of the Heaton et al. (1991) published norms in a very negative review. Heaton, Grant, Matthews, and Avitable (1996) responded with the unconvincing argument that the tables are based on a regression analysis of the entire sample rather than on just the individual cells of age, education, and gender permutations. This particular rejoinder is unconvincing as the tables are presented as comparisons to substantial collections of subjects complete with percentiles and T-scores. Other suggestions by Heaton et al. (1996), such as that the scores on the 60-item version of the Boston Naming Test be prorated to use the 85-item experimental version represented in the comprehensive norms, also are not convincing. Heaton et al.'s (1996) replies to other criticisms raised by Fastenau and Adams (1996) are reasonable. It is important to not lose sight of the fact that the Heaton comprehensive norms are superior in some aspects to those provided in the original publications and therefore represent a substantial contribution to the resources available to clinicians who use the HRNB. However, it should also be said that clinicians would be wise to not rely exclusively on this data base in the interpretation of HRNB scores. Fastenau (1999) examined the use of the Heaton norms in evaluating the performance of 63 healthy older adults in interpreting scores from the TMT-A, TMT-B, and Boston Naming Test. Unfortunately, the Heaton norms resulted in the creation of education effects in the sample. There was overcorrection of age influences. Clearly, caution should be used, at least in this age range (over 60 years old).

Reitan and Wolfson (1995a) argued against the use of these demographic corrections. Their point is that the effects of cerebral impairment will largely overcome the effects of age, education, or gender. Reitan and Wolfson (1995a) marshalled evidence that the influence of age and education are much stronger for normal subjects than for impaired subjects. In their sample of 100 individuals equally divided between control subjects and subjects with documented brain damage, the General Neuropsychological Deficit Scale (GNDS) clearly separated the two groups of subjects. In addition, the GNDS was correlated with age and education only for the control group. The use of demographic correction factors may not affect the sensitivity of the HRNB to neurological impairment, but it might affect the specificity by increasing the false-positive rate in subjects with advanced age or low education. Moses, Pritchard, and Adams (1999) evaluated the Heaton et al. (1991) demographic corrections in a sample of 290 neurological and 346 psychiatric patients. Although these researchers concluded that the norms were helpful in reducing the effect of age and education on HNRB performance, they warned against interpreting the scores as reflecting the same levels of impairment on different tests because they were generated on a sample of only normal individuals.

It is not just the use of demographic corrections that is at issue here. The choice of normative groups and standards has extremely important implications for the interpretation of data. Kalechstein, van Gorp, and Rapport (1998) found very different conclusions in a set of Monte Carlo data when the fictitious test scores were compared to different sets of published norms. There is much variability in test performance even among normal subjects. It is extremely important to understand the characteristics of the normative sample and compare them to the subject at hand in choosing a normative set of data for interpretation purposes.

The GNDS is another method suggested for interpretation of the HRNB. The GNDS (Reitan & Wolfson, 1993) is a sum reflecting four different areas of information from the HRNB; namely, level of performance, pathognomonic signs, patterns and relationships among test results, and right–left differences. There are 42 different factors comprising these areas. In addition, it is impossible to calculate a Left Neuropsychological Deficit Scale (LNDS) and Right Neuropsychological Deficit Scale (RNDS). The GNDS was intended as an improvement on the Halstead Impairment Index and the Average Impairment Index and as a way to detect diffuse neuropsychological impairment.

Reitan and Wolfson (1993) reported that the GNDS could separate impaired from intact subjects using a cutoff of 26 points. Sherer and Adams (1993) found that although the GNDS could identify neurologically impaired subjects in their sample, it had a fairly high misclassification rate for pseudoneurologic subjects. Reitan and Wolfson (1995b) later cross-validated their original classification study and criticized Sherer and Adams (1993) for using subjects with low GNDS scores in their pseudoneurologic group. Then again, that appears to be the point of using pseudoneurologic subjects, to examine sensitivity in subtle cases.

Collingwood and Harrell (1999) examined the GNDS in a sample of psychotic and substance abusing patients with and without a history of closed head injury. The majority of the patients exhibited GNDS scores above the cutoff of 26 points, but there were no significant differences in comparisons of the patients with and without head injury. The GNDS may be sensitive to diffuse involvement. Sweeney (1999) found that the GNDS was more sensitive to the effects of nonimpact acceleration injuries from motor vehicle accidents than was either the comparison of subtest performance to the original cutoffs or the translation of raw scores to demographically corrected T-scores. All of the individuals in this study had subjective complaints of cognitive difficulty, and 94% were involved in litigation. Because there was no external criterion, it can be concluded only that the GNDS was more sensitive, not that it was more accurate. Rojas and Bennett (1995) examined the GNDS in two groups of fairly well matched subjects in which one group had experienced mild traumatic brain injury and the other group had not. The GNDS was superior to the HII in accurately identifying subjects and the HII was superior to any subtest of the HRNB in isolation, although the difference between the accuracy of the HII (.80) and the Category test (.72) was small. The GNDS was superior to the HII in discriminating among learning-disabled, head-injured, and normal subjects (Ostreicher & O'Donnell, 1995).

Effect of Age

The restricted age range of the normative group for the HRNB merits serious concern, especially because many cognitive functions are known to vary with age, and older individuals may be likely to receive neuropsychological evaluations. The subjects ranged from 14 to 50 years of age; the average age was 28.3. However, as noted by Lewinsohn (1973), Prigatano and Parsons (1976), and Bak and Greene (1980), performance on most of the subtests decreases with age. As a result, erroneous diagnostic conclusions may be reached with older adults (Ehrfurth & Lezak, 1982; Price, Fein, & Feinberg, 1979). In general, the research literature indicates that HRNB tests that are more complex measures of cognitive skills show stronger age effects than measures of specific motor or sensory skill (Fitzhugh, Fitzhugh, & Reitan, 1964; Golden & Schlutter, 1978; Reed & Reitan, 1963; Reitan, 1967). Older subjects tend to demonstrate greater deficits on tasks requiring immediate adaptive ability, and to perform better on tasks requiring use of stored information or previous experience. There are some age-related norms to address this problem. Pauker (1977), for example, supplied means and standard deviations for five age levels (for subjects between the ages of 19 and 76) for the seven commonly used HRNB scores and the Impairment Index using WAIS Full Scale IQ as a covariate. Harley et al. (1980) provided T-score conversions based on a sample of veterans for five age ranges from 55 to 79. Schludermann, Schludermann, Merryman, and Brown (1983) provided an excellent review of the neuro-psychological changes associated with aging using Halstead's data from older subjects.

Effect of Education

The patient's educational level can be a confounding variable in performance on the HRNB (Finlayson, Johnson, & Reitan, 1977). Well-educated subjects with neurological deficits may attain relatively high scores, whereas less educated, neurologically intact subjects may obtain low scores indicative of neurological impairment. Vega and Parsons (1967) reported that the Speech Sounds Perception Test and the Seashore Rhythm Test are most susceptible to this effect. Finlayson et al. (1977) reported that education is a confounding variable across all of the HRNB subtests.

Effect of Sex

Male–female differences have been reported on the HRNB. For example, in a study using a matched-subjects design for a sample of 47 nonneurological subjects and a sample of 47 neurological patients, Dodrill (1979) found that males obtained significantly higher scores on tasks containing a strong motor and/or spatial component (e.g., Finger Tapping; dynamometer; and Wechsler Memory Scale, Visual Reproduction). On the WAIS, females performed better on the Digit Symbol subtest, whereas males performed better on the Arithmetic, Picture Completion, and Block Design subtests. No significant differences were noted on the WAIS summary measures (Verbal IQ, Performance IQ, and Full Scale IQ). In their evaluation of the Finger Tapping Test, the Form Board, and the State–Trait Anxiety Test, King, Hannay, Masek, and Burns (1978) found a sex effect on the Finger Tapping Test: females performed slower. In females, trait anxiety was also found to be negatively correlated with finger tapping performance and to be positively correlated with the time used to complete the Form Board.

Reliability

Only a limited number of reliability studies have been reported that have assessed the HRNB in its entirety. The focus of the majority of this research has been test–retest reliability. Typically, research in this area has involved calculating the traditional psychometric index of reliability, that is, Pearson's coefficient of correlation (r).

Test–Retest

Investigators have generally reported significant correlations (Dodrill & Troupin, 1975; Klonoff, Fibiger, & Hutton, 1970; Matarazzo et al., 1974; Matarazzo, Matarazzo, Wiens, Gallo, & Klonoff, 1976) in studies assessing the test–retest reliability of the HRNB. Klonoff et al. (1970), for example, demonstrated test–retest correlations for the complete battery that ranged from .87 on Part B of the Trail Making Test to .59 on the Localization component of the TPT. The more complex measures on the HRNB are subject to statistically and clinically significant practice effects. Dodrill and Troupin (1975) reported that the Category Test; the Tactual Performance Test (TPT), Location; and the Impairment Index are most sensitive to practice effects. Dodrill and Troupin (1975) reported that a group of chronic epileptic patients showed a 10-point gain on the second administration of the Category Test. The mean score on the Category Test improved another 10 points for the epileptic subjects by the fourth testing. Significant improvement, as noted previously, was also noted on the Location score of the Tactual Performance Test. Overall score improvements lowered the average Impairment Index from .60 to .45 by the fourth administration.

In a test–retest study (20 weeks apart) of 29 healthy young males, Matarazzo et al. (1974) obtained results consistent with Dodrill and Troupin's findings (1975) regarding the Category Test and the TPT Location score. However, Matarazzo et al. (1974) interpreted the results of this study as supporting the reliability of the HRNB. In their discussion of this research, these authors made an important distinction between psychometric and clinical reliability. For example, whereas a Pearson test–retest coefficient of reliability of .08 (not significant) was obtained for the Halstead Impairment Index, perfect clinical reliability was demonstrated in terms of correctly classifying all 29 subjects as being "normal" on both test and retest. The results of this study were extended by the addition of a comparison group of 16 older subjects with cerebrovascular disease (Matarazzo et al., 1974), and later by the addition of a sample of 35 chronic schizophrenic patients and a sample of 15 organically brain injured patients who had undergone endarterectomy (Matarazzo et al., 1976). The subjects varied considerably across samples in terms of age, education, IQ, and intertest interval.

As noted previously, a high degree of clinical as well as psychometric reliability for most of the tests comprising the HRNB was reported by Matarazzo et al. (1976). The results of these studies were extended further by comparing the performance of a drug-free alcoholic sample ($n = 91$) with a nonalcoholic medical inpatient sample ($n = 20$) (Eckardt & Matarazzo, 1981). The drug-free alcoholic group had been evaluated within 7 days of their last drink, and again 17 days later. The nonalcoholic medical inpatient group was reported to be similar in terms of education, age, and socioeconomic characteristics. This group was reevaluated 2 to 3 weeks after the first administration. Both groups were judged to be stable neuropsychologically. Significant correlations between test–retest scores were obtained. An evaluation of the stability in the binary classification scheme (abnormal vs. normal), however, revealed less than desirable clinical reliability.

In the largest study of test–retest reliability of the HRNB, Dikmen, Heaton, Grant, and Temkin (1999) reported higher correlations for the composite measures (AIR—.92 and HII—.81) than for the individual tests (e.g., TPT Location—.60 and Seashore Rhythm—.70), although some of the tests had intermediate values (e.g., Category Test—.85 and Trails B—.89). This sample consisted of 384 control subjects from various studies tested twice across approximately 2-month to 15-month intervals. Because of the size of the sample, practice effects were statistically significant for all tests except the Seashore Rhythm test, although most practice effects are likely to be clinically insubstantial, for example, an average improvement of four seconds on Trails B. Temkin, Heaton, Grant, and Dikmen (1999) then used these data to examine the ability to detect change in single clinical subjects and found that the best method was a multiple regression model where the predictors included initial score on the test of interest, initial value for AIR, and age.

In evaluating the research literature as a whole, it would appear that mildly to moderately impaired persons with stable brain conditions are likely to have test–retest reliabilities that are different from those of normal or severely impaired subjects. The performance of normal subjects, for example, may be more subject to the relative ceiling effects of these test instruments. Severely impaired subjects would be expected to demonstrate a reduced capacity for new learning and therefore may not demonstrate significant practice effects. Conversely, patients with stabilized, mildly to moderately impaired brain functions may demonstrate changes in scores as a function of practice effects. Consistent with the research of Dikmen and her colleagues, clinicians should be sensitive to the initial level of performance when evaluating changes in test performance.

Internal Consistency

Aside from the test–retest studies discussed previously, other measures of the reliability of the HRNB as a whole are lacking. A slightly greater number of studies have been conducted to assess the internal consistency of the individual instruments. Shaw (1966) reported a split-half reliability on the Category Test of .98, while Bornstein (1983b) has reported split-half reliability coefficients of .74 and .77 for two different combinations of items from the Seashore Rhythm Test. Moses (1985a) reported internal consistency values (coefficient alpha) of .61 for the Speech Sounds Perception Test, .96 for the Category Test, and .76 for the Seashore Rhythm Test. In addition, Moses (1985a) reported a coefficient alpha value of .95 for the short form of the Category Test involving only the first four subtests (Caslyn, O'Leary, & Chaney, 1980). Charter, Adkins, Alekoumbides, and Seacat (1987) presented internal consistency reliabilities values for the HRNB tests and summary indices using the split-half method and using coefficient alpha in a mixed sample of 300 individuals with and without cognitive impairment. These values ranged from .51 for the TPT Memory score to .95 for Trail Making A (using alternate forms). Charter and Webster (1997) reported that the three subtests of the Speech Sounds Perception Test have low reliabilities, whereas the total test has an adequate internal consistency coefficient of .78.

Because many of the scoring procedures of the HRNB are relatively objective, there have been few interscorer reliability studies reported. The TPT does contain some element of judgment and subjectivity in scoring the drawings of patients for memory and localization. Charter, Walden, and Hoffman (1998) reported .98 interscorer reliability for the Memory score and .98 for the Localization score of the TPT.

Validity

A contrasted groups design has been used in the development of many of the tests comprising the HRNB. No major studies have addressed the issue of content validity per se.

Validational research has traditionally focused on discriminative validity. There are some studies that provide evidence of the concurrent validity of the HRNB, even though the original focus of these studies was more typically concerned with the comparative effectiveness of different neuropsychological instruments and their ability to differentiate between different neuropsychological conditions. Predictive validity studies have not been a major focus of neuropsychological research except in attempts to relate performance on neuropsychological tests to future adaptive functioning (e.g., McSweeny, Grant, Heaton, Prigatano, & Adams, 1985). Traditionally, neuropsychological testing has been used primarily to describe a patient's relative strengths and weaknesses, relating patterns of the patient's neuropsychological deficits to either known neuropathological disease processes or concomitant behavioral manifestations. Also, few incremental and factorial studies have been performed. The studies that have addressed the issue of incremental validity (Goldstein & Shelly, 1984) have been the result of research focused on the discriminative ability of the HRNB versus another neuropsychological procedure.

Concurrent Validity

Attempts have been made to establish the validity of the HRNB by correlating test findings with certain neuropathological conditions associated with cerebral dysfunction. For example, Matthews and Booker (1972) demonstrated that a relationship exists between the size of the ventricles and performance on neuropsychological tests. This relationship became evident, however, only when the extremes of the distribution (subjects with the largest ventricles and subjects with the smallest ventricles) were compared. In this study, 15 cases with the largest right- over left-ventricle measurement ratios and 15 cases with the largest left- over right-ventricle measurement ratios were compared. A statistically insignificant relationship was found between ventricular dilation and lateralized neuropsychological deficits.

Klove (1959, 1963) has attempted to demonstrate the unique contribution that neuropsychology—and more specifically, the HRNB—has made to the neurodiagnostic process. For example, Klove (1959) demonstrated that this battery is sensitive to behavioral deficits related to impaired brain functions in brain-damaged patients who have either a normal or an abnormal EEG, and that patients with severely abnormal EEGs tend to be more neuropsychologically impaired than patients with normal EEGs. Finally, Klove (1963) demonstrated that brain-damaged patients may be correctly identified on the HRNB independent of the patients' performance on neurological examination.

Filskov and Goldstein (1974) evaluated the diagnostic validity of the HRNB in comparison to such medical procedures as the brain scan, cerebral blood flow studies, the EEG, the angiogram, the pneumoencephalogram, and the X-ray study. These procedures were compared in terms of their hit rates for a sample of 89 patients with confirmed diagnoses of seizure disorder, neoplasms, degenerative neurological disease, subdural hematoma, cerebrovascular accident, specific cerebrovascular disease, and arteriosclerotic cerebrovascular disease. Overall, the HRNB was found to be superior to these medical procedures in terms of the identification, lateralization, and determination of the neuropathological process (100%, 89%, and 85% correct, respectively).

In a somewhat different approach, Swiercinsky and Leigh (1979) used CT scans as the criterion for determining the presence or absence of neurological impairment, as well as the lateralization of the deficit, in a sample of 62 patients. Clinical decisions based on the results of neuropsychological testing (essentially the HRNB) were found to agree with the criterion measure more often than did conclusions based on electroencephalographic results, routine neurological examination, or the results of the Russell et al. (1970) neuropsychological keys.

Discriminative Validity

The HRNB is effective in discriminating a variety of neurological conditions (Klove, 1974; Wheeler, Burke, & Reitan, 1963). There is a significant amount of variability in the reported effectiveness of this battery in diagnosing the presence, the lateralization, and the localization of brain dysfunction. Wheeler et al. (1963), for example, reported an average lateralization classification rate of 93.56%, whereas Swiercinsky and Warnock (1977) reported lateralization classification rates of only 42.7% when the Russell et al. (1970) neuropsychological keys were used, 51.9% when key variables in a discriminant function were used, and only 56.9% when a maximum set of variables in a discriminant function were used.

An initial validation of the test procedures comprising the Halstead battery was reported by Reitan in 1955. This study presented a cross-validation of Halstead's work. An excellent early review of the validity of the HRNB can be found in Halgrim Klove's "Validation Studies in Adult Clinical Neuropsychology" (1974). The tests comprising the HRNB have generally been found to be sensitive to the effects of neurological dysfunction. In a study using 50 pairs of subjects (brain-damaged and non-brain-damaged), Reitan (1955c) found, with the exception of two measures based on the critical-flicker-fusion test, significant differences between the two groups on all instruments. Comparable results were reported by Vega and Parsons (1967) in their cross-validation study. Support for the statistical and clinical validity and utility of these procedures has also been reported by other researchers in a variety of geographical and neuropsychological settings (Chapman & Wolff, 1959; Goldstein, Deysach, & Kleinknecht, 1973; Klonoff et al., 1970; Klove, 1974; Matthews, Shaw, & Klove, 1966; Schreiber, Goldman, Kleinman, Goldfader, & Snow, 1976; Vega & Parsons, 1967).

Using a discriminant function technique, Wheeler et al. (1963) reported prediction rates ranging from 90.7% to 98.8% correct for a group of 140 subjects assigned to groups with: (1) no cerebral damage; (2) left cerebral damage; (3) right cerebral damage; and (4) diffuse cerebral damage. The subjects were assigned to these groups based on "independent neurological criterion information." Wheeler and Reitan (1963) attempted to cross-validate these results by using the discriminative weights derived in the aforementioned study in an evaluation of a sample of 304 subjects. A 10% to 20% reduction in accuracy was obtained for all comparisons, except for the right-damage versus the bilateral-damage groups, where the discrimination was essentially no better than chance. These results may be attributable, in part, to the fact that the neurological evidence used for group inclusion was not as distinct in the cross-validation study.

The diagnostic accuracy of the HRNB is partly function of the disease process being assessed and the area of the cortex involved. Reitan (1955c) and Klove (1974), for example, have shown that different performance patterns exist in patients with left- and right-hemisphere lesions where the sensory examination contributes significantly to the discriminatory power of the HRNB. Wheeler and Reitan (1963) and Schreiber et al. (1976), for example, have reported that, without the sensory examination, right–left hemisphere differences are not identified with sufficient consistency to warrant basing clinical decisions regarding lesion localization on the HRNB test scores alone. Goldstein and Shelly (1973) found that the presence of suppressions (i.e., extinction and unilateral inattention) is the single best discriminator of left- and right-hemisphere lesions. Lateralized motor and tactile recognition dysfunctions are fairly accurate lateralization indicators.

To summarize, there is evidence that the HRNB can predict, to a high degree, right- versus left-hemispheric involvement (Reitan, 1955b, 1966); focal diffuse or bilateral focal damage (Reitan, 1959); lobular localization (Reitan, 1966); static versus rapidly growing lesions (Fitzhugh, Fitzhugh, & Reitan, 1961); and the disease process, including cerebro- vascular disease, neoplasm, trauma, or degenerative disease (Reitan, 1966). In general, the diagnostic accuracy would appear to be greatest in cases involving primary and secondary functional systems (Parsons, 1970).

Differentiation between Psychiatric and Neurological Presentations

Watson, Thomas, Anderson, and Felling (1968) attempted to differentiate patients diagnosed as schizophrenic from those diagnosed as "organics" by (1) assessing the statistical differences in the performance of these two groups versus (2) a "clinical" evaluation of the test data, but neither method succeeded in differentiating the two groups. Klove (1974) criticized this study for failing to provide appropriate evaluations before classifying a subject as "organic" or schizophrenic. The confounding influence of medica- tion effects and prior electroconvulsive treatment (ECT) treatments also limits the conclu- sions that we can draw from this study.

Lacks, Colbert, Harrow, and Levine (1970), in a study of 64 male patients (predomi- nantly veterans), found the Bender–Gestalt to provide greater predictive accuracy in differentiating between organic and nonorganic patients (schizophrenics and general medi- cal patients) than did the Halstead–Reitan. Unfortunately, the authors did not separate the hit rates for the two groups composing the nonorganic group. Similarly, it does not appear that any medical or testing evaluations were conducted to rule out the existence of neurological deficits in the schizophrenic group. This is especially important given the chronicity of the schizophrenic group (their mean length of hospitalization was 36.7 months). Finally, from the brief description of Lacks et al. (1970), it would appear that the organic group was comprised primarily of individuals who presented with diffuse brain damage (e.g., encephalitis or Pick's disease) and whose clinical presentation most likely had a psychiatric overlay.

In contrast to the above research, Golden (1977), in a study using a mixed psychiatric and brain-injured sample of 116 patients, found the HRNB 90% effective in identification and localization, according to a discriminant function analysis. These results are generally consistent with reports from Watson, Thomas, Felling, and Andersen (1969); Klonoff et al. (1970); Barnes and Lucas (1974); and Malec (1978).

The research literature indicates that the predictive accuracy of making a differential diagnosis of "organic" versus "schizophrenic" is contingent on whether chronic or acute populations are evaluated. Neuropsychological instruments in general have been found to be more accurate in differentiating acutely psychotic patients from neurologically impaired subjects than for comparison with normal subjects. For example, Wheeler et al. (1963) found the Category Test to be the HRNB test most sensitive to the presence of brain dysfunction, with a hit rate of nearly 90% in differentiating brain-injured and normal subjects. However, even after raising the cutoff point for the Category Test from 51 to 64 errors, Golden (1978a) was able to obtain only a 70% hit rate when using an acute schizophrenic control group.

In addition to chronicity, several other variables may account for the results obtained in the study of psychiatric and neurologically impaired subjects. The selection of the tests from the HRNB was not consistent across studies. Different base rates for different disorders may exist from study to study. Similarly, medication effects were rarely controlled. Finally, the process of patient selection and the method of test analysis may create a confounding variable.

Pseudoneurological Studies

Matthews et al. (1966) compared the performance of 32 patients with unequivocal evidence of brain damage with that of 32 patients who presented symptoms strongly suggestive of organic brain damage (e.g., headache, nausea, paresthesia, motor weakness, and gait disturbance), but whose neurological and medical examinations were negative. The subjects were matched for age, sex, and years of education. Even though the groups were deliberately composed to attenuate rather than to maximize differences in performance, a number of significant differences were found by the authors. It would have been further interesting to have as a comparison group individuals who did not have any signs or symptoms to see if the pseudoneurological patients scored in the intermediate range.

Detection of Malingering

Goebel (1983) obtained a hit rate of 94.4% in the blind interpretation of neuropsychological test data from a sample of neurologically impaired patients ($n = 46$) and a group of nonimpaired subjects who were instructed to fake brain damage ($n = 149$). Heaton, Smith, Lehman, and Vogt (1978) correctly classified 100% of a sample of 16 volunteer malingerers from a group of 16 head trauma patients via a discriminant function. The diagnostic accuracies of 10 neuropsychologists who interpreted the test data blind, however, ranged from chance-level prediction to about 20% better than chance. Overall, these results indicate that the HRNB is sensitive to the effects of faking brain damage. The issue of malingered performance or less than optimal effort has received much scrutiny recently and is detailed in another chapter. However, a few comments relevant to the HRNB are appropriate here. Reitan and Wolfson (1995c) have suggested an index related to the consistency of performance across time. A subsequent examination of this index indicated that there was no overlap between the distribution of scores obtained by individuals involved in litigation versus individuals not involved in litigation (Reitan & Wolfson, 1996a). Unfortunately, the index requires that the entire HRNB be administered at least twice.

Heaton et al. (1978) had developed a discriminant function to separate malingerers from truly impaired subjects, but the subject-to-predictor ratio was inadequate, resulting in an unstable solution. Mittenberg, Rotholc, Russell, & Heilbronner (1996) used the same method to derive a discriminant function on a larger sample and then cross-validated it on published data sets with 84% true positives and 94% true negatives. McKinzey and Russell (1997a) found a 23% false-positive rate in a sample of 796 subjects administered the HRNB for reasons other than forensic referral where no litigation was involved.

Because there may be dissociation among the effects of poor effort on different tests, it is important to develop indices of poor effort on the tests themselves as well as using tests specifically designed to evaluate level of effort. The HRNB has been examined in this manner. Two indices of consistency across time have been reported. The Retest Consistency Index (Reitan & Wolfson, 1997) examines scores on the Comprehension, Picture Arrangement, and Digit Symbol subtests of the WAIS or WAIS-R as well as the Category Test, Trail Making Test B, and the Localization scores of the TPT. The Response Consistency Index (Reitan & Wolfson, 1995c) examines responses to individual items on the Information, Comprehension, Arithmetic, Similarities, and Vocabulary subtests of the WAIS or WAIS-R across two different test administrations. These two indices can be combined into a Dissimulation Index. A limitation of this method includes the fact that it appears that all three indices (Retest Consistency, Response Consistency, and Dissimulation Index) were developed using the same sample of subjects. In addition, the method used in the research differentiated between people involved in litigation and people not involved in litigation. The critical question is the identification of malingered effort, and the indices need to be examined in the context of known malingerers or analog malingerers. Reitan and Wolfson (1996b) report no overlap in the distribution of scores on the Dissimulation Index between a group of 20 subjects with head injury not involved in litigation and 20 subjects with head injury involved in litigation. The method requires serial evaluations separated by several months, limiting the practical utility.

Trueblood and Schmidt (1993) developed a key system for the detection of malingering in HRNB. There are seven signs or cutoff scores for various indices of the HRNB. When two or more of the cutoffs are exceeded, then malingering is suspected. In an attempt to cross-validate this system, there was a false-positive rate of 32% (McKinzey & Russell, 1997b).

The Halstead Category test may lend itself to the detection of malingered effort. Two strategies are to either examine for less than chance performance or to examine the protocol for subjects who miss easy items while passing more difficult items. Tenhula and Sweet (1996) examined and cross-validated these two strategies using the Booklet Category Test in separate samples of neurologically impaired and normal subjects. Because the strategies were equivalently effective, the authors combined the two strategies into a single decision rule that will now need to be cross-validated.

Statistical and Actuarial Models

Several studies have been conducted to assess automated interpretations of the HRNB as opposed to clinical interpretation. Heaton, Grant, Anthony, and Lehman (1981) compared interpretations by two relatively experienced clinicians with those generated by the Key Approach (Russell et al., 1970) for accuracy of classification along the dimensions of presence, chronicity, and laterality of brain damage. Although the ratings of severity were highly correlated ($r = .95$), the clinicians made significantly more accurate classifications of both the presence and the laterality of brain damage. Neither the Key Approach nor the clinicians were able to predict chronicity better than base rate.

Anthony, Heaton, and Lehman (1980) investigated the diagnostic effectiveness of automated interpretations by comparing the Key Approach (Russell et al., 1970) and a Fortran IV program called BRAIN 1, which was devised to simulate clinical inference. The prediction rates for both programs surpassed chance levels but were lower than had been predicted by their authors. Both programs failed to provide clinically useful predictions of localization or recency of damage. Goldstein and Shelly (1982) and Adams, Kvale, and Keegan (1984) also reported significant shrinkage in accuracy rates for cross-validation efforts using the Key Approach. The Key Approach may not be applicable in all settings. Goldstein et al. (1996) suggested that the Key may be most applicable among stroke patients in instances of recent thrombotic/hemorrhagic stroke. Of course, this represents limits in terms of the overall generalizability of the approach.

Moses et al. (1996) have developed a set of modal profiles of the HRNB in a sample of 678 patients. These researchers used the Q-sort metholodgy and principal-components analysis to determine clusters of similar profiles. The solution contained 18 modal profiles of which 12 could be replicated in patients with differing diagnoses. The next step would be to explicate the psychometric characteristics of these clusters and to identify external correlates to determine the clinical utility of assigning individual patients to one of the clusters based on maximum similarity.

Concurrent-Discriminative Studies

Several reported studies have compared the discriminative validity of the HRNB to that of the Luria–Nebraska Neuropsychological Battery (LNNB). Kane, Sweet, Golden, Parsons, and Moses (1981) compared the differences in accuracy of these two batteries in discriminating a heterogeneous group of neurological patients ($n = 23$) from a mixed group of psychiatric patients ($n = 22$). Two expert clinical neuropsychologists were used as raters in the study, one of whom administered the HRNB, and one of whom administered the LNNB. The results of this study revealed a nonsignificant tendency for the HRNB rater to correctly identify a higher percentage of the psychiatric patients (86% vs. 77%). The LNNB rater identified a greater percentage of the brain-damaged patients (87% vs. 70%). This latter difference was reported as being statistically significant. Overall hit rates of 78% and 82% were obtained for the Halstead–Reitan and the LNNB, respectively. The two raters were found to agree with each other's classifications in 82% of the cases.

Similar results were reported by Golden et al. (1981b), in which a discriminant analysis found the HRNB and the LNNB equally effective in identifying brain damage, with hit rates over 85%. In this study, 30 patients diagnosed as schizophrenic, 48 as brain-damaged, and 30 as normal were used. No significant differences in age or education existed in the three groups. The patients diagnosed as schizophrenic had been evaluated with a CT scan to rule out the existence of structural changes indicative of organicity. The brain-damaged patients had confirmed evidence of organicity as evidenced by CT scan, angiogram, EEG, or history of a coma of at least 24 hours' duration following head trauma. The HRNB yielded a hit rate of 90% in the neurological group and 84% in the control group; the overall hit rate was 86%. The LNNB classified 87% of the neurological patients and 88% of the controls; the overall hit rate was 88%. Complete agreement between the batteries was obtained in 89% of the cases. Hit rates for the schizophrenic patients were similar for both batteries (23/30 for the HRNB and 24/30 for the LNNB). Using a combination of all 14

LNNB scales through multiple regression analysis, Golden et al. attempted to predict 14 Halstead variables. Predictions of the LNNB scale scores were made by the HRNB in a similar manner. The multiple R values for the Halstead tests ranged from .71 to .96. The multiple R values for the LNNB scores ranged from .77 to .94.

These results also support the concurrent validity of these instruments. For an excellent overview of the HRNB, as well as a discussion of the relationship between this instrument and the LNNB, see Incagnoli, Goldstein, and Golden (1986). Diamant (1981) also reported that the HRNB and Luria's Neuropsychological Investigation (LNI) (see Christensen, 1979) generated comparable conclusions concerning the presence of brain dysfunction, its lateralization, and its localization in a sample of 31 psychiatric inpatients suspected of having brain dysfunction.

Sherer, Scott, Parsons, and Adams (1994) reported that although the HRNB was able to discriminate between brain-damaged subjects and normal controls matched for age and education, it was not incrementally better than the use of the WAIS-R IQ and subtest scores. Furthermore, when subjects were matched for IQ, the differences between the two groups disappeared. The effect of brain impairment on HRNB scores is most probably not independent of its effects on IQ, despite Ward Halstead's criticisms of Wechsler IQ as being largely social and the proposal that the HRNB tests reflect biological intelligence.

The high correlations reported between various neuropsychological measures such as the HRNB and the LNNB have been attributed to the confounding effects of intelligence, and when one partials out the effect of intelligence, these correlations are substantially reduced (Chelune, 1982). Golden, Gustavson, and Ariel's response (1982c) to this criticism emphasizes the importance of partialing out the effects of education when interpreting neuropsychological test data (as a control for premorbid level of functioning) but argues against the partialing out of postmorbid intelligence, as postmorbid measures of intelligence may reflect the effects of brain damage (the very thing that neuropsychological batteries attempt to assess).

In their reviews of the literature on the HRNB, Parsons and Prigatano (1978) and Hevern (1980) concluded that at least five variables may moderate the outcomes of past validational studies: the age of the subjects, possible different educational levels, gender performance differences, different levels of socioeconomic status, and inexperienced or poorly trained examiners. An additional moderator variable that should be considered in this area of research is the criteria used to define brain dysfunction (e.g., the use of different medical testing procedures such as the CT scan, EEG tracings, studies of regional cerebral blood flow, and physical neurological findings).

Klesges, Fisher, Pheley, Boschee, and Vasey (1984), in a study that addresses many of these methodological shortcomings, conducted a validational study of the HRNB with a sample of 224 subjects (83 normal and 141 brain-damaged) who did not differ in age, education, sex, and socioeconomic status. All the subjects were assessed by trained examiners. Brain damage was determined by a CT scan evaluation that was read independently by both a radiologist and a neurologist and by at least one additional diagnostic evaluation (i.e., a pneumoencephalogram, an angiogram, or an EEG). Both procedures had to agree on the presence, absence, and site of the dysfunction. The brain-damaged sample was evaluated approximately 9 months after injury (median = 9.18; SD = 80.9) and consisted of subjects with heterogeneous injuries: occlusions ($n = 26$), tumors ($n = 22$), hematomas ($n = 18$), contusions ($n = 16$), and aneurysms ($n = 12$). In this study, an overall correct classification rate of 64% was achieved (67% of all normals and 62% of all brain-damaged subjects). These results are disappointing because the base rate for brain damage in this study was 63% (141 of 224 subjects). The most correctly classified group was left-hemisphere-damaged subjects (71%), whereas subjects with diffuse damage were classified correctly 33% of the time. When those subjects with diffuse brain damage were excluded from the statistical analyses, the overall correct classification rate increased to 66%. The authors noted that, when only left- versus right-hemisphere cases were compared (as in other reported validational studies—e.g., Wheeler et al., 1963), the classification rate improved to 81%. In terms of localization, 60% of left anterior injuries, 65% of right anterior injuries, 50% of posterior left injuries, and 37% of posterior right injuries were correctly classified via a discriminant function. The overall correct classification rate for this sample was 55%. When normals were excluded from the analysis, correct classification improved to 71%. The HRNB may have greater positive than negative predictive value.

It should be noted that, in the Klesges et al. (1984) study, the classification rates for lateralization and localization noted earlier were significantly lower than those reported in other published studies on the HRNB (Boll, 1981). However, as illustrated earlier, with the exclusion of certain groups (i.e., normals and those subjects with diffuse brain damage), the classification rates compared favorably with those in other studies of the HRNB. The marginal rate of discrimination between neurologically impaired and normal subjects deserves additional comment. One hypothesis proposed by Klesges et al. (1984) for this finding was related to the fact that the "normal" group used in this study consisted of subjects who had initially been referred for testing because they were suspected of having "some type of problem." When a similar group of normal subjects was evaluated by Swiercinsky and Warnock (1977), disappointing discrimination rates were obtained. However, in contrast, Matthews et al. (1966) reported that "pseudoneurological" subjects were successfully discriminated from subjects with definitive brain damage. A more plausible explanation for the results noted in the Klesges et al. (1984) study may have to do with the sensitivity of neuropsychological test procedures, such as the HRNB, and their ability to assess subtle changes in brain function following an insult or a disease process. Neurodiagnostic medical procedures such as the CT scan may prove to be inadequate as criterion measures in this area of research. Future research would fruitfully investigate whether the more advanced neurodiagnostic techniques such as positron emission tomography (PET), Spect or magnetic resonance imaging (MRI) and fMRI might provide a greater agreement with the HRNB.

Factor-Analytic Studies

Halstead proposed his concept of "biological intelligence" based on a factor analysis of 13 tests developed in Halstead's laboratory. Halstead (1947) summarized his four-factor theory of biological intelligence as follows:

1. A central integrative field factor C. This factor represents the organized experience of the individual. It is the ground function of the "familiar" in which the psychologically "new" is tested and incorporated. It is the region of coalescence of learning and adaptive intelligence. Some of its parameters are probably reflected in measurements of psychometric intelligence, which yield an intelligence quotient.

2. An abstraction factor A. This factor concerns basic capacity to group to a criterion as in the elaboration of categories and involves the comprehension of the central similarities and differences. It is the fundamental growth principle of the ego.

3. A power factor P. This factor reflects the undistorted power factor of the brain. It operates to counterbalance or regulate the affective forces and thus frees the growth principle of the ego for further ego differentiation.

4. A directional factor D. This factor constitutes the medium through which the process factors, noted here, are exteriorized in any given moment. On the motor side, it specifies the "final common pathway," while on the sensory side, it specifies the avenue or modality of experience.

Royce, Yeudall, and Bock (1976) performed a factor analysis of the data obtained from 176 patients with heterogeneous neurological impairment. Unfortunately (for our purposes), the results are clouded because the researchers included 21 other variables of cognitive test data along with the 15 Halstead–Reitan variables. Newby, Hallenbeck, and Embretson (1983) performed a confirmatory factor analysis on data from 497 subjects. The variables were a modified HRNB. The confirmatory factor analysis sought to determine which of four models provided the best fit with the data. The four models included Royce's model of the structure of intellect (eight first-order factors and three second-order factors), Swiercinsky's model of nine factors, Lezak's model of a two-factor (verbal and nonverbal) structure, and Luria's model of 10 intercorrelated factors. None of the models fit the data adequately, although three of the models provided a fit somewhat better than chance.

Fowler, Richards, Berent, and Boll (1987) factor analyzed the subtests of the HRNB as a way of data reduction in investigating the relationship of lateralized EEG results and neuropsychological test results in 108 epileptic subjects. The five factors identified in that analysis were interpreted as Verbal Comprehension, Perceptual Organization, Selective Attention, Motor Skills, and Abstract Reasoning from variables that included WAIS subtest scores. This factor structure was essentially replicated in a sample of general neuropsychiatric patients (Fowler, Zillmer, & Newman, 1988). We are still in need of a major factor-analytic study of the HRNB.

Individual Subtests

Some of the subtests from the HRNB have been used individually or in conjunction with other tests. Perhaps the Category Test and the Trail Making Test are the subtests most frequently used in this manner. The Category Test and Trail Making Test B (TMT-B), in particular, are frequently hypothesized to be indices of frontal lobe functions. However, although frontal impairment may result in deficits specifically on these two tests, the tests are probably also sensitive to cortical impairment of other locations, and poor performance on either test should not be interpreted as reflecting frontal impairment without a more general consideration of other test scores. Reitan and Wolfson (1995d) report that although a group of frontal lobe patients performed poorly on the TMT-B and the Category Test, there were no significant differences found in a group of frontal lesion patients and a group of nonfrontal lesion patients when the two groups were matched for age, education, and type of lesion (intrinsic vs. extrinsic tumors, vascular disease, traumatic injury). Similarly, Anderson, Bigler, and Blatter (1995) reported no association between volume of frontal lobe lesion and score on either the Category Test or TMT-B in a sample of closed head injury patients. Lorig, Gehring, and Hyrn (1986) reported that performance on the TMT is associated with activation of multiple brain areas as measured by EEG in normal subjects.

Performance on the TMT-B may partly reflect cultural variables. Manly et al. (1998) reported poorer performance on TMT-B with use of black English among African-American healthy and intact individuals. Taylor (1998) administered the TMT in typical and reversed order to a group of 50 consecutive patients. He found that the order of administration resulted in a somewhat higher ratio of TMT-B/TMT-A, but this difference did not seem to affect clinical utility, indicating that the TMT-B may be used in isolation. Further research is needed to evaluate whether the diagnostic accuracy is changed when only TMT-B is administered. LoSasso, Rapport, Axelrod, and Reeder (1998) reported that clinical implications of scores on the TMT are basically unchanged regardless of whether the preferred or nonpreferred hand is used.

The TMT requires a short amount of time to administer and is an accurate index of brain impairment. The TMT administered to head injury patients at the time of emergence from posttraumatic amnesia predicted psychosocial outcome at 1 year post-injury whether outcome was measured by self-report (Millis, Rosenthal, & Lourie, 1994) or by the report of significant others (Ross, Millis, & Rosenthal, 1997). Performance on the TMT also appears to be related to driving skill in individuals who have experienced closed head injury (Schmidt, Brouwer, Vanier, & Kemp, 1996). There are multiple sets of "normative" information regarding the TMT. Soukup, Ingram, Grady, and Scheiss (1998) have combined these data into three sets of norms based on age of the subject.

The construct validity of the TMT is in need of greater explication. Its utility as a screening procedure is probably related to the complex set of skills required for successful performance. Apart from organic etiologies, TMT-B appears to be sensitive to depression (Veiel, 1997a). In addition, an important component skill may be cognitive speed, at least in relation to head injury patients (Spikman, van Zomeron, & Deelman, 1996). Although the TMT is usually thought to be very sensitive to neurological impairment, at least one study (Cicerone, 1997) did not find a difference between individuals who had received mild closed head injuries and control subjects. On the other hand, TMT-B is correlated with arterial oxygen pressure and arterial carbon dioxide pressure in subjects with chronic obstructive pulmonary disease (Stuss, Peterkin, Guzman, Guzman, & Troyer, 1997).

The TMT is frequently used as a screening device for impairment and has great utility for the assessment of the elderly. The significant age effects make it necessary to have different cutoffs for different age groups. Rasmusson, Zonderman, Kawas, and Resnick (1998) found that TMT-B but not -A showed significant slowing in a group ($n = 385$) of normal elderly tested over a 2-year interval, especially for subjects in their 80s and 90s. For the entire group a cutoff of 172 seconds for TMT-B showed the best combination of sensitivity and specificity.

The TMT is so frequently used that repeat evaluations in the same patient are likely. As a result alternate forms, called TMT-C and TMT-D have been proposed (desRosiers & Kavanaugh, 1987). It appears that the alternate forms of A and B have similar classification and score patterns (Franzen, Paul, & Iverson, 1996) as well as similar relationships to other frequently used neuropsychological tests in factor analytic designs (McCracken & Franzen, 1992). LoSasso et al. (1998) found that TMT-D is slightly more difficult than TMT-B, but that this difference is not clinically meaningful when TMT-D is used in a retest situation rather than being administered first. Yet another alternate form of the TMT is available for individuals with visual or motor impairment. The ratio of scores on the Oral Trail Making Test (Ricker & Axelrod, 1994) to scores on the original version does not differ as a function of age, motor speed, or score on TMT-B (Abraham, Axelrod, & Ricker, 1996). Yet another form of the TMT is actually an extension with Forms X and Y. In Form X, the subject is asked to connect clocks in ascending order of time portrayed, and in Form Y, the subject is to connect dots in increasing order of size. Davis, Adams, Gates, and Cheramie (1989) report that Forms X and Y can successfully discriminate learning disabled and normal children. Forms X and Y correlate with Forms A and B and discriminate between normal and brain-damaged subjects as defined by at least two neurodiagnostic tests (Stanczak, Lynch, McNeil, & Brown, 1998).

Performance on the TMT does not appear to be affected by anxiety level, at least not in normal control subjects (Waldstein, Ryan, Jennings, Muldoon, & Manuck, 1997). It is necessary to examine this potential relationship both in a sample of individuals with anxiety disorders and in individuals with neurobehavioral disorders who experience anxiety because clinical anxiety can be very different phenomena from self-reported levels of non-clinical anxiety.

The Category Test has been used in examinations of the cognitive characteristics of schizophrenic patients (Goldstein & Shemansky, 1997), substance abuse patients (Peters, Lewis, Dustman, Straight, & Beck, 1976), and individuals with a propensity for psychotic symptoms (Porch, Ross, & Whitman, 1995). Choca, Laatsch, Wetzel, and Agresti (1997) suggested that high error scores on the Category Test are more easily interpreted than low error scores.

Multiple short forms are available for the Category Test (Caslyn et al., 1980; Charter, Swift, & Blusewicz, 1997; Golden, Kuperman, MacInnes, & Moses, 1981; Gregory, Paul, & Morrison, 1979; Russell & Levy, 1987; Wetzel & Boll, 1987; Wood, & Strider, 1980). It should be noted that only the Wetzel and Boll (1987) and the Charter et al. (1997) short forms have normative information specifically derived from the use of their respective forms. Because the relationship between these short forms and the original form of the Category Test is generally correlational, interpretation of the short forms should be more conservative than that of the long form. In addition, with exception of the short form developed by Labreche (1983), which was cross-validated by Kozel and Meyers (1998), and the short form developed by Caslyn et al. (1980), which was cross-validated by Golden et al. (1980), few of these short forms have been investigated in subjects other than the original derivation samples.

The Category Test is also available in a booklet form (DeFillipis, McCampbell, & Rogers, 1979) and a computerized form (DeFillipis, 1992). One study indicated that the original form, the booklet form, and a computerized form were all equivalent in their ability to differentiate neurologically impaired individuals from control subjects (Mercer, Harrell, Miller, Childs, and Rockers, 1997). Choca et al. (1997) suggested that high scores are more easily interpreted than are low or moderate scores on the Category Test. This is probably true of most neuropsychological tests, especially the component tests of the HRNB. Clinical neuropsychology has concerned itself with the identification of pathology and not with the measurement of superior or normal performance.

The Finger Tapping Test correlates with cerebellar size (approximately .21 correlation) when corrections for overall brain size are made (Paradiso, Andreason, O'Leary,

Arndt, & Robinson, 1997). This correlation was not observed for size of the temporal lobe, suggesting specificity in the relationship of this test to brain structures.

A short form of the Speech Sounds Perception test has been proposed (Crockett, Clark, Labreche, Lacoste, & Klonoff, 1982) in which only the first 30 items are used. Moses (1985a) reported an internal consistency reliability of .80 for this short form compared to .92 for the long form. Charter and Dobbs (1998) provided age and education corrections and a regression formula to transform short test scores into long form scores.

Adult HRNB—Summary

There is considerable disagreement in the literature about which tests in the HRNB are the best predictors of cerebral dysfunction. Klove (1963), for example, reported that the best predictors of brain damage were the Category Test, the TPT (Time, Memory, and Location), the Rhythm Test, the Speech Sounds Perception Test, and the Time Sense Test. Swiercinsky and Warnock (1977), however, found the Finger Tapping Test scores for the dominant and nondominant hands, TPT left-hand time, Trails A, and Tactile Dysfunction (hand and face) to be the best predictor variables. Although identification of the more sensitive test was not the purpose of Reitan and Wolfson (1996b), these researchers found that a general test of complex function (TPT Total Time) was more sensitive that was a specific test of simple function (Finger Tapping Test). The order effects of testing also need to be addressed. Further research in these areas is extremely important to retain the utility of the HRNB. A further serious problem is in the aging normative data base of the HRNB, which has been only partially ameliorated by the publication of the Heaton et al. (1991) norms, which have their limitations.

Children's Forms of the HRNB

The children's forms of the HRNB (Reitan, 1969; Reitan & Wolfson, 1992) have received less empirical scrutiny until relatively recently. The reliability appears to be adequate (Brown, Rourke, & Cicchetti, 1989) when measured across various intervals, with the mean value being a little over 2½ years. Byrd and Ingram (1988) reported a split-half reliability of .92 for the Intermediate Category Test (booklet form). Livingston, Gray, and Haak (1999) reported on the internal consistency reliability of certain subtests of the HRNB for Older Children by calculating coefficient alpha in a sample of 334 patients referred for evaluation. The Speech Sounds Perception Test had a reliability coefficient of .82, the Seashore Rhythm Test had a reliability coefficient of .69, and the Aphasia Screening Test had a coefficient of .81. Strom, Gray, Dean, and Fisher (1987) reported that the HRNB for Older Children accounts for a substantial increase over the WISC-R in predicted variability of WRAT-R scores. Livingston et al. (1997) have provided a typology based on modal profile analysis which is promising and in need of further validation.

Tramontana, Klee, and Boyd (1984) presented correlations of the HRNB for Older Children and the WISC-R in a sample of 39 psychiatric inpatients. The highest correlations with the HRNB tests were found with FSIQ, and the highest correlations with WISC-R variables were found with the sum of scaled scores for the HRNB subtests. None of the correlations exceeded .62, indicating that although there is shared variance, there is also unique variance such that the use of both procedures would not be redundant.

Livingston, Gray, Haak, and Jennings (1997) conducted a factor analysis of the HRNB for Children and concluded that a nine-factor solution best explained the structure. They provided methods for estimating factor scores in individuals and suggested that these factors may be helpful in interpretation. Although this suggestion is intriguing, further empirical work is needed before confident application of the factor scores to clinical work can be made.

The Children's HRNB is being increasingly used in published research reports, adding to the sparse information available previously. For example, Livingston, Mears, Marshall, Gray, and Haak (1996) reported that medicated and unmedicated children with ADHD scored similarly in terms of level of performance as well as pattern of performance on the age-appropriate version of the HRNB. Horton (1996) developed a shorter form of the children's Neuropsychological Deficit Scale for Older Children (Reitan & Wolfson, 1992) which he termed the Children's Alternative Impairment Index. Unfortunately, cross-validation resulted in only 50% correct classification. Development of a Short-Form Screening Index (Horton, 1998) resulted in somewhat better classification accuracy in a limited sample of 20 children, but this new index is in need of cross-validation in a larger sample. Performance on neuropsychological tests is affected by intellectual status, and the identification of impairment in subjects with above-average IQ may be limited. McIntosh, Dunham, Dean, and Kundert (1995) reported that only one child in a sample of 68 children with high IQ and learning disability obtained impaired scores on five or more subtests of the HRNB-C. However, the Tactual Performance Test-Memory score and Trail Making-B were most likely to show impairment in the same sample. In fact, one half of the children were impaired on the TPT-Memory, indicating different classification rules, involving only the most sensitive subtests may be useful in this population.

Of the component tests of the children's HRNB, perhaps the test most frequently used individually is the Category Test (Boll, 1993), which is actually a reduced item version of the Adult Category Test. Donders and Strom (1995) suggest profile analysis of the subtest performance on the Children's Category Test. This is an intriguing notion, but it is in need of cross-validation. Both the Children's Category Test and the California Verbal Learning Test-Children's Version were standardized on the same sample of 920 subjects. Donders (1998) calculated the standard error of difference between the Children's Category Test and the Total Correct score from the California Verbal Learning Test-Children's Version at each age level between 5 and 16 years. Using the standardization sample, he also calculated the abnormality of the scores. Although a difference of only about 9 points was required for a reliable difference, more than 50% of the standardization sample exhibited a difference that large, indicating the need for additional information before the reliable differences can be interpreted. A booklet form is available, just as there is a booklet form available for the Adult Category Test. Reeder and Boll (1992) offered a shortened form of the Category Test by comparing three possible versions. Donders (1996) cross-validated the optimal short form of the Children's Category Test in a sample of 87 children with closed head injury, and found that it discriminated between mild/moderate TBI and severe TBI subjects.

D'Elia and Satz (1989) developed a different form of the Trail Making Test for children. In this version, Part 1 consists of numbers embedded in pink circles for the odd numbers and yellow circles for the even numbers. The child is asked to connect the numbers in sequence. In Part 2, all of the numbers are duplicated in pink and yellow circles and the child is asked to connect the numbers in sequence, first the pink circles and then the yellow circles, alternating between the two colors. Color Trails correlates highly with the Children's Trail Making Test and discriminates between normal children and children with neurological impairment (Williams et al., 1995). The use of Color Trails may reduce the impact of language deficits on the assessment of general cortical functioning.

THE LURIA–NEBRASKA NEUROPSYCHOLOGICAL BATTERY

The Luria–Nebraska Neuropsychological Battery (LNNB) is an attempt to provide a comprehensive neuropsychological assessment technique that combines features of Alexandr Luria's neuropsychological theory of brain organization and function with the North American psychometric tradition. Administration of the LNNB can be learned in approximately 1 to 2 weeks. However, interpretation is extremely complex, relying on complicated notions of test theory as well as on an understanding of the neuropsychological theory of Alexandr Luria. Although the items in the LNNB are based on procedures used by Luria and published by Anne Lise-Christensen (1979), the LNNB should not be confused with Luria's Neuropsychological Investigation or with Lurian methodology.

The LNNB is divided into 11 subscales: Motor, Tactile, Rhythm, Visual Processes, Receptive Speech, Expressive Speech, Reading, Writing, Arithmetic, Memory, and Intellectual Processes. (Form II of the LNNB has 12 subscales, with the addition of an Intermediate Memory scale.) Consistent with Lurian theory, none of the items are presumed to measure only a single function. Therefore, in more recent versions of the test, the names of the scales have been dropped in favor of numbers. However, the items in Scale C1, for example (formerly the Motor scale), measure mainly motor functions.

Lurian theory specifies that observable behaviors are the result of combinations of molecular skills and that the successful performance of a behavior depends on cooperation among several brain areas. These brain areas are linked in a functional chain that eventuates in the behavior. Therefore, according to Lurian theory, there is no such thing as a pure point-to-point localization of molar skills as measured by overt tasks. Failure to perform a given task successfully can be the result of an impairment in any of the component molecular (nonobservable) skills that comprise the functional chain. By comparing performance across similar items that differ in their single-task requirements, we can isolate the dysfunctional unit.

Although the scale construction and item and scale score generation methods of the LNNB are developed from psychometric theory, the scales themselves are not traditional psychometric entities. The scale scores are more consistent with the behavioral tradition of assessment in which the scale score is not assumed to reflect a certain specified construct. In traditional psychometric theory, the usual presumptive theory of measurement is Representational (Michell, 1986), that is, the number resulting from use of the assessment system is assumed to reflect an underlying skill. Movements along the scale values are furthermore assumed to reflect differences in the skill level. In behavioral assessment theory, the theory is Operational. Here the measurement operation is assumed to produce a number that can be interpreted only in relation to other information, typically information regarding external relationships. Such is the case with the LNNB clinical scale scores, where an underlying construct is not assumed for each of the clinical scales. Although the early publication referred to the clinical scales by name (Motor, Memory, etc.), later editions used only the alphanumeric titles (C1, C2, etc.). High scores on the C1 scale are not automatically interpreted as reflecting motor impairment, although certainly that would be one hypothesis to evaluate. The clinical scales can be fruitfully conceptualized as indices of ability in broad classes of topographically related behaviors. For example, an elevated score on the C1 scale would suggest hypotheses related to some form of motor impairment such as slowness, dysmetria, or frontally based executive control deficits. On the other hand, certain of the empirically derived scales such as the factor analytic scales are consistent with the Representational theory of measurement. An elevated score here may be reflective of impairment in a specific cortical function such as tactile recognition.

From the prior discussion, it can be seen that the LNNB is a synthetic instrument. It is a blend between the European Behavioral Neurology tradition and the North American psychometric tradition. Its interpretation involves a blend of representational (item scores and factor analytic scores) and operational (clinical scales) theories. Furthermore, interpretation can be based on a sign approach (qualitative scores) and a multivariate approach (modal profiles, actuarial rules). It is a rich instrument with multiple levels of interpretation possible. Because of its similarity to behavioral assessment, it would seem that ecological validity would be enhanced, especially for more complex behaviors. There have been few studies to investigate this issue, but the findings have been encouraging. For example, McKay and Ramsey (1984) reported that sociometric data on patients in group therapy for alcohol-related problems was correlated with factor analytic scales from the LNNB for those factor scales that had a strong conceptual relationship to nonverbal aspects of communication. Heinrichs (1989) found that the LNNB provided statistically significant, if moderately sized, increases in prediction of employment status over demographic and medical data.

The LNNB material consists of several visual stimuli and a set of audiotaped rhythm and pitch stimuli. In addition, the examiner provides a few common items (a rubber band, a key, a nickel, a protractor, a rubber eraser, and a large paper clip) for use in the tactile and visual recognition items. The procedures are interactive: the examiner gives verbal instructions and then observes and, in some cases, times the responses of the subject. The test is portable and can be performed at the bedside. Forms I and II of the LNNB are intended to be used with subjects over the age of 15. The LNNB can be used with most levels of neuropsychological functioning, although the reliability of the test is attenuated in the normal range of ability. Because of ceiling effects, the accuracy of the LNNB is limited in the superior range of functioning.

Each item is given a score of 0, 1, or 2, where 0 corresponds to a normal performance, 1 corresponds to a borderline performance, and 2 corresponds to an impaired performance. The manual contains explicit rules for the assignment of item scores. The item scores are then summed to provide scale raw scores, which are translated to standardized T-scores with a mean of 50 and a standard deviation of 10 points. Besides the original 11 clinical scales, there are a Right and Left sensorimotor scale and a Pathognomonic scale. The Right and Left scales can be used to help lateralize the area of dysfunction. The Pathognomonic scale is composed of the items that best differentiated between neurological and psychiatric subjects. Recent work has developed two additional scales, which are comprised of items drawn from items on the original clinical scales (Sawicki & Golden, 1984b). These scales can provide useful information about the recency of the injury, the severity of the impairment, and the degree of the predictable compensation. Moses (1985b) subsequently presented data regarding the relationship of these two scales to neurological status.

All of the scales are presented as standardized T-scores with a mean of 50 and a standard deviation of 10. There are several steps in interpretation. The first step involves calculating the critical level, which is the score beyond which the obtained scores represent impaired performance (Golden, Hammeke, & Purisch, 1980b). The critical level is one standard deviation above the average scale score expected from a person with a given age and level of educational attainment. The critical level is determined by substituting values for age and education in a regression formula that was empirically derived. In this way, interpretation is more individualized than would be the case with absolute cutoff points. The critical level can be adjusted to reflect the amount of scatter in the scale scores. If there is more than a 30-point difference between the highest and the lowest scale score, the critical level can be lowered to 25 points above the lowest scale score (Moses, Golden, Ariel, & Gustavson, 1983a).

In addition, items can be summed to provide factor scale scores and localization scale scores, which are also standardized T-scores. The factor scales were derived from separate principal-components factor analyses for each of the clinical scales. The localization scales were empirically derived from an examination of those items that are able to discriminate groups of subjects with localizable deficits.

After the clinical scales are compared against the critical level, scatter among scale scores is examined. The localization scales are also examined against the critical level, as are the factor-analytic scales, although there are no rules regarding the interpretation of scatter on these two sets of scales. Next, performance on items across scales is examined to reveal whether any patterns consistent with neuropsychological theory exist. Last, the qualitative aspects of performance are examined. Although interpretation can be terminated at any level (and should be terminated early by inexperienced examiners), the battery gives the most amount of information and the most accurate information when the five interpretive steps are followed (Golden, Ariel, Wilkening, McKay, & MacInnes, 1982a). Other explications of interpretation can be found in Golden and Maruish (1986) and Moses (1997).

Goldstein, Shelly, McCue, and Kane (1987) reported that cluster analysis of the LNNB in subjects with left- or right-hemisphere damage, diffuse damage, or learning disability resulted in a normal mean profile cluster; a language impairment cluster; a nonverbal skill, memory, and intellectual impairment cluster; and a generalized impairment cluster. However, these clusters were not significantly related to external criteria of diagnosis. Katz and Goldstein (1993) found that although statistically significant differences exist between learning disabled adults and control subjects, the LNNB was unable to correctly classify individual cases.

Moses, Pritchard, and Faustman (1994) developed a set of 22 modal profiles. Seven of these profiles were associated with single criterion diagnoses in a cross-validation. In their system the scales scores were classified as low, medium, or high and the resulting system was therefore not dependent upon simple level of performance, but was instead related to actual configuration differences. Subsequent research indicated that modal profiles on the LNNB were related to modal profiles on the WAIS-R in a way that made conceptual sense; that is, sensorimotor profiles corresponded to Performance subtest profiles (Moses, Pritchard, & Adams, 1997). The basic rationale of modal profile analysis is that individuals with similar diagnoses will have profiles that are more similar to each other than they are to profiles of individuals with other diagnoses. Therefore, an individual's test profile can be interpreted by determining which modal profile his or her profile is most like. Notice this is not an average profile. It is not simply summing and finding the arithmetic mean for each scale. Modal profile analysis involves examination of the multivariate space defined by the relationship of scale to each other and not just the relationship to the Critical Level (CL). Identifying the modal profile most similar to the obtained profile will help inform decisions regarding differential diagnosis as well help generate initial interpretative hypotheses.

Reliability

Golden, Berg, and Graber (1982b) evaluated the test–retest reliability of the LNNB in a study of 27 patients who had diagnoses of static injuries. These individuals were tested twice; the average test–retest interval was 167 days. The resulting correlation coefficients ranged from .77 for the Right Hemisphere scale to .96 for the Arithmetic scale. These results were subsequently replicated by Plaisted and Golden (1982), who evaluated 30 psychiatric subjects.

Interscorer reliability was evaluated on a sample of five patients. For each patient, a different pair of examiners scored the responses while simultaneously observing the patient. The agreement between raters ranged from 92% agreement for one patient to 98% for another patient. Overall, there was a 95% agreement rate (Golden, Hammeke, & Purisch, 1978). These percentages may be inflated because approximately two thirds of the items are trichotomously scored and the remaining one third of the items are dichotomously scored.

Bach, Harowski, Kirby, Peterson, and Schulein (1981) addressed the deficiencies of the aforementioned study by evaluating the interrater agreement on a sample of borderline performances by two subjects and five raters. Bach et al. used Cohen's kappa as an uninflated measure of agreement and reported values ranging from .79 to 1.00. The subjects in this study were normal confederates who were instructed on how to respond to the items so as to produce borderline performance on a random set of items. The identities of the items that had been performed in a borderline manner were unknown to the examiners.

To evaluate and extend these findings, Moses and Schefft (1985) used two examiners to evaluate 16 neurological patients, 15 psychiatric subjects, 3 subjects with a history of substance abuse, and 2 normal medical patients (a total of 36 subjects). The authors found that the correlation coefficients for the summary score ranged from .97 for the Intellectual Processes scale to .99 for the Receptive Speech scale, with mean differences in total scores of 1.47 and 0.00 1-score points, respectively. The localization scales' correlation coefficients ranged from .96 to .99. The authors also evaluated the agreement on decisions regarding whether the scales exceeded the critical level. Agreement levels ranged from 33/36 for the Receptive Speech scale and the Writing scale to 36/36 for the Expressive Speech, Tactile, Arithmetic, and Intellectual Processes scales. Analyses of the same data using the chi-square and Kendall's tau resulted in similar results. In examining agreement on individual item scores, the authors found complete agreement on 95.71%, disagreement of 1 point value on 3.5%, and disagreement of 2 points on 0.78% of the individual item scores.

Under Lurian theory, the battery was constructed so that the scales are not completely homogeneous. Therefore, one would expect moderate degrees of internal consistency in the scales. Golden, Fross, and Graber (1981a) evaluated the split-half reliability of the clinical scales using an odd–even split in a sample of 338 patients. The sample constituted 74 normal controls, 83 psychiatric patients, and 181 neurological patients. The split-half reliability correlation coefficients ranged from a high of .95 for the Reading scale to a low of .89 for the Memory scale. Once again, these values may have been inflated by the restricted range of the scoring procedure. However, the values do represent acceptable degrees of consistency.

The internal consistency reliability of the summary, localization, and factor-analytic scales was evaluated for a heterogeneous group of subjects by Moses, Johnson, and Lewis (1983b). These evaluations were also conducted separately for a sample of 451 neurologically impaired, 414 schizophrenic, 128 mixed psychiatric, and 108 normal subjects. The values for the normal subjects ranged from .54 to .78, and for the remaining subjects, they ranged from .83 to .93. The relatively lower values for the normal subjects were probably due to restriction of range in those subjects and underline the problems encountered in using the LNNB to describe neuropsychological functioning in normal subjects.

Internal consistency reliability was again evaluated for the summary and for localization in a sample of 451 brain-damaged subjects, 414 schizophrenic subjects, 128 subjects with mixed psychiatric diagnoses, and 108 normals (Maruish, Sawicki, Franzen, & Golden, 1985). With the use of Cronbach's coefficient alpha, which is a conservative estimate of internal consistency reliability, the values were moderately high. In the brain-damaged subjects, the values ranged from .93 (for three of the scales) to .84 (for four of the scales). For the schizophrenic subjects, the values ranged from .93 (for three of the scales) to .83. For the mixed psychiatric subjects, the values ranged from .92 to .82. For the normal subjects the values ranged from .54 to .78.

Validity

The original attempts to provide validational evidence for the LNNB focused on its accuracy in discriminating neurological patients from normal subjects. Golden, Hammeke, and Purisch (1978) reported that all of the summary scales were successful in discriminating brain-damaged from normal subjects at the .001 level of significance. Other studies have investigated the discriminative ability of the LNNB for elderly subjects (Spitzform, 1982), for psychiatric populations (Golden, Graber, Moses, & Zatz, 1980; Golden et al., 1982e; Puente, Heidelberg-Sanders, & Lund, 1982; Shelley & Goldstein, 1983; Silverstein, McDonald, & Meltzer, 1988), for alcoholics (Chmielewski & Golden, 1980), for patients with AIDS (Ayers, Abrams, Newell, & Friedrich, 1987), and for epileptics (Berg & Golden, 1981). It should be mentioned that later research by Hermann and Melyn (1985) indicated that the success of the LNNB in discriminating epileptic subjects from control subjects may have been partly due to the use of severely affected inpatient epileptics, and that with outpatient epileptics, the LNNB is no better than the HRNB or other neuropsychological instruments. Scores on the LNNB are related to size of cortical ventricles in schizophrenic patients (Kemali et al., 1986).

Of particular interest is the finding that the LNNB can successfully discriminate between the effects of aging and of alcoholism (Burger, Botwinick, & Storandt, 1987).

These studies have reported varying levels of success, but they generally support the utility of the LNNB in discriminating neurologically impaired subjects from normal subjects. As with many test of cognitive function, there may be differential effects of psychiatric diagnosis and symptoms on score level, including depression (Newman & Sweet, 1986). The LNNB appears to be specific to the cognitive effects of mild closed head injury and insensitive to the effects of headache during the evaluation of these patients.

A difficult question in neuropsychological assessment is the differential diagnosis of patients who present ambiguous or inconclusive symptoms and who consequently represent difficult diagnostic problems. Using the rule of classifying as impaired those subjects who have three or more clinical scales above critical level, Malloy and Webster (1981) found 80% agreement between the LNNB and noninvasive neurodiagnostic techniques in subjects with mild cortical impairment. It is also important to know about the effects of medication on neuropsychological test performance. At least for schizophrenic patients receiving neuroleptic medication, there does not appear to be a significant effect (Moses, 1984a).

To evaluate the validity of the LNNB as a technique for measuring specific neuropsychological tasks, a series of factor analyses were undertaken (McKay & Golden, 1981a,b; Moses, 1983, 1984c,d,e). These analyses were conducted in a scalewise fashion. To provide a partial test of the stability of the factors, Moses (1986a) conducted the analysis again, this time with a larger subject sample and using items grouped in construct related bands (i.e., sensorimotor items, speech items, and conceptual items) rather than using groups of items based on scale membership. The results of the analyses were similar to those analyses conducted using scale membership as a grouping variable. Several studies that were conducted present general support for this idea, but too little is known about the temporal stability of these scales to allow them to be recommended for clinical use in retest situations (Golden et al., 1982d).

The concurrent validity of the LNNB has been assessed by correlating its results with that of the HRNB Neuropsychological Battery, with encouraging results. (See earlier discussion in section on the HRNB.) Golden et al. (1981b) reported that, when the summary scores of the LNNB were correlated with the summary scores of the HRNB, the minimum value was .71. Chelune (1982) objected that the large correlations may have been due to shared overlap of the two batteries with the Wechsler Adult Intelligence Scale (WAIS). Golden et al. (1982b) responded to this criticism with a conceptual argument, namely, that postmorbid IQ will reflect neurological impairment. Golden et al. (1982b) then partialed out level of education as an estimate of premorbid IQ and still found moderate correlations between the two batteries. Shelley and Goldstein (1982) reported that, in a sample of 137 subjects, correlations between the LNNB and the HRNB scores ranged from .60 to .96. They also conducted a factor analysis and found that both batteries contributed substantially to the extracted three-factor solution, a finding indicating shared sensitivity to the same neuropsychological variables. Moses (1985c) reported that the WAIS subtests accounted for approximately 50% of the variance in LNNB scale scores;* however, this relationship appeared to consist of performance level predictions rather than specific construct predictions.

Another factor to consider is whether the use of the LNNB and the HRNB results in a similar classification of subjects. Golden et al. (1980a) found that a discriminant function analysis of the two batteries resulted in approximately 85% accurate classification for each.

Goldstein and Shelley (1984) reported similar rates of accuracy in diagnosis for the two batteries, as did Kane, Parsons, and Goldstein (1985). Berg et al. (1984) reported that the LNNB and the HRNB had equivalent diagnostic accuracy in the assessment of idiopathic epileptics.

Some of the original research involving the validity of Form 1 used the number of clinical scales above CL as a guide to the determination of an organic etiology. This is a simple test for the presence of organic impairment and is the least sophisticated use of the instrument. However, it is also a method that can be used by nonspecialists or used in the beginning stages of a sophisticated analysis and interpretation. Although simple, this method is powerful. Moses, Csernansky, and Leiderman (1988) found that using the criterion of two or more clinical scales above CL (excluding the academic skills related C7 or C9) identified cognitive deficit in 75% of a sample of patients with limbic epilepsy. This identification rate was not significantly changed by examining the range or scatter among scales. The suggested method is to compare clinical scale scores, including the Pathognomonic scale, to the CL. If at least three scales exceed the CL, the probability of acquired neurological impairment is fairly high. This hypothesis is modified by examination of the scales related to academic skills (C7, C8, and C9). Elevation of these scales may be related to academic experience. The interpretation of this rule can be conducted with more confidence when acquired neurological impairment is ruled out than when it is detected. Application of the rules suggested for interpretation of neurological impairment resulted in a 3% false-positive rate in a sample of 241 normal individuals which increased to a 13% false-positive rate in a sample of older individuals (McKinzey, Roecker, Puente, & Rogers, 1998). This may be partly due to the fact that the demographic values for the critical level regression formula have a ceiling at age 70 years. Since increasing age has the effect of raising the CL and therefore reducing the probability that a given score will be found to be impaired, there may be more older people incorrectly diagnosed as being neurologically impaired. This is an important issue for all of neuropsychology and can be best addressed by acquisition of adequate normative information from older individuals.

The manual suggests that scatter greater than three standard deviations (or 30 T-score points from lowest to highest clinical scale score) is suggestive of neurological impairment. Subsequent empirical investigations have generally supported this guide (McKinley et al., 1998).

The interpretation of individual scale scores is complicated by the fact that none of the clinical scales is actually homogeneous. However, scales scores can be interpreted by reference to their external correlates as demonstrated in the empirical literature. For example, Macciocchi, Fowler, & Ranseen (1992), by conducting a multitrait–multimethod matrix analysis and confirmatory factor analysis, provide useful information regarding interpretation of the C1, C10, and C11 Scales. An excellent review of various construct validity studies can be found in Moses and Maruish (1988a,b). Other attempts to evaluate the concurrent validity of the LNNB have correlated the results of the Peabody Individual Achievement Test with appropriate scales of the LNNB in 100 neurological, psychiatric, and normal subjects, with acceptable results (Gillen, Ginn, Strider, Kreuch, & Golden, 1983).

Because of the heterogeneity of the scale composition, interpretation of the LNNB must not be limited to scale interpretation, although that is a necessary first step. Full interpretation must also take into account scores on the empirically derived localization scales, the factor-analytic scales, comparisons of items across scales, and a consideration of the qualitative aspects of the subject's performance. Interpretation is best left to individuals who have received specialized training in neuropsychological assessment and who are familiar with Lurian theory.

The LNNB has been the subject of various attempts to develop scales from either a conceptual or an empirical methodology. The Pathognomonic Scale is an example of the empirical methodology and the Right and Left Sensorimotor Scales are examples of the conceptual, theoretical methodology. The Pathognomonic Scale consists of those items that best differentiated between patients with central nervous system dysfunction and people without central nervous system involvement. This scale is also useful for differentiating between patients with neurologic disorders and patients who have psychiatric disorders even when those disorders have central nervous system concomitants. The Pathognomonic Scale may also be sensitive to recency of injury. Therefore Sawicki and Golden (1984a,b) developed two scales, using an empirical strategy, to partial out the effects of recency. The Profile Elevation Scale was derived by examining those items that best correlated with the mean scale scores and the Profile Impairment Scale was derived by examining those items that best correlated with the number of clinical scales above CL. The manual suggests that in cases of acute injury, the Profile Elevation scale will exceed the Profile Impairment Scale and as time progresses and compensation is developed by the individual, the two scales tend to become equal in elevation.

Evaluation of the construct validity of the individual scales has been conducted on a limited basis. Moses (1984e,f) examined the relationship of LNNB results in subjects with and without sensorimotor deficits and with and without forms of cognitive impairment. He reported that the Motor, Tactile, Receptive Speech, Pathognomonic, and Left and Right Sensorimotor scales were able to discriminate the four groups of subjects formed by crossing the two conditions of sensorimotor and cognitive deficits. This finding lends limited support to the construct validity of these particular scales.

Prifitera and Ryan (1982) compared the performance of the LNNB Memory scale with other memory assessment techniques. Larrabee, Kane, Shuck, and Francis (1985a) examined the construct validity of the Memory factor scales. They found that the two LNNB Memory factor scales loaded highly on the factor on which the Benton Visual Retention Test and portions of the Wechsler Memory Scales also loaded. However, they concluded that there may not be much clinical utility in the Memory factor scales because of item heterogeneity and short scale length. Prifitera and Ryan (1981) compared the LNNB Intellectual Processes scale with the WAIS. Pheley and Klesges (1986) evaluated the relationship of the LNNB Memory scale score to various laboratory memory tasks. They found a correlation between the LNNB and the laboratory tasks of paired associates and face–name association but not the laboratory tasks of digit span and trigrams with distraction. The lack of a significant correlation may have been due to the small sample size and the restricted range of scores. These studies represent a start on the necessary task of evaluating the specific concurrent validity of the components. However, more research needs to be done before definite conclusions can be reached.

Studies evaluating the accuracy of the localization scales of the LNNB have been conducted and have resulted in a generally accurate identification of the site of lesion. The use of the localization scales resulted in a 89% correct classification rate in the derivation sample and a 74% correct classification rate in the cross-validation sample (Golden et al., 1981c). However, these results need to be replicated because of the inclusion of closed-head injury subjects in the sample. Closed-head-injured patients may be injured in sites other than the site of the main injury because of contrecoup effects, which can contaminate these characteristics of the experimental sample.

The localization scales are perhaps the most problematic of the derived scales for the LNNB. It is unclear whether the original samples on which the scales were derived were pure localization cases. Attempts to cross-validate the accuracy of the scales have not been encouraging. Misuse of the scales has been reported (Klein, 1993). The most promising use of these scales is to lateralize structural brain impairment using the two out of three rule. Examining the three highest localizations scales, two of these scales will be related to the same hemisphere which is likely to be the laterality of the structural neurological impairment. This method results in approximately 90% accuracy in cases of lateralized damage.

Like many new tests, the LNNB has been the subject of criticism. And as with many new tests, there have been replies to these criticisms in the literature. The exchange of criticisms and answers has helped to assess the limits of the utility of the LNNB. Adams (1980a) criticized the LNNB on the basis of the methodology of its development, stating that multiple *t*-tests were an inappropriate means of deciding which items to retain in the battery. He similarly criticized the use of a small subject sample in the discriminant function analysis. Although Golden (1980) replied that the derived discriminant function had an acceptable ratio of predictors to subjects, the fact remains that the number of tested potential predictors exceeded the number from which safe conclusions can be reached, given the sample size. Golden's reply to the criticism of multiple *t*-tests is more to the point. *T*-tests were used in an apparent attempt to minimize the probability of Type I errors, an acceptable practice in the early stages of test development. The items have subsequently been evaluated, and this methodology has apparently had little effect on the accuracy of the battery as a whole. Adams (1980b) replied by questioning the veracity of the reports of the accuracy of the battery, calling into question the scientific background of the test's developers. Empirical evidence is needed to validate the relevance of these doubts.

Spiers (1981) published a few conceptual criticisms of the LNNB. He stated that the idea of a battery was antithetical to the methods of Luria, and that the availability of MMPI-like graphs on which to plot results may increase the probability that insufficiently trained psychologists will use the battery clinically. The first criticism is undeniable. The use of the name "Luria–Nebraska" is honorific because of its reliance on the contributions of Luria to the field of neuropsychology and the reliance of the battery on his theory. The second criticism is directed more at the users of the battery than at the battery itself, and it is well taken. Unless the users of the LNNB have had specific training in neuropsychological assessment, they would do better to limit themselves in interpretation.

Spiers (1982) further criticized the LNNB on the basis of the intent of the items. In the same paper, he criticized the standardized, quantified approach in general because of its reliance on average scores, which mask individual differences. Hutchinson (1984) criticized Spiers (1982) on a factual basis, stating that there are discrepancies between Spiers's reading of the manual and verbatim quotes from the manual. Hutchinson further accused Spiers of misunderstanding the intended use of the battery. Spiers (1984) replied that Hutchinson (1984) had misinterpreted his (Spiers's) statements and accused Hutchinson of misreading his article. Stambrook (1983) also criticized the LNNB in the literature; how-ever, his article repeats concerns raised by Adams (1980a,b) and by Spiers (1981, 1982) and will therefore not be discussed here.

At least two conclusions can be drawn from this discussion. First, some of the contro-versy surrounding the LNNB is actually related to disagreements between the proponents of the standardized, quantified approach to neuropsychological assessment and the propo-nents of the intuitive, qualitative approach. Second, the controversy has degenerated into personal accusations. Theoretical arguments may be necessary in the evaluation of any assessment technique, but they are insufficient without direct empirical evidence.

The LNNB does not have a universally valid utility for all populations. The LNNB should be used with reference to the experimental literature regarding the population in question. Further, the LNNB is not totally comprehensive, as it does not assess reading comprehension or memory, other than short-term, mainly verbal memory.

Because of its reliance on Lurian theory and on Luria's emphasis on the verbal mediation of behavior, valid use of the LNNB depends largely on language skills. Crosson and Warren (1982) criticized the use of the LNNB for aphasic populations. Delis and Kaplan (1982) presented a case in which the use of only the clinical scales for an aphasic would result in a misunderstanding of the subject's deficits. Golden et al. (1982c) reexam-ined the data regarding the case reported by Delis and Kaplan and found that the LNNB had been inappropriately used, as the primary language of the subject was Spanish. Golden et al. (1982a) also found evidence in the subject's history of chronic alcohol abuse, a seizure disorder, bilateral atrophy, and a left temporal–parietal infarct, indicating that the conclu-sions of the LNNB were in closer agreement with the actual deficits of the subject than had been implied by Delis and Kaplan (1982). Despite this foray into personal aspects of the controversy, the heavy dependence on language may limit the utility of the LNNB in language-impaired individuals.

Because the LNNB cannot distinguish between average and superior performance, it may be inappropriate in the assessment of normal neuropsychological functioning, except to rule out the possibility of impairment. As stated earlier, the reliabilities of the scale scores are attenuated in normal subjects. Partly in response to this issue Moses and Pritchard (1999) have developed performance scales for the LNNB. In this methodology, age and education were separately regressed for each clinical scale using data from both normal subjects and medical patients; next the raw scores for the clinical scales were translated to z-scores using only the normal subjects' data. Next each of the z-scores for the clinical scales were averaged and the age- and education-corrected raw scores were regressed against the average z-scores to produce new scores that reflected normal performance at the low ends of the scale and impaired performance at the higher ends. The scales range in value from 0 to 16. Although psychometrically superior to the original T-score scales, these new scales are in need of further empirical validation.

Finally, although the LNNB relies on an understanding of Lurian constructs for its most effective use, these constructs have yet to be conclusively validated. In short, despite the many studies conducted to date, because of the complexity of the battery there is still a need for more research to fully evaluate each aspect of the LNNB. For example, the construct validity of the clinical scales is in need of empirical investigation. The LNNB can be recommended for clinical use, but only in the hands of a trained psychologist who is familiar with the research regarding the question to be answered and the population from which the subject is drawn. The LNNB seems to have applicability in both research and clinical settings.

LURIA–NEBRASKA NEUROPSYCHOLOGICAL BATTERY FORM II

The Luria–Nebraska Neuropsychological Battery Form II is an attempt to provide both an alternate to Form I and some improvements over the original form. The organization of Form II is similar to the organization of Form I except that there is an additional scale: C12 (Intermediate Memory). Partly in response to criticism regarding the relationship of the names of the scales to the content validity of the scales, the names have been removed and replaced with numbers, C1 through C11 for the clinical scales, S1 through S4 for the supplementary scales, L1 through L8 for the localization scales, and alphanumeric characters for the factor scales. The LNNB relies heavily on the subject's ability to comprehend verbal instructions and may therefore have limited utility in assessing subjects with receptive language impairments. However, revised administration instructions allowing for alternate response modalities extend the utility of the instrument for assessing subjects with expressive language impairments.

As in the case of Form I, Form II combines features of Alexandr Luria's theories of brain function with a standardized approach to assessment. Therefore, many of the comments made with regard to Form I also apply here and are not repeated in great depth. For a discussion of the particulars, the reader is referred to the discussion of Form I in the earlier parts of this chapter.

The stimulus materials for Form II are similar to those for Form I. The visual stimuli have been bound into a single booklet arranged in the chronological order required for administration, an improvement over the separately bound portions of Form I. The visual stimuli were enlarged so that subjects with poor vision would not be penalized for peripheral impairment reasons. The audiotape stimulus for the C2 (Rhythm) scale is identical to the audiotape for Form I.

In some instances, entirely new stimuli have been devised for Form II, using the same rationale as was used in devising the original items. For example, the C8 scale (Reading) shares no items across the two forms, nor does the C11 scale (Intellectual Processes). As mentioned earlier, the C12 scale (Intermediate Memory) is a new development in Form II, not having existed in Form I. In other instances, items were retained across the two forms, as in the case of the C2 scale (Rhythm), where 92% of the items originally appeared in Form I. The additional scale on Form II is Scale 12, which is conceived of as a measure of intermediate or delayed memory. In the C12 (Intermediate Memory) scale, the examiner questions the subject about aspects of items that were previously given in the test. Therefore, this scale can be seen as tapping incidental memory as well as delayed memory with interference.

Because of the great similarity between the two forms of the LNNB, the information regarding administration and scoring can probably be assumed to be equivalent. Research regarding the amount of training necessary to achieve reliable scoring indicates that approximately 40 hours of training will produce adequate administration by a B.A.-level technician. The tests are administered from test protocols that contain the administration instructions as well as the basic scoring criteria. More detailed scoring instructions are contained in the manual. In addition, a patient response booklet contains space for the written and drawn responses of the subject, as well as the printed stimuli for two of the C4 scales. In both forms, scores are represented in the form of standardized T-scores with a mean of 50 and a standard deviation of 10 points. A critical level is computed with a regression formula using the age and level of education of the subject as predictors.

There is a new manual to accompany Form II (Golden, Purisch, & Hammeke, 1985). Actually, it is a combined manual for both forms. The new manual is substantially larger than the original manual and it includes information regarding new derived scales, such as the Impairment and Elevation scales. These scales contain items that were drawn from across the various scales, the patterns of which provide information regarding the acuteness of an injury as well as the probability that behavioral compensation will still occur. There are also a power scale and a speed scale composed of items that were hypothesized to be related to those constructs. T-score conversions are available for the Impairment and Elevation scales, based on a normative sample of approximately 800 cases. T-score conversions for the Speed and Power scales are based on a normative sample of 45 medical patients. Initial empirical studies suggest that a relatively higher Elevation scale (over the Impairment scale) is related to recency of injury and the probability of compensation, and that a relatively higher Speed scale (over the Power scale) is related to a posterior focus of the injury. More research is needed before these rules can be strongly recommended for clinical use.

Other changes in the manual include decomposing the C7 scale (Writing) into a Spelling and a Motor Writing scale. Hopefully, users of the LNNB were already making that distinction in formulating an interpretation of results, but this change helps to ensure that process. The new manual also describes the development of a set of qualitative categories that can be scored independently of the quantitative scores. These categories can be summed, and the frequency counts can be compared with the frequency of occurrence in the normative sample ($n = 48$). Because of the limited size of the normative sample, interpretation of the qualitative information is best conducted with reference to neuro-psychological theory. At present, the qualitative scores have the potential to serve a useful function by helping the assessor to systematize his or her observations. To make the qualitative scores more useful, one would need a larger normative sample as well as a comparison sample of impaired subjects.

The expanded administration instructions in the new manual provide guides for administering the LNNB to individuals with peripheral sensory losses. The manual also contains a set of 25 cases written by James A. Moses. There are also discussions of illustrative profiles for different localizations. Although these features can be an aid in learning interpretation, they should not be used as a substitute for supervised learning experiences.

The appendices to the manual contain information regarding the factor structure of Form I, as well as item difficulty indices and information regarding mean performances for each item. Similar information regarding Form II is needed.

Form II was developed and standardized on a sample of 73 subjects who were given both forms of the test. There were no significant differences in the raw scores for any of the scales. Scale scores for Form II were then derived by regressing the raw scores for Form II against the raw scores for Form I and applying the linear solution to l-score transformations for Form II. Form II was then administered to a sample of 125 normal subjects, 140 subjects with central nervous system dysfunction, and 34 schizophrenic subjects. A MANOVA conducted on the data resulted in significant differentiation among the groups. Subsequently, Form II was administered to 100 normal subjects and 100 neurologically impaired subjects. Use of the clinical rules stated in the manual resulted in classification accuracy rates equivalent to those for Form I. Although these studies help us to evaluate the validity of Form II, much of the research originally conducted on Form I now needs to be conducted on Form II. Also needed is a separate normative sample for the derivation of T scores for Form II. Although the above-mentioned research indicates that Form I and II appear to be equivalent, a separate normative sample will help to ensure the accuracy of estimates of the precision of scores obtained by the use of Form II.

Wong, Schefft, and Moses (1990) published additional normative observations on the LNNB-II which were then included in the sample used by Moses, Schefft, Wong, and Berg (1992) to calculate T score transformations of raw scores for the clinical scales. Moses et al. (1992) also derived a critical level formula for the LNNB-II. Wong and Gilpin (1993) correlated select scales of the LNNB-II with index scores from the WMS-R and concluded that the C10 scale was primarily a measure of verbal memory.

Overall, Form II of the LNNB shows promise as a clinical neuropsychological assessment instrument. The initial research supports its basic comparability with Form I. However, more recent research has indicated that the two forms are not entirely equivalent (Blackerby, 1985; Moses & Chiu, 1993) and the specific interpretations should be conducted with reference to whether the validational studies used Form I or Form II. Kashden (1994) examined the interrater reliability of the qualitative scoring system and found that although there was some variability, there was generally excellent reliability. Future investigations can address the comparative validity. The empirical base for LNNB-I is greater than it is for LNNB-II. There are well over 200 published studies using the LNNB Form I. Not all of this research needs to be replicated on Form II, but the basic reliability and validity studies are in need of replication. For example, Garmoe, Schefft, and Moses (1991) reported that the LNNB-II is able to discriminate between neurologically impaired and control subjects.

In addition, the LNNB has been translated into other languages including Greek (Donias, Vassilopoulou, Golden, & Lovell, 1989) and Chinese (Yun, Yao-Xian, & Matthews, 1987) and modified into short forms (Golden, 1989; Horton, Anilane, Puente, & Berg, 1988). The discussion here has been restricted to the full-length forms of the English language versions.

Children's Form

A form of the LNNB appropriate for children or the LNNB-C has been published. Just as with the children's forms of the HRNB, less information is available about the children's form of the LNNB than about the adult form. Karras et al. (1987) reported the results of factor analysis in a sample of 719 children, but these factor scales are in need of external validation for interpretation purposes. Tramontana et al. (1984) found that the WISC-R correlated moderately with the LNNB-C summary scale scores. This was true especially for correlations between the LNNB-C variables, which required greater abstract thought and higher cortical functioning, and the FSIQ.

There were lower correlations between the LNNB-C scales measuring simpler sensory–motor functioning and the VIQ. This pattern of intercorrelations is consistent with that expected on the basis of theory. Carr, Sweet, and Rossini (1986) reported significant agreement between the WISC-R and LNNB-C in the identification of cognitive impairment, but later reported that there were few significant correlations among the scales of the two tests (Sweet et al., 1986), indicating that the two tests may be not redundant but complementary.

The LNNB-C may also be useful in the assessment of learning disabilities. The LNNB-C can discriminate between reading disabled children and academically normal children (Myers, Sweet, Deysach, & Myers, 1989; Teeter, Boliek, Obrzut, & Malsch, 1986).The LNNB-C Pathognomonic Scale predicted reading and spelling achievement but not arithmetic achievement over and beyond that variance predicted by the WISC-R (McBurnett, Hynd, Lahey, & Town, 1988). Similarly, the adult LNNB discriminated between learning disabled and normal adolescents (Lewis & Lorion, 1988). However, the LNNB-C may not be useful in discriminating among different types of learning disabilities (Morgan & Brown, 1988).

In a study of children and adolescents with idiopathic epilepsy, the LNNB-C and the HRNB for Children agreed regarding the presence of cognitive impairment 91% of the time, indicating reasonable concurrent validity (Berg et al., 1984).

Malingering

Mensch and Woods (1986) offered suggestions for evaluating the results of the LNNB in determining the possibility of malingering. The suggestions involve examining the pattern of easy versus difficult items missed. Because the items in the LNNB are arranged in increasing order of easy to difficult and simple to complex, this process is somewhat simplified. However, the examiner should also consult tables of item difficulty indices in the manual.

McKinzey, Podd, Krehbiel, Mensch, and Trombka (1997) identified items on the LNNB that were either more likely associated with malingered performance or more likely to be associated with true impairment. These items were summed into two scales and a decision rule was developed. When this decision rule was cross-validated on a separate sample of 51 malingerers and 202 patients there was an 88% accuracy of classification rate. Although promising, this method is in need of cross-validation in an independent sample. In a concatenated set of data from normal control subjects across different settings, McKinzey, Roecker, Puente, and Rogers (1998) found that use of the malingering formula with normal profiles resulted in a false-positive rate of 26%; however, when the impaired profiles produced by normal individuals were examined, there was only a 6% false-positive rate. Therefore, less confidence can be placed in findings of malingering indices in an otherwise normal profile. Luckily, it is rare that a normal profile might be questioned as to the possibility that it reflects malingered performance. McKinzey et al. (1997) developed and validated a formula for detecting malingering on the LNNB and cross-validated with an overall hit rate of 88%.

LNNB—Summary

The LNNB has been shown to be reliable and valid in several settings and populations. There is continued research among a group of psychometrically sophisticated investigators and this research will likely enhance the utility of the instrument. As with any instrument, continued examination of the psychometric properties and continual updates of the normative base are necessary to the continued use of the LNNB in a clinical setting. Validational research using the newer neurodiagnostic techniques such as the functional imaging techniques will help articulate the construct validity of the LNNB.

Benton's Neuropsychological Assessment

Even a quick look at this book would indicate that the largest areas of development have been in the construction of new tests and procedures. That is not true for the various tests associated with Arthur Benton. Additional and updated normative information has been made available (Sivan, 1992), but there have been no new tests or procedures. All the same, the Benton procedures continue to be used both clinically and in research settings. The continued utilization of the tests reflects the sound design and the fact that not many tests have been developed focusing on the functions of the right hemisphere.

Arthur Benton has made several large contributions to the field of neuropsychological assessment in terms of test constructions, the understanding of right-hemisphere function, in training, and in professional development. Benton's approach to test construction is to take laboratory tasks that had been found to be sensitive to differences in cortical integrity and to apply them in a clinical setting. Although not all of Benton's tasks actually derive from the laboratory, the construction of all of the tasks has the spirit of laboratory investigations. In addition, the procedures are well defined and standardized. Scoring is described explicitly, and the results are summarized in a quantitative score. A third characteristic of Benton's tests is the use of norms that represent the influence of age and education. Benton was perhaps the first clinical neuropsychologist to have paid more than mere lip service to the confounding effects of age and education in the assessment situation. Finally, Benton was not bound by the left-hemisphere bias of traditional neuropsychology. Many of his tests are either sensitive to the effects of right-hemisphere impairment or, as in the case of the Tactile Form Perception Test, are designed to partial out the linguistic (left-hemisphere) effects from the more purely perceptual (right-hemisphere) effects.

Benton may be the person in this country most responsible for the rise of the flexible approach to neuropsychological assessment. His tests do not constitute a battery. Instead, the tests to be used in each assessment are chosen on the basis of presenting complaints, the type of referral question, or the results of previous testing. Therefore, a different set of assessment techniques is likely to be used on each subject. The tests were not normed on the same set of normative subjects, and therefore comparisons of scores across tests of the same individual are limited. However, the tests are extremely useful for the assessment of particular functions or when administered in conjunction with other assessment devices.

The tests included in the Benton conglomeration are the Benton Visual Retention Test; the Multilingual Aphasia Examination; and the tests of Temporal Orientation, Right–Left Orientation, and Serial Digit Learning. Benton's perceptual and motor tests include Facial Recognition, Judgment of Line Orientation, Visual Form Discrimination, Pantomime

Recognition, Tactile Form Perception, Finger Localization, Phoneme Discrimination, Three Dimensional Block Construction, and Motor Impersistence. These tests are considered singly.

RIGHT–LEFT ORIENTATION

Right–left orientation has been interpreted as indicative of spatial impairment and as being associated with linguistic impairment. The Benton Test of Right-Left Orientation requires the patient to respond with rudimentary motor responses, a requirement that minimizes the influence of aphasic symptoms on the test results. The test consists of 20 commands that are presented in increasing order of complexity. The first set of commands requires the patient to point to right or left parts of his or her own body. The second set of commands requires the patient to point to lateralized parts of his or her body with either the right or the left hand. The third set of commands requires the patient to point to lateralized parts of the examiner's body. Finally, the fourth set of commands requires the patient to point to lateralized parts of the examiner's body with the right or left hand.

There are alternate forms of the test. Form B is identical to Form A except that the words right and left are interchanged. The responses are scored for whether the patient uses the correctly lateralized body part or the correct body part. In addition, errors are separated on the basis of whether the command required the subject to point to his or her own body or to the body of the examiner. Formal investigations of the alternate-forms reliability of the test have not been conducted. However, because of the similarity between the two forms, equivalency can probably be safely assumed. Form R is for patients who cannot use their right hand, and Form L is for patients who cannot use their left hand. Because Forms R and L are sufficiently different, the alternate-forms reliability of these two forms needs to be investigated.

The test was normed on a sample of 234 male and female subjects who had no history of brain impairment. Statistical analyses indicated no significant differences due to age, sex, or level of education. Distributions of scores for the impaired subjects are also presented in the manual (Benton, Hamsher, Varney, & Spreen, 1983). The impaired subjects consisted of 34 patients with bilateral brain impairment, 20 patients with right-hemisphere lesions, 20 aphasic patients with left-hemisphere lesions, and 20 nonaphasic patients with left-hemisphere lesions. The interpretation of results is based on the similarity of the type of error made by the patient in reference to the normative data. Although interpretations of Forms R and L are referred to the normative data, formal evaluations of the validity of these two forms need to be conducted.

Knowledge about relationships to other tests (concurrent validity) will help us to understand the nature of the deficit underlying poor performance on this test. Information regarding the internal consistency reliability and the test–retest reliability would also enhance the clinical utility of the test.

SERIAL DIGIT LEARNING

Benton's Serial Digit Learning Test is a standardized form of digit supraspan. (The reader is referred to the discussion of supraspan procedures elsewhere in this book.) One of the advances in Benton's Test of Serial Digit Learning is that normative data are available for different levels of education and for different age groups. Another advance is that scoring is sensitive to the degree of error manifested by the patient. Nearly correct responses (an error involving only 1 digit in the series) are scored 1 point, and perfectly correct responses are scored 2 points.

There are two forms of this test. Form SD9 can be given to patients between the ages of 16 and 64. Form SD8 can be given to subjects up to the age of 74. Normative data are available for 500 medical patients without a history of brain disease. The quantitative score is converted to different percentiles for the age and the education level of the patient. There were no statistically significant differences due to sex in the normative sample. Therefore, there are no corrections for sex in the scoring procedures.

Hamsher, Benton, and Digre (1980) found that, in a sample of 100 patients with diagnosed brain impairment, use of the Serial Digit Learning Test was more likely to result in a correct diagnosis than was the use of the Digit Span subtest of the WAIS. The increase in diagnostic accuracy was greatest for subjects with bilateral lesions. The increase in diagnostic accuracy was least for patients with left-hemisphere lesions. Despite this difference in accuracy as related to laterality of the lesion, it does not appear that the Test of Serial Digit Learning would be useful in lateralizing brain lesions.

FACIAL RECOGNITION

Benton's Test of Facial Recognition is an evaluation of the patient's ability to recognize unfamiliar faces from black-and-white photographs. (The reader is referred to the discussion of other tests of familiar and unfamiliar faces elsewhere in this book.) This test has three parts. The first part requires the subject to identify the face in a stimulus photograph from a choice of six front-view photographs. The second part requires the patient to identify the person in the stimulus photograph from a series of six three-quarter view faces, three of which are of the stimulus face. The third part requires the patient to identify the face in the stimulus photograph from a series of six photographs under different lighting conditions. Again, three of the faces are the same as the stimulus face. The test has a short and a long form. The long form differs only in having a larger number of items. The photographs are organized into a spiral-bound booklet.

The normative data are available in the manual based on a sample of 196 medical inpatients with no history of brain disease, psychiatric disorder, or childhood mental deficiency, and on a sample of 90 normal subjects. All 286 subjects were between the ages of 16 and 74. Significant differences due to age were found. Significant differences due to education were found only in the 55- to 74-year-old group. Therefore, a correction factor for age was added for the subjects in the 55- to 64-year-old and the 65- to 74-year-old groups. A correction for education was added for the same two groups.

Normative data are also available for patients between the ages of 6 and 14. These data are based on a sample of 266 schoolchildren. The IQ score of all of the children was in the 85 to 116 range as measured by the WISC.

The relationship between the short and long forms has been investigated by correlating the scores of the items in the short form with scores of all of the items. The correlation coefficient for 151 of the control subjects was .88, and the correlation coefficient was .92 for the brain-damaged subjects. Overall, a correlation coefficient of .93 was obtained for the entire sample of 336 subjects. Based on these data, short-form scores can be converted to long form scores by the use of a table in the manual (Benton et al., 1983).

After the appropriate age and education corrections have been made, the scores are converted to percentiles. Percentile conversions using age conventions are also available for the child sample.

Hamsher, Levin, and Benton (1979) investigated the performance of brain-impaired subjects on the Test of Facial Recognition. The overall sample of 286 subjects consisted of 196 controls, 23 subjects with right anterior lesions, 36 subjects with right posterior lesions, 15 nonaphasic subjects with left posterior lesions, 5 aphasic subjects without comprehension deficits but with left anterior lesions, 8 aphasic subjects without comprehension deficits but with left posterior deficits, 17 aphasic subjects with comprehension deficits and left anterior lesions, and 27 aphasic subjects with comprehension deficits and left posterior lesions. Poor performance appeared to be related to right-hemisphere lesions as well as to left-hemisphere lesions in the presence of comprehension deficits. Levin, Grossman, and Kelly (1977) found that closed-head injury was associated with poor performance on the Test of Facial Recognition only when patients had been comatose for longer than 24 hours. There were no relationships with the presence of abnormal EEGs or the presence of depressed skull fracture. Furthermore, the Facial Recognition Test does not appear to be related to subcortical white matter hyperintensity as measured by magnetic resonance imaging (MRI) in healthy older individuals (Tupler, Coffey, Logue, Djang, & Fagan, 1992). However, the Facial Recognition Test does correlate with P300 latency in auditory evoked potentials (Dywan, Segalowitz, & Unsel, 1992). The relationship of the Facial Recognition Test to physiological variables needs to be better explicated.

Levin and Benton (1977) investigated the performance of 44 psychiatric patients whose symptoms implied the presence of cortical impairment and found that their scores were all in the normal range, with the exception of the score of one paranoid schizophrenic. The authors therefore recommended the Test of Facial Recognition as being useful in differential diagnosis. However, these recommendations need to be tempered in light of the results of Kronfol, Hamsher, Digre, and Waziri (1978), who found that, of 18 severely depressed psychiatric inpatients, 3 performed in the impaired range.

All aspects of the reliability of this test need to be evaluated. In addition, it would be instructive to compare the internal reliability of the short and long forms. More information is needed regarding the validity of this test in psychiatric populations. The relationship of receptive aphasic symptoms to performance on the Test of Facial Recognition needs to be more clearly delineated.

JUDGMENT OF LINE ORIENTATION

The Test of Judgment of Line Orientation (JLO) resulted from Benton's earlier investigations into the effects of right-hemisphere lesions on spatial orientation skills. His earlier investigations involved the tachistoscopic presentation of two lines that may or may not differ in angle. Because of the difficulty in using tachistoscopic presentation methods at the bedside, a booklet form of this procedure was devised in which the stimulus items are presented as incomplete lines to approximate the level of difficulty when full length lines are presented tachistoscopically (Benton, Varney, & Hamsher, 1978).

There are two forms of the test, which actually contain the same items presented in slightly different order. There are 30 items in this test. Each item contains two lines of angles varying from the horizontal. For each item, there is also the same template stimulus of a collection of lines in an arrangement with 18-degree increments. The task presented to the patient is to identify the lines in the constant template stimulus that match the angles of the two incomplete lines.

The normative data are available in the manual based on a sample of 137 adult control subjects who ranged in age from 16 to 74 years. Significant differences due to age and sex were found. Therefore, corrections are suggested on the basis of these two variables. There was no systematic effect of level of education, so no corrections for this variable are suggested. However, a larger sample may result in systematic differences due to level of education, and this possibility needs to be investigated. Normative data are also available based on a sample of 221 children aged 7 to 14 years. Corrected scores are converted to percentiles for the purpose of interpretation. Additional normative information is available stratified by age and corrected for level of education is a sample of 750 normal adults between the ages of 55 and 97 years (Ivnik, Malec, Smith, Tangalos, & Petersen, 1996).

The split-half reliability of Form H, corrected for attenuation, was found to be .94 in a sample of 40 subjects. The split-half reliability of Form V was found to be .89 in a sample of 124 subjects. The split-half reliability of the test (the form used was not identified) was found to be .84 in a sample of 221 children (Lindgren & Benton, 1980).

Although test–retest reliability has not been evaluated separately for the two forms, it was evaluated when first one form and then the other was administered to a sample of 37 patients. The interval varied from 6 hours to 21 days. The reliability coefficient was .90, and there were no significant differences between the two scores.

Short forms of the JLO have been developed. Vanderploeg, LaLone, Greblo, and Schinka (1997) reported the results of investigating the psychometric properties of four short 15-item forms of the JLO. The odd-item and even-item versions possessed adequate reliability. Doubling the scores obtained from the two short forms resulted in mean scores and standard deviations similar to those in the original form in a sample of 81 patients. Adequate psychometric properties are necessary but not sufficient to recommend clinical use of the short forms. Woodard et al. (1996) reported the correlations between both the original and the short forms of the JLO and WAIS-R IQ values, Block Design scores, and Mattis Dementia Rating Scale scores. There were no significant differences among the correlations in comparisons of the short forms with other and with the original form. In addition, classifying a sample of 386 patients using the JLO categories of impairment from the manual resulted in good agreement between each of the short forms and the original form. Weingarden, Yates, Moses, Benton, and Faustman (1998) examined different short forms of the JLO, and based on examination of internal consistency as well as correlation with the full form, recommended a short form composed of items 11 to 30 of Form V for clinical use. Woodard et al. (1998) examined the distributions of scores on odd- and even-item versions of Form V of the JLO in a sample of healthy elderly subjects. They found nearly equal mean scores and equivalent distributions as well as equivalent relationships with the Beery Visual Motor Integration test and suggested that these two short forms be used in conducting screening evaluations or serial evaluations of the elderly.

The sensitivity of the test to lateralized impairment was investigated in a sample of 50 subjects with left-hemisphere lesions and 50 subjects with right-hemisphere lesions.

None of the subjects were aphasic. Although both groups contained subjects with a wide range of scores, the right-hemisphere lesioned subjects were much more likely to perform in the impaired range. The test therefore appears to be sensitive to lateralized impairment. However, much more knowledge is needed regarding the construct validity of the test. Preliminary investigations of this type are promising. Benton et al. (1983) reported that, at least for children, there is a low partial correlation of this test with the Test of Facial Recognition (when age and Verbal IQ are corrected for), indicating that the two tests measure separate constructs. As another way of examining the construct validity of the JLO, Kempen, Kritchevsky, and Feldman (1994) investigated the impact of visual impairment (refractive error) on performance on the JLO and found that although visual impairment affected scores on the Facial Recognition and Visual Form Discrimination tests, there was no effect on the JLO.

Trahan (1998) reported that twice as many right cerebrovascular accident (CVA) patients exhibit impaired performance on the JLO as left-hemisphere CVA patients. This result was supported by the findings of York and Cermak (1995) in a smaller sample of patients with either right- or left-hemisphere CVA. Another method of investigating the laterality of JLO performance involves the use of functional imaging techniques in non-clinical subjects. Deutsch, Bourbon, Papanicolaou, and Eisenberg (1988) reported that regional cerebral blood flow shows right-sided asymmetry when 19 subjects were administered the JLO. Hannay et al. (1987) reported similar results when specifically looking at the right temporo-occipital region. Therefore the JLO appears to be related to right-hemisphere activity in the noninjured brain. Scopolamine, a drug that interferes with cholinergic activity, has a negative effect on JLO performance (Meador et al., 1993).

Although the JLO has norms available for both adults and children and has been suggested for use in both sets of subjects, there may be differential validities in the two age groups. Riccio and Hynd (1993) reported that although the JLO correlates with the visual–spatial measures of the WISC-R and with math ability (WRAT-R), the JLO did not differentiate among groups of psychiatric, learning disabled, and normal control children.

Yet another way to interpret results of the JLO is related to types of errors exhibited by the subjects. Ska, Poissant, and Joanette (1990) reported that certain types of errors were specific to patients with Alzheimer's dementia. However, another set of researchers failed to replicate this finding and instead reported that patients with Parkinson's disease exhibited a specific set of errors types (Finton, Lucas, Graff-Radford, & Uitti, 1998). This second set of results is in need of replication, but the approach of error analysis holds promise for future applications of the JLO.

VISUAL FORM DISCRIMINATION

The Test of Visual Form Discrimination (VFD) is an attempt to assess the ability of a patient to perceive and recognize complex visual patterns. The test stimuli are spiral-bound in a booklet. Each item consists of a target stimulus and four choices, one of which matches the target exactly. Each stimulus consists of two major figures and a peripheral figure. Aside from the correctly matching stimulus, one of the alternate stimuli involves the rotation of a major figure, one involves the rotation of the peripheral figure, and one involves the distortion of a major figure. Qualitative information about the type of error made can be derived from this multiple-choice test.

Originally, there were 64 items in the test. A pilot study based on a sample of children (sample size unspecified) provided estimates of item difficulty. Sixteen items representing a wide range of difficulty levels were chosen to comprise the final test. The items are presented in increasing order of difficulty.

Scoring is based both on a record of the type of error and on a numerical system in which correct responses are assigned values of 2 points, peripheral errors are assigned 1 point, and the major rotations and major distortions are assigned 0 points. In this way, scores are potentially sensitive to the degree of visual impairment.

The normative information is available from the manual (Benton et al., 1983; Benton, Sivan, Hamsher, Varney, & Spreen, 1994) on a sample of 85 subjects (medical inpatients and normal subjects with no history of brain disease). The subjects ranged in age from 19 to 74 years. There were no significant differences in performance due to age, sex, or education; therefore, no corrections were recommended. Most of the normative sample achieved nearly perfect scores. It should be noted that a later study indicated that in a sample of 184 elderly patients, equally divided between cognitive impaired and nonimpaired classifications, the VFD was correlated with age and education (Nabors, Vangel, & Lichtenberg, 1996). However, even in this sample of heterogeneous subjects, classification rates were similar to those obtained in the original research reported in the manual.

A short form of the VFD has been suggested for use in screening situations both for patients with closed head injury (Iverson, Slick & Smith-Seemiller, 1997b) and for patients with dementia of various etiologies (Iverson, Sherman, & Smith-Seemiller, 1997a). In both instances, there was a fairly high correlation between scores on the short form and scores on the long form and classification of the subjects into impaired and nonimpaired categories results in high concordance rates.

As with the other Benton tests, interpretation is conducted by reference to the normative distribution as well as to the distribution of scores of a sample of impaired individuals. Fifty-eight patients with a diagnosis of lateralized brain dysfunction constituted the sample of impaired individuals. Of these subjects, 19 had right-hemisphere dysfunction, 23 had left-hemisphere impairment including aphasic symptoms, 9 had left-hemisphere impairment but no aphasic symptoms, and 7 had bilateral neurological impairment. Although there is some overlap in the two distributions, none of the normal subjects scored below 23 points, whereas 50% of the neurologically impaired subjects scored in that range. Impaired performance was therefore defined as a score lower than 24 points. When that value was used as a cutoff point, there were no false-positive scores in the original sample, and 53% of the brain-damaged subjects were classified as presenting impaired performance.

With use of the recommended cutoff value, the manual reports a study in which patients classified as presenting defective performance were examined for the impaired sample broken down by laterality of lesion, for anterior or posterior site of lesion, and (for the left-hemisphere subjects) for the presence and absence of aphasic symptoms. When the effects of laterality were investigated, 47% of the left-hemisphere subjects, 58% of the right-hemisphere subjects, and 71% of the bilateral-diffuse subjects were classified as having impaired performance. A higher percentage of left anterior (58%) than left posterior (47%) subjects were classified as impaired. However, the opposite pattern was found in the right-hemisphere subjects: 43% of the anterior subjects and 78% of the posterior subjects were classified as impaired. Left-hemisphere nonaphasic subjects (56%) were more likely to present impaired performance than were left-hemisphere aphasic subjects (43%).

Because no specific information was provided about the etiology or the degree of brain lesion on these subjects, it is difficult to interpret the construct validity of this test. Because the group of bilateral-diffuse subjects had the highest percentage of impaired individuals, it may be that the VFD is sensitive to a wide range of corticobehavioral skills, with a slightly higher loading on right-hemisphere skills. The degree of impairment in the bilateral-diffuse subjects may also reflect sensitivity of the test to impairment in attention and concentration, in which case one would expect closed-head-injury patients to perform poorly. In a sample of 104 children with various neuropsychological diagnoses, the Benton Visual Retention Test (BVRT) loaded on factor related to general visuospatial–motor skills. The VFD is sensitive to the visual–spatial impairment that accompanies even the early stages of Alzheimer's dementia (Becker, Lopez, & Boller, 1995; Kaskie & Storandt, 1995). In addition, Lichtenberg, Millis, and Nanna (1995) found that the VFD was useful in the evaluation of general cognitive impairment in elderly patients. It is likely that the VFD is sensitive to a broad variety of cognitive skill impairments, making it useful in screening situations, but also making it less useful in specifying the nature of the impairment.

The relationship between aphasic symptoms and performance on this test also needs to be better investigated. Varney (1981) reported a relationship between performance on the test and alexia. However, the larger percentage of left-hemisphere nonaphasic individuals with impaired performance and the interaction of laterality with caudality represent areas where further research is needed to explain the results. Research is also needed to determine the different forms of reliability of the test. Visual refractive error impairment may affect performance on this procedure (Kempen et al., 1994) and patients should wear their corrective eyewear.

PANTOMIME RECOGNITION

The Test of Pantomime Recognition grew out of investigations that seemed to show that some aphasic patients demonstrate an impairment in their ability to comprehend the symbolic meaning of activities. There is a long tradition of the conceptualization of aphasia as an impairment in symbolic functions, and this test was devised to allow a partial assessment of the degree to which nonlinguistic symbolic functions may be impaired in aphasics.

The test consists of 30 videotaped pantomimed activities. Although the use of the videoplayer required for this test is cumbersome and expensive, videotapes represent an important advance in the standardization of pantomime assessment techniques. The tape reduces the possibility of variability in the presentation of the stimulus items. The subject is shown the pantomime of an object's use and is then asked to choose the picture of the correct object from among four alternatives. The four alternatives are the correct object, an incorrect object drawn from the same semantic class as the correct choice, an object that would be the correct choice elsewhere in the test, and an object that is not suitable for pantomime. The subject is asked to point to the correct object; thus, the need for a linguistic response is obviated. The test is scored on the basis of the total number of correct answers, as well as the total of the different types of errors (e.g., the number of times an object from the same semantic class is chosen).

The normative information in the manual was derived from a limited sample of 30 hospitalized inpatients who did not show evidence of brain disease. Nearly all of the subjects gave perfect performances, although two of the subjects did make four errors. Data were also collected on 105 aphasic patients. Of these subjects, 30% gave perfect performances or performances with only one error. Altogether, 60% of the aphasic individuals gave performances in the normal range. The performances of the remaining aphasics ranged down to 20 errors. Most of the errors made by the aphasic patients were in choosing objects from the same semantic class as the correct choice. Varney and Benton (1982) found that, in a sample of 40 aphasic patients with impaired performance on this test, 36 made the largest number of their errors in the semantic class.

Although it appears that aphasia plays a role in impaired performance on this test, investigations using neurologically impaired individuals without aphasic symptoms have not been conducted. The only investigation of the construct validity of this test indicates that poor performance on this test in aphasic patients is not related to poor performance on the Block Design subtest of the WAIS.

The Test of Pantomime Recognition appears to have great promise in the clinical setting. However, a much larger normative base is required. There is no information regarding the reliability of the test. More information regarding the diagnostic validity as well as the construct validity is needed before this test can be recommended for unlimited clinical use.

TACTILE FORM PERCEPTION

Tests of sensory impairment have a long history in neuropsychology. However, in many of these tests, the assessment of tactile sensation is confounded with linguistic ability, as in the case of the naming tests or the fingertip letter-drawing tests. Benton's Test of Tactile Form Recognition requires only the skills of tactile-information processing that allow the subject to identify a line drawing of an object that is presented tactilely. Because the stimulus items are cards with geometric designs cut from sandpaper, verbal encoding is not required. However, in the case of the simple figures, such as the star and the circle, linguistic encoding is possible. The subject is told to feel the design on the card, which is kept out of sight. The subject then identifies the object from a card that contains 12 line drawings of the figures. After one form of the test is given to one hand of the subject, the second form is given to the other hand. There is a 30-second limit for each item. Scoring is based on the total number of correct responses for each hand separately and for the two hands together. The manual encourages the examiner to record the response latency but does not provide normative data for these time scores.

The manual (Benton et al., 1983, 1994) states that the two alternate forms are equal in difficulty. The alternate-forms reliability of the two was investigated by administering the two forms to a sample of 56 normal right-handed individuals. The order of the tests was counterbalanced, as was the first use of either the right or the left hand. There were no significant differences due to the form of the test used, the hand used first, or the order of test administration.

Normative information is available from the manual on a sample of 90 normal subjects between the ages of 15 and 70 years. Because performance appeared to decrease with age and with lower levels of education, there are corrections for these variables. Further normative information has been based on data from a group of 25 subjects between the ages of 71 and 80 years. Spreen and Gaddes (1969) presented normative information based on the performance of 404 children between the ages of 8 and 14 years.

Data from a sample of 104 patients with brain dysfunction indicate that brain dysfunction is related to poor performance on this test, especially brain dysfunction that results in motor or sensory impairment. In addition, although left-hemisphere dysfunction can result in poor performance, right-hemisphere dysfunction is more likely to result in poor performance. Bilateral brain dysfunction resulted in the highest percentage of patients with poor performance.

The Test of Tactile Form Recognition appears to be another promising tool in the assessment of spatial functions. However, more information is needed regarding its temporal reliability, its concurrent validity, and the actual construct underlying performance.

FINGER LOCALIZATION

Finger recognition is an important aspect of many different forms of neuropsychological assessment. Behavioral neurologists have long used some form of finger recognition task when assessing clients for parietal lobe damage. The Luria–Nebraska Neuropsychological Battery contains a finger recognition section as part of its assessment of tactile functions. Acknowledging that finger localization may have more than one component skill, Benton's Test of Finger Localization presents the stimuli in three different modalities.

The test consists of 60 items; each of the 10 fingers are touched individually two times in each of the three touches. The first touch allows visual as well as tactile output. The second touch is done without the benefit of visual information. For the remaining 20 items, two fingers are touched simultaneously. In each case, the subject is asked to identify the fingers touched by name, by pointing, or by referring to a chart on which the fingers are assigned numbers.

Normative information is available on a sample of 104 medical inpatients who had no history of brain dysfunction or psychiatric disorder. These subjects ranged in age from 16 to 65 years. Sixty-two of these subjects made two or fewer errors on the test. Of the errors made by these normative subjects, 82% were on simultaneous stimulation. No significant differences were found due to age, sex, or education. The normative scores were converted into percentiles for each hand separately, as well as for the difference between the scores for the two hands.

Normative information has been provided for children based on earlier studies conducted by Benton (1955a,b, 1959) and Wake (1956, 1957, cited in Benton et al., 1983). In all of these cases, the section using simultaneous stimulation consisted of only 5 trials instead of 10. These scores were therefore doubled so that they could be consistently prorated with the adult data. There are also normative data derived from a sample of 61 right-handed individuals with diagnosed brain dysfunction. The ages of these subjects ranged from 18 to 64 years.

Interpretation is suggested on the basis of patterns of scores, including such categories as left and right unilateral impairment, bilateral asymmetrical impairment, and normal performance. There are different relationships between different diagnostic categories and score patterns; however, the safest conclusion regarding poor performance is that the subject has some form of brain impairment. The manual suggests a relationship between finger recognition scores and later reading skills in children; however, this question needs to be more thoroughly addressed.

Data are needed about the different forms of reliability, as is information regarding the validity of the different score patterns. Concurrent-validity and predictive-validity studies also need to be conducted.

PHONEME DISCRIMINATION

The manual describes this test as a brief screening measure for the assessment of phonemic decoding. The test consists of a taped set of sound pairs that the subject is asked to identify as being either the same sounds or different sounds. There are 10 single-syllable pairs and 20 two-syllable pairs, for a total of 30 items. The scoring is based on the number of correct "same" and "different" responses and the number of incorrect "same" and "different" responses. A summary score is obtained from the total number of correct responses.

Normative data are available on the scores attained by 30 inpatients who did not have signs of brain dysfunction. There was no evaluation of the effects of age, sex, or education. There is also information regarding the distribution of the scores attained by 16 nonaphasic patients with right-hemisphere lesions, as well as the distribution of the scores attained by 100 aphasic left-hemisphere-lesioned subjects. Because none of the normal subjects scored lower than 22, that value was chosen as the cutoff point. Only one of the right-hemisphere-lesioned subjects scored lower than the cutoff, but 24% of the left-hemisphere aphasic patients scored lower than the cutoff.

Because oral comprehension skills may be seen to be partially dependent on phonemic discrimination skills, this test holds much promise for the evaluation of subjects with receptive aphasic symptoms. However, more information is needed regarding the different forms of reliability, as is a more complete understanding of the relationship of performance on this test to performance on other tests of receptive language skills.

THREE-DIMENSIONAL BLOCK CONSTRUCTION

Constructional apraxia is assessed in many different ways. Constructional practice skills are components of the Bender–Gestalt Visual Motor Test as well as of the Block Design subtest of the WAIS-R. Benton's test attempts to assess constructional practice skills without the confound of the fine-motor response required in drawing tests, and with a three-dimensional element not found in the Block Design test.

There are two forms of the test, each consisting of three stimuli. For each item, the subject is shown a photograph of a block model and is asked to reconstruct the model from a set of loose blocks. In an investigation of the alternate-forms reliability of this test, the test was administered to 120 subjects who were equally divided among three diagnoses (Benton et al., 1983): one third of the subjects had no evidence of brain impairment, one third of the subjects had evidence of left-hemisphere dysfunction, and the remaining one third had evidence of right-hemisphere dysfunction. These subjects were divided into four groups: one half received Form A and one half received Form B; furthermore, one half received the photographic stimuli and one half received actual models of the designs from which to complete their models. There were no significant differences among the groups. This finding indicates not only that Form A and Form B are equivalent, but also that the photographic-model method is equivalent to the actual-model method of administration.

The scoring is based on the type of errors made by the subject. The errors are classified as omissions, additions, substitutions, or displacements. In addition, the total number of correctly placed blocks is counted, and if the subject takes more than 380 seconds to complete the test, 2 points are subtracted from her or his score.

Normative data for the block model presentation method are available on a sample of 100 medical patients with no evidence of neurological impairment, as well as on a sample of 20 individuals with left-hemisphere dysfunction and a sample of 20 individuals with right-hemisphere dysfunction. Normative data are also available on the same number of similar patients who received the photographic-presentation method.

Normative data for children were taken from Spreen and Gaddes (1969). In this study, the test was administered to 259 children between the ages of 6 and 12 years. These scores were transformed to percentiles for the purpose of interpretation. The children's scores generally increased with age, although there was great variability within age groups. Benton et al. (1983) estimated that, at age 14, the children's performance would approximately equal adult performance.

Validational studies have found that the test is sensitive to brain dysfunction in general (Keller 1971, reported in Benton et al., 1983). Benton (1973) found that, although about 35% of 14 right-hemisphere-lesioned subjects and about 32% of 34 left-hemisphere-lesioned subjects gave impaired performances, there was an interesting relationship of aphasic symptoms to performance. Of the 18 left-hemisphere-lesioned subjects with aphasic symptoms, 59% gave impaired performances. Of the 9 subjects with severe aphasic symptoms, 67% gave impaired performances. This relationship needs to be better elucidated in future research. In addition, reliability information is needed.

MOTOR IMPERSISTENCE

The inability to maintain a motor activity on command has been associated with right-hemisphere disease. However, the relationship is far from clear and is not universally accepted. The Test of Motor Impersistence is an attempt to provide a standardized assessment of the phenomenon. There are eight different tasks in this test, and in each case, the subject is asked to continue the activity until he or she is told to stop. The score is some variant of the time in seconds during which the behavior is persistently engaged in or the number of times the subject ceases to follow the instructions. The tasks range from telling the subject to keep her or his eyes closed (up to a limit of 20 seconds) to instructing the subject to retain central fixation during confrontation testing of visual fields.

Impersistence is scored somewhat differently for each task, and the total score for the test is the number of subtests on which impersistence is demonstrated. Normative data are available on a sample of 106 medical inpatients with no history of brain dysfunction. Based on these data, moderate impersistence is defined as defective performance on two or three subtests, and marked impersistence is defined as defective performance on four or more subtests. Normative data are also available on a sample of 140 normal children between the ages of 5 and 11 years. Because there was great variability in impersistence across the tasks in the child sample, and because the tasks sample such a wide range of motor skills, it is important that the internal consistency reliability of this test be evaluated. Other forms of reliability also need to be evaluated.

Earlier studies investigated the association between brain dysfunction and impersistence, but only the studies that used the Benton test are considered here. Levin (1973) found that 44% of patients with unilateral lesions demonstrated impersistence; however, no hemispheric differences were found. Garfield (1964) found that 68% of a sample of children with brain dysfunction exhibited impersistence on two or more tasks, but that only 3% of a sample of normal children exhibited impersistence on two or more tasks.

Benton, Gaffield, and Chorini (1964) showed that, on each task of the test, mentally retarded children demonstrated a larger degree of impersistence than did normal children, a finding that was supported by Rutter, Graham, and Yule (1970). Garfield, Benton, and MacQueen (1966) compared the performance of retarded children with brain damage to that of retarded children with equivalent IQ scores but without other signs of brain damage; these authors found that the brain-damaged children had a greater degree of impersistence. Domrath (1966) reported that schizophrenics exhibited a greater degree of impersistence than did normals, but a smaller degree than did neurological patients. Impersistence appears to be related to mental impairment, but this relation is unclear, especially in light of the Garfield et al. (1966) study.

Age appears to play a role in performance on this test, and this variable needs to be better investigated. Reliability data would enhance the clinical utility of this instrument, as would a greater understanding of the test's diagnostic validity and its concurrent validity.

THE BENTON VISUAL RETENTION TEST

The Benton Visual Retention Test (BVRT) is perhaps the most famous and most frequently used of all of the assessment procedures that have come out of the Neuropsychological Laboratory at the University of Iowa. Arthur Benton's large contributions to neuropsychological assessment included his approach of adapting laboratory procedures to the purposes of clinical assessment. The BVRT involves several complex cognitive–behavioral skills and is therefore sensitive to organic impairment in these areas: visual motor construction, visual–spatial perception, immediate memory, and visual conceptualization. In addition, because some of the items have verbal referents, the test also taps verbal conceptualization. However, it is not appropriate as an individual screening device.

The BVRT exists in three forms: C, D, and E. These are alternate forms, although there is evidence that Form C is a little less difficult than the other two forms under conditions of immediate recall (Benton, 1974). There are three forms of administration. In Administration A, the subject is shown the stimuli for 10 seconds and is then asked to reproduce them. In Administration B, the subject is shown the stimuli for 10 seconds and is asked to reproduce them after a delay of 5 seconds. In Administration C, the subject is allowed to copy the stimuli directly.

The original manual (Benton, 1974) presents normative data for all three forms and administrations. Although it is not clear which of the alternate forms were used to yield these norms, from the alternate-forms studies it is apparent that each of the forms may be referred to the norms. Performance on the BVRT is positively correlated with IQ and negatively correlated with age. Therefore, the norms are for the expected correct responses and the expected number of errors for each of three adult age groups (15 to 44, 45 to 54, and 55 to 64 years) crossed with each of six IQ groups (corresponding to the diagnostic groups of very defective, defective, borderline, low average, average, and superior). In addition, norms are available for five IQ groups (high average is combined with superior) crossed with the ages of 8, 9, 10, 11, 12, and 13 to 14 years. The revised manual (Sivan, 1992) also contains normative information for children down to kindergarten which is separated by IQ level and age. In addition, the revised manual summarized additional normative information for older adults up to the age of 102 years. Further normative information is available with both age and education corrections (Youngjohn, Larrabee, & Crook, 1993). Giambra, Arenberg, Zonderman, Kawas, and Costa (1995) reported that the age-related changes in performance on the BVRT are especially prominent between the ages of 65 and 74 years. This is consistent with the normative information provided for Indian subjects (Prakash & Bhogle, 1992). Norms have also been developed for Chinese subjects (Tan & Jun, 1992).

Another important consideration is related to potential cultural differences. Manly et al. (1998) reported that there were differences between older Caucasian and African-American subjects on the BVRT even when education was matched. It may be that separate norms are needed for different cultural groups at least in the elderly. These differences may not exist in younger subjects whose experience may be somewhat more homogeneous. Although cross-cultural comparison was not involved, Zappala et al. (1995) reported normative information related to the performance of 701 healthy Italian subjects between the ages of 20 and 79 years. Nielsen, Lolk, and Kragh–Sorensen (1995) reported normative information derived on a sample of 130 Danish subjects between the ages of 64 and 83 years. Normative data are available for elderly Japanese subjects (Shichita, Hatano, Ohashi, Shibata, & Matuzaki, 1986).

There may be an interaction between type of error and age. Resnick, Trotman, Kawas, and Zonderman (1995) reported that although woman tend to make more omission errors, men show a steeper rate of increase with age.

The norms for Administration B were generated from the performance of 103 medical patients who had no history of brain disease and who were between the ages of 16 and 60 years. On the basis of these data, the manual proposes that subtracting the number 1 from the normative scores for Administration A will provide norms for Administration B.

Norms for Administration C were derived from the test protocols of 200 medical patients with no history of brain disease. The children's norms for Administration C were obtained from the performance of 236 schoolchildren between the ages of 6 years, 6 months and 13 years, 5 months. All of these children had IQ scores between 85 and 115. In addition, norms were obtained from a group of 79 children in the same age groups who had IQ scores higher than 115. Norms are not available for more detailed divisions by IQ value. There is no normative information for Administration D.

There is yet another alternate form of the BVRT. Form 1 is an attempt to remove the motor component of the BVRT to assess a more purely visual skill. In this form, the subject is asked to pick out the original form from a series of four alternatives (Benton, 1950; Benton, Hamsher, & Stone, 1977). Unfortunately, this form of the test may be solved by a logical strategy not related to visual memory. Blanton and Gouvier (1985) pointed out that, by simply picking the alternative that does not have the characteristics shared by the other three, one can answer all items correctly even if one has not seen the original stimulus. Therefore, when this form is used, the examiner should interview the subject afterward to see if the logical strategy was used.

Reliability

The Benton (1974) provides an estimate of the test–retest reliability of Administration A based on the equivalent-forms reliability coefficient. This value is .85, and it appears to overestimate, according to the values reported by Lezak (1982). Lezak administered Forms C and E to a small group of normal males on three occasions. The intertest intervals varied from 6 months to 1 year, and not all of the subjects received each administration. For Form E, the correlation between the first and second occasions was .50. Between the first and third occasions, the correlation was .79. For Form C, the value of the correlation between the first and second occasions was .58. Between the first and third occasions, the correlation was .60. Because Lezak (1982) did not report which administration was used, it is difficult to interpret these data. However, it does appear that the values reported in the manual may overestimate the actual value. Brasfield (1971) reported a correlation coefficient of .75 when Administration C was given twice to a group of 194 kindergarten children, with an interval of 4 months.

Wahler (1956) investigated the interscorer reliability and reported that, for Form C, interscorer agreement for the total number of errors was .95. Egeland, Rice, and Penny (1967) found that in a group of three raters, the average interscorer reliability coefficient for Form A was .94 for the Total Error score and .90 for the Total Number Correct. Similar values were found in a sample of healthy elderly (Swan, Morrison, & Eslinger, 1990) and in a sample of depressed individuals (Engelsmann, Katz, Gharidian, & Schacter, 1988).

Alternate-forms reliability has been more extensively evaluated. When the BVRT is given under Administration A, Forms D and E appear to be easier than Form C (Breidt, 1970). However, for normal children, under Administration C, Form D appears to be easier than Form C (Benson, Spreen, Fangman, & Carr, 1967). For mentally retarded children, there appear to be no differences among the forms (Brown & Rice, 1967). Although there are moderately high correlations between the different administrations of the same form, the correlations between the different administrations of the different forms tend to be low (Breidt, 1970).

Validity

The concurrent validity of the BVRT was examined by correlating the performance of 100 neurologically impaired patients on Administration C of the BVRT with their performance on a three-dimensional block-construction test, a stick-construction test, and the WAIS Block Design subtest. The BVRT was found to be related to the construction tasks, but less than the construction tasks were related to each other (Benton, 1967). In the same study described under Reliability, Breidt (1970) correlated the BVRT with various subtests of the WAIS and reported that the higher correlations were obtained with the visual–spatial subtests of the WAIS.

Discriminative validity was examined by giving Administration A to a group of normal, organically impaired, depressed, and schizophrenic subjects. Only the difference between the normal subjects and the depressed subjects was statistically significant, although the normal subjects performed better than each of the clinical groups (Velborsky, 1964). Cronholm and Schalling (1963) reported that the BVRT was able to discriminate between subjects with focal brain injury and normal subjects even when the influence of IQ was statistically partialed out. Watson (1968) reported that the BVRT was able to discriminate between schizophrenic and organically impaired subjects when neither the Bender–Gestalt nor the Memory for Designs was able to do so. Marsh and Hirsch (1982) reported that, in a sample of 100 neurological patients, the BVRT was able to correctly classify more of the subjects as impaired than was the Memory for Designs. However, the results of this investigation cannot be interpreted strongly because of the lack of a control group and the high base rate (100%) of impairment. Crockett, Clark, Browning, and MacDonald (1983) found that a background interference procedure, such as that used for the Bender–Gestalt, increased the discriminative ability of the BVRT in separating psychiatric subjects from brain-damaged subjects. These authors stated that they used Form C, but they did not specify which administration was used. The different administration forms may have different constructs. Rasmusson, Carson, Brookmeyer, Kawas, and Brandt (1996) reported that better scores on the delayed reproduction form of the BVRT are associated with rapid decline in Alzheimer's dementia whereas worse scores on the copy condition of the BVRT are associated with rapid decline. The BVRT loaded on more than one factor related to everyday memory indicating that the underlying construct may be multifactorial (Tomer, Larrabee, & Crook, 1994). In addition, the BVRT may be related to some aspects of personality functioning (Kirkcaldy, 1987), a point that warrants further investigation.

Benton (1967, 1968) investigated the construct validity of the BVRT and reported that poor performance was associated with lesions in the right hemisphere. Nehil, Agathon, Greif, Delagrange, and Rondepierre (1965) reported that performance on the BVRT was associated with diagnoses as determined by EEG tracings. The manual (Benton, 1974) also suggests interpretations of qualitative aspects of performance that had been validated by Poitrenaud and Barrere (1972). However, cross-validation of these results is necessary. Silverstein (1962, 1963) concluded that there was a complexity of factors involved in performance on the BVRT, at least for mentally retarded subjects. Larrabee et al. (1985a) investigated the construct validity of the BVRT by factor-analyzing the data from 102 subjects. The variables included in the analysis were the Wechsler Memory Scale (WMS) Logical Memory Score, Paired Associates, Visual Reproduction, Administration A of Form C of the BVRT, and the two-factor scales of the Luria–Nebraska Neuropsychological Battery. Two factor analyses were conducted, one using the immediate recall administration of the WMS and the second using the delayed recall of the WMS. In both cases, the BVRT loaded more heavily on a visual–perceptual motor factor and secondarily on the memory factor. A factor analysis of test data in alcoholic subjects indicated that the BVRT loaded on a visual–spatial factor in which the Block design loaded an almost equivalent amount (Bobic, Pavicevic, & Drenovac, 1997).

Moses (1986b) performed a factor analysis of the BVRT, the BVRT Multiple Choice Form, the Benton Visual Form Discrimination test, Digit Span, and the Rey Auditory–Verbal Learning Test in a sample of 97 VA neuropsychiatric patients. The copying and recall procedures emerged as separate factors, but the BVRT was found to have a significant loading on factors interpreted as being verbal. These results were replicated by the same researcher (Moses, 1989). The exact construct measured by the BVRT needs to be specified.

In a sample of learning disabled and normal children a factor analysis of the BVRT resulted in a significant loading on a factor reflecting visual memory and processing, supporting the construct validity of the BVRT in this population (Williams & Dykman, 1994).

The BVRT is sensitive to the effects of substance abuse in Arabic subjects (Amir & Bahri, 1994) Robinson-Whelan (1992) reported that although the BVRT summary scores can separate healthy from demented older individuals, the qualitative scores do not separate as well. Vakil, Blachstein, Sheleff, and Grossman (1989) reported that using the immediate reproduction administration of the BVRT can identify general neurological impairment, but using the delayed reproduction administration can also separate right-hemisphere-lesioned from left-hemisphere-lesioned subjects with the right-hemisphere subjects performing more poorly. Other data suggest that, at least for subjects with multiple sclerosis, performance on the BVRT is more highly associated with diffuse brain damage than with localized lesions.

There is a set of information regarding the BVRT that had been unique in the area of clinical neuropsychological assessment; it regards subterfuge and dissimulation (see chapter on measures of malingering). This is a problem faced by clinical neuropsychologists who work in a forensic setting or who must evaluate individuals who might be motivated to manipulate the data. Benton and Spreen (1961) compared the performance of 48 subjects with moderate and severe neurological impairment with 47 college students and 23 medical inpatients with no history of neurological impairment. The neurologically impaired subjects were given Administration A of Form C under normal conditions. The normal subjects were first given Administration A of Form E under normal instructions and were then given Form C with instructions to perform as if they had moderate brain damage from a car accident 3 months before. The simulators exhibited more errors overall than did the real neurologically impaired subjects. Qualitatively, the simulators gave more distortions, fewer perseverations, and fewer omissions than did the neurologically impaired subjects. Spreen and Benton (1963) followed this finding with a study of the performance of subjects who were instructed to simulate moderately low IQ (the mind of a 10-year-old). The same design as above was used, with similar quantitative and qualitative results. Therefore, the BVRT is one of the few neuropsychological tests for which patterns of dissimulation are known.

THE SENTENCE REPETITION TEST

The Sentence Repetition Test (Spreen & Benton, 1963) is a series of sentences that increase by single-syllable increments, resulting in a final sentence of 26 syllables. The subject is asked to repeat the sentence. The score on this test is the number of syllables in the final sentence that has been accurately repeated. Spreen and Gaddes (1969) presented norms for the test for children aged 6 to 13 years. Carmichael and MacDonald (1984) subsequently published norms for children between the ages of 3 and 13 years, using a much larger sample than was used in Spreen and Gaddes (1969). This test has also been used as part of the Multilingual Aphasia Examination. Hinshaw, Carte, and Morrison (1986) administered the Sentence Repetition Test to a sample of 74 children who had been diagnosed as reading disabled. The subjects were divided by median split into a group aged 6.5 to 8.5 years and a group aged 8.5 to 11 years. All of the subjects had an IQ of at least 80 and a difference between IQ and standardized reading scores of .6 standard deviations. There was no relationship between performance on the Sentence Repetition Test and performance on either the Reading Comprehension scale of the WRAT-R or the Gates–MacGinitie reading test. This finding indicates that the Sentence Repetition Test may not be related to academic aspects of reading. Relatively little is known about the reliability and validity of the Sentence Repetition Test, although Davis, Foldi, Gardner, and Zurif (1978) presented some data that suggest that the test may be useful in the diagnosis of transcortical aphasia.

The Minnesota Multiphasic Personality Inventory and Personality Assessment Inventory

The Minnesota Multiphasic Personality Inventory (MMPI) and its revision the MMPI-2 have been the subjects of well over 10,000 published studies investigating their use and properties. There are many summary studies of validity and reliability issues (Cottle, 1950; Dahlstrom & Welsh, 1960; Dahlstrom, Welsh, & Dahlstrom, 1975; Gravitz & Gerton, 1976; Hathaway & McKinley, 1942; Hathaway & Meehl, 1951; Holzberg & Alessi, 1949; Horn, Wanberg, & Appel, 1973; Johnson, Klingler, & Williams, 1977; Kroger & Turnbull, 1975; McKinley & Hathaway, 1942, 1944; Mehlman & Rand, 1960; Ritter, 1974), including meta-analytic studies (Atkinson, 1986; Hiller, Rosenthal, Bornstein, Berry, & Brunell-Neulieb, 1999; Parker, Hanson, & Hunsley, 1988). Although the MMPI is one of the most frequently used and researched instruments, psychometric weaknesses have been identified such as those discussed in David Rogers' review of the original MMPI in *The Seventh Mental Measurements Yearbook* (1972).

The focus of the present review is on evaluating the existing literature regarding the use of the MMPI in neuropsychological assessment as well as to review literature regarding other constructs such as dissimulation, substance abuse, and psychological diagnoses when these are potentially at question in neuropsychological assessment. Interpretation research in general is also reviewed. Specifically, the MMPI has been used by researchers as an objective measure of personality for the purpose of delineating the relationship between brain function and personality. Four general research approaches have been used in this endeavor. In the first approach, a localizationalist approach is used in an attempt to relate differences in personality (as demonstrated on the MMPI) to specific areas of brain dysfunction. With the MMPI-2, this approach has taken the form of trying to identify MMPI profiles associated with specific disorders, such as cerebrovascular accident (CVA) patients or head injury patients. The second research approach attempts to differentiate neurologically impaired subjects from some other group of subjects (e.g., schizophrenics) by identifying the differences in their response patterns. The third research approach uses deficits on neuropsychological tests as a means of defining group inclusion. Those subjects whose performance falls at the brain-damaged level are compared for personality differences on the MMPI. The fourth design involves the use of correction factors for the overlap of neurological symptoms with psychiatric symptoms. Yet another use of the MMPI, primarily the MMPI-2, is to identify those subjects whose neuropsychological test performance is influenced by psychological factors, especially by response bias characteristics.

The MMPI lends itself to research of this type on theoretical grounds and on the basis of the nature of its test items and its scale composition. For example, as Lezak and Glaudin (1969) noted, among the 51 items of the 357 scored items on a short form of the MMPI (omitting scale Si and all items normally not scored) that are referable to symptoms of physical disease, 26 relate to central nervous system diseases and 8 describe problems associated with being ill. Many of the "neurological symptom" items have double and triple MMPI scale loadings.

With the advent of the MMPI-2, one might expect that use of the MMPI would decline. While a decline may certainly be present, the MMPI is still marketed by its publisher, and is still in current use. There are several reasons for this dual usage. First, the MMPI has been available and in near universal use for nearly 40 years; old habits are the hardest to break. Second, the amount of research available to inform the interpretation of the MMPI is quantitatively superior to that of the MMPI-2, although this will certainly change. Third, initial research indicates that although there are substantial similarities between the MMPI and the MMPI-2, there are also substantial differences, such as in the concordance of 2-point codes. Some clinicians may feel more confident using the earlier version. Therefore, this chapter includes discussion of both versions of the MMPI.

MMPI

Reliability

Although there has been research on the development of new scales to assess neuropsychological impairment by recombining items, there have been no investigations regarding the forms of reliability of these new scales. However, because some of the research has concerned the use of the clinical scales of the MMPI, the reliability investigations for the clinical scales are relevant here. It must be noted that none of these studies involved individuals with organic brain impairment. Dahlstrom et al. (1975) collected data from different studies into a data base related to the reliability of the MMPI scales. Many of the reliability studies were conducted on college students. In a study using 288 male and 33 female college students, the test–retest reliability coefficients with a 1-day interval ranged from .97 for the F Scale for males to .71 for Scale 6 for females. In a sample of 42 college males and 55 college females, and with test–retest intervals of 1 to 2 weeks, the reliability coefficients ranged from .49 for Scale 6 in males to .92 for both the K Scale and Scale 7 in the females. Internal-consistency reliability coefficients ranged from $-.05$ for Scale 1 in 97 college students to .90 for Scale 1 in 220 VA patients. In certain code types (Spike 4, 2–4/4–2, 2–7/7–2, and 6–8/8–6), there is remarkable stability of both validity scales and clinical scales across a 40-year period (Greene, 1990).

Hunsley, Hanson, and Parker (1988) reviewed the reliability research and concluded that individual scales have acceptable stability and internal consistency. The Spanish translation of the MMPI has parallel temporal reliability (Traub & Bohn, 1985). The high-point, 2-point, and 3-point codes of the MMPI have low temporal consistency, but it is unclear as to whether this is related to instability of the instrument or behavioral change in the subjects (Graham, Smith, & Schwartz, 1986).

Validity

Localizationalist Paradigm

As noted previously, researchers have speculated on the relationship between personality changes and the location of the cerebral insult. Anderson and Hanvik (1950), for example, attempted to characterize the differences between patients with parietal lobe damage and those with frontal lobe damage, but there were no tests for statistical significance of the differences between groups. In addition, the groups were not pure, as the parietal group contained subjects with damage to the temporal and occipital lobes.

Friedman (1950) developed a 132-item parietal–frontal (PF) scale with reasonable success (Dahlstrom & Welsh, 1960). Williams (1952) constructed a similar scale, the Caudality (Ca) scale, in which 40% of Friedman's scale was reproduced. Williams's 36-item scale was reported to significantly differentiate patients with parietal and temporal lesions, as a group, from those with frontal lesions (Dahlstrom & Welsh, 1960; Meier, 1969). Reitan (1976), however, reported that later research did not support these earlier findings.

Black (1975) and Templer and Connolly (1976) attempted to separate the associated personality variables within a laterally dichotomized (left- vs. right-hemisphere) brain-damaged population. In Black's study, for example, differential effects were found in the two groups. On the F, K, D, Pa, Sc, and Si scales, the left-hemisphere-damaged subjects scored significantly higher ($p < .05$) than did the right-hemisphere-damaged subjects and had greater cognitive and neurosensory deficits.

Using the lesion localization paradigm, Vogel (1962) attempted a global study of effects on the MMPI. Vogel (1962) investigated whether left-hemisphere-lesioned subjects would show a more pathological profile than right-hemisphere-lesioned subjects, and whether subjects with parietal and temporal lobe damage would show a more pathological profile than those with frontal lobe damage. The overall index of MMPI pathology was operationalized as the number of scales greater than 70. The study results did not support the original hypotheses. Dikmen and Reitan (1974b) failed to demonstrate personality changes as a result of medically conclusive locations of brain damage along rostrocaudal as well as lateral dimensions. These investigators concluded that the MMPI was a poor measure of personality changes when groups were derived according to the location of brain damage, but it might also be that reliable changes in personality secondary to localizable injury are minor compared to individual variation in psychological response. In a study using subjects with mixed organic diagnoses (Flick & Edwards, 1971) and in a study of patients with temporal lobe epilepsy (Meier & French, 1965), similar negative results were reported. Consistent with the foregoing discussion, Lezak (1995) described lateralization research results as being equivocal.

In summary, little reproducible evidence has been generated by the localizationalist approach to the study of brain–personality relationships. The problem may be related to the different effects of lesions even within the same broad area of the brain because of differences in their etiology, the time since onset, the medical treatments, their pressure effects, and their exact location (Luria, 1966; Reitan, 1966). Finally, observed personality differences may relate more to differences in the behavioral deficits suffered by individuals than to the area of the damage.

Differential Performance Paradigm

The second approach taken to delineate the personality patterns characteristic of brain damage is to compare the performance of brain-injured subjects with that of nonneurologically impaired subjects to identify differentiating scales or items on the MMPI. Studies have included investigations of the MMPI scores of patients diagnosed with multiple sclerosis (Dahlstrom & Welsh, 1960; Gilberstadt & Farkas, 1961; Schwartz & Brown, 1973), epilepsy (Klove & Doehring, 1962; Kristianson, 1974; Matthews, Dikmen, & Harley, 1977; Meier, 1969; Small, Milstein, & Stevens, 1962; Stein, 1972), Huntington's disease (Boll, Heaton, & Reitan, 1974; Norton, 1975), and Guillain–Barré syndrome (Sziraki, 1978). Similarly, traumatically brain-injured subjects have been compared with normals (Hovey, 1964), neurotics (Reitan, 1955a), schizophrenics (Ayers, Templer, & Ruff, 1975; Holland, Lowenfeld, & Wadsworth, 1975a; Markowitz, 1973; Neuringer, Dombrowski, & Goldstein, 1975; Russell, 1977; Watson, 1971), and psychiatric patients in general (Shaw & Matthews, 1965).

The MMPI has been found to differentiate between organically impaired and psychiatric or normal subjects (Matthews et al., 1966; Reitan, 1955a; Watson & Thomas, 1968), but no profile unique to one group has emerged. For example, in the study by Reitan (1955a), a heterogeneous brain-damaged group scored higher on the F, Pa, Pt, Sc, and Ma scales of the MMPI than did the control group. The experimental subjects varied according to the type, extent, and location of the brain lesion and were matched for sex, age, and education with members of a control group that contained normal and neurotic subjects with no known brain damage. The experimental group yielded a wide range of personality profiles.

In contrast to the Reitan study, Watson and Thomas (1968) compared neurological patients with schizophrenic patients on the 10 MMPI scales and found significant differences on the Hs, D, Mf, Pt, Sc, and Si. Four decision rules were developed (a strategy to be discussed in detail later) that yielded a 69% correct classification. Three validation studies yielded classification rates of 71%, 79%, and 45%. Norton and Romano (1977) conducted a cross-validation study of the Watson–Thomas rules on a sample of 14 neurological patients, 14 alcoholic patients, 14 married schizophrenic patients, 14 unmarried schizophrenic patients, and 14 patients with mixed psychiatric diagnosis who lacked neurological symptoms. These authors reported generally good levels of accuracy of classification for all except the unmarried schizophrenic patients. However, the accuracy of their classification rates may have been inflated by their use of "pure" cases and by the use of equal frequencies of subjects in all groups. The most consistent finding in these studies, aside from being unable to generate a common patient profile, was that the Sc scale can differentiate psychotic patients from organically impaired patients (e.g., Russell, 1977).

The second approach to diagnosis with the MMPI has been to establish organicity scales that can discriminate between experimental and control groups (Hovey, 1964; Shaw & Matthews, 1965; Watson, 1971; Watson & Plemel, 1978). The results of these studies have been highly variable, because of the use of populations that varied widely in severity, chronicity, type of injury, age, education, and duration of hospitalization (Ayers et al., 1975; Holland et al., 1975a; Neuringer et al., 1975; Pantano & Schwartz, 1978; Ruff, Ayers, & Templer, 1977; Russell, 1977; Sand, 1973; Siskind, 1976; Upper & Seeman, 1966; Zimmerman, 1965). Few studies have attempted to compare any combination of these scales on a single population to eliminate much of the interpretive problem in the current literature.

In the Hovey (1964) study the five items were chosen from the MMPI that appeared to be most able to discriminate brain-injured patients and controls. Items 10, 51, 192, and 274 are marked false, and Item 159 is marked true. The cutoff score for organicity is 4. Hovey recommended that, to minimize the possibility of false-positive errors, this scale be used only when the K-scale raw score is 8 or above. Using these five items, Hovey correctly classified 50% of the brain-damaged subjects; there was a 9% to 18% misclassification rate of the normal subjects. Upper and Seeman (1966) cross-validated Hovey's scale using a non-brain-damaged schizophrenic control group and found similar differences between groups. Overall, however, the Hovey five-item scale has met with only limited success. This scale was found to be ineffective in discriminating patients with organic impairment from groups of organically intact patients with functional disorders (Dodge & Kolstoe, 1971; Maier & Abidin, 1967; Schwartz & Brown, 1973), schizophrenic patients (Watson, 1971), and normal control subjects (Weingold, Dawson, & Kael, 1965). A classification of chronic alcoholic patients by the Hovey scale was not found to bear any systematic relationship to cognitive indices of organic impairment (Chaney, Erickson, & O'Leary, 1977). Jortner (1965) also reported a failure to replicate Hovey's results.

Watson (1971) abandoned his attempt to develop a profile indicative of neuropsychological impairment in favor of developing a new MMPI scale, the Schizophrenia-Organicity (Sc-O) scale, for differentiating brain-damaged patients from schizophrenic patients. Eighty items were initially identified and combined to form the scale. Two other scales were derived from the original 80 items by first weighting all of the items according to their power of discrimination, and then by weighting only the 30 most powerful items. Using these scales, Watson reported 85% accuracy; on cross-validation with a similar patient population, the scale yielded 76% accuracy. However, there were later failures in attempts to cross-validate the findings (Halperin, Neuringer, Davis, and Goldstein, 1977; Holland et al., 1975a).

Watson (1973) noted that the Sc-O Scale does not separate nonschizophrenic functional groups from organically impaired groups. Therefore, he developed the Psychiatric-Organic (P-O) Scale. This scale consists of 56 items that were found to differentiate 40 brain-damaged subjects from a group of 60 psychiatric patients (all subjects were male veterans). The group of functionally disordered patients consisted mostly of alcoholics (35). The P-O scale correlates positively with age (R = .30). The internal consistency of the scale, as reported by Watson and Plemel (1978), was .90 for the organics, and only .68 for the control. Additional research is needed before one can use this scale with additional populations.

Shaw and Matthews (1965) also addressed the problem of differentiating between organic and psychiatric deficits by developing a neurological impairment scale—with two important differences. Here, the subject-sampling procedure included "pseudoneurological" patients who were diagnosed as being psychiatric patients but who also manifested "soft" neurological symptoms. This study also differed in the procedure it used to identify the items to be included in the scale: 17 items, 5 of which are marked true (38, 47, 108, 238, and 253) and 12 of which are marked false (3, 8, 68, 171, 173, 175, 188, 190, 230, 237, 238, and 243), were chosen from only those scales that, as a whole, differentiated between the two groups (Hy, Hs, and Pt). Items on other scales that may or may not have differentiated between the groups were excluded from analysis. A cutoff score of 7 was established for the scale.

Originally, an accuracy of 78% was reported. A cross-validation sample yielded 73% correct classifications, with misclassifications 33% of the time in the psychiatric group and 22% of the time in the neurological group. Again, the scale failed to meet the criterion normally expected of a clinical diagnostic device.

The final strategy within this research design entails the use of the MMPI in the development of decision rules for diagnosing organicity. In this approach, an algorithm or decision tree with a hierarchy of rules is used to differentiate the diagnostic categories. Major systems of this type have been proposed by Watson and Thomas (1968) and Russell (1975b, 1977). Limited success has been reported for these approaches. For example, in a study of 20 brain-damaged, 21 schizophrenic, and 24 clinically depressed subjects, Trifiletti (1982) found that Russell's MMPI key correctly identified 85% of the brain-damaged subjects and 0% of the schizophrenics, and only 33% of the depressed subjects; the overall hit rate was 68%. Overall, it must be concluded that additional cross-validation is needed for decision-tree-algorithm approach to the differential diagnosis of organicity.

Golden, Sweet, and Osmon (1979) compared each of the above approaches in their study of a single population consisting of 30 schizophrenic, 30 brain-injured, and 30 hospitalized normal patients. Their results indicated that the most effective diagnostic device was the use of the Sc scale alone or in conjunction with the remaining clinical scales and the F scale. The result of this study does not support the existence of a unique organic profile. The study does support the effectiveness of the Sc and Pa scales in the diagnosis of brain damage. These results were identical to those reported by Russell (1977). These findings suggest that the greater the degree of psychosis present, the less likely is the presence of an organic brain syndrome. However, as noted by Golden et al. (1979), even this limited conclusion is questionable. The Golden et al. (1979) study did not include individuals with brain damage who were also psychotic. It is likely that such a group would show high elevations on the Sc, Pa, and other MMPI scales equal to those shown by the schizophrenic group without brain damage. Thus, when a diagnosis of organic brain syndrome with psychosis is considered, even the presence of psychosis cannot rule out the presence of brain damage.

Although the second research design (differentiating groups by their performance on the MMPI) shows that personality differences do exist between brain-damaged and non-brain-damaged psychopathological groups, it has been unable to produce clinically useful diagnostic devices, with large differences found among brain-injured subjects (Reitan, 1955a).

The difficulty of cross-validating research in this area may also be attributable to the fact that those general pattern tendencies that characterize the responses of the neurologically impaired subject may only be an artifact of the test items and the scale composition of the MMPI. For example, a confounding factor in research of this type is that many of the "neurological symptom" items appear on the Sc scale, and many have double and triple scale loadings, particularly on scales Hs, D, and Hy. As a result, nonpsychiatric patients with central nervous system disease tend to have an elevated "neurotic triad" (Hs, D, and Hy) (Dikmen & Reitan, 1974b) and higher-than-average Sc scores. Pt is also among the scales most likely to be elevated in an organic population (Mack, 1979). Schwartz (1969) examined both the 1–3–9 and the 2–9 profiles in a sample of 50,000 consecutive medical outpatients. Using the 1–3–9 rules resulted in a sample of 24 subjects. Using the 2–9 rules resulted in a sample of 23 subjects. There were no differences in the independently determined degree of organic impairment between these subjects and control subjects with 1–3/3–1 profiles who were matched for age, sex, and date of clinic appointment. In addition, only one of the 1–3–9 subjects and five of the 2–9 subjects had been diagnosed as organically impaired. These results seriously question the accuracy of the rules.

The 2–9 and 1–3–9 scale elevations once thought to represent organic patterns have not been validated (Russell, 1977). However, Casey and Fennell (1981) reported elevations on Scales 2, 8, and 1 that characterized the MMPI profiles of traumatically injured patients: Heaton et al. (1978) also observed that head-injured patients tended to have elevated scores on Scales 2 and 8. In general, elevated MMPI profiles tend to be common among brain-damaged populations, a finding reflecting the relatively frequent incidence of emotional disturbance in these patients (Filskov & Leli, 1981). The tendency of Sc to be one of the highest scales has been noted for epileptic patients (Klove & Doehring, 1962; Meier, 1969). High scores on the neurotic triad have characterized the MMPI profiles of patients with multiple sclerosis (Dahlstrom & Welsh, 1960). Huntington's disease patients, too, have abnormally high score profiles, but these profiles are indistinguishable from the profile pattern of heterogeneous groups of brain-damaged patients (Boll et al., 1974; Norton, 1975).

Thus, for brain-damaged patients, acknowledgment of specific symptoms accounts for some of the elevation of specific scales. Premorbid personality tendencies and the patient's reactions to his or her disabilities also contribute to the MMPI profile. The combination of the symptom description, the anxiety and distress occasioned by central nervous system defects, and the need for adaptive psychological measures probably accounts for the frequency with which brain-damaged patients produce neurotic profiles.

Neuropsychological Functioning as a Means of Defining Group Inclusion

The third paradigm was developed in response to the failure of the first two approaches. This paradigm assumes that behavioral deficits specifically related to a brain lesion can be used to create more exact definitions of brain-injured groups, and therefore to make more homogeneous samples possible. As a result, a group with similar behavioral deficits can be identified. In such groupings, one need not presuppose an all-encompassing personality profile of brain damage.

In an early study by Doehring and Reitan (1960), behavioral deficits were used to define three groups of diagnoses: brain-damaged aphasic dysfunction, brain-damaged nonaphasic dysfunction, and intact neurosis, but no significant differences were found for the MMPI scales.

It was later suggested by Dikmen and Reitan (1974a) that the failure of the Doehring and Reitan (1960) study to find personality differences between the three groups was probably due to the heterogeneity of the personality deficits in the neurotic group, which masked any intergroup differences that might have existed and to the method of data analysis. When the neurotic group was eliminated and the data were reanalyzed using t ratios, significant differences on the Pd and Sc scales were found between the two brain-damaged groups.

In a similar study, Dikmen and Reitan (1974a) successfully demonstrated personality differences within a brain-damaged population by assigning their subjects to brain-damaged aphasic and brain-damaged nonaphasic groups. These subjects were matched for age, education, and type (but not location) of lesion. The dependent variables were the regular MMPI clinical and validity scales, as well as six additional indices created from combinations of the scales.

A discriminant analysis found significant multivariate differences in MMPI profiles. An analysis of the individual scales using the student's t test yielded a significant difference on the Pd and Sc scales. The groups were similar on the neurotic triad scales (Hy, D, and Hs); however, the aphasic group had substantial elevations relative to the nonaphasic group on the psychotic scales (Pd, Pt, and Sc); only the Sc scale achieved statistical significance. No significant differences between the groups were found with the six derived scales, although the scores were somewhat higher for the aphasic group on the indices for anxiety, psychosis, cognitive slippage, and acting-out impulsiveness.

From these results, one can conclude that, among those who are brain damaged, there is considerable variation of personality patterns. Dikmen and Reitan (1974a) demonstrated with the Welsh (1956) composite profile code that the aphasic group peaked on Sc scales, whereas the nonaphasic group yielded a more normal profile. Furthermore, Dikmen and Reitan (1974a) concluded that, in studies of the effects of brain injury on personality, behavioral deficit identification may more efficiently define groups than locus of injury.

As noted earlier, the results of the Dikmen and Reitan (1974a) study suggest that the behavioral deficits of the individual may be more important to personality than is the location of the lesion that is responsible for the deficits. Osmon and Golden (1978) hypothesized that, if this is true, one would expect patients with different patterns of impairment to demonstrate different personality structures. In a study of 50 subjects with medically verified brain lesions, Osmon and Golden investigated the relationship between various neuropsychological deficits and patterns of personality variables. This study attempted to examine how behavioral deficits are related both to individual personality variables and to patterns of personality variables. Whereas the Dikmen and Reitan (1974a) study revealed that different individual personality variables, as well as profiles, exist within a brain-damaged population, the Osmon and Golden (1978) study attempted to extend this earlier research on aphasic and nonaphasic symptomatology to an investigation of the role of other major cognitive processes, such as sensory perception, concept formation, cognitive interference, concentration, planning, learning, and memory. This study also investigated the effect of behavioral deficits other than aphasia on personality variables.

The relationship between the subjects' responses on the MMPI and their performance on a selected battery of tests taken from the Halstead–Reitan Neuropsychological Battery was evaluated. Although a relative lack of individual relationships was found between cognitive and personality variables, strong predictive relationships between the MMPI and the presence or absence of neuropsychological deficit were obtained. Hit rates of 78% to 86% were reported.

Erlandson, Osmon, and Golden (1981) investigated further the relationship between brain function and personality by extending both the Dikmen and Reitan (1977) and the Osmon and Golden (1978) studies to a psychiatric population. The neuropsychological instrument used in this study was the Luria–Nebraska Neuropsychological Battery. Using a population of 73 schizophrenic subjects with medically verified brain damage, Erlandson et al. found, with the exception of the F scale, a relative lack of individual relationships between the cognitive and the personality variables. Relatively strong correlations, however, were found between neuropsychological performance and overall patterns of personality variables for 11 of the 14 neuropsychological variables. The traditional personality differences associated with lesion laterality were replicated. In a sophisticated approach to this issue, Gass and Ansley (1994) reported that verbal impairment on the Halstead–Reitan Neuropsychological Battery (HRNB) was associated with the F and Hy scales and that sensorimotor deficits were associated with scores on the Pt scale in left-hemisphere CVA patients but not right-hemisphere patients.

These findings suggest that the relationship between personality and neuropsychological functions is not a simple one-to-one relationship. Instead, each neuropsychological deficit may be associated with a complex personality change that can be investigated only by use of all of the MMPI scales. One could conclude that intellectual deficits underlie the overall personality changes associated with brain damage.

The results of the Erlandson et al. (1981) and the Osmon and Golden studies are consistent with the discriminant analysis results in Dikmen and Reitan (1974a, 1977). Again, these results pointed out the necessity of looking at the overall personality pattern rather than the simple relationship of individual neuropsychological deficits to individual personality variables. Individual neuropsychological deficits can be associated with personality profiles when the entire MMPI pattern is taken into account. A future avenue of research would be to examine the relationship of sets of neuropsychological variables to the set of MMPI variables.

Several limitations of these studies should be pointed out. These studies were conducted with relatively small ratios of subjects to predictors. These circumstances can result in unstable least-squares solutions, limiting the generalizability of the results. Cross-validation is a necessary precondition before reasonable conclusions can be reached. Also, because of the correlational nature of the designs, we cannot make causative, etiological statements regarding the role of the neuropsychological deficits in producing the MMPI patterns. We do not even know if the MMPI profiles represent a change or stable functioning. The use of this particular multivariate methodology limits the clinical utility of the results.

As for any proposed typology, there are some exceptions. In the present case, there are at least two studies that do not fit neatly into the tripartite division we have proposed. These two studies examined the amount of variance shared by MMPI information and evaluations of neuropsychological functioning. This correlational design does not fit into any of the three paradigms, but its logic pervades each of them. The logic posits a relationship between neuropsychological functioning and relatively stable patterns of behavioral functioning.

To investigate this premise, Wiens and Matarazzo (1977) administered the HRNB, the MMPI, the Cornell Medical Index, and the Taylor Manifest Anxiety Scale to two separate samples of healthy, normal young males. Each sample contained 24 individuals, and the second sample was used as a cross-validation sample for the first. There were no significant correlations between any of the Halstead–Reitan variables and any of the personality variables. Because normal individuals were tested, the lack of correlations might at first be ascribed to restriction of range. However, there was sufficient range to allow the Halstead–Reitan variables to correlate among themselves in the range of .50 with a similar pattern of results among the personality variables.

Morgan, Weitzel, Guyden, Robinson, and Hedlund (1972) examined the relationship between information derived from a standardized 120-question mental status exam and items on the MMPI. The authors judged 174 of the MMPI items to overlap with the mental status exam and 48 of the mental status exam items to overlap with the MMPI items. In the cases of total overlap, there was only 50% to 60% agreement in the information derived from the two sources. In the cases of partial overlap, there was more variable agreement. Unfortunately, the authors did not specify their criteria for overlap, either total or partial.

All of this calls into question the existence of robust relationships between standard measures of neuropsychological functioning and MMPI results. It does not mean, however, that no relationship exists between neuropsychological functioning and behavioral functioning. Because of the MMPI's origin as an instrument to perform the psychological assessment of psychiatric patients, it may be inappropriate in diagnosing organic impairment. This inappropriateness does not undermine its utility in describing psychological functioning in individuals who have been diagnosed as organically impaired by the use of standard neuropsychological assessment instruments.

Conclusions Regarding the MMPI

In general, the research reviewed does not support the existence of a specific personality style or profile per se that is unique to brain damage. A body of research does exist, however, that indicates that the relationship between personality and neuropsychological functioning is not simply one-to-one. Neuropsychological deficits have been associated with certain complex personality changes.

From the literature reviewed, it can be concluded that the localization paradigm has failed to relate personality to brain function, as evidenced by the conflicting data accumulated to date. Even if brain damage is confined to one cerebral lobe, there is far too much variability in the resultant behavioral deficits for a consistent personality type to emerge. It also seems unlikely that one personality profile is common to all types of brain damage. Although research in defining the brain-damaged group by behavioral deficits is promising, additional study appears warranted.

An alternative paradigm not discussed, but worthy of mention, is one modeled after the notion of incremental validity (Sechrest, 1963); it is concerned with how much knowledge of a test's outcome (an MMPI profile, for example) contributes to the prediction of a criterion (a correct diagnosis or treatment decision). Schwartz and Wiedel (1981) reported the use of the MMPI in neurological decision-making. In a review of 13 cases representing a range of different neurological and psychiatric diagnoses, it was found that knowledge of the MMPI results increased the diagnostic accuracy of a group of neurology and psychiatry residents. The actual hit rates were not reported, nor were the diagnostic groups used. The importance of this study lies in the recognition that information generated by the MMPI, as by any other psychometric instrument, should not be used in isolation. More appropriately, results from the MMPI should be integrated with other test data, as well as with information derived from clinical observation, and from a review of the patient's history.

Reliability data are lacking for neuropsychologically impaired subjects. Although interscorer reliability is moot in the case of the MMPI, test–retest and internal-consistency reliability remain important issues that have not been addressed.

MMPI-2

The standardization sample of the MMPI-2 differed from the census standardization sample in a few ways, mainly related to the average level of education. To investigate the consequence of such a difference, Schinka and LaLone (1997) pulled 1000 subjects from the original standardization sample of 2600 on the basis of congruence to the characteristics of the United States population. These researchers found no significant differences in T-score transformations with the exception of Hy, which differed by 3 T-score points. Although this information is encouraging, the fact that the 1000 subjects contributed to the transformation equations of both solutions may have contributed to the lack of differences. Examination of this point in a separately collected sample would be necessary to investigate this point more fully.

Based on the lessons learned with the MMPI and secondary to a higher level of sophistication regarding the relationship of neuropsychological and general psychological assessment, there have still been no published studies attempting to diagnose neurological impairment or localize lesions based on the MMPI-2. There have been several studies conducted using nonneurological subjects, but addressing assessment questions that might be frequently encountered in a neuropsychological setting, and this discussion will focus on those studies.

An extremely important question us related to the effect of ethnic identification on MMPI-2 scale scores. Clinical lore holds that ethnic differences result in elevations on certain scales in non-Caucasian individuals. McNulty, Graham, Ben-Porath, and Stein (1997) reported no differences in the accuracy of MMPI-2 results for African-American and Caucasian patients when therapist ratings were used as the criterion. In reviewing 50 studies of the MMPI and MMPI-2 in African-American, Hispanic, and Caucasian subjects, Hall, Bansal, and Lopez (1999) concluded that although statistically significant differences exist, these differences may not be clinically important. Still, these researchers called for additional studies before definitive statements can be made.

The MMPI-2 may be administered either in the standard booklet or in a computerized form. The manual states that the two forms are equivalent, which is supported by Pisoneault (1996) using a sample of 30 graduate students and by Roper, Ben-Porath, and Butcher (1995). Handel, Ben-Porath, and Watt (1999) reported no differences between the computerized normal version and the computerized adaptive testing version. A dissenting view is presented, at least for the Japanese version of the MMPI. It is unclear why this may be true, although specifics of the language may be responsible here (Sukigara, 1996). Although different studies have produced somewhat variable results, a meta-analysis of the research comparing the computerized and booklet forms of the MMPI and MMPI-2 indicated psychometric equivalency (Finger & Ones, 1999).

The publishers of the MMPI-2 also offer a computerized scoring and interpretation system. This interpretation system offers suggestions regarding the validity of the resulting profiles. Shores and Carstairs (1998) instructed three sets of graduate students to complete the MMPI-2 by portraying themselves in an unrealistically negative fashion, portraying themselves in an unrealistically positive fashion, or portraying themselves in an accurate fashion. The correct classification rates for the different groups were as follows: 94% fake-good, 100% fake-bad, 78% normal. The remainder of the normal responders were classified as fake-good. The computerized report system may be more accurate in classifying symptom magnification than symptom minimization.

Reliability

The MMPI-2 measures both state or condition-specific characteristics and historical features of diagnostic entities. Therefore, the temporal stability of the resulting profiles of clinical subjects may be questionable. Test–retest reliability of normal subjects should be fairly high. Matx, Altepeter, and Perlman (1992) reported adequate temporal and internal consistency reliability in a sample of college students similar to the results reported by Butcher, Graham, Dahlstrom, and Bowman (1990) using a similar sample. Putnam, Kurtz, and Houts (1996) reported that the stability of results in normal clergy tested across a 4-month period is acceptable, with the majority of scales exhibiting increases or decreases of between 3 and 6 points. Although the individual scales may show temporal stability, the reliability of interscale relationships or profiles may be limited. Ryan, Dunn, and Paolo (1995) found that although test–retest coefficients were significant across both a 5-month and 13-month interval, agreement for high-point, 2-point, and 3-point code in a sample of substance abusers was low.

Validity Scales and Response Bias

Putzke, Williams, Daniel, and Boll (1999) reported that the K scale is related to the number of item endorsements on the K-sensitive scales of 2, 4, 7, and 8 in a sample of medical inpatients, lending support to the use of the K correction. In an experiment to investigate the capacity of the MMPI-2 validity scales to discriminate malingerers from individuals undergoing pretrial evaluations, the F scale and the F–K difference both performed better than the other validity indicators. However, in discriminating defensive responding from actual responding, the F–K difference was less effective than the S (Superlative Self) scale (Nicholson et al., 1997). In a comparison of schizophrenic patients who completed the MMPI-2, once under standard instructions and once under instruction to conceal their symptoms, the Edwards Social Desirability scale and the L scale were best at discriminating the two conditions. Of greater interest is the fact that even individuals with clinical training can be detected as malingerers using the MMPI-2, at least when the disorder to be malingered is schizophrenia (Bagby et al., 1997b). It remains to be seen if the same accuracy of detection applies to neurological disorders.

Much of the research investigating the MMPI-2 in relation to malingered performance has focused on the fabrication of psychiatric symptoms. For our purposes, it would also be important to investigate the effect of malingered symptoms of closed head injury (CHI). Greiffenstein, Gola, and Baker (1995) examined the ability of the MMPI-2 validity scales to discriminate among patients with known head injury, patients who were suspected of probable malingering, and patients with persistent post-concussive syndrome. The study additionally examined the relationship of the MMPI-2 scales to measures specifically aimed at detecting less than optimal effort in neuropsychological evaluations. All five of the neuropsychological instruments separated the three groups. Only the F scale and the Subtle-Obvious scale were able to discriminate between the brain-injured and the probable malingering subjects, but not the persistent post-concussive syndrome subjects. The

MMPI-2 validity scales may have the greatest utility in detecting exaggerated complaints of emotional or behavioral difficulties following neurological injury or disease rather than detecting exaggerated complaints of cognitive difficulties.

As a self-report instrument, the MMPI-2 is sensitive to dissimulation attempts. The traditional and new validity scales are designed to detect such efforts, but it is important to evaluate the integrity of interpretations for specific disorders. Wetter and Deitsch (1996) found that although individuals faking posttraumatic stress disorder (PTSD) showed stability on profiles across a 2-week interval, individuals faking closed head injury showed significantly lower stability than either the PTSD group or individuals completing the MMPI-2 under standard instructions. In addition, knowledge about the presence of the validity scales may reduce the effectiveness of the validity scales to detect underreporting (Baer & Sekirnjak, 1997). The L scale was able to discriminate between schizophrenic patients completing the MMPI-2 under normal and fake-good conditions (Bagby et al., 1997b).

Gallen and Berry (1997) reported that the F and Fb scales are helpful in determining whether random responding occurred in the first two thirds of the test, in which case the clinical scales should not be interpreted or in the last third of the test, in which case the supplementary and content scales should not be interpreted. These researchers also proposed a set of subscales of the VRIN scale which were sensitive to random responding to items in the latter part of the test in their sample of simulating college students. Cross-validation and generalization to clinical samples would be necessary before these subscales can be used clinically. Archer, Fontaine, and McCare (1998) reported that MMPI-2 protocols with valid VRIN scales have higher correlations between MMPI-2 scales and both self-report and clinician ratings of psychopathology than do the protocols with high (invalid) VRIN scores.

Another potentially useful validity index was developed in reaction to the presence of possibly confounding severe psychopathology symptoms on the F scale. The F(p) scale does not contain those items from the F scale that are related to severe distress and psychopathology. An initial examination of this scale in 308 male psychiatric inpatients indicated that the F(p) scale score was lower than either the F or the Fb scale and was not related to diagnosis (Arbisi & Ben-Porath, 1997). The effectiveness of this scale in separating psychiatric inpatients who either answered honestly or under instruction to exaggerate symptoms was cross-validated in a sample of 74 VA patients (Arbisi & Ben-Porath, 1998). The Fp scale demonstrates hypothesized relations with other measures of psychopathology in a sample of 180 subjects being treated for substance abuse (Ladd, 1998). Further examination of this scale may support what is now potential utility in neuropsychological populations.

The Subtle/Obvious items distinction has been suggested as an index of the validity of the clinical scale. However, empirical research has usually failed to support such a use (Franzen, Iverson, & McCracken, 1990). Boone (1994) reported that the internal consistency of the Obvious scales is high while that of the Subtle scales is low, and that furthermore, inclusion of the subtle items in the clinical scales reduces the reliability of the clinical scales. In general, use of the subtle/obvious distinction cannot be recommended.

Gallen and Berry (1996) reported that the F, Fb, and VRIN scales all differentiated between random and "actual" responding in a sample of 804 undergraduate students who had received instructions to respond accurately or randomly with different start points for random responding (items 100, 200, 300, 370, 400, and 500), although VRIN and the index suggested by Greene (1991) of VRIN + |F − Fb| showed the best positive predictive power, negative predictive power, and hit rates across three base rates.

An important consideration in interpretation of the MMPI-2 validity scales is the relationship to neuropsychological invalidity. The F, F–K, and Lees-Haley Fake Bad scales from the MMPI-2 correlate moderately with the results of the Victoria Symptom Validity Test, but there was no such relationship for the Subtle-Obvious scales (Slick, Hopp, Strauss, & Spellacy, 1996). Larrabee (1998) reported that the Lees-Haley Fake Bad Scale (FBS) identified individuals in neuropsychological evaluation who had exhibited objective evidence of malingering whereas the F scale was elevated in only 3 of the 12 subjects.

Paul Lees-Haley has developed and evaluated a scale (Fake Bad Scale or FBS) to evaluate exaggeration specifically in personal injury litigants. The original study found 96% sensitivity and 90% specificity (Lees-Haley, English, & Glenn, 1991). A subsequent evaluation using subjects claiming PTSD found a sensitivity of about 75% and a specificity of 94%; however, the cutoff needed to be adjusted for optimal classification (Lees-Haley, 1992b). Larrabee (1998) examined the Lees-Haley FBS in 12 litigants with normal medical and neurological findings and objective evidence of malingering using the Rey Fifteen Item Test, the PDRT, or the Warrington Recognition Memory Test. Larrabee (1998) found that the FBS was elevated in 11 of the 12 subjects whereas the F scale was elevated in only three of the subjects.

The presence (or absence, depending upon one's point of view) of omitted items on the MMPI-2 may reduce the validity of interpretations. Berry et al. (1997) reported that up to 30 items can be deleted without affecting 2-point codes, although small decreases in scale elevation will occur.

Validity Studies

The authors of the MMPI-2 originally stated that there was sufficient similarity to the MMPI that the same interpretation strategies might be used and Ben-Porath and Butcher (1989) reported good agreement in the MMPI and MMPI-2 profiles of college students. However, Vincent (1990) reported only modest agreement of 2-point codes across the two instruments in a clinical sample.

One of the interpretation systems for the MMPI involved classifying individuals on the basis of scale elevations, slope, patterns of high and low scores, and differences between selected theoretically relevant scales. This system was used to classify prison inmates (Megaree & Bohn, 1979; Megaree & Dorhut, 1977; Meyer & Megaree, 1972), but the general classification system has broader implications regarding differences between the MMPI and MMPI-2. Megaree (1997) subsequently found that using the original classification system on data from the MMPI-2 that had been scored to both provide MMPI-2 profiles and to estimate MMPI profiles resulted in 69% agreement in classification. However, using new classification rules derived on the MMPI-2 resulted in 76% agreement. Consistent with the general trend of other research, although there is some similarity in results obtained by use of the MMPI-2 and MMPI, there are sufficient differences to support the development of new classification and interpretation systems.

There are three scales on the MMPI-2 that are purported to assess substance abuse problems, an area that is of considerable concern in evaluating neuropsychological patients.

The Addiction Acknowledgement Scale appears to be superior to the Addiction Potential Scale and the MacAndrews Alcoholism Scale-Revised when the criterion is a rating of substance abuse problems made by intake workers (Stein, Graham, Ben-Porath, & McNulty, 1999). The best assessment combination appears to be Addiction Acknowledgement Scale and the MacAndrews Alcoholism Scale-Revised, at least when the criterion is rating provided by outpatient therapists (Rouse, Butcher, & Miller, 1999).

The conceptualization of the original MMPI was based on a psychiatric nosology system fairly consistent with Axis I-type diagnoses of the DSM system. The utility of the MMPI-2 in diagnosing Axis-II conditions may be limited. In a comparison of the MMPI-2 with the Personality Assessment Inventory (PAI), the MMPI-2 was more accurate in identifying normal subjects—77% for the PAI versus 95% for the MMPI-2—but was much less accurate in identifying the subjects with borderline personality disorder—82% for the PAI versus 9% for the MMPI-2 (Bell-Pringle, Pate, & Brown, 1997). The MMPI-2 has three personality disorder scales that have been suggested for use in the identification of anti-social, borderline, and narcissistic personality disorders. Castlebury, Hilsenroth, Handler, and Durham (1997) found that the narcissistic personality disorder scale should be used only for negative predictive purposes only, but that the other two scales could be used to screen for the presence of their respective personality disorders. O'Maille and Fine (1995) reported that the personality disorder scales of the MMPI-2 have reasonable convergent validity when the Personality Diagnostic Questionnaire-Revised was the criterion, but discriminant validity was only modest.

The Mf scale was originally designed to detect "sexual inversion" but has been consistently found to be inaccurate in identifying individuals with homosexual inclinations. The scale has been suggested as a measure of identification with traditional gender roles, but little data exist to support such a suggestion. Johnson, Jones, and Brems (1996) reported that the MMPI-2 Feminine Gender Role (GF) and Masculine Gender Role (GM) scales lack similar concurrent validity when various measures of gender role are used as criteria. The interpretation of the GF and GM scales should be conducted very cautiously.

Because of the potential presence of PTSD symptoms in closed head injury patients, the PTSD scales of the MMPI-2 may have relevant information in the assessment of these patients. Herman, Weathers, Litz, and Keane (1996) found that the embedded PTSD scale and a standalone version had comparable psychometric properties in Vietnam veterans.

In addition to the basic clinical scales, there are 15 content scales available on the MMPI-2. These scales are relatively homogeneous with regard to intent and substance of the item and are purported to evaluate constructs such as fears, anxiety, anger, cynicism, and type A behavior. Less is known about the interpretation of these scales as compared to the clinical scales. By ranking items in the entire MMPI-2 based on social desirability and constructing 21 scales of 27 items each in increasing desirability, Jackson, Fraboni, and Helmes (1997) attempted to examine the desirability of the content scales. These desirability scales were factor analyzed and the resulting circumplex structure was superimposed on the structure of the content scales, indicating substantial correlation between the two structures. Furthermore, the internal consistency estimates of the content scales (coefficient alpha) were greatly reduced when the desirability variance was partialled out.

It is important to know whether the content scales provide additional information over and beyond the clinical scales. A study of outpatient subjects using therapist ratings as criteria indicated that for men the Anger, Anxiety, Health Concerns, Depression, Antisocial

Practices, Low Self-Esteem, and Family Problems scales and for women the Bizarre Mentation, Antisocial Practices, and Family Problems provided incremental information over the corresponding clinical scales in a regression analysis. The amount of additional variance accounted for ranged from 1% to 8%, and these values are relatively small (Barthlow, Graham, Ben-Porath, & McNulty, 1999). Interpretation of the content scales should be more conservative than that of the basic scales.

As with the MMPI, there are supplementary scales for the MMPI-2. These supplementary scales include measures of ego strength, social responsibility, substance abuse, and PTSD, among other constructs. Archer, Elkins, Aiduk, and Griffin (1997) conducted a set of hierarchical multiple-regression analyses to determine whether the supplementary scale contributed variance in prediction of Symptom Checklist-90-Revised scales, Brief Psychiatric Rating Scales, and the Global Assessment Scale in a sample of 597 psychiatric inpatient subjects. The supplementary scales contributed only marginal variance and therefore may be of limited utility. The Low Self-Esteem (LSE) scale demonstrates reasonable internal consistency and agreement with other measures of self-esteem (Brems & Lloyd, 1995).

Recently, there has been a spate of published papers addressing the use of both the MMPI and the MMPI-2 in neurologically impaired subjects. This increase in publications probably reflects the twin trends of adapting the MMPI to special populations and the increased awareness among neuropsychologists regarding emotional factors. Although there have been attempts to associate different emotional profiles with lateralized lesions, especially when those lesions are epileptogenic, Trenerry et al. (1996) reported that side of seizure onset had a lower association with MMPI profile characteristics than did amount of seizure control afforded by surgical intervention.

Many of the items contained in the scales related to psychopathology are also related to symptoms of neurological disturbance. For example, the presence of IQ, memory, or attention impairment may result in elevations of the validity scales, although these effects may be clinically significant only in cases of severe cognitive impairment (Mittenberg, Tremont, & Rayls, 1996). As a result interpretation of MMPI-2 results may need to be somewhat different in a nonpsychiatric population (Gass & Russell, 1991). Gass (1991) developed a correction factor derived from the collection of 14 items on the MMPI-2 that are related to neurological disturbance. These items are summed into a correction factor. Subsequent research indicated that when a sample of 54 patients with CHI were compared to the normative sample for the MMPI-2, the CHI group could be differentiated on the basis of 13 of the 14 correction factor items. A similar finding was reported by the same researcher in a sample of stroke patients (Gass, 1996a; Gass & Lawhorn, 1991). The next step would be to evaluate the accuracy of interpretations of the MMPI-2 in these subjects when the correction factor has been used. Derry, Harnadek, McLachlan, and Sontrop (1997) did not find difference in interpretation of the MMPI-2 profiles for patients with epilepsy when items related to seizure content were removed. Other correction factors have been suggested by Alfano, Paniak, and Finlayson (1993). Brulot, Strauss, and Spellacy (1997) examined these two sets of correction factors as well as a set proposed in a dissertation of Artzy (1994) and found that there was a greater relationship between the correction factors and score on the 2 (D) scale than between the correction factors and measures of severity of head injury or scores on neuropsychological tests. These researchers therefore questioned the utility and accuracy of such correction factors. Cripe (1996) discussed some of the difficulties and complexities in interpreting the MMPI profiles of neurologically impaired individuals. He suggested that interpretation be restricted to a description of the awareness of emotional difficulties evidenced by the patient.

The use of the MMPI-2 in neuropsychological populations should entail a consideration of both organic and psychological variables in interpretation. Youngjohn, Davis, and Wolf (1997) found that mild head injury patients, all of whom were involved in litigation, had elevations on the Hs, D, Hy, and Pt scales relative to patients with severe head injury, regardless of whether the severely head-injured patients were involved in litigation or not. Gass (1996b) reported significant relationships between MMPI-2 variables and measures of attention and memory and suggested that the MMPI-2 is helpful in examining the relative contribution of psychological factors to performance on these neuropsychological measures. An examination of the MMPI and MMPI-2 profiles that were administered to a small ($n = 10$) group of amnesic patients across a period of "several weeks" indicated that there was great similarity and stability between the two forms. Furthermore, consideration of the profiles in the context of the history of neurological injury indicated that the interpretation was more highly related to the effects of the amnesia than to premorbid personality dysfunction (Bachna, Sieggreen, Cermak, Penk, & O'Connor, 1998). The correction factors were not found to have a relationship to performance on neuropsychological tests, duration of loss of consciousness, or posttraumatic amnesia in closed head injury patients, although there was a relationship to Scale 2 (Brulot, Strauss, & Spellacy, 1997) indicating limitations in the use of these correction factors.

Because the MMPI is interpreted in multiple ways (scale elevations, profile analysis, actuarial), it is important to investigate the similarity between the MMPI and the MMPI-2 in these multiple ways. Two-point code analysis is one of the methods frequently used in interpretation. Miller and Paniak (1995) administered the items of the MMPI and the MMPI-2 to a sample of 53 brain-injured patients. They found little difference in single scale elevation code types (45 out of 53 agreed) and moderate differences in 2-point codes (28 out of 53 agreed). However, there were significant differences in profiles. In an interesting research design, amnesic patients were administered the MMPI and MMPI-2 across a mean interval of 20 days in counterbalanced order to 10 patients with severe memory impairment. There was 50% concordance between 2-point codes and no significant differences among scale elevations (Bachna et al., 1998).

The Spanish translation of the MMPI-2 has only moderate correlation with symptoms elicited by the Diagnostic Interview Schedule and does not have good agreement with the diagnoses of alcohol abuse, depression, schizophrenia, or anxiety disorders using the same criteria (Fantoni-Salvador & Rogers, 1997). The Spanish MMPI-2 is better used for the description of symptom correlates and should not be used for diagnosis.

MMPI-A

Before the MMPI-A was available, the MMPI was administered to adolescents and age-appropriate norms were used. The best compilation of research studies and clinical applications can be found in Archer (1987). The MMPI-A was meant to be used in subjects between the ages of 14 and 18 years old. Archer (1992) has provided norms to be used with 13-year-old subjects. Janus, de Groot, and Toepfer (1998) compared the protocols of 56

13-year-old psychiatric inpatients with 85 14-year-old psychiatric inpatients and did find differences in scale elevation related to age. However, the use of the Archer (1992) 13-year-old norms resulted in lower scale elevations than did the original norms. The evaluation of 13-year-old subjects should involve a careful choice of normative base.

In the past, therapist observations and clinical judgment regarding the presence of psychopathology were felt to be less sensitive to response style and bias than were self-report instruments for the detection of psychopathology. However, Pogge, Stokes, Wong, and Harvey (1997) found that for adolescents completing the MMPI, therapist ratings and clinical scales reported higher levels of depression in the presence with higher F scale scores than in the presence of low F scale scores. In addition, confirmatory factor analysis indicated that validity scales were related to both self-report of depression and therapist ratings, but that there was no difference between the subtle and the obvious items of scale 2.

The manual reports acceptable temporal reliability values for the basic scales as well as for the content and supplementary scales. Stein, McClinton, and Graham (1998) reported that those values were approximated in a separate sample of 61 adolescents who were evaluated across a 1-year period.

Stein and Graham (1999) reported that the 11 and K scales were able to differentiate between adjudicated adolescents instructed to fake good and those incarcerated adolescents instructed to respond normally. In addition, the clinical scales were significantly lower in the fake-good subjects.

The use of the MMPI in adolescents may be problematic with regard to the frequently encountered condition of conduct disorder which may mask signs of depression in those adolescents with both characteristics (Herkov & Myers, 1996). The use of Rorschach variables did not contribute to the classification of adolescents with depression whereas the MMPI-A Scale 2 and DEP scale did (Archer & Krishnamurthy, 1997). In general, there are few and only small correlations between Rorschach and MMPI-A variables (Archer & Krishnamurthy, 1993).

An interesting approach to the interpretation of the MMPI-A has involved factor analyses of the scales to provide more content consistent entities. Archer, Belevich, and Elkins (1994) uncovered an eight-factor solution in an analysis of the 69 basic scales and subscales of the MMPI-A derived on the standardization sample. Later, using a clinical sample of 358 adolescents, Archer and Krishnamurthy (1997) determined that a nine-factor solution had great similarity to the original solution. This finding is in need of statistical testing via confirmatory factor analysis. In addition, the validity of the scales in terms of their interpretative meaning should be supported by empirical evaluations.

Selected content scales of the MMPI-A (Health Concerns, Alienation, Anger, Conduct Problems, and Social Discomfort) fared well in an examination of their convergent and discriminant validity, although the Depression and Anxiety scales did not discriminate well (Arita & Baer, 1998).

The MMPI-A contains a scale not found in the MMPI-2, namely the immaturity scale (IMM). The IMM is thought to measure ego development and maturation. Imhof and Archer (1997) reported that the IMM scale correlates with projective measures of ego development as well as with measures of intelligence and reading ability. Zinn, McCumber, and Dahlstrom (1999) reported a cross-validation of the IMM scale of the MMPI-A using a projective technique as the criterion measure. Archer and Slesinger (1999) reported that certain scale patterns on the MMPI-A are associated with endorsement of the suicidal ideation items on the MMPI-A, although the relationship to external criteria such as independently endorsed suicidal ideation or actual suicidal behavior needs to be better explicated.

Gallucci (1997) reported that ACK and PRO scales of the MMPI-A correlated well with therapists' rating of behavior undercontrol and substance abuse in adolescents in treatment for substance abuse.

Conclusions Regarding the MMPI-A

The empirical evidence related to the MMPI-A is more sparse than that available for the MMPI-2. However, it is also true that there is no other personality assessment instrument for adolescents that has been as well studied as the MMPI-A. The reading level may limit which subjects may be able to complete the MMPI-A. As with the MMPI-2, interpretation of results from subjects in a neuropsychological population should be more conservative than the interpretation of results from subjects in a psychiatric population.

PERSONALITY ASSESSMENT INVENTORY

The Personality Assessment Inventory or PAI (Morey, 1991) was designed to be a general clinical assessment instrument related to psychological clinical issues. The instrument is aimed at providing information related to the psychiatric nosological system, although trait descriptors are also part of the results. One of the reasons why the PAI may be becoming popular among neuropsychologists is that it is somewhat briefer than the MMPI-2 (344 items vs. 567 items), which makes it a less onerous task for neuropsychological clients who may be prone to fatigue or attentional lapses. In addition, the reading level of the items on the PAI is at the fourth grade, so that it may be more applicable among individuals with cognitive impairment. Instead of answering only True or False, the PAI allows a range of four responses (False, Slightly True, Mainly True, and Very True). Four validity scales (Inconsistency, Infrequency, Negative Impression, and Positive Impression) are used to evaluate the utility and accuracy of the resulting profile. Clinical scales involve 11 clinical entities such as Borderline Features or Anxiety. The five treatment scales evaluate aspects of personal characteristics such as aggression and treatment rejection. Finally, two interpersonal scales, Dominance and Warmth, are used to assess interactional style.

Reliability

Internal consistency reliability using Cronbach's alpha in a sample of 111 psychiatric inpatients are similar to those reported in the manual for the standardization sample (Boone, D., 1998). Furthermore, Alterman et al. (1995) reported similar internal consistency reliability values in a sample of 160 low-socioeconomic African-American and Latino patients enrolled in a methadone maintenance program. However, not all researchers are in agreement regarding the reliability of the PAI. Boyle and Lennon (1994) reported that in an Australian sample, the PAI test–retest reliability and internal consistency reliability do not match the values reported in the manual, and a factor analysis of the data was inconsistent with the original factor structure. Boyle, Ward, and Lennon (1994) reported that a confirmatory factor analysis of the PAI does not fit the factor structure reported in the manual. Morey (1995) responded with criticisms of the researchers' methods , and Boyle (1996) responded with his own criticisms. Conger and Conger (1996) provided a balanced discussion of the relevant factors. Deisinger (1995) had replicated the factor structure. One option is that the factor structure may vary with different cultural groups, although this variability does not appear to be present for Spanish-speaking subjects living in the United States (Rogers, Flores, Ustad, & Sewell, 1995). The factor structure was only slightly different in a sample of alcohol abusing subjects (Schinka, 1995).

Response Bias

Response style is an important component of self-report instruments and has generated much interest among neuropsychologists. Morey and Lanier (1998) examined six different indices of distortion on the PAI and reported that all six of them were able to discriminate between analog responders told to malinger or to present a positive image, in contrast to college students responding accurately. Fals-Stewart (1996) used the PAI to classify subjects into a group of substance abusing individuals instructed to answer forthrightly, a group of subjects instructed to answer defensively, and a group of suspected substance abusing subjects referred by the criminal justice system. In an attempt to cross-validate those findings, Fals-Stewart and Lucente (1997) applied the classification equation to a new sample of substance abusing subjects and suspected substance abusing subjects. There was shrinkage from 82% correct classification to only 68% correct classification. When naive and sophisticated (doctoral psychology students) were compared on their ability to malinger schizophrenia, depression, and generalized anxiety disorders, the validity scales were less successful in detecting the sophisticated subjects (Rogers, Sewell, Morey, & Ustad, 1996), but a discriminant function analysis was fairly successful in separating clinical patients from even the sophisticated malingerers. Rogers, Ornduff, and Sewell (1993) reported that the Negative Impression Management scale detected subjects attempting to malinger schizophrenia and to a lesser extent depression, but not anxiety. In this study sophistication did not allow greater success in escaping detection of malingered performance. An examination of the validity scales in correctional and forensic settings was conducted by comparing the scores of known malingerers to patients (Rogers, Sewell, Cruise, Wang, & Ustad, 1998). Both the Negative Impression Management and the Malingering Index were found to separate the two groups.

In a sample of 111 undergraduate students, the Positive Impression Management scale and the Defensiveness Index were both able to identify subjects who had completed the scales with instructions to positively bias their responses (Peebles & Moore, 1998). Baer and Wetter (1997) administered the PAI to a group of college students under standard instructions and to two groups under instructions to provide positive impression management. One of these two groups was given information about the presence of the validity scales, and that group was somewhat more successful in escaping detection. Cashel, Rogers, Sewell, and Martin-Cannici (1996) examined the profiles of students and criminals who completed the PAI twice, once under standard instructions, and once under instructions to respond defensively, and found that a discriminant function separated the two conditions with 84% accuracy.

Validity

Rogers, Ustad, and Salekin (1998) reported good agreement between the PAI and three other instruments specifically designed to evaluate for schizophrenia, affective disorders, suicidal tendencies, and feigned symptoms in a sample of corrections patients. Using a similar population, Wang et al. (1997) reported good agreement with measures of feigned symptoms, suicidal tendencies, and overt aggression.

One difference with the MMPI-2 is that the PAI may have greater sensitivity to the presence of personality disorders because its items were written specifically to correspond with DSM-IV nosology whereas the MMPI-2's items were written with the goal of detecting the major Axis I diagnoses. In a comparison with the MMPI-2, the PAI was more accurate in diagnosing the presence of borderline personality disorder (Bell-Pringle et al., 1997).

Spanish Language PAI

Rogers et al. (1995) reported good temporal stability in monolingual Spanish-speaking subjects and equivalence between the Spanish and the English versions in bilingual subjects. Furthermore, the internal consistency was adequate in both versions. Fantoni-Salvador and Rogers (1997) reported that the Spanish translation of the PAI correlates only moderately with clinical symptoms derived from use of the Diagnostic Interview Schedule. Furthermore, the Spanish PAI did have greater agreement with the diagnoses of depression, schizophrenia, anxiety disorders, and alcohol abuse disorders than did the Spanish MMPI-2.

Conclusions Regarding the PAI

The PAI has potential utility in the assessment of emotional functioning of individuals with neuropsychological impairment. Because it is slightly shorter than the MMPI-2 (approximately 60% of the length) and because the required reading level is lower, its use in the total assessment of the individual bears further investigation. Research directly involving neuropsychological populations is necessary to more completely actualize this potential.

The Rorschach Inkblots

The use of the Rorschach as a neuropsychological instrument remains an issue of controversy. Despite the extensive clinical and theoretical literature related to the Rorschach, those individuals critical of this instrument maintain that the validity of the Rorschach has not been established according to strict psychometric standards. Proponents of the Rorschach maintain that the functional utility of this instrument relies on the clinical skills and sensitivities of the clinician using it. The past few years have seen a great increase in the number of research studies investigating the reliability and validity of the Rorschach. However, the controversy continues. Regardless of one's bias toward the use of this instrument, there is a paucity of research on its validity and reliability when it is used with neurologically impaired clients. The utility, or the potential utility, of this procedure, however, continues to be of interest (see the symposium listing for the Eighth European Conference of the International Neuropsychological Society, Costa & Rourke, 1985). The proponents of the Rorschach defend its use and conclude that the Rorschach has an adequate empirical base to allow its use in a forensic context (McCann, 1998). The courts seem to agree, as a review of legal cases in which the Rorschach was involved in legal testimony indicates that the findings of an evaluation using the Rorschach were allowed in testimony the majority of times in which the Rorschach was used (Meloy, Hansen, & Weiner, 1997). However, the true test of the Rorschach needs to be conducted in the context of expert research psychologists published in peer-reviewed journals (Exner, Colligan, Boll, Stischer, & Hillman, 1996; Wood, Nezworski, & Stejskal, 1996).

A recent article by Wood, Nezworski, Stejskal, Gerven, and West (1999) raises several pertinent points regarding validity studies of the Rorschach. First, it is essential to realize that no conclusive studies regarding the validity of the Rorschach can be made. Instead, validity questions need to address the validity of individual scores obtained from the Rorschach. Second, each study should use its own control group instead of relying on comparisons to the normative base of the Exner system. Finally, contrasted extreme group designs have limited utility for clinical application of the Rorschach. Statistical power may be artificially inflated in such studies, although comparisons of diagnostic groups may be informative.

The Rorschach research has been summarized multiple times during its history (Baker, 1956; Goldfried, Stricker, & Weiner, 1971; Klebanoff, Singer, & Wilensky, 1954). It continues to be difficult to assess the Rorschach in terms of the experimental and statistical models typically used in psychology. Similarly, the methodological shortcomings discussed in the aforementioned reviews continue to cause problems (Viglione, 1997). Despite these problems, Parker, Hanson, and Hunsley (1988) concluded that the Rorschach had sufficient convergent validity when used for the purposes for which it was designed. Weiner (1996) also supported the use of the Rorschach and argued that misunderstanding of the instrument had led to the criticisms.

There have been a few meta-analyses conducted on studies of the Rorschach. Garb, Florio, and Grove (1998) criticized these meta-analyses as being flawed and reevaluated the data with the result that the Rorschach appears to explain only 8% to 13% of the variance in the criteria of these studies. As a point of comparison, the MMPI appears to explain 23% to 30% of the variance in criteria.

The Rorschach is used as an indicator of brain pathology, both because there may be direct effects of brain damage brain on emotional functioning and because there can be secondary effects of the emotional reaction to the neurocognitive changes. The implied assumption is that tests of personality functions should therefore be sensitive to the existence of an "organic" personality. One research approach has been to determine which Rorschach scores (signs) are found in cognitively impaired individuals, and to use these signs in predicting the presence of brain pathology. This simplistic approach has not been proven to be highly successful, however, in part because it rests on the erroneous assumption that brain damage is a unitary construct. Furthermore, brain lesions are likely to produce both general and specific effects, and signs constructed from a heterogeneous group of neurologically impaired subjects can be sensitive, at most, to the general effects. The Rorschach is a complex visual–perceptual task requiring such cognitive processes as attention, recognition, integration, naming, and the ability to formulate an oral–verbal expressive response. Lesions affecting any one of these processes may therefore be manifested on the Rorschach.

Before we discuss the various sign approaches that have been used with the Rorschach, it is important to provide a general overview of the Rorschach, as the various sign approaches are often interpreted in the context of the entire Rorschach protocol. An evaluation of the utility of the Rorschach is complicated by the fact that a number of scoring systems have been developed for use with this instrument (e.g., Beck, Beck, Levitt, & Molish, 1961; Exner, 1974). Most of these systems share such common scoring categories as location, determinants, and content. The analysis of a Rorschach protocol is based on the relative number of responses falling into the various categories, as well as on certain ratios and interrelationships among different categories (Exner, 1974). The Exner Comprehensive System is probably best suited to empirical evaluation and may be the most likely to be used in research (Ganellen, 1996).

NORMATIVE DATA

Putatively normative data have been provided by a number of researchers on the various scoring systems for the Rorschach (Ames, 1966; Ames, Metraux, Rodell, & Walker, 1973; Beck et al., 1961; Cass & McReynolds, 1951; Klopfer & Davidson, 1962). Ames and her associates, for example, collected and published Rorschach norms on children between the ages of 2 and 10, on adolescents between the ages of 10 and 16, and on adults 70 and older (Ames, Learned, Metraux, & Walker, 1954; Ames, Metraux, Rodell, & Walker, 1974;

Ames, Metraux, & Walker, 1971). Combining data from 15 studies, Levitt and Truumaa (1972) compiled a summary of the published normative data for children and adolescents up to 16 years old. The means of various quantitative Rorschach indices were provided by age and intellectual level.

However, a general, adequate normative data base has not been established for the Rorschach (Goldfried, et al., 1971). Often, there has been a failure to ensure that the data base is representative of the sample on which the data are based. Similarly, a review of the literature reveals that there has been a general failure to control or assess the effects of age, sex, IQ, and educational level in the development of these data bases. Finally, norms have not been established to control for the effects of varying response totals on the Rorschach.

Because of the many shortcomings in earlier "normative" studies, Exner (1974) developed the Comprehensive System. The Exner Comprehensive System, which is an integration of the five major Rorschach systems, synthesizes, according to psychometric criteria, the most reliable and useful indices from the other Rorschach scoring systems. Exner (1974, 1978) has compiled a substantial data base for this scoring system based on a nonpatient group ($n = 325$) and four psychiatric groups: an outpatient nonpsychotic group ($n = 185$), an inpatient character-problems group ($n = 90$), inpatient depressives ($n = 155$), and inpatient schizophrenics ($n = 210$). Means and standard deviations are provided for the following categories: responses, location features, determinants, and ratios and derivations. According to Exner (1978), the five samples of subjects were closely monitored to ensure that various socioeconomic strata would be proportionally represented in accordance with the 1970 U.S. Census figures. All five of the patient samples were reported to be essentially equivalent in terms of sex. Normative data for older adults were not differentiated, nor was information regarding education or level of intellectual functioning provided. As noted previously, education and intelligence have been found to be a confounding variable with the Rorschach, especially in such variables as the number of responses produced on a protocol (R). Awareness of this fact is important in that the number of responses produced has a direct bearing on a number of ratios that are derived from the patient's protocol. A low number of responses severely limits the usefulness of many of these ratios.

It should be noted, however, that normative data ($n = 1870$) have been collected and reported for nonpatient children across 12 age groups (ages 5 through 16). Gender, socioeconomic, and geographical differences have also been discussed (Exner, 1982).

RELIABILITY

There have been a very limited number of reliability studies conducted on the Rorschach. Hertz (1934), for example, reported that, in a study of 100 junior high school students, an "odd–even" procedure was used that resulted in reliability coefficients ranging from .66 to .97. Following essentially the same approach used by Hertz, but using records of younger children, Ford (1946) obtained comparable split-half reliabilities. The Oral Dependency Scale has been shown to have internal consistency similar to other Rorschach scales (Bornstein, Hill, Robinson, Calabrese, & Bowers, 1996); however, this may not be adequate in comparison to other psychological assessment methods.

There have been a few temporal reliability studies. The use of test–retest measures, however, is inherently limited to those traits that one would expect to be stable over time.

For example, developmental scorings, or measures of transitory depression or anxiety, would be inappropriate, as changes would be expected on these measures over time.

The findings from temporal reliability studies have been relatively positive. Ford (1946) reported reliabilities for scoring determinants ranging from +.38 to +.86 for a group of young children retested after 30 days. Kerr (1936), however, reported substantially lower reliabilities for young children retested after 1 year, results that may logically be attributed, in part, to developmental issues. Using a schizophrenic sample, Holzberg and Wexsler (1950) reported significant reliabilities across most scoring variables. Kelley, Margulies, and Barrera (1941) found very little change in the "psychograms" of 12 patients retested 2 hours after having received electroconvulsive therapy. These subjects demonstrated total amnesia for the first testing, which had been completed just before treatment. Perry, McDougall, and Viglione (1995) reported that the 5-year stability of the Ego Impairment Index has moderate levels. Bornstein (1996) reviewed the studies related to the Rorschach Oral Dependency scale and found very few studies examining temporal reliability or predictive validity. Studies of the internal consistency reliability have been inconclusive. Bornstein, Rossner, and Hill (1994) found that the Rorschach Oral Dependency Scale has adequate stability in college students over a 16-week period, but not in longer periods.

Exner (1978) assessed the temporal stability of the Comprehensive System by evaluating the performance of several different groups of subjects at varying intervals. Three nonpatient groups consisting of 25, 25, and 100 subjects were retested after 7 days, 60 days, and 3 years, respectively. Data from the following four psychiatric groups was also assessed: 30-day retest of 25 outpatients waiting for treatment assignment; 20 patients diagnosed as schizophrenic who were retested on day 10 of a 10-day evaluation period (without treatment); 35 outpatients retested after a 90-day interval, during which brief treatment had occurred; and 30 long-term outpatients, who were retested 180 days later. The results of the aforementioned seven studies (including the study of the schizophrenic group) provide support for the temporal stability of the Rorschach. In the three studies involving nonpatients, for example, 17 of the 19 variables correlated were found to be stable over time (having correlation coefficients of .70 or higher).

Interrater reliability is an important consideration for Rorschach research because scoring involves a fair amount of clinical judgment. Because of the categorical nature of the data generated, the best statistic to describe interrater reliability would seem to be Cohen's kappa (McDowell & Acklin, 1996). Unfortunately, interrater reliability studies are nonexistent.

The Exner Comprehensive System was critiqued by Wood, Nezworski, and Stejskal (1996), who found great fault with the reliability and validity reports. The reliability of the Exner Comprehensive System for scoring the Rorschach was subsequently reviewed by Meyer (1997a), who concluded that temporal reliability is adequate. Wood, Nezworski, and Stejskal (1997) criticized the methods and logic of Meyer (1997a) and came to exactly opposite conclusions. Their criticisms focused on Meyer's representation of item level versus aggregated data, the role of chance agreement in temporal reliability studies, a confusion between temporal and interrater reliability, and Meyer's (1997a) method of using one study to estimate base rates in other studies in which this information is not reported. Meyer (1997b) replied with critiques of the criticisms. However, both Meyer (1997b) and Wood, Nezworski, and Stejskal (1997) seem to be in agreement regarding the need for rigorous validity studies using the Rorschach and the conclusion that those studies have yet to be completed. The fact that there is still considerable controversy regarding the psychometric basis of the Rorschach should serve as caution to potential users.

VALIDITY

Content validity for the Rorschach has proved difficult to demonstrate. Goldfried et al. (1971) suggested that the Rorschach may not be amenable to such an evaluation because it has not been shown that the Rorschach is, indeed, representative of those personality and cognitive variables that it purports to measure. Although they involve problems, measures of criterion-related validity and construct validity appear to be more promising in terms of establishing support for the Rorschach as a psychometric procedure. Two major approaches, which are somewhat divergent but not mutually exclusive, have been used to establish the validity of the Rorschach: the empirical sign or psychometric approach and the conceptual approach. The following discussion of Exner and his colleagues' research on the Comprehensive System represents an example of the empirical sign approach.

Most validation studies of the Comprehensive System have revolved around the "four-square" interrelationships (Viglione & Exner, 1983). The four-square incorporates the basic scores and ratios thought to be characteristic of one's problem-solving style, and it forms the foundations for Exner's Comprehensive System. The four indices of the four-square are: (1) Erlebnistypus (EB, the ratio of human movement to weighted color responses); (2) Experience Actual (EA, the sum of human movement and weighted color responses); (3) Experience Base (eb, the ratio of nonhuman movement to shading and gray–black responses); and (4) Experience Potential (ep, the sum of nonhuman movement, shading, and gray–black responses). According to Exner and his colleagues, these four variables taken as a whole incorporate the fundamental information about the psychological habits and capacities of an individual and represent the crucial interpretive departure from previous Rorschach systems (Lerner & Lerner, 1986).

Research conducted by Exner and his colleagues involving temporal consistency data indicates that the EA/ep ratio stabilizes through development and achieves permanence by adulthood (Exner, 1982). Normative data indicate that EA increases relative to ep as children mature, and that ratios in which EA is greater than ep are associated more often with normal subjects than with patients. Collectively, these findings demonstrate that the EA/ep relationship represents a stable personality characteristic that indicates the "amount" of psychological activity organized and available for "coping purposes" as opposed to more immature experiences that impinge on the subject. Treatment studies reveal increases in EA, both alone and in relationship to ep, among patients who have shown improvement in psychotherapy (Exner, 1978). For subjects beginning treatment with ep greater than EA, a reversal has been demonstrated in most cases; that is, EA becomes greater than ep when intervention is not short term (Exner, 1978). All of these suggestions and studies are in need of independent empirical examination.

In contrast to the psychometric or sign approach to the Rorschach, the conceptual approach addresses issues of construct as opposed to criterion-related validity. Construct validity therefore addresses the extent to which a theoretical formulation can account for relationships between selected aspects of a Rorschach protocol and some condition or behavior (see Lerner & Lerner, 1986).

Empirical findings have also been reported that provide support for the concept of construct validity. Hall, Hall, and Lavoie (1968), for example, reported differences between right- and left-hemisphere-damaged patients on a variety of Rorschach variables. Similarly, three studies have assessed the performance of epileptics on the Rorschach: Vagrecha and Sen Mazumadar (1974); Delay, Pichot, Lemperier, and Perse (1958); and Loveland (1961).

Exner, Colligan, Boll, Stischer, and Hillman (1996) reported that among closed head injury (CHI) patients Rorschach results indicate a lower level of available resources, simplistic functioning in reference to detail, inconsistent decision-making and coping, and an unwillingness to deal directly with the emotional stimulation around them. However, this was based on a limited sample of 60 individuals who had experienced a CHI 3 to 5 weeks prior to testing. The conclusions were based on comparison to published normative information on the Rorschach and did not evaluate premorbid characteristics. Using a much more severely injured sample of 35 patients who had experienced an average of 34 days in a coma, Ellis and Zahn (1985) report significantly lower mean number responses, as well as lower X+% and F+% scores and significant cognitive disarray. However, all of these results may have been due to the perceptual and cognitive dysfunction attendant upon such a severe level of injury.

Meta-analyses have been conducted to examine the different validity studies of the Rorschach in comparison to the MMPI. Atkinson (1986) and Parker et al. (1988) examined the relative validity coefficients of the Rorschach and MMPI and both concluded that the two instruments were equivalent. These two studies have been criticized. For example, the effect size estimates of the Atkinson (1986) assumed only positive values so that studies with positive values would have the same indices as studies with negative validity coefficients. The Parker et al. (1988) meta-analysis has been criticized on the basis of study inclusion because of possible bias of the journal (*Journal of Personality Assessment*) used as a source. Hiller, Rosenthal, Bornstein, Berry, and Brunell-Neulieb (1999) attempted to remediate these deficiencies through a more representative choice of study sources and the use of a more sensitive effect size estimate. These researchers concluded that there were approximately equivalent validity indices. However, the MMPI had somewhat larger validity coefficients for studies using self-report criteria and psychiatric diagnoses. The Rorschach exhibited somewhat greater validity indices using suicide, hospitalization, or other objective measures as criteria. The Rorschach depression index was not effective in identifying adolescents with depression whereas both the MMPI and the Beck Depression Inventory were able to do so (Carter & Dacey, 1996). Krishnamurthy, Archer, and House (1996) found that there were minimal correlations between the Rorschach and MMPI-A even when the response frequency index was used as a moderator variable, as suggested by Meyer (1993) or when subjects were classified by diagnosis.

ORGANIC SIGNS

Although numerous sets of Rorschach signs have been developed for the purpose of assessing brain damage (see Aita, Reitan, & Ruth, 1947; Dorken & Kral, 1952; Evans & Marmorston, 1963b, 1964; Hughes, 1948; Piotrowski, 1937, 1940; Ross & Ross, 1944), it is questionable whether any system has demonstrated sufficient validity to warrant their use clinically (Goldfried et al., 1971).

Piotrowski Signs

Piotrowski (1937) developed the most notable of these systems, which consists of 10 signs dealing with both the response style and the content of the response. Piotrowski's research indicates that organic patients tend to give Rorschach protocols with fewer than 15 responses, long latencies for each response, perseveration, perplexity (the patient demonstrates a distrust of her or his own ability and seeks reassurance), poor form, little movement, color naming, and impotency (the patient recognizes an unsatisfactory response but does not change or improve it). Piotrowski (1937, 1940) cautioned, however, that, although the presence of five signs suggests neurological impairment, a qualitative analysis of the patient's performance is necessary before a diagnosis of brain damage can be made.

However, this system results in a high number of "false negatives" or nonconclusive diagnoses and does not differentiate chronic schizophrenics from organically impaired patients. Furthermore, the most effective of the Piotrowski signs are actually behavioral observations that might also be elicited by many other psychometric techniques. Perplexity, impotence, perseveration, and automatic phrases are ways of dealing with a stimulus situation rather than unique Rorschach variables.

Although the Piotrowski signs have been researched more than any other system, the efficacy of these signs has yet to be proved (Birch & Diller, 1959; Goldfried et al., 1971; Hertz & Loehrke, 1954). The Piotrowski signs continue, however, to be the Rorschach signs most commonly used in the assessment of brain damage. The utility of this approach is exemplified in Shukla, Tripathi, and Dhar (1987), in which only three of the signs were found associated with organic impairment in a comparison of 35 female subjects with documented brain lesions, 35 patients with schizophrenia, and 35 control subjects.

Other Sign Systems

The Hughes system (1948) consists of 14 signs derived from a factor analytic investigation. Of the 14 signs that were derived, 7 are identical to Piotrowski's signs. The score on the Hughes signs can range from −7 to +17, with a recommended cutoff of +7 being used to define brain damage (Goldfried et al., 1971). Research has not shown the Hughes signs to provide an appreciable advantage over the Piotrowski signs.

The Dorken and Kral (1952) system consists of seven signs, whose presence is considered contraindicative of organicity. The method by which the signs were chosen was unspecified. The signs were weighted according to their incidence in a criterion population (Goldfried et al., 1971). The Dorken and Kral (1952) system has the most false positives and a large number of false negatives. The signs suggested by Aita et al. (1947) for the diagnosis of organicity were not proposed as a formal sign system. No cutoff point was suggested for the nine signs as indicating the presence or absence of brain pathology

Evans and Marmorston's system (1963b, 1964) represents a compilation of signs suggested by other researchers. Their initial 46-item list includes the 9 signs of Aita et al., as well as the 10 signs composing Piotrowski's system. A number of cutoff points have been suggested for the 46-item list, depending on the type of comparison being made. The use of this system has been restricted primarily to the authors, in research with patients with cerebral thrombosis and acute myocardial infarctions.

Normative Data for the Sign Systems

Adequate normative data have not been established for any of the major Rorschach sign systems. There has been a general failure to provide adequate control or assessment of such variables as age, sex, intelligence, or level of education. Sample sizes have also tended to be inadequate. For example, in a review of 24 studies in which the Piotrowski signs were used, the median sample was found to be made up of fewer than 30 subjects (Goldfried et al., 1971). These samples have tended to be heterogeneous, and the method of diagnosis of brain injury in almost half the cases was unspecified.

Reliability Studies

Aside from interscorer reliability measures, essentially no research has been conducted regarding the reliability of the various Rorschach sign systems. In a study using selected signs from Piotrowski's system (impotency, automatic phrases, perplexity, and repetition), and from the Hughes system (contamination, color shock, and shading shock), Forar, Farberow, Meyer, and Tolman (1952) reported interscorer reliability, both between independent scorers and between the same scorer on two different occasions, for the Piotrowski signs to be consistently in the 80s. In the Hughes system, the color shock sign was found to be unreliable, and the shading shock sign was found to be of questionable validity. The contamination sign was found to be consistently reliable.

Additional reliability data have been reported by Evans and Marmorston (1963a,b, 1964), using their 46-item list. Test–retest correlations of .97 (for the same evaluator) were obtained following an intertest interval of 6 months. The test–retest reliability was recorded as .77.

A review of the research literature indicates that research on test reliability is needed. There has been only a limited amount of research on interscorer or test–retest reliability, and additional research is warranted as well.

Validity of the Sign Systems

The majority of the validity studies reviewed have been criterion-related studies. The Piotrowski system is the only major system on which sufficient data have been published to permit an adequate assessment of its validity. These signs have proved to be able to differentiate brain-damaged and control groups about 50% of the time. The call rate (the percentage of subjects diagnosed as brain-damaged) is considered low, and as a result, few false positives are produced. In contrast, these signs are liable to produce false negatives. The impotency sign has been found to be one of the best predictors of neurological impairment, whereas more traditional Rorschach variables have proved to be relatively poor predictors.

In validity studies using the Piotrowski and the Hughes systems (Fisher, Gonda, & Little, 1955; Hertz & Loehrke, 1954), the Piotrowski signs have been found to be slightly superior. Fisher et al. (1955) also compared the Piotrowski and Hughes systems to the Dorken and Kral signs. This study found the Piotrowski system the most effective and the Dorken and Kral system the least effective of the three systems evaluated.

Construct Validity

A systematic approach to establishing the construct validity of any of the major Rorschach systems has not been reported. Independent studies have been conducted on a variety of patient populations and have provided some support for several of the Rorschach systems. For example, Allison and Allison (1954) used the Dorken and Kral signs in a study of the effect of transorbital lobotomies; Evans and Marmorston (1963a, 1965) studied the effects of Premarin therapy by randomly dividing groups of cerebral thrombosis and myocardial infarction patients and administering Premarin to half and a placebo to half; Grauer (1953) selected 18 improved paranoid schizophrenics and 18 unimproved paranoid schizophrenics and compared their Rorschach protocols. No differences in Piotrowski signs were found between the two groups in this last study.

As noted previously, the research methodology most used in evaluating the Rorschach's ability to assess the neuropsychological changes associated with brain damage has been the sign approach. A number of methodological problems become obvious as one reviews the research literature in this area. A second methodological problem that is common in the research on the various sign systems is that not one of the major systems of Rorschach indicators has controlled for such variables as age, intelligence, education, sex, race, or socioeconomic status. Third, there has been a general failure to cross-validate the signs, as well as a failure to take base rates into account when assessing the signs' ability to discriminate between different groups.

Detection of Response Bias

Although the Rorschach does not have any index of response bias, it does not appear to be sensitive to the effects of negative response bias, at least in terms of malingering psychosis. When two groups of individuals who had been accused of serious crimes were administered both the MMPI and the Rorschach and then classified as malingerers or honest responders based on the MMPI validity scales, there were no differences on Rorschach indices thought to be reflective of psychosis (Ganellen, Wasyliw, Haywood, & Grossman, 1996). In general, the Rorschach can not be reliably used to determine the extent of response bias. Ganellen et al. (1996) reported that the Exner scores cannot reliably detect exaggeration of psychopathology in criminal subjects. On the other hand, when MMPI validity scales indicated defensive responding in airline pilots following treatment for alcohol abuse, their Rorschach responses indicated emotional distress, indicating that positive response bias may not affect results (Ganellen, 1994). Freuh and Kinder (1994) found that both the Rorschach and the MMPI were susceptible to malingered symptoms of posttraumatic stress disorder (PTSD). Wasyliw, Benn, Grossman, and Haywood (1998) reported that the Rorschach is essentially useless in detecting minimization of psychopathology in a sample of clergy and laity referred for evaluation as the result of allegations of sex offenses.

CONCLUSIONS

There are many problems with the research related to the Rorschach in the diagnosis of organicity. There has not generally been an adequate definition of the nature of the organic impairment, the researchers typically fail to exclude organic involvement in the control subjects, and there is a lack of adequate reliability studies. Frank (1991) concluded that the Rorschach should not be used to detect organic impairment.

Goldfried et al. (1971) concluded that, although several of the Rorschach indices surveyed have demonstrated enough validity to justify their use in research, their suitability for clinical use has not been sufficiently established. The Rorschach does not lend itself easily to split-half reliability studies, nor is there any satisfactory parallel form for the test. Rorschach reliability studies must therefore focus on the temporal stability of this instrument.

Future studies will need to define the subject groups on the basis of preestablished diagnostic guidelines. There is also a need for normative data for specific populations. Future researchers should discard the unitary concept of brain damage, given the problems with the heterogeneity of the effects of brain damage and the need to separate groups according to the characteristics of the lesion and of the affected person. It may be possible to provide multiple sets of relevant signs and norms that control for age, sex, intelligence, and level of education. All of this research should be conducted with cross-validation, and attention should be paid to base-rate information.

The Rorschach may be affected by visual–spatial difficulties or perceptual problems that suggest emotional problems that may not be present. Certain frontal disorders or disorders such as dementia may reflect the client's inability to process information cognitively rather than provide a measure of the patient's personality style.

One of the principal problems has to do with defining the term *brain damage*. Birch and Diller (1959) argued that a distinction should be made between brain damage, which is an anatomical occurrence, and organicity, which is possibly a behavioral consequence. Of necessity, the Rorschach can be expected to be sensitive only to organicity. Organicity is not, however, a necessary sequel to brain damage. Lesions can exist with no apparent sensory, motor, mental, or emotional symptoms, and lesions can produce sensory or motor symptoms without accompanying mental or emotional difficulties. Every case in which a lesion exists without a cognitive or emotional symptom—in other words, in which brain damage exists without organicity—will produce a false negative, in that it would be impossible for the Rorschach to detect the brain damage in the absence of organicity.

The Rorschach continues to be a source of controversy with greater support coming from the clinical than from the empirical contingent. Given that the use of the Rorschach with general and with psychiatric populations is still controversial, its use with neuropsychological populations should be even more circumscribed. In general, it is not efficient as an instrument to diagnose cortical impairment. It may also be limited as an instrument to diagnose psychological dysfunction, at least in a neuropsychological population.

The Wechsler Memory Scale and its Revisions

The Wechsler Memory Scale consists of seven subtests, which were designed to measure different aspects of memory. It exists in two forms (I and II). The subtests, Personal and Current Information, Orientation, Mental Control, Logical Memory, Digit Span, Visual Reproduction, and Associate Learning comprise a structure that is largely replicated with some changes in the subsequent revisions, the Wechsler Memory Scale-Revised (WMS-R) and the Wechsler Memory Scale-Third Edition (WMS-III). These subtests are scored for the number of correct responses, which are then summed. The summed score is age-corrected and converted to a Memory Quotient, which has a mean of 100.

The WMS is still in use despite the criticism that it does not discriminate well between intact and brain-damaged subjects (Prigatano, 1978) and despite two subsequent revisions. Because of the criticisms raised, it is very important that a clinician interested in using the instrument be familiar with the research regarding the reliability and the validity of the WMS. In addition, because these criticisms helped inform the later revisions, the Wechsler Memory Scale-Revised and the Wechsler Memory Scale-Third Edition, a brief review of the WMS literature can help the clinician in understanding these later manifestations.

THE WECHSLER MEMORY SCALE

Normative Data

The original standardization sample consisted of 200 normal subjects who ranged in age from 25 to 50 years. The proportion of males to females was not given in the manual (Weschler & Stone, 1973). The small size of the standardization sample and the un-availability of important descriptive statistics regarding the sample detract from the useful-ness of this instrument. Ivison (1977) presented some normative data derived from a sample of Australian subjects. Using some of the same sample, des Rosiers and Ivison (1986) reported normative data regarding the difference between performances on the high asso-ciative word pairs and on the low associative word pairs. Ivinskis, Allen, and Shaw (1971) examined performance on the WMS in 30 younger (10 to 14 years) subjects and 44 somewhat older subjects (16 to 18 years). The proportion of males and females was not given. Compared with the subjects used in Wechsler's original sample, the younger sample of Ivinskis et al. (1971) performed more poorly on each of the subtests except Associate Learning, on which they performed better than the older subjects. This sample was also too limited in size to allow confidence in generalizing the results. However, the results do point out the differences in WMS performance that may be attributed to the effects of age.

Cauthen (1977) looked at the WMS in 64 people over age 60. The effects of both age and IQ were examined in this study. Although the older subjects did more poorly on all of the subtests, only Visual Reproduction showed a statistically significant decline with age.

Reliability

Reliability information on the WMS is scarce. Ryan, Morris, Yaffa, and Peterson (1981) performed a test–retest experiment on Form I with both a normal ($n = 34$) and a mixed psychiatric-neurological inpatient sample ($n = 30$), but the intertest interval was not equivalent for the two groups. All of the normals were retested after 14 days, but the patients were retested after 5 days to 37 months with a mean interval of 14.2 months. Pearson product–moment correlation coefficients were calculated separately for the two groups with a value of .75 for the normals and a value of .89 for the patients. Although there were gains in some subjects and losses in others, on the average there was a gain in Memory Quotient (MQ). The normals gained an average of 7.2 points ($t = 3.95$, $p < .001$), and the patients gained an average of 4.0 points ($t = 2.32$, $p < .05$). These results suggest that, although there is adequate reliability in terms of the stability in position in group distribution, individual subjects are likely to manifest a gain in scores across time.

Stinnett and DiGiacomo (1970) administered Form I to 15 psychiatric inpatients before electroconvulsive therapy (ECT) and Form II sometime after ECT, with a mean interval of 18.9 days. In examining the data, Prigatano (1978) computed a correlation coefficient of .80. It should be noted that, because of the time that intervened between the two tests and the procedure that was performed (ECT), it may be that this is a lower estimate of what the test–retest reliability may actually be in this sample. The small sample size limits confidence in the stability of the solved coefficient. In reviewing the unsystematic studies that have been performed on the WMS, Prigatano (1978) concluded that its test–retest reliability is fairly stable and that its alternate-forms reliability is probably adequate. Over short intervals, MQ scores will increase, and that, with longer intervals (and with age), the MQ scores will decrease.

The WMS produces both a single MQ score and scores for the seven subtests. A reasonable question regards the degree of internal consistency in the test as a whole as well as in the subtests. No internal consistency data are reported in the manual. Ivinskis et al. (1971) reported that the split-half reliability of the WMS is .75. with no information on the type of split that was used or whether or not the Spearman–Brown formula was used to correct for the length of the test.

In addition, there is only one report of an examination of the internal consistency of the subtests. Hall and Toal (1957) reported low Cronbach's coefficient alpha values for two of the WMS subtests: .383 for Mental Control and .368 for Associate Learning. The values for the other subtests were more moderate: .814 for Logical Memory, .647 for Digit Span, and .634 for Visual Reproduction. Cronbach's coefficient alpha for the whole test was .686. No values were reported for the Information or Orientation subtests. Hall and Toal (1957) reported low intercorrelations among the subtests, a result that Ivinskis et al. (1971) supported, using their sample of younger subjects.

Ivison (1977) adapted the WMS for use with Australian people. Although Australians share the English language with citizens of the United States, there are enough cultural differences to imply that restandardization is necessary. After changes were made to reflect differences in culture and language (e.g., changing "president" to "prime minister" in the Information section and "took up a collection" to "made up a purse" in the Logical Memory section), the Australian WMS was normed on 500 hospitalized subjects. Slightly different norms were obtained, underscoring the importance of restandardization for clinical interpretation.

However, it is instructional for us to examine the intercorrelations among these translated subtests to glean whatever useful information may be contained there. Clement (1966) administered the French WMS to 477 males and 276 females who ranged in age from 16 to 100 years. He did not correlate the Personal Information, the Orientation, or the Mental Control subtests with the other four subtests, and he entered the Digits Backward score separately from the Digits Forward score. The correlation coefficients ranged from $-.05$ to $.41$. Although the analysis was conducted on a French translation, its results agree with the English language version, lending further support to the notion of meaningful subtest interpretation. In the same study, the subtests were correlated with the total WMS score ranging from $.36$ to $.71$, which do not support the notion of high internal consistency in the test as a whole. Pershad and Lubey (1974) calculated intercorrelations among the WMS subtests in a sample of 150 subjects in an Indian translation. They reported correlations that ranged from $.31$ to $.73$, again adding limited support to the notion of subtest interpretability over MQ interpretability.

Factor structure is an area that has been more adequately, if still somewhat sparsely, investigated. The question of unidimensionality can be partially addressed by a factor analysis of the instrument. The first published account was given by Davis and Swenson (1970). This study evaluated 622 mixed psychiatric and neurological patients. The authors performed a centroid factor analysis with an oblique rotation, and they interpreted the resulting two factors as memory and freedom from distractibility. It must be remembered that the results of factor analysis are influenced by the sample as well as by the structure of the instrument.

Dujovne and Levy (1971) conducted separate factor analyses for 276 normals and 158 patients, 81 of whom had been diagnosed as organic, and the rest of whom had psychiatric diagnoses. In a preliminary examination of the data, it was determined that a large majority of all the subjects had passed all of the items in the Personal and Current Information and the Orientation scales of the WMS. The authors therefore removed these scales from further analysis. The remaining WMS items were then submitted to factor analysis, along with the WAIS Full Scale, Verbal, and Performance IQ scores and the classification of patient or normal, all of which were used as reference variables. A principal-axis solution with varimax rotation was used. The authors interpreted the three factors for the normal group as general retentiveness, simple learning, and associative flexibility. The three solved factors for the patient group were mental control, associative flexibility, and cognitive dysfunction, indicating both some similarity and some disparities in the structure of the WMS in subjects with different characteristics. There are two problems in interpreting these results as indicative strictly of the internal structure of the WMS. First, the use of the WAIS variables as references very likely modified the factor analysis results. Second, the removal of the Personal and Current Information and the Orientation variables from the analysis means that only a partial view of the structure could be afforded by the analysis.

Kear-Colwell (1973) performed a factor analysis on all of the WMS variables, as well as a separate analysis, using the same subjects, on the WMS factor scores, the WAIS variables, and the age and the sex of the subjects as a comparison. The sample included 161 males and 89 females. All of the subjects had been referred for neuropsychological evaluation, and 66 had organic deficits, as confirmed by neurological or neurosurgical exam. The factor analyses were performed by the principal-components method, the scree test was used as the criterion for stopping extraction, and oblimin rotation was used to model factor interrelationships. The analyses were conducted separately for the 66 confirmed organically impaired patients and the 184 suspected organically impaired patients. In the case of the WMS only analysis, both groups produced highly similar factors that were not significantly different when Harmon's psi congruence coefficient was used. The two groups were combined, and the combined analysis produced an almost identical factor structure, which produced three factors. These were interpreted as learning and recall of novel material, attention and concentration, and orientation and long-established verbal information. The analyses that included the WAIS and demographic data were again similar and were again combined. The combined analysis was similar to both of the separate analyses and produced three factors, which were interpreted as intellectual ability, verbal-performance discrepancy, and age. Kear-Colwell (1973) concluded that the factor structure of the WMS was identical in subjects with confirmed lesions and in subjects without confirmed lesions. Together, these three factors accounted for 77% of the variance in the WMS. Kear-Colwell (1977) attempted a replication, in which he again found three factors that, when compared by use of the Harmon psi coefficient, were similar to the factors in the original study.

One of the factors extracted in the analysis that used demographic data was age, raising the possibility that the factor structure of the WMS is influenced by age. To investigate this question, Arbit and Zagar (1979) used a data set of 2500 hospitalized and non-hospitalized patients with suspected neurological disorders. There were 1322 males and 1178 females. The subjects were divided into three groups on the basis of age (13 to 39, 40 to 59, and 60 to 88 years). In each group, both the males and females were divided into two randomly assigned groups, for a total of 16 samples. The analyses performed were principal components, with oblique rotation, and an eigenvalue criterion of .92 for factor extraction. In each analysis except for the 60- to 88-year-old group, similar solutions of two factors were obtained. The differences between the solutions in the above studies may be related to differences in the types of analyses conducted: oblique versus varimax rotation (Sawicki & Golden, 1984a) and the scree test versus the eigenvalue criterion for the extraction of factors (Franzen & Golden, 1984a).

Dye (1982) performed a factor analysis on 99 older males (average age, 63.43 years). The type of factor analysis was not reported, but the rotation method (varimax) and the factor extraction criterion (eigenvalues > 1.0) were reported. The three obtained factors were interpreted as general retentiveness, attention and concentration, and orientation. The author concluded that the factor structure of the WMS is indeed stable over age. However, the sample size was probably too small to allow much confidence in the stability of the solution, the method of factor analysis differed from that of the earlier studies, and no similar concurrent analysis was conducted on younger age groups with which to compare these results.

Skillbeck and Woods (1980) conducted two parallel factor analyses. One was on a sample of 150 neurological inpatients, and the second was on a sample of 156 geriatric subjects. Both times, the method used was principal-factor analysis with oblimin rotation, and the scree test was used for the number of factors. The neurological patient sample yielded three factors, which were interpreted as learning-recall, attention-concentration, and information-orientation, similar to the earlier analyses of neurological patient analyses. The geriatric sample yielded three factors, which were interpreted as learning-recall, attention-concentration, and visual-short-term memory. With the use of Harmon's psi coefficient, the first two geriatric factors were congruent with the first two factors of the neurological sample; however, the third factor was not congruent. The safest conclusion in considering all of these studies together is that the factor structure of the WMS does change with age, especially after 60.

Other characteristics of the sample may also influence the factor structure of the WMS. Kear-Colwell and Heller (1978) attempted to replicate the earlier results found in neurological inpatients in a normal sample of 116 subjects. They found a three-factor solution that did not replicate the earlier solutions. When they forced a four-factor solution, they found that the first, second, and fourth factors roughly agreed with the earlier solutions. They concluded that the factor structure of the WMS was stable, a statement that is not borne out by the data. Age and neurological status are two variables that can affect the structure.

Ernst et al. (1986) investigated the factor structure of the WMS in a sample of 70 psychiatric inpatients. They used principal-factors analysis with varimax rotation on the raw data of scores from the delayed-recall variant of the WMS. This procedure resulted in a four-factor solution. The first two factors were interpreted as attention-concentration and rote memory. The third and fourth factors were labeled minor factors and were not interpreted. The rote memory factor appeared to be similar to earlier factors labeled retentiveness. In general, the different factor solutions seemingly related to sample characteristics can be seen in the studies of the WMS-R and may also be found in the future in studies of the WMS-III. The use of confirmatory factor analysis methods will help test this hypothesis, but it will be important to analyze the role of these variables in future research to avoid some of the ambiguity in these studies.

Validity

Just as there has been little direct research on the reliability of the WMS, there has been little direct research on the validity of the WMS. From an examination of the instrument, arguments regarding its construct validity can be raised. Although it supposedly measures memory as a whole, the WMS is seemingly weighted toward the assessment of verbal memory. There are no tests of delayed memory or of memory with interference. The existence of the MQ begs the question of whether memory is actually a unitary construct.

Originally, Wechsler saw the WMS as a test of organic impairment when used in conjunction with the Wechsler–Bellevue (at first) and later with the Wechsler Adult

Intelligence Scale. The MQ was developed to have the same meaning as the IQ. It was supposed to represent the memory ability of an individual in comparison to the memory ability of other people of roughly the same age. An individual was assumed to have roughly the same IQ as MQ. If there was a discrepancy between the two scores (e.g., if IQ was sufficiently higher than MQ) then a memory deficit was present. In addition, it was thought that all brain damage would result in memory impairment and, as a consequence, would result in a large IQ–MQ discrepancy. These assumptions exist in a somewhat more sophisticated version in the WMS-III which has been co-normed with the WAIS-III to allow comparisons with index scores of both instruments. The empirical validity of these differences still needs to be addressed.

The diagnostic validity of the IQ–MQ split has not been supported by studies in the literature. MQ was found to be slightly but not significantly lower than IQ in a group of mixed neurological patients, but the same pattern was found in the normal subjects who served as controls in the study (Parker, 1957). Cohen (1950) had earlier reported similar results, but without a control group. Fields (1971) also reported a failure to support this clinical interpretation guide in a sample of 126 neurological patients. Norton (1979) examined the IQ–MQ split in 95 neurologically normal and 87 abnormal patients who had been referred for neuropsychological evaluation. He found no relationship between the IQ–MQ split and the eventual finding of neurological abnormality as defined by the results of noninvasive neurodiagnostic techniques. McCara (1953) examined the MQ–IQ split in adults of average and superior intelligence and found that the size of the split was related to IQ. The subjects in the superior group (mean IQ = 134.4) had a significantly larger MQ–IQ split than did the subjects in the average IQ group (mean IQ = 105.3). These results should have a sobering effect on attempts to clinically interpret WMS- III/WAIS-III discrepancy scores without empirical examination.

Bachrach and Mintz (1974) examined the usefulness of the WMS in separating individuals whom neurologists had diagnosed as impaired from individuals who had not been so diagnosed. These authors found that, in a discriminant function analysis, the seven subtest scores were able to discriminate between the two groups of subjects. Unfortunately, the authors did not report the percentage of correct and incorrect classifications that resulted from the application of the discriminant function, nor did they attempt a cross-validation; both kinds of information are necessary for us to judge the accuracy of the variables in discriminating between the two groups (Franzen & Golden, 1984b). An interesting result of this study is the fact that the Visual Reproduction subtest alone had a zero-order correlation that was almost identical to the multiple correlation relating all of the WMS subtest scores and group membership, indicating that nearly all of the discriminatory power in the WMS is actually contained in the Visual Reproduction subtest.

Kljajic (1975) examined the accuracy of detecting organicity in a sample of 19 neurologically impaired and 18 neurologically nonimpaired subjects, using two different formulas for the interpretation of WMS scale scores, and reported a 70% accuracy rate. The need for cross-validation is obvious because of the small sample. Prigatano (1978) exam- ined the diagnostic accuracy of three methods including the Kljajic (1975) method in a sample of mixed brain-dysfunction patients and 26 matched controls. He concluded that there was no support for the use of the WMS in diagnosing neurological impairment when any of the methods were used.

Black (1973a) found slightly lower but not statistically significant scores on the WMS for 100 subjects with penetrating missile wounds to the head when they were compared with 50 normal subjects. Black (1974a) compared the WMS scores of 50 subjects with closed-head injuries and 50 subjects with penetrating missile wounds and found that those with closed head injuries had significantly more impaired scores on the WMS. This finding is an indication that the WMS is not sensitive to neurological impairment in general but is sensitive to certain forms of brain damage. Further evidence is found in Kear-Colwell and Heller (1980) and in Brooks (1976); both reported significantly impaired WMS performance following closed head injury.

If IQ and MQ do not actually differ much following brain damage, do they measure the same thing? Fields (1971) reported a correlation of .83 between the two Wechsler quotients, indicating a fair amount of shared variance. As noted earlier, McCara (1953) found that, although IQ is highly related to MQ at normal IQ levels, the relationship deteriorates as IQ increases. Fish and Sinkel (1980) correlated IQ with MQ in 10 alcoholic subjects and 10 matched controls and concluded that the WMS measures an ability separate from IQ in alcoholics, but not in normals.

Libb and Coleman (1971) correlated the WMS, the Quick Test, and the Revised Beta with the WAIS in a sample of 30 clients from a rehabilitation center. Sixteen of the clients were diagnosed as retarded. The WMS correlated .80, the Quick Test correlated .84, and the Revised Beta correlated .83. Because both of the other tests are used for estimates of IQ, it would seem from these results that the WMS may actually measure IQ. Similar results have been reported by other researchers (Black, 1973b; Ivinskis et al., 1971; Kear-Colwell, 1973).

Because there is some inconsistency in reported correlations between IQ and MQ, it appears that each instrument offers information that is independent of the other. Larrabee, Kane, and Schuck (1983) conducted a factor analysis of the WMS and the WAIS combined to address the question of unique information from each. They used a maximum-likelihood solution with orthogonal factors. They found a factor structure that replicated earlier factor-analysis research into the WMS and the WAIS separately. The factors were interpreted as perceptual organization, verbal comprehension, attention and concentration (with loadings from both WAIS and WMS subtests), verbal learning and recall, and orientation and information. They concluded that the previously reported correlations between the WMS and the WAIS were the result of shared procedures (the Digit Span) and a shared factor (attention and concentration). The discrimination of IQ from MQ is important in the evaluation of construct validity. However, it is also necessary to demonstrate that the variance not shared with intelligence actually does measure memory.

The WMS as a Measure of Short-Term Verbal Memory

By face validity, the WMS is a measure of short-term verbal memory. As a test of verbal short-term memory, we would expect the WMS to be sensitive to disturbances of physiology and structure in the deep posterior left hemisphere and to be sensitive to disturbances as a whole. Alcoholism is a disorder that is often associated with memory disorders. Rausch, Lieb, and Crandall (1978) correlated WAIS and WMS measures with EEG spike activity in 12 patients with intractable temporal lobe epilepsy. Total spike activity was correlated with IQ, but lateralization of the spike activity was correlated with MQ. This finding is consistent with the hypothesis that the WMS is sensitive to dysfunctions in deep posterior dominant-hemisphere activity.

In a study to test the effect of alcoholism and a history of blackouts, Tarter and Schneider (1976) examined the effect of blackouts on memory function by using the WMS, consonant trigrams, the retention of temporal sequencing, and Hebb's number-recall test. There was no relationship between low- and high-incidence blackout subjects and any of the measures. These results may speak more to the construct underlying blackouts more than to the sensitivity of these memory assessment instruments. Advanced Huntington's disease subjects demonstrated deficits on several measures of neuropsychological functioning, but the subjects with recently diagnosed Huntington's disease demonstrated deficits only in memory (Butters, Sax, Montgomery, & Tarlow, 1978).

Earlier, we discussed the nonsignificant findings in the attempts to relate penetrating missile wounds to WMS scores. The experimental group of missile-wound victims was a heterogeneous group in terms of the location of the wound. Black (1973b) found significant deficits on the WMS when left-hemisphere missile-wound subjects were compared with normal controls, but not when right-hemisphere missile-wound subjects were compared with normals. Bornstein (1982a) examined the relationship between location of lesion and performance on the WMS. Although there were no significant differences in MQ or IQ–MQ split between the two groups, the left-hemisphere subjects performed more poorly on the Logical Memory and the Paired Associates subtests, and the right-hemisphere subjects performed more poorly on the Visual Reproduction subtest. These findings once more underline the insensitivity of the MQ as compared to the sensitivity of the subtests themselves.

Jackson (1978) reported that bilateral ECT produced the largest effect on WMS performance, unilateral left ECT the next largest, and unilateral right ECT the smallest effect. Fraser and Glass (1980) reported that both unilateral right ECT and bilateral ECT eventually improved memory to the same degree. Unfortunately, there was no attempt to examine the effects of unilateral left ECT. Likewise, Stromgren (1973) and Stromgren, Christensen, and Fromholt (1976) reported that unilateral right ECT eventually improved WMS scores, without a comparison with unilateral left ECT. When memory was assessed the day following the last ECT treatment, unilateral right ECT improved MQ scores, whereas bilateral ECT decreased MQ scores. There was no information on recovery on follow-up.

Attempts at Improving the WMS

Many criticisms have been leveled at the WMS directed at the adequacy of the standardization sample, at the reliability of the instrument, and at the validity of the scores obtained. Some of the criticisms have also been directed at the adequacy of the scoring system. For example, the manual (Wechsler, 1945; Wechsler & Stone, 1973) states that the Logical Memory section should be scored for each reiteration of an idea as marked on the protocol. Unfortunately, the marked ideas often contain more than one word, and confusion results when, for example, the subject correctly reiterates the first name of the story's protagonist but gives incorrectly the last name of the protagonist. Sweet and Wysocki (1982) suggested that the ideas be scored for equivalence of meaning rather than for verbatim performance. These authors presented a table of acceptable equivalents and stated that the interscorer reliability for their scoring system is .97. This is a good start in the right direction, but it may be inadequate to remedy other aspects of the WMS that have been criticized. The scoring instructions of the WMS-R and WMS-III help reduce these problems.

Osborne and Davis (1978) attempted another improvement on the WMS by suggesting that the subtests be given standardized scores. By examining the standard deviation and the means of Mental Control, Logical Memory, Visual Reproduction, and Associate Learning reported in Davis and Swenson (1970), these authors gave formulas for calculating standardized scores with a mean of 10 and a standard deviation of 3 from raw scores on the subtests. Unfortunately, there are no data on the usefulness of these scores. The translation of raw subtest scores into standardized scores has been conducted on the WMS-III, facilitating the empirical investigation of this concept.

Russell's Revision of the WMS

Russell (1975a) identified some of the shortcomings of the WMS. These shortcomings were partly based on the assumptions underlying the construction of the battery. One of those assumptions is that memory is a unitary construct that has verbal and visual implications, but not verbal and visual components. The ramification of this assumption is that memory deficits are deficits in both verbal and visual memory, and that a deficit in one area is always associated with a deficit in the other. Second, the WMS assumes that brain damage is a unitary construct that can be determined by a single test. Citing both experimental work on memory and factor analyses of the WMS, Russell concluded that a more precise, multidimensional scoring system for the WMS would increase its utility.

After consideration of the factor analysis studies and the validity studies of the WMS, Russell (1975a) decided on two subtests for the WMS: Verbal (consisting of the Logical Memory subtest of the WMS) and Figural (consisting of the Visual Reproduction subtest of the WMS). In addition, Russell added what he termed a long-term memory factor, although it could more accurately be termed a delayed-memory factor. This factor is produced by asking the subjects to recall the material in the test one half hour following the original administration. Six scores are available: short-term verbal, long-term verbal, the difference between the two, short-term figural, long-term figural, and the difference between the two. This conceptualization is reflected in the WMS-R and WMS-III.

Russell (1975a) administered his revised WMS to 30 normals and 75 brain-damaged inpatients at a VA medical center. When corrected for test length by the Spearman–Brown formula, the split-half reliability of the six scores obtained ranged from .88 for the long-term verbal score to .51 for the figural difference score. No other forms of reliability were reported in this study. The validity of the Revised WMS (RWMS) was assessed by examining the effect of an organic diagnosis on the RWMS subtest scores. The organics had significantly worse performance on each of the subtests. The subtest scores correlated with each subject's HRNB Average Impairment Rating (AIR), ranging from −.49 to −.76, indicating moderate relationships between memory scores and general neurological impairment, and these correlations were always lower for the normal subjects (Russell, 1975a).

Using the same sample, Russell (1975a) translated the raw subtest scores on the RWMS to a 5-point scale by transforming both AIR and RWMS scores to z scores and using the AIR 5-point scale as a reference for the determination of the 5 points in the RWMS scale. Drawing the lateralized subjects from the original sample of brain-damaged individuals, Russell examined the effect of a lateralized diagnosis on the subtest scores and concluded that the subtest scores could be used, in conjunction with each other, to lateralize damage. He further concluded that long-term memory subtests were more sensitive to lateralized damage than were the short-term subtests.

This was a noble effort to improve the utility of the WMS, but it fell short of its goal for several reasons. The standardization sample of 105 subjects was even less sufficient than Wechsler's sample of 200 subjects. The fact that Russell's study was conducted in a VA setting means that few of the subjects were female; thus, the applicability of the RWMS to a broad population is severely limited. The most significant shortcoming was that all of the above analyses were conducted on the same sample of 105 subjects. We can have very little confidence in the generalizability of the results beyond the sample. Sound scale-construction methodology dictates that separate samples be used at each step of the study.

Further research would be needed before any conclusions regarding the utility of this instrument could be reached. Along those lines, Brinkman, Largen, Gerganoff, and Pomara (1983) provided evidence that the subtest scale scores significantly differentiated between 31 healthy elderly and 25 elderly with diagnoses of probable Alzheimer's disease.

In an attempt to provide additional evidence regarding the RWMS, McCarty, Logue, Power, Ziesat, and Rosenstiel (1980) administered two forms of the RWMS to 25 female residents of a nursing home for the elderly. The two forms of the RWMS were composed from the alternate forms of the WMS. The alternate-form reliability estimates ranged from .74 for short-term verbal scores to .40 for verbal difference scores. However, because of the differences in the level of scores for individual subjects, it appears that a comparison of the two forms should not consist of raw scores.

Following up on this study, Keesler, Schultz, Sciara, and Friedenberg (1984) administered the alternate forms of the RWMS in counterbalanced order. The subjects for these two studies were drawn from two different populations: a group of 48 inpatient alcoholics and a group of 60 normal volunteers drawn from the staff of a private psychiatric hospital. Consistent with the results of McCarty et al. (1980), these authors found that these groups performed differentially on the two forms.

These results have two implications for the RWMS. The first is that the use of the alternate forms of the RWMS to perform serial testing is likely to eventuate in inaccurate conclusions regarding the improvement or the deterioration of the subject's memory, depending on which form is administered first. The second implication involves the danger of making even slight changes in a test without renorming the revised form. One should not assume that the equivalence of the alternate forms of the WMS will carry over to the revised scoring system of Russell. Instead, what is needed is an evaluation of the equivalence of the two revised forms. In considering the differences in scores on the two forms, Schultz, Keesler, Friedenberg, and Sciara (1984) recommended two possible solutions. Their first suggestion was to raise the scores obtained from the form with the lower performance by the percentage by which the stimuli for the two forms were judged to be more difficult. In other words, they suggested that the score obtained on the Immediate Figural Memory scale of Form I be increased by 10%. Although such a linear transformation of scores would not affect the distribution of the scores obtained by a sample or affect the reliability of Form I, it would have effects on the validity of the interpretation of the obtained scores. Therefore, we cannot recommend the practice.

The second recommendation of Schultz et al. (1984) was to reverse the stimuli across forms, that is, to administer Figure 1 from Form I and Figure 2 from Form II, and so on. This suggestion would result in even more undesirable effects, two brand new tests with unknown psychometric and clinical properties. Although it is possible that this approach might result in equivalent forms, that conclusion cannot be reached without extensive empirical investigation. A more direct method of dealing with this problem would be to convert the raw scores obtained on the two forms to standardized scores by means of a linear transformation. This transformation would not affect the reliability of the instrument and would permit a comparison of the scores obtained from the two forms.

There is no study that examines the factor structure of the RWMS by itself. Russell (1982) did examine the structure in conjunction with the WAIS and the Halstead–Reitan and interpreted the factors as immediate verbal memory, recent verbal memory, recent memory, figural learning, and verbal learning storage. It is difficult to interpret the results of this analysis because of the inclusion of the WAIS and the Halstead–Reitan, and because of the existence of a substantial loading of nonmemory tasks on factors that Russell interpreted as memory factors.

A few validation studies exist for the RWMS. Logue and Wyrick (1979) reported that the RWMS discriminated between 29 normal older and 29 demented older subjects. Prigatano, Parsons, Wright, Levin, and Hawryluk (1983) reported that 100 chronic obstructive-pulmonary disease patients performed significantly worse on the RWMS than did 25 normal controls. Crosson and Trautt (1981) presented case study evidence that the RWMS is a sensitive indicator of recovery from brain stem infarction. These are all indications that the RWMS may be a useful instrument for the assessment of memory functions. However, much more work, such as the elderly norms reported by Haaland, Linn, Hunt, and Goodwin (1983), is needed before the RWMS can be recommended for clinical use. Evidence supporting the need for further work, especially in establishing a normative base, can be found in Crosson, Hughes, Roth, and Monkowski (1984), who found that, when Russell's norms were applied to data from previous studies, a large proportion of subjects were misclassified as memory-impaired, when the Logical Memory subscale, but not the Visual Memory subscale, was used. Wallace (1984) presented a valuable gathering of the available data in a single location, but the Logical Memory and the Visual Reproduction subtests are still based on a sample of only 66 normal subjects, who ranged in age from 10 to 94.

Conclusions

The Wechsler Memory Scale is a widely used instrument that has little empirical evidence to support its clinical application. Originally construed as a unidimensional measure of brain damage when the MQ is used in conjunction with the IQ, it has been shown to be neither a good index of brain damage in general nor a single indicator of memory impairment. Although it has failed to stand up to its initial conceptualization, there is evidence that it may be useful as a measure of particular forms of memory impairment. Although it remains in limited current usage, the most important role of the WMS is as the precursor of the later revisions, WMS-R and WMS-III.

WECHSLER MEMORY SCALE-REVISED

In 1987, the long-awaited revision of the Wechsler Memory Scale was published (Wechsler, 1987). Currently, the WMS-R is in very wide usage whether the context is clinical (Guilmette, Faust, Hart, & Arkes, 1990) or forensic (Lees-Haley, Smith, Williams,

& Dunn, 1996). The Wechsler Memory Scale-Revised (WMS-R) has several intended improvements over the original WMS. The WMS-R has age-related norms for nine age groups: 16 to 17 years, 18 to 19 years (estimated), 20 to 24 years, 25 to 34 years (estimated), 35 to 44 years, 45 to 54 years (estimated), 55 to 64 years, 65 to 69 years, and 70 to 74 years. Because of criticisms regarding the loss of information in using a single memory quotient (MQ), the WMS-R has five composite scores: General Memory (GMI), Attention/ Concentration, Verbal Memory, Visual Memory, and Delayed Memory (DMI). Each of these composite scores has a mean of 100 and a standard deviation of 15. There were also new subtests added to obtain nonverbal information (related to figural, spatial, and visual associative memory) analogous to the verbal information obtained on the original WMS. A delayed recall procedure was added, and scoring procedures were revised to make them more reliable. The items related to Information and Orientation were deleted from the computation of index scores because of the controversy regarding whether they reflected memory or not.

The scorable subtests of the WMS-R consist of Mental Control, Figural Memory, Logical Memory, Visual Paired Associates, Verbal Paired Associates, Visual Reproduction, Digit Span, Visual Memory Span, and delayed procedures for the Logical Memory, Visual Paired Associates, Verbal Paired Associates, and Visual Reproduction subtests. The scores for the Digit Span and Visual Memory Span subtests can be converted to percentiles by age, separately for the forward and the backward procedures. Percentile equivalents are also available for the Logical Memory and the Visual Reproduction subtests separately by age for both the original administration and the delayed recall procedures.

Normative Information

A nationally stratified sample of 316 individuals was used to standardize the scoring system. There were approximately 50 individuals in each of the six aforementioned age groups. The sample was approximately one half male and one half female. The racial composition of the sample was proportionate to information derived from the 1980 U.S. Census. Subjects were stratified across four geographic regions according to the 1980 Census data. Subjects were also stratified across three educational groups: 0 to 11 years, 12 years, and 13 or more years of education. The number of subjects in each educational group was proportional within age groups, based on 1980 Census data. Finally, each subject was administered all or a portion of the WAIS-R to help ensure that the distribution of IQ of subjects in each age group was equivalent to the distribution of IQ in the general population. Scoring weights for the arithmetic combination of subtests were decided upon by comparing the methods of simple unweighted combination, weighting the subtests proportional to the inverse of the standard deviation of each subtest, and weighting the subtests inversely proportional to the standard error of measurement of the subtests. The comparison was based on the criteria of optimal reliability and maximum discrimination between a normal sample and a clinical sample. The best overall method of combination was based on the third method (inverse proportion of standard error of measurement).

The interpolation procedure resulted in early criticism and a suggestion to use the WMS in the age groups where interpolated scores were given in the manual (D'Elia, Satz, & Schretlen, 1989), although other authors recommended the continued use of the WMS-R (Bowden & Bell, 1992). Although the procedure of estimating standardized scores for some groups may seem reasonable because of the known monotonic decreasing relationship between age and memory performance, the relationship may not be linear as is assumed by the interpolation procedure. In a sample of 50 residents of Florida who otherwise matched the standardization sample criteria in the WMS-R manual, the differences between interpolated and actual standardized scores for the WMS-R indexes were 2 points for Attention/Concentration (lower for the Florida sample) and less than 1 for Verbal Memory (lower for the Florida sample) and General Memory (higher for the Florida sample). However, for Visual Memory and Delayed Recall, the differences were 4 and 3 points, and in both cases the Florida sample exhibited higher scores (Mittenberg, Burton, Darrow, & Thompson, 1992). Therefore caution should be applied when using scores derived from interpolated normative information.

The stratification and sampling strategy used by the test developers appears to have been successful in obtaining accurate normative information and transformation formulae. In one study, the use of the WMS-R tended to result in a lower proportion of clinical subjects being classified as impaired than did the use of the California Verbal Learning Test (CVLT). In addition, for normal control subjects, the WMS-R standardized scores are more consistent with the scores expected on the basis of the education and intellectual level of the subjects, whereas the CVLT scores are more likely to be in the impaired range for the control subjects (Randolph, Gold, Kozora, & Cullum, 1994).

There have been some additional data for a wider normative base for the WMS-R. Because of increasing memory complaints with age, it is important to have normative information beyond that given in the manual since the standardization sample contained no people over the age of 74 years. Clinical neuropsychologists at the Mayo Clinic have published a series of studies involving data from healthy older individuals who were administered a variety of tests of cognitive function, including the WMS-R. These authors subsequently provided factor scores for the entire battery used (Wechsler Adult Intelligence Scale-Revised, WMS-R, and Rey Auditory Verbal Learning Test) and replicated the covariance structure in a clinical sample (Smith, Ivnik, Malec, & Tangalos, 1993). Smith, Wong, Ivnik, and Malec (1997) published information related to norms separately for the Logical Memory (I and II) stories based on a sample of 349 normal individuals between the ages of 56 and 93 years. Marcopulos, McLain, and Giuliano (1997) provided normative information for rural older subjects (over the age of 55 years) with less than 10 years of education. Lichtenberg and Christensen (1992) also provided information related to performance on the WMS-R by elderly subjects. Although the WMS-R was not originally intended for use with children, the relative dearth of standardized tests for this population has led some individuals to apply it in this population. To aid this application, Paniak, Murphy, Miller, and Lee (1998) provided norms for the Logical Memory and Visual Reproduction subtests based on a sample of 714 children. Scores on both the Logical Memory and Visual Reproduction immediate and delayed recall improved with age. Percent retained improved with age for Visual Reproduction, but not for Logical Memory.

Reliability

The manual provides test–retest reliability information for the Mental Control subtest ($r = .51$) as well as for both the initial ($r = .58$) and the delayed recall ($r = .58$) procedures of the Visual Paired Associates subtest and the initial ($r = .60$) and the delayed recall ($r = .41$)

procedures of the Verbal Paired Associates subtest. The intertest period ranged from 4 to 6 weeks. Bowden, Whelan, Long, and Clifford (1995) investigated the test–retest reliability of the WMS-R index scores in a sample of alcoholic subjects with a somewhat longer intertest interval (4 months) than was used in the manual. They found slightly higher test–retest correlations for the index scores for 20- to 24-year-olds and 55- to 64-year-olds than those presented in the WMS-R manual, and comparable coefficients as compared to the 70- to 74-year-olds.

Internal consistency reliability estimates are provided for the Figural Memory ($r = .44$), the initial Logical Memory ($r = .74$), the delayed recall of Logical Memory ($r = .75$), the initial Visual Reproduction ($r = .59$), the delayed recall Visual Reproduction ($r = .46$), the Digit Span ($r = .88$), and the Visual Memory Span subtest ($r = .81$). Moore and Baker (1997) provided internal consistency estimates based on a sample of 181 patients diagnosed with epilepsy. The Cronbach's alpha values ranged from .68 for Attention/Concentration to .81 for Delayed Recall.

Because the scoring criteria for most of the subtests are objective, interscorer reliability was computed only for the Logical Memory and Visual Reproduction subtests. Two trained scorers rated a set of 60 protocols. The interscorer reliability coefficient was .99 for Logical Memory and .97 for Visual Reproduction. Sullivan (1996) corroborated the high reliability coefficients when undergraduate students scored the Logical Memory subtest. O'Carroll and Badenoch (1994) reported similarly high interrater reliability coefficients for the Visual Reproduction subtest (greater than .92) regardless of whether the protocols were scored by experienced psychologists or relatively inexperienced trainees. Interrater reliability coefficients have been replicated in clinical samples for both the Logical Memory and Visual Reproduction subtests (Woloszyn, Murphy, Wetzel, & Fisher, 1993). Interscorer reliability may be affected by administration style. Shum, Murray, and Eadie (1997) reported that higher scores were associated with slower presentation of the stories in Logical Memory. It is important to use a consistent medium speed rate of delivery of the stimuli.

The manual reports the standard error of measurement as ranging from 4.86 for the Attention/Concentration index to 8.47 for the Visual Memory index. Bowden et al. (1995) administered the WMS-R twice over a 4- to 5-month interval to a sample of subjects with a diagnosis of alcohol dependence. At the second test occasion, 73% of the subjects admitted to having had a drink during the interval. Only the Attention/Concentration Index (14%) and Delayed Memory Index (16%) scores had a significant proportion of subjects whose change in scores exceeded the standard error of prediction.

The standard error of difference for three pairwise comparisons were computed and reported in the manual. The standard error of difference for comparing General Memory with Attention/Concentration is 16.38. The standard error difference for comparing Verbal Memory with Visual Memory is 21.89. The standard error of difference for comparing General Memory with Delayed Memory is 19.75. These suggested values have been elaborated and complemented by Atkinson (1991e) and Alkinson (1992c). Mittenberg, Thompson, and Schwartz (1991) calculated and reported confidence intervals for intratest scale comparisons. There is no empirical evidence for interpreting the differences, and they are best interpreted in terms of abnormality of the difference. Early reports suggested that laterality may be reflected in Visual–Verbal Memory Index comparisons (Chelune & Bornstein,

1988); however, Loring, Lee, Martin, and Meador (1989) demonstrated the difficulties in interpreting Visual–Verbal Memory Index scores as reflecting laterality of brain damage.

The WMS-R is frequently administered in conjunction with the WAIS-R, under the assumption that clinical conditions may differentially affect these cognitive abilities; for example, persons with Korsakoff's disease may show major memory impairment with relatively preserved intellectual functioning (Parkin & Leng, 1993). Therefore, IQ–MQ discrepancy scores may be useful for understanding clinical conditions and planning rehabilitation activities. If the history of the IQ–MQ difference in the WMS can be used as a guide, WMS-R IQ–MQ discrepancy scores may have little diagnostic value. Atkinson (1991d) used reliability data from the WAIS-R and the WMS-R manuals to calculate the standard error of differences between various IQ and Index scores. These standard error of differences were multiplied by 1.96 to create a 95% confidence interval for the various difference scores. This provides the clinician with an estimate of measurement error for the IQ–Index difference scores. The statistically reliable difference scores ($p < .05$) between the FSIQ and the Indexes, on average for all age groups, were 11 points for Attention–Concentration, 15 points for Verbal Memory, 17 points for Visual Memory, 14 points for General Memory, and 15 points for Delayed Recall.

Bornstein, Chelune, and Prifitera (1989) computed the base rates of various IQ–MQ difference scores in normal controls from the standardization sample and in clinical patients. As a group, the patients demonstrated larger FSIQ–Delayed Memory Index difference scores than the normal control subjects. These data are very helpful to the clinician. A difference score of 15 points is unusual in the general population (i.e., experienced by 10% or less) and a difference score of 22 points is rare (i.e., experienced by 5.5% or less of the general population). No patient in the general population had a difference score of 28 points or more. The base rates of these difference scores in the clinical subjects were 32.5% (15 points), 18.8% (22 points), and 11.5% (28 points).

The relationship between WAIS-R IQ and WMS-R scores can best be described as monotonic and roughly correlated. Individuals with low-average IQ score lower on the WMS-R than people with average and high-average IQ scores (Rapport et al., 1997). Furthermore when both the WAIS-R and WMS-R were repeated after a 2-week interval, all three groups of IQ level subjects increased their scores, but the differences among the groups remained. WAIS-R IQ at initial testing accounted for up to 41% of the variance in retest memory scores. Clearly, there is a relationship between IQ and memory performance, but the clinician would be wise to not strictly interpret small or moderate differences between IQ and memory scores. A confirmatory factor analysis of the WAIS-R and WMS-R in a normal healthy sample found that the best fitting model involved a five-factor model with verbal comprehension, perceptual organization, attention–concentration, verbal memory, and visual memory as factors (Bowden, Carstairs, & Shores, 1999). The WMS-R appears to provide information beyond that obtainable from the WAIS-R.

Detecting Improvement or Decline

The WMS-R is often used in serial assessments for the purpose of detecting improvement or decline in functioning. Unfortunately, relatively limited data are available to assist the clinician in this matter. A few important considerations, however, are known. First, persons from the general population and some clinical groups are known to show practice effects, especially over relatively brief retest intervals (Bowden et al., 1995; Chelune, Naugle, Lueders, Sedlak, & Awad, 1993; Wechsler, 1987). Second, the stability coefficients for the Index scores, and for the subtest scores, are relatively low. Therefore, the reliable change difference scores are large. Calculation of reliable change difference scores is a method for estimating the probability that a given test–retest difference score is not within the probable range of measurement error. Reliable change difference scores are estimated from the standard error of difference (S_{diff}); the S_{diff} is an estimate of measurement error relating to both test and retest scores. The S_{diff} is derived from the standard error of measurement (SEM) from both the test and retest scores. Essentially, each SEM is squared, and these products are added together. The S_{diff} is equal to the square root of the latter sum. The S_{diff} is then multiplied by a z-score to provide a confidence interval for possible measurement error (e.g., $S_{diff} \times 1.64 = .90$, or $1.28 = .80$). Jacobson and Truax (1991) advocated this approach for psychotherapy research, and Chelune and colleagues have applied this methodology to the evaluation of change following temporal lobectomies (Chelune et al., 1993; Sawrie, Chelune, Naugle, & Luders, 1996). It is important to realize that previous researchers have used an estimated (i.e., prorated) S_{diff}, as opposed to the "obtained" S_{diff}. That is, their calculational formulas used the SEM from time 1 only, as opposed to separate SEMs for test and retest.

One clear advancement in the use of the WMS-R subtest scores is the calculation of retention rates (i.e., savings scores). This issue, although rather obvious, may be neglected by rapid, routine interpretations of subtest performance. For example, imagine if a 36-year-old man with a closed head injury recalls 9 bits of information on Logical Memory I and 8 bits of information on Logical Memory II. These raw scores correspond to the 3rd and 9th percentiles, respectively. The clinician may then suggest that the patient's immediate memory and delayed memory for stories is in the borderline range. However, the patient retained 89% of the originally recalled information, which is perfectly normal for his age. Thus, his problem is in the initial acquisition of the material, not in the encoding or later recall of that material.

Retention rates were initially studied on the WMS (e.g., Bornstein, 1982b; Delaney, Rosen, Mattson, & Novelly, 1980; Russell, 1975a). Unfortunately, these rates were not included in the WMS-R manual but were later presented at a conference (Prifitera & Ledbetter, 1992). Subsequently, researchers have reported retention rate information from multiple clinical populations, including schizophrenia, traumatic brain injury, Alzheimer's disease, and Huntington's disease (Gass, 1995; Gold, Randolph, Carpenter, Goldberg, & Weinberger, 1992; Tröster et al., 1993). Interpretation of retention rates is strongly recommended. Failure to consider these can result in misinterpretation of delayed recall scores on Logical Memory and Visual Reproduction.

Validity

Discriminative Validity

Contrasted groups designs were used to evaluate the validity of the WMS-R. There were significant differences between the standardization sample and the clinical memory impaired samples of mixed psychiatric, schizophrenic, alcoholic, closed head injury, stroke, tumor, seizure disorder, multiple sclerosis, and neurotoxin exposed patients (Wechsler, 1987). Subsequent reports have focused on patients with Alzheimer's disease and Huntington's disease (Butters et al., 1988), patients with multiple sclerosis (Fisher, 1988), alcoholics (Ryan & Lewis, 1988), and patients exposed to industrial solvents (Crossen & Wiens, 1988).

Of particular note is a study by Chelune and Bornstein (1988). These researchers investigated WMS-R performance in patients with unilateral lesions. They found that although there was a significant multivariate difference between the two groups of patients, there was a significant univariate difference only for the Verbal Memory score. On the other hand, comparison among subtests in the same individuals indicated that patients with left-hemisphere lesions performed better on the subtests of visual memory than on the subtests of verbal memory, and that patients with right-hemisphere lesions performed better on the subtests of verbal memory than on the subtests of visual memory. There were no differences between left- and right-hemisphere epilepsy patients on the Visual Reproduction scores (Barr et al., 1997), although this lack of difference may reflect the difficulty of devising a right-hemisphere memory task more than it reflects construct validity of the WMS-R visual memory indices. Similar information is provided by Barr (1997), who found that using the receiver operating characteristic curves of the WMS-R resulted in near chance separation of right- and left-hemisphere temporal lobe epilepsy patients using the subtests of the WMS-R. Loring et al. (1989) reported similar inconsistent patterns of Visual/Verbal Memory Index score differences in unilateral temporal lobectomy patients. Apparently, the distinction between the subtests that comprise the Visual Memory Index and the subtests that comprise the Verbal Memory Index may not reflect laterality.

Reid and Kelly (1993) reported that the WMS-R indexes discriminated between patients with closed head injury and matched control subjects. In addition, all of the indexes were related to severity of everyday memory impairment, but only the Visual Memory Index correlated with severity of injury as measured by duration of posttraumatic amnesia. Gass and Apple (1997) demonstrated that performance on the Logical Memory but not the Visual Reproduction subtest was found to be significantly related to subjective complaints of memory disturbance in a sample of closed head injury patients.

O'Mahony and Doherty (1993) demonstrated that alcoholic subjects show a pattern of nonspecific memory impairment on the WMS-R. In addition, the WMS-R has been used to study aspects of schizophrenia (Hawkins, Sullivan, & Choi, 1997) and the effects of aging on memory processes (Fastenau, Denburg, & Abeles, 1996).

Concurrent Validity

Nestor and colleagues (1993) reported a positive correlation between magnetic resonance imaging (MRI) measures of temporal lobe volume and WMS-R verbal memory tasks, but not visual memory tasks, in a small sample of patients with schizophrenia. Gale, Johnson, Bigler, and Blatter (1995) reported that measures of brain atrophy, especially fornix atrophy, correlated with WMS-R performance in a sample of patients with closed head injury.

The WMS-R has been compared to other tests as a means of investigating concurrent validity. The earliest concurrent validity study published investigated the relation between the WMS-R and the California Verbal Learning Test (CVLT). This study (Delis, Cullum,

Butters, & Cairns, 1988) indicated that there are significant correlations between the two tests. A total of 460 correlations were computed, of which 341 were significant at the .01 level. The WMS-R has been recommended in combination with the Kaufman Adolescent Intelligence Test to evaluate the role of general memory functions when evaluating learning disabled individuals (McIntosh, Waldo, & Koller, 1997). The WMS-R was found to be similar to the Rivermead Behavioural Memory test in its relations to estimates of everyday memory function (Koltai, Bowler, & Shore, 1996). This point is especially interesting because the Rivermead has been promoted as an instrument with greater ecological validity than typical psychometric tests of memory. In contrast, the Memory Assessment Scales (MAS; Williams, 1991) produced lower standard scores than the WMS-R for the constructs of visual memory, verbal memory, general memory, attention, and delayed memory in a small sample of 30 adults. Even though the standard scores are generally lower for the MAS, there were still modest correlations between the standard scores derived from the two tests.

A concurrent validity study investigated the relation between the WMS-R and the CVLT. This study (Delis et al., 1988) indicated that there are significant correlations between the two tests. There were a total of 460 correlations computed, of which 341 were significant at the .01 level. The WMS-R has also been correlated with the Memory Assessment Scales or MAS (Hilsabeck, Dunn, & Lees-Haley, 1996). This study found that the WMS-R resulted in significantly higher standardized scores than the MAS for verbal memory, visual memory, attention, and general memory. The MAS had a greater relationship to self-report in this sample of 30 patients referred for outpatient evaluation.

Construct Validity

There are multiple reasons why there have been a number of factor analytic studies conducted on the WMS-R. Perhaps the most relevant reason is that the WMS-R is composed of subtests that are summed into subscale scores as well as a general score (the General Memory Index). The composition of the indexes was determined on the basis of a conceptual theoretical analysis. The factor analytic studies can therefore help evaluate whether the assignment of subscales to indexes is correct as well as determine whether the indexes are in fact separate, discriminable, and appropriate for independent interpretation.

The manual reports the results of a principal-components factor analysis conducted on the standardization sample in which two factors seemed to emerge; a General Memory and Learning factor and an Attention/Concentration factor. Principal-components factor analysis of a mixed clinical sample provided similar results. Roid, Prifitera, and Ledbetter (1988) reported the results of a confirmatory factor analysis on the data from the normative sample, indicating that the two-factor solution provided the best fit to the data.

Bornstein and Chelune (1988) subsequently reported a series of principal-components factor analysis of data derived from 434 patients referred for neuropsychological evaluation. When the initial administration subtest scores were included, a two-factor solution similar to that obtained with the standardization sample was obtained. When WAIS-R Verbal IQ (VIQ) and Performance IQ (PIQ) were included in the analysis, the factor structure of the clinical sample remained unchanged; however, in the normal sample, the two factors switched places with the attentional factor being extracted first. When the delayed recall subtests were included in the analysis with the initial administration subtests, a three-factor solution emerged: verbal memory, nonverbal memory, and attention. When PIQ and VIQ were included in the analysis, they tended to load on the third factor. Apparently, the factor structure of the WMS-R differs slightly in a normal versus a clinical sample. Moore and Baker (1997) reported that a three-factor solution (Visual Memory, Verbal Memory, Attention) described the data in a sample of patients with epilepsy. On the other hand, Bowden et al. (1997) reported a three-factor solution of attention/concentration, immediate recall, and delayed recall best fit their data obtained from a sample of patients recovering from alcohol dependence. These researchers used maximum likelihood confirmatory factor analysis and included a spatial memory measure as a marker variable.

The factor structure of the WMS-R has been investigated in various samples and using various methodologies. One reason lies in the utility of the index scores. Franzen, Wilhelm, and Haut (1995) investigated the factor structure of the WMS-R in the context of other neuropsychological screening instruments. These researchers found that when the index scores were used as variables, a general memory factor, a cognitive efficiency factor, a visual motor speed factor, and an attention factor were extracted. When the subtest scores were used as variables, an attention factor, a verbal memory factor, a visual memory factor, a visual motor speed factor, a cognitive efficiency factor, and a freedom from distractibility factor were extracted. Jurden et al. (1996) found that although the factor structure of the WMS-R may vary across clinical samples, the index scores have relatively stable characteristics across clinical samples.

The construct validity of the Attention/Concentration Index has been investigated separately from the WMS-R memory indexes. The Attention/Concentration Index may not be independently related to other measures of attention, although it is related to other measures of memory (Johnstone, Erdal, & Stadler, 1995). Schmidt, Trueblood, Durham, and Merwin (1994) reported the results of a factor analysis of various measures purported to measure attention and found that although the Digit Span and Visual Span measures from the WMS-R seemed to form a separate factor interpreted as Visual/Auditory Spanning, this factor was weak and may not have been robust. On the other hand, when examining the sensitivity of the various instruments in the sample, it appeared that the Attention/Concentration Index was among the most sensitive of the measures in identifying cognitive impairment.

Ecological Validity

The ecological validity of the WMS-R was evaluated by comparing its ability to predict patients' self-ratings and relatives' ratings on the Everyday Memory Questionnaire (Koltai, Bowler, & Shore, 1996). The WMS-R General Memory Index correlated −.55 with the patient self-ratings and −.56 with the relative ratings. There was no difference between the predictive ability of the WMS-R and the Rivermead Behavioral Memory Test.

Detecting Biased Responding

The WMS-R has also been used to evaluate patterns of performance related to biased responding and attempts to malinger. Although the diagnosis of malingering requires much more than simply a pattern of test scores, it appears that the WMS-R often possesses a distinctive pattern associated with biased responding (Mittenberg, Azrin, Millsaps, &

Heilbronner, 1993). The two most common findings in the literature relate to the Digit Span subtest and a particular pattern of index scores.

The Digit Span subtest of the WAIS-R and WMS-R has been used in several studies involving analog malingerers, who, when asked to simulate cognitive impairment, significantly suppressed their performance on the Digit Span procedure (Bernard, 1990; Binder & Willis, 1991). Other studies have found that analog malingerers drawn from undergraduates, federal prison inmates, and psychiatric inpatients performed much more poorly on Digit Span than patients with acquired brain damage and documented memory impairment (Iverson & Franzen, 1994, 1996). As a marker for nonoptimal performance, the basic premise is that potential malingerers may not realize that Digit Span abilities often are relatively preserved in patients with neurological impairment (Baddeley & Warrington, 1970; Black, 1986; Cermak & Butters, 1972, 1973; Drachman & Arbit, 1966; Warrington & Weiskrantz, 1973). Therefore, severely deficient performance may be indicative of exaggeration, especially when this performance is obtained from an individual with a mild head injury.

Mittenberg and colleagues used discriminant function analysis to develop a "malingering index" for the WMS-R (Mittenberg et al., 1993). These investigators found that experimental malingerers had a distinctly different pattern of WMS-R Index scores from nonlitigating patients with head injuries. Subjects given instructions to malinger suppressed their Attention/Concentration Index relative to their General Memory Index ($M = 71$ vs. 85, respectively). The patients with head injuries showed the opposite pattern (i.e., the mean Attention/Concentration Index was 96 and the mean General Memory Index was 85). A discriminant function analysis using the General Memory-Attention/Concentration (GM-A/C) difference score as the independent variable yielded an 83% correct classification rate, with 10% false positives and 23% false negatives. A table was developed reflecting the probability that a given difference score will be consistent with the performance of experimental-malingerers (Mittenberg et al., 1993, p. 37, Table 4). Slick, Iverson, and Franzen (1996) examined the base rate of the GM-A/C difference score in a large sample of nonlitigating individuals from an inpatient substance abuse program ($N = 332$).Only a small percentage of patients showed large General Memory-Attention/ Concentration difference scores (i.e., 22 or more points).These results provide further support for the validity of this difference score as a marker for nonoptimal effort.

The GM-A/C difference score as an index of nonoptimal effort is supported on theoretical grounds. Since learning new information requires a certain degree of attentional functioning, a person with normal memory should not demonstrate significantly impaired attentional abilities. Therefore, it should be possible to have significantly impaired memory with relatively intact attention, but not the converse. This theoretical position, of course, is limited by the construct validity of the index scores. In other words, the theory is persuasive to the degree to which the Attention/Concentration Index is a valid measure of "attentional functioning."

Martin, Franzen, and Orey (1998) presented a new way of looking at forced choice procedures. Because it is becoming increasingly well known that chance performance levels can be one method of detecting less than optimal effort on forced choice procedures, different methods of scoring the data may be helpful. These researchers used expert opinion to assign likelihood of endorsement or magnitude of error to recognition procedures for the Logical Memory and Visual Reproduction subtests of the WMS-R. There were three choices for each item in the Logical Memory and five choices for each item in the Visual

Reproduction item. Summing the magnitude of error scores for each endorsed item resulted in greater accuracy in identifying analog and clinical malingerers in discrimination from clinical patients not involved in litigation. This is a promising method for further research.

Short Forms

Woodard and Axelrod (1995) developed three subtest linear formulas to predict the General Memory Index (GMI) and the Delayed Memory Index (DMI) which were successfully cross-validated (Axelrod, Putnam, Woodard, & Adams, 1996) when 94% of the 258 subjects had predicted GMI scores within 6 points of obtained scores and 97% had predicted DMI scores within 6 points of obtained scores. Similar results were reported by Hoffman, Scott, Tremont, Adams, and Oommen (1997). Subsequently, van den Broek, Golden, Loonstra, Ghinglia, and Goldstein (1998) found somewhat lower agreement values of 86% for the GMI and 85% for the DMI. These researchers then shortened the form even further by using only two subtests (using only Logical Memory and Visual Reproduction and not Visual Paired Associates) for each index and found that 59% of their subjects agreed within 6 points.

Demsky, Mittenberg, Quintar, Katell, and Golden (1998) investigated the possibility of using a Spanish translation of the WMS-R. They reported that the use of English-speaking norms resulted in lower scores for Spanish-speaking subjects even on the visual subtests and recommended that use of the Spanish translation be postponed until norms involving Spanish speaking subjects be generated.

Criticisms

The WMS-R is a vast improvement over its predecessor. However, there are a few shortcomings in the WMS-R. One potentially serious problem is the fact that scores bottom out at 50; therefore, there is likely to be overestimation of memory function in individuals with marked or severe memory deficits. There is no verbal recognition test even though there is a test of visual recognition. Fastenau (1996) attempted to remedy this lack with recognition procedures for the Logical Memory and Visual Reproduction subtests, but the sample of 81 individuals is limited. Although the transformation of raw scores to standardized scores is stratified by age group, there are no normative data available for subjects in the age groups 18 to 19 years, 25 to 34 years, and 45 to 54 years, and scores for these subjects are consequently estimated. Finally, the WMS-R is not standardized for subjects older than 74 years. This last point is unfortunate because older individuals are overrepresented in the population of people with memory complaints.

One obvious limitation of the WMS-R is the lack of recognition memory subtests. All procedures relate to free recall, and these procedures are often too difficult for lower functioning patients. Gass (1995) has published multiple-choice recognition procedures to allow interpretation of results related to deficits in retrieval versus deficient storage. Most useful is his 21-item five-option multiple-choice procedure for Logical Memory; this procedure is administered in paper–pencil format after Logical Memory II. He also employed a cuing procedure for the designs, where the examiner slowly draws a portion of the "forgotten" design until the patient remembers, then the patient completes the drawing (in a different color of pencil). The drawing is scored, according to the criteria in the manual, for only those parts completed independently by the patient. Gass (1995) reported that a sample of veterans with mixed psychiatric disorders performed better on the recognition procedures than a sample of veterans with either traumatic brain injuries or strokes.

Performance on the Visual Reproduction subtests requires several component skills. Haut, Weber, Wilhelm, and Keefover (1994) demonstrated empirically what is a "clinical assumption": a person must be able to perceive and draw geometric designs for the clinician to interpret Visual Reproduction subtest performance as reflective of memory. These researchers have added tasks designed to assess perception (i.e., multiple-choice matching task) and visual-construction (i.e., straight copy of each design). Patients with Alzheimer's disease performed more poorly on both the copy and matching tasks than patients with frontal lobe lesions and elderly control subjects (Haut et al., 1994). In a second study, these researchers reported a scoring methodology for controlling the effects of constructional dysfunction on memory performance on the Visual Reproduction subtests (Haut, Weber, Demarest, Keefover, & Rankin, 1996). These studies illustrate that it is important to determine whether perceptual or constructional problems are adversely affecting "visual memory" performance.

Although the WMS-R is a vast improvement over its predecessor, the scale does have shortcomings. The minimum score available for the indexes is 50; therefore, there is likely to be overestimation of memory function in individuals with severe memory deficits. Although the transformation of raw scores to standardized scores is stratified by age group, there are no actual normative data available for subjects in the age groups 18 to 19 years, 25 to 34 years, and 45 to 54 years. Instead, scores for these subjects are estimated. Loring (1989) criticized the WMS-R for not separating delayed memory into visual and verbal components. The most serious limitation of the WMS-R, as noted by Elwood (1991), is the low reliabilities of the subtests and indexes. These low reliabilities seriously limit measurement accuracy.

Another limitation involves the interpretation of the Index scores. The various factor analytic studies discussed previously in this chapter do not lend confidence in the ability to state which aspects of memory may be reflected in the scores even though these scores may be generally sensitive to cognitive impairment and to diagnostic categories. Alternately, the interpretation of subtest scores may be more easily conducted because the subtests do not have the same degree of heterogeneity that is present in the Indexes. The factor analytic studies do support the distinction between visual and verbal memory as well as the distinction between immediate recall and delayed recall. What is uncertain is whether the calculation procedures specified in the manual as well as the exact components of the constructs are related to these distinctions.

The main asset of the WMS-R is that it allows measurement of different aspects of memory in a single composite instrument. This feature is especially useful when comparisons of different forms of memory are necessary for diagnosis or for treatment planning. Another major asset of the WMS-R is the large number of empirical studies that have been conducted and that inform our clinical use of the test. The fact that it has been utilized in several different populations is another positive attribute. In a curious way, the various studies that determine the shortcomings of the WMS-R are also assets because these studies help define the proper applications of the instrument. Researchers have enhanced the clinical usefulness of the WMS-R by studying retention rates, expanding the norms for the elderly, developing procedures for partialling out the effects of constructional problems on Visual Reproduction, and developing a recognition procedure for Logical Memory.

A serious problem with the clinical interpretation of WMS-R scores is related to the low reliabilities of several of the subtests and the Index scores. This was elaborated by Elwood (1991) in his critique of the psychometric characteristics of the scale. Essentially, the reliabilities are so low that the confidence intervals for the obtained scores (or the estimated true scores) are very broad. For example, the 95% confidence interval for the General Memory Index is ±14 points. If a patient scores 87, then the confidence interval surrounding the obtained score ranges from borderline to average. Assessing memory functioning with the WMS-R is less reliable than assessing intellectual functioning with the WAIS-R. In general, it is best to interpret the Index scores, as opposed to individual subtest scores. If the entire WMS-R is not administered, it is notable that the most reliable subtest scores are derived from Logical Memory, Digit Span, and Visual Memory Span (average coefficients for all ages ranging from .74 to .88). Although it is common practice among many neuropsychologists to administer only the Logical Memory and Visual Reproduction subtests, relatively little is known about the reliability and validity of this approach to memory assessment.

Conclusions

Despite its drawbacks, the WMS-R is one of the best instruments available for the overall evaluation of memory functions. It has already generated a fair amount of research interest that is likely to increase multiplicatively. It may very well become the standard for the clinical evaluation of nonseverely memory impaired, nonelderly patients.

WECHSLER MEMORY SCALE-THIRD EDITION

Introduction

The Wechsler Memory Scale-Third Edition (WMS-III; Wechsler, 1997b) is meant to be more than a revision of the WMS-R. It is meant to reflect a contemporary conceptualization of memory and its disorders. The WMS-III consists of six primary and five optional subtests. According to the manual, the primary subtests can be administered in 30 to 35 minutes. The normative sample consists of 1250 adults between the ages of 16 and 89 years. Thirteen age bands were used for the normative tables; the first 11 have 100 subjects each and the oldest two bands have 75 subjects each. Information on the standardization sample and norms development is available in the technical manual (Wechsler, 1997b).

In the development of the WMS-III, there were substantial revisions of the WMS-R subtests, administration and scoring procedures, and index configurations. Specifically, new subtests were added, and stimulus materials were revised. Scoring procedures have become much more sophisticated. Subtests now are individually normed with, and presented as, scaled scores; and there are more specific index scores. Although extensive details of these revisions are provided in the manual (Wechsler, 1997), some of the highlights are reviewed in this chapter.

The changes in the WMS-III were made for various reasons. Some changes were brought about in response to criticism of the WMS-R. Some changes were meant to reflect current theories of memory as involving stages of processing, as being relatively independent in modalities, and as involving both retrieval and recognition aspects. The WMS-III is integrated with the WAIS-III with a sample of individuals in the standardization samples being shared across the two instruments. Two of the subtests, Digit Span and Letter-Number Span, are shared across the two instruments, so that when both the WAIS-III and the WMS-III are given, those subtests need be administered only once.

Eight index scores are derived from age-adjusted scaled scores. The indexes have been named to more accurately represent how the information is presented and the presumed underlying ability. For example, the Auditory Immediate Index is comprised of Logical Memory I and Verbal Paired Associates I, and the Visual Delayed Index is comprised of Faces II and Family Pictures II.

Psychometric Properties

In general, the reliability of the WMS-III is higher than the reliability of the WMS-R. This is true for both estimates of internal consistency and stability. The average internal consistency coefficients for all age groups ranged from .74 to .93 for the primary subtest scores. All of the primary indexes have average internal consistency estimates of .82 or greater, with the exception of the Auditory Recognition Delayed Index ($r = .74$). The average test–retest reliability coefficients, for all age groups, ranged from .62 to .82 for the primary subtest scores, and .75 to .88 for the primary indexes (with the exception of the Auditory Delayed Recognition Index of .70).

The validity of the WMS-III was examined through special group studies. In these studies, independent researchers collected data on small groups of clinical subjects. For a sample of 35 patients with mild Alzheimer's disease, most of the mean primary index scores fell in the range from 60 to 71, with the exception of Working Memory ($M = 80.4$). The lowest primary index scores for the sample of patients with traumatic brain injuries were Visual Immediate, Immediate Memory, Visual Delayed, and General Memory (i.e., 74.3 to 81.9). Results from small samples of patients with Huntington's disease, Parkinson's disease, multiple sclerosis, temporal lobe epilepsy, chronic alcohol abuse, Korsakoff's syndrome, schizophrenia, Attention Deficit Hyperactivity Disorder (ADHD), and learning disabilities also were reported. In general, the clinical subjects performed more poorly than did the standardization subjects. The next step would be to see if the pattern of performances on subtests matches theories regarding the specific types of memory impairment seen in these different diagnostic groups.

Assets and Limitations

The WMS-III shows great promise because of its greater theoretical underpinnings and standardization data. Perhaps its greatest contribution is the co-norming with the WAIS-III. However, the promise of the WMS-III is in need of independent empirical evaluation. Lessons learned from experiences with the WMS-R include the fact that not all theoretical assumptions are eventually supported under the light of careful scrutiny. Furthermore, based on experience with the WMS-R, clinicians are likely to use only selected subtests of the WMS-III. Availability of percentile translations for subtests will facilitate this process, but may also detract from use of the entire instrument. An area of research would then be the decision rules related to choice of subtest procedures and interpretations possible when the entire battery is not given.

The length and complexity of the WMS-III can be seen as both an asset and a limitation. These two features of the WMS-III will allow a more finely grained examination of memory processes than would be possible with either the WMS-R or with most other memory assessment instruments. However, these two features may also discourage clinicians from using the instrument or may limit the appropriate use and interpretation of the instrument.

Future research directions include examining the relationship of WMS-III scores to everyday functioning. This is an important question not only for the WMS-III, but also for memory instruments in general. However, given the relative stature of the WMS-III, it is especially important that it be evaluated. Furthermore, empirical investigations of the theoretical bases of the WMS-III and the interpretative strategies suggested in the manual are warranted. Viewing the explosion of studies following publication of the WMS-R, the possibility of these investigations can almost be guaranteed.

Intelligence–Memory Discrepancy Analyses

Interpretation of IQ–MQ discrepancies is much more accurate and sophisticated on the WMS-III, versus the WMS-R, given that the WAIS-III and WMS-III were co-normed. As such, it is possible to determine if a given IQ–MQ discrepancy is reliable, unusual, and/or abnormal. The reliable splits on the WMS-III (i.e., discrepancies that are not due to measurement error) range from 9 points on the Auditory Immediate Index to 16 points on the Auditory Recognition Delayed Index. On average, for all ages, the clinician could conclude that a General Memory Index that is 10 points lower than the individual's FSIQ represents a reliable difference ($p < .15$), indicating that memory is a *relative weakness* for the person. However, a split of this magnitude is common in the general population, so it is not until the split reaches a magnitude of 13 points to 16 points that the clinician should conclude that the difference is both reliable and "unusual" (i.e., the split occurs in less than 15% or 10% of the general population, respectively). A FSIQ–General Memory Index discrepancy score of 22 points occurs in 5% or less of the general population (i.e., a statistically "abnormal" split), and should be considered rare. These psychometrics are now in need of empirical guides for interpretation.

In interpreting the WMS-III results, impaired performance on the percent retention score is likely to be the result most sensitive to the types of everyday memory impairment subjectively reported by many individuals. This is likely to be true regardless of the etiology of the memory impairment. Poor performance on the Logical Memory subtest also has conceptual relationships to subjective memory complaints, as a frequent index of everyday memory is the ability to follow and remember textual narratives spoken by other people.

The Visual Reproduction subtest of the WMS-III is an optional subtest. There have been some concerns from colleagues regarding the length of the subtest and the complexity of the scoring which may result in decreased use of this subtest in clinical practice. However, the subtest is now more sophisticated than ever before, allowing the neuropsychologist to make inferences regarding basic visual perception, visual-construction, immediate and delayed recall, percent retention, and recognition memory for geometric designs. These refinements emerged out of the literature relating to percent retention, perception, and construction on the WMS-R (e.g., Haut et al., 1994; Tröster et al., 1993). For example, to "remember" the designs the patient must accurately perceive them. The Discrimination procedure is a simple matching task, where the subject is asked to select the target design from a set of distracters. The vast majority of persons in the standardization sample scored either 6/77 or 7/7 on this task. Scores of 5/7 or less occur in 5% or less of persons under the age of 75 (thus, scores in this range may be indicative of a perceptual problem). Normative data also are available for straight copy of the designs. Scores range from 0 to 104, and scores falling in the very low 90s for persons under the age of 65 *may* be a reflection of visual-constructional problems. It should be noted that other tests of visual construction and memory also have complex scoring and less sophisticated norms (e.g., Rey–Osterrieth Complex Figure), so the complexity of the scoring should not be a deciding factor for whether to include this subtest in a comprehensive neuropsychological evaluation.

Conclusions

The WMS-III is likely to attract as much controversy and even more research attention than either of its predecessors. It is likely to become the predominant method for evaluating memory in adults. For that reason, it is extremely important that the research be completed. The WMS-III has much promise and will probably prove to be a real advancement.

Tests of Memory

THE REY–OSTERRIETH COMPLEX FIGURE TEST

The Rey–Osterrieth Complex Figure Test (ROCF) involves both an assessment of copy accuracy and recall accuracy. This chapter considers only the memory or recall condition, and the reader is referred to the chapter on visual and construction functions for information related to the copy condition. The immediate recall condition of the Rey–Osterrieth may not be a pure visual memory test, as it tends to correlate with the Block design subtest of the WAIS-R, Trail Making Test Part B, and the Category Test (Cornell, Roberts, and Oram, 1997) and loads on a visuospatial perceptual/memory factor (Berry, Allen, & Schmitt, 1991). The Rey–Osterrieth has been administered in a variety of manners, and the relationships among these different manners is not entirely understood. The most frequently used methods are: a, copy, immediate recall, 30-minute delay; b, copy, 3-minute recall, 30-minute recall; c, copy, 30-minute recall; and d, copy, immediate recall, 3-minute recall, 30-minute recall. In addition, a 45-minute recall is used instead of a 30-minute recall. Meyers and Meyers (1995a) reported no difference in 30-minute recall scores regardless of whether the immediate or 3-minute recall methods was used.

Percent retention of recall scores on the Rey–Osterrieth tends to correlate better with left hippocampal atrophy than with right hippocampal atrophy following head injury (Bigler et al., 1996). Silverstein, Osborn, and Palumbo (1998) reported that chronic schizophrenics exhibit worse recall scores than acute, outpatient schizophrenics or patients with other psychotic disorders. Because of the complexity of the design and the heterogeneity of most scoring systems, memory for the ROCF may be related to both left- and right-hemisphere function. Although they used a nonconventional administration method (copy with a 20-minute unwarned recall), Breier et al. (1996) found that when the scoring system was divided into figural (accuracy of rendering the details) and spatial (accuracy of placement of details) aspects, the spatial and figural scores were associated with right- and left-hemisphere dysfunction; the figural score was less sensitive. Qualitative scoring systems have generally been developed and evaluated in the interpretation of the copy condition, but at least one qualitative scoring system has its greatest utility in evaluating the recall condition (Loring, Lee, & Meador, 1988).

Meyers and Meyers (1995b) developed a comprehensive scoring system for the ROCF that includes aspects of accuracy and placement. In addition, their methods utilize a delayed recognition procedure, as previous research had indicated this method as a source of

230

clinical information (Meyers & Lange, 1994). Meyers, Bayless, and Meyers (1996) developed a system of classifying types of protocols based on errors and scores using their scoring system. This system identifies subjects as exhibiting primarily retrieval, storage, encoding, or attention problems. Meyers and Volbrecht (1998a) confirmed the types using cluster analysis and examined the external correlates of the clusters and provided base rates of the different error profiles in 601 normal subjects.

Younger subjects between the ages of 6 and 12 years show a trend toward improvement in immediate recall memory for the Rey–Osterrieth (Akshoomoff & Stiles, 1995a). There is an age-related difference in memory score in children between the ages of 7 and 14 years, even when copy score is covaried out, indicating development of spatial memory itself (Anderson & Lajoie, 1996). These authors also provide tables of mean values by age in a sample of 376 normal Canadian children.

An opposite trend is seen at the other end of the developmental spectrum. Advanced age is associated with decreases in performance on the immediate recall condition (Ostrosky, Jaime, & Ardila, 1998; Rosselli & Ardila, 1991); however, these are not strictly due to decreases in memory as the accuracy of copy, immediate recall, and delayed recall all decrease at similar rates after the age 70 years (Chiulli, Haaland, La Rue, & Garry, 1995). In general, age has a greater effect on memory than it does on copy performance (Chervinsky, Mitrushina, & Satz, 1992) and the relationship is particularly strong over the age of 60 years (Berry, Allen, & Schmitt, 1991). The effect of aging on Rey–Osterrieth recall scores may be related to a loss of detail (Mitrushina, Satz, & Chervinsky, 1990) and does not appear to be solely related to changes in visual–spatial construction or organization (Hartman & Potter, 1998). Using a copy, immediate unwarned recall, and 30-minute delayed recall procedure, Chiuli et al. (1995) found that the copying organization strategy, although related to recall accuracy, did not show age-associated declines in healthy elderly individuals.

The Taylor Figure is sometimes suggested as an alternate form of the Rey–Osterrieth. Although it appears that the copy scores are similar when both are administered to the same subjects, there may be important differences in immediate recall (Peirson & Jansen, 1997) and in percent recall memory scores (Kuehn & Snow, 1992). Therefore, it would be preferable to develop separate norms for the Taylor rather than rely on the attractively extensive Rey data base.

It is extremely important to consider the method of administration of the Rey–Osterrieth as well as the scoring system when choosing a normative base or study on which to base interpretation of individual results. Although Berry and Carpenter (1992) reported that the delay period did not have an effect on performance, it is difficult to generalize beyond the age group of this study since developmental trends tend to moderate other group differences. The delayed recall score was the only measure to discriminate between patients with Alzheimer's dementia and patients with frontotemporal dementia, indicating utility in this sometimes difficult diagnostic decision (Pachana, Boone, Miller, Cummings, & Berman, 1996).

The ROCF may not be a measure of visual memory so much as a measure of memory per se. In a large-scale, multicenter study of left- and right-hemisphere seizure disorder patients, there were no significant differences between right- and left-hemisphere patients on the ROCF (Barr et al., 1997). However, an alternative qualitative scoring system resulted in significant differences between right- and left-hemisphere foci of temporal lobe epilepsy patients (Piguet, Saling, O'Shea, Berkovic, & Bladin, 1994). In addition, scores on the

ROCF, especially the copy score, are related to measures of constructs other than memory, notably the Category Test and the Trail Making Test (Cornell et al., 1997).

THE CALIFORNIA VERBAL LEARNING TEST

The California Verbal Learning Test or CVLT (Delis, Kramer, Kaplan, & Ober, 1987) is currently one of the most frequently used and investigated tests of memory. The expansion in use of the CVLT since the publication of the first edition of this book has been nothing short of phenomenal. Its popularity is partly due to its relationship to cognitive neuroscience. The CVLT consists of a list of 16 words organized into four semantic categories. The list is read to the subject five times with a free recall condition after each repetition. Then a competing list of 16 words is read to the subject with a free recall condition. Next the subject is asked to recall the original list first under a free recall procedure and then a recall condition in which the subject is cued as to the four categories. After a 30-minute delay, the subject is again asked for a free recall and again given a cued recall. Finally, a recognition procedure is used in which a longer list of words is read to the subject, some of which were on the competing list and some of which were not on either list. The CVLT therefore provides a number of indices related to memory including indices related to both retroactive and proactive interference and related to the tendency of the subject to use either a serial position strategy or a semantic organization strategy in recalling the words. Elwood (1995) provides an excellent review of the psychometric properties of the CVLT.

Normative information is provided for individuals between the ages of 17 and 80 years separately for females and males. Because of its standardization sample characteristics (relatively high functioning individuals), the CVLT may result in a greater likelihood of conclusions of impairment than the Rey Auditory Verbal Learning Test (Stallings, Boake, & Sherer, 1995). Performance on the CVLT is related to intelligence both at an initial administration of the CVLT and at a retest after 2 weeks (Rapport, Charter, Dutra, Farchione, & Kingsley, 1997), and IQ scores should be taken into consideration when interpreting the results of the CVLT. Paolo, Troster, and Ryan (1997a) reported normative data for older subjects that help increase the utility of the CVLT in that age group. Keenan, Ricker, Lindamer, Jiron, and Jacobson (1996) reported a significant relationship between scores on the WAIS-R Vocabulary subtest and the CVLT. In fact, Vocabulary score and age accounted for 31% of the variance in some CVLT scores. Education did not produce a similar relationship, and Vocabulary-based norms may increase the utility of the CVLT.

Reliability

Significant practice effects and associated low test–retest reliability are commonly assumed in memory tests. The effects of prior exposure may be greater in memory impaired subjects than in normal control subjects for multiple reasons. If the memory impaired subjects are initially tested soon after the etiological injury, increase in score may partly reflect improvement in memory skill. Since the initial scores of impaired subjects may exhibit greater deviations from the population mean, improvement at the second test occasion may also reflect regression toward the mean. In addition, normal control subjects may exhibit initial scores that are at the ceiling of the available scores; therefore, significant improvement may be limited by psychometric considerations. Novack, Kofoed, and Crosson (1995) presented evidence of significant improvement in several scores on the CVLT in a sample of individuals with severe traumatic brain injury when those individuals were tested initially less than 5 months post-injury and then again after an additional 6 months. To reduce the potential effects of the high functioning standardization sample, a matched control group was used for comparison. However, the control group was tested only once, and a comparison of score changes was not possible. This study also demonstrated lower levels of efficient memory strategy in the traumatic brain injury subjects. Paolo, Troster, and Ryan (1997b) reported reasonable test–retest reliability in a sample of 151 healthy elderly subjects tested twice across somewhat more than 1 year's time. The highest correlation was .76 for the Total Recall of Trial A and for the Long Delay Free Recall scores. There were significant improvements in List A, Trial 1, List A Total Score, Long Delay Free Recall, the Semantic Clustering Ratio, and Discriminability; however, these differences were not clinically meaningful. Of course, retest across a shorter interval is likely to result in greater improvement.

Validity

The manual describes six factors in normal subjects based on a principal-components factor analysis. Wiens, Tindall, and Crossen (1994) found five to seven factors in normal subjects in different age groups, consistent with the findings of Vanderploeg, Schinka, and Retzlaff (1994) in clinical samples. Elwood (1995) critically reviewed the various factor analytic studies and concluded there were between one and three major components and between two and three minor components. The factor structure is in need of more definitive explication.

The recall measures of the CVLT correlate with the general memory index of the WMS-R (Schear & Croft, 1989). The serial clustering score does not appear to differentiate between subjects with dementia and normal subjects (Bondi et al., 1994; Cullum, Filley, & Kozora, 1995), nor is it sensitive to the presence of AIDS (Peavy et al., 1994). The semantic clustering index may be sensitive to a variety of clinical conditions (Elwood, 1995). The delayed recall index appears to be sensitive to the effects of closed head injury (Cross, Novack, Trenerry, & Craig, 1988; Haut & Shutty, 1992). The CVLT allows the calculation of indices of recognition, cued recall, and interference effects. These are all promising variables, but further research is needed to specify the clinical interpretations.

Artiola I Fortuny, Heaton, and Hermosillo (1998) reported that performance on the Spanish translation of the CVLT is related to socioeconomic status and bilingualism. Bilingual subjects and higher socioeconomic status subjects generally performed better.

The CVLT results in several different indices based on the initial conceptualization of learning derived from cognitive neuroscience. Factor analysis of the CVLT with other neuropsychological measures in spinal cord injury patients indicates that the indices for total words recalled and delayed recall loaded on the same factor as the Immediate and Delayed Recall scores on the WMS-R but not measures of attention, measures of visual spatial processing, or the Warrington Recognition Memory Test-Faces (Dowler et al., 1997). Millis and Ricker (1994) reported that the CVLT indices could discriminate among three types of memory difficulty in closed head injury patients. These results were partially replicated by Deshpande, Millis, Reeder, Fuerst, and Ricker (1996) who also reported an additional two types of learning and memory difficulties using a wider variety of clustering methods. The various indices of the CVLT are in need of separate validational studies. Stout et al. (1999) reported that atrophic changes in the mesial temporal lobes in subjects with Alzheimer's dementia, as measured by MRI, is associated with poorer learning scores, but not with delayed recall or recognition. Wilde, Boake, and Scherer (1995) reported that the CVLT delayed recall-delayed recognition discrepancy is not an accurate index of retrieval deficits as suggested by the test's authors, at least in a sample of individuals who have experienced moderate and severe closed head injury. Although Veiel (1997b) later challenged these conclusions, further examination of the study upheld the original conclusions (Cicchetti, 1997; Fuerst, 1997; Wilde, Boake, & Sherer, 1997).

Owing to the large number of scores available from administration of the CVLT, there is interest in the factor structure. Delis, Freeland, Framer, and Kaplan (1988) reported a five-factor solution in neurologically impaired individuals and a six-factor solution in normal control subjects. Vanderploeg et al. (1994) reported a similar five-factor solution in their sample of neurological patients. The six-factor solution emerged in a sample of individuals with moderate and severe closed head injury (Wilde & Boake, 1994). Millis (1995) factor analyzed the data from a sample of 75 patients with moderate and severe closed head injury and reported a six-factor solution interpreted as General Verbal Learning, Response Discrimination, Learning Strategy, Proactive Effect, Self-monitoring, and Serial Position. Only the first factor, General Verbal Learning, correlated with other neuropsychological measures, namely Delayed Recall Logical Memory, COWAT, and the Warrington Recognition Memory-Words and Faces. It would be helpful to clarify the factor structure in different populations and to determine the construct validity of the factors.

The various scores may also be helpful in discriminating among different types of diagnoses. For example, Diamond, DeLuca, Johnson, and Kelly (1997) reported that subjects with anterior communicating artery aneurysm tend to score lower on Trial 1 and Trial 5 than subjects with multiple sclerosis (MS) and also scored lower on the recognition score than did the subjects with MS, whereas the subjects with MS scored lower than control subjects on the acquisition trials but not on the recognition score. Polysubstance abusing subjects score lower than alcohol abusing subjects on the recall scores but not on the recognition score (Bondi, Drake, & Grant, 1998). Adults with residual ADHD tend to score lower on the delayed free recall index than adults who had current complaints of attentional difficulties but without the history of childhood symptoms of ADHD.

The relationship between MS and performance on the CVLT may be related to a deficit in conceptualization rather than being directly related to deficits in memory processes per se (Troyer, Fisk, Archibald, Ritvo, & Murray, 1996). Kareken, Moberg, and Gur (1996) reported that the degree of semantic clustering is significantly less in schizophrenic patients than in controls. When divided into groups with severe and mild hypoxia, patients with COPD differed only on the List B score (Stuss et al., 1997).

There is published information regarding the performance of depressed adults (Otto et al., 1994) and depressed adolescents (Horan, Pogge, Borgaro, Stokes, & Harvey, 1997). In general, depression tends to exert a general downward effect on scores, which is somewhat greater for adolescents than for adults. Interestingly, Otto et al. (1994) found that although the depressed individuals had scores up to 1.5 standard deviations below average, there was no relationship between severity of depression as measured by a 17-item Hamilton depression rating scale; there was a significant relationship between self-assessment of cognitive difficulties and level of depression. King, Cox, Lyness, Conwell, and Caine (1998) reported that depressed elderly subjects have lower scores on all indices except retention, and the presence of depression tended to accelerate the effects of aging. Perhaps because of its sensitivity to depression, the CVLT may not be able to discriminate between adults with ADHD and adults with depression (Katz, Wood, Goldstein, Auchenbach, & Geckle, 1998).

There is a shorter (nine words) version of the CVLT specifically for use with the elderly. Libon et al. (1996) reported that factor analysis in a normal sample resulted in a three-factor solution and that the tests discriminated between healthy elderly and individuals with either ischemic vascular dementia or Alzheimer's dementia. This version may be useful when assessing individuals with considerable impairment. However, in those cases the diagnosis is not usually at issue. Future research could address whether change is reliably measured using this version.

The CVLT is significantly related to both occupational status and job performance in closed head injury patients 1 year or more post-injury (Kibby, Schmitter-Edgecombe, & Long, 1998).

Detection of Malingering

The CVLT contains a recognition memory procedure that can be examined for the presence of malingered memory deficits (Millis, Putnam, Adams, & Ricker, 1995). In particular, an optimal cutoff on the Discriminability index correctly classified 93% of a sample of individuals with moderate or severe closed head injury versus individuals with suspected response bias. Coleman, Rapport, Millis, Ricker, and Farchione (1998) found that a simple set of coaching instructions reduced the accuracy of the index, although these same researchers suggested that the index might still be used, albeit with less confidence.

CVLT for Children

There is also a children's form of the CVLT (Delis, Kramer, Kaplan, & Ober, 1994). This form roughly parallels the adult form, with the exception of a slightly shorter wordlist and fewer semantic categories. The CVLT-C is sensitive to the effects of closed head injury in children (Jaffe et al., 1993). Interestingly, children with mild closed head injury do not show the impairment in semantic clustering strategy that is shown by adults on the CVLT (Yeates, Blumenstein, Patterson, & Delis, 1995). Donders (1998) has calculated the standard error of difference as well as the abnormality of difference scores for comparing the CVLT-C with the Children's Category test. The manual reports small difference related to gender and subsequent research indicated that there were significant but small differences at all age levels between 5 and 16 years, with girls generally outperforming boys (Kramer, Delis, Kaplan, O'Donnell, & Prifitera, 1997). However, the magnitude of these differences does not seem sufficient to warrant separate norms. All the same scores near cutoff points should be reexamined for the potential influence of gender. Roman et al. (1998) reported that children with severe closed head injury exhibit lower scores than children with traumatic non-central-nervous system injuries on the immediate recall, delayed recall, and recognition measures of the CVLT. Children with mild to moderate closed head injuries did not differ from the control subjects.

MEMORY FOR DESIGNS TEST

The Memory for Designs (MFD) Test was written in 1946 and revised in 1960 (Graham & Kendall, 1960). It is a series of designs that the subject examines and then draws from memory. It is suggested for use in subjects older than 8 years. The original derivation sample consisted of 140 subjects equally divided between brain-damaged and normal control subjects. The brain-damaged subjects had a variety of diagnoses. No information is given regarding the ages of the subjects. Further normative data from 225 subjects aged 15 to 40 years old are provided by Yeudall, Fromm, Reddon, and Stefanyk (1986). In the manual, the two authors evaluated the test's protocols separately for each of the 140 subjects; the interscorer reliability coefficient was .99. Howard and Shoemaker (1954) reported an interscorer reliability of 93% agreement with less sophisticated scorers. Riege, Kelly, and Klane (1981) reported an interscorer reliability coefficient of .82.

In the original derivation sample, the split-half reliability was reported as .89 (Graham & Kendall, 1960). In a sample of 32 children and 180 adults, the test–retest reliability was .89 when the retest occurred after less than 24 hours. (The retest intervals varied from immediately afterward to approximately 24 hours afterward.) However, there was a consistently lower score on the second test occasion, indicating the presence of practice effects. The difference was not significant, but it was most marked in the brain-damaged sample. This issue needs to be further explored before the MFD can be recommended as a serial test instrument for a neurologically impaired population.

The original validation evaluation examined the difference in scores between the 70 neurologically impaired subjects and the 70 normal controls. There was a significant difference in scores between the two groups, a finding that was replicated in a sample of 168 normal controls and 33 neurologically impaired subjects. There were no differences due to the type of impairment, nor were there any differences due to anterior versus posterior location of the lesion. There were no significant differences between the performance of neurologically impaired subjects and that of psychotic subjects. However, the authors recommended retesting to differentiate these two groups, as organic subjects can be expected to improve and psychiatric subjects can be expected to present variable performances. This recommendation is in need of empirical validation. As well as being sensitive to psychiatric diagnoses, scores on the MFD are significantly related to age (Riege, Kelly, and Klane, 1981).

Grundvig, Needham, and Ajax (1970) compared different strategies of presentation and scoring. They found that the most accurate classification of 114 subjects into three groups of increasing neurological impairment occurred with the use of the original Graham–Kendall scoring system, when the stimuli were presented tachistoscopically.

Marsh and Hirsch (1982) administered the MFD and the Benton Visual Retention Test to 100 subjects who had been referred for evaluation. The Benton Visual Retention test misclassified 29% of the impaired subjects. The MFD misclassification was much larger: 61% of the impaired subjects. The problem with false negatives in screening instruments is widespread; however, Marsh and Hirsch's data (1982) cast serious doubt on the utility of the MFD. Black (1974b) reported similar problems with false-negative results in evaluating subjects with penetrating head injuries. Kljajic (1976) examined the MFD by using a sample of 15 impaired and 15 nonimpaired subjects. The impairment had been determined from the results of pneumoencephalography or EEG. The two groups showed a large amount of overlap in scores, resulting in no significant differences.

To assess the efficiency of the MFD in separating organically impaired psychiatric inpatients from psychiatric inpatients who were not organically impaired and from normals, Shearn, Berry, and Fitzgibbons (1974) administered the instrument to inpatients at the Institute for Living. The patients had been rated as suspected organically impaired or not, both at admission and 4 months later. The ratings had been performed by the attending physicians for each subject and were based on clinical judgment. The MFD scores, taken at admission, did not separate the groups at admission, but did separate the suspected organic from the psychiatric patients who were not suspected of organicity and the normals after the 4-month interval. The authors concluded that the MFD was an effective predictor of organicity judgments after 4 months but not at admission. It is difficult to see the utility of being able to predict clinical judgment when the purpose of testing is to provide objective information.

In studying patients with borderline intelligence and mild retardation, Mandes, Massimino, and Mantis (1991) reported that the MFD was more highly related to intelligence than to organicity. In another examination of the relationship of the MFD to neurological impairment, 178 subjects with different numbers of other indications of organic deficits were administered the MFD. The MFD scores did not discriminate well among the different levels of indicators and did not demonstrate a relationship to the other indicators (Mandes & Gessner, 1989). When the study is confined to patients with epilepsy, error rate on the MFD is associated with lower scores on the verbal scales of the WAIS-R, but not the performance scales (Mandes & Gessner, 1988). There does appear to be some relationship to cortical integrity, as Jones-Gotman (1986) reported that right temporal lobectomy patients scored lower than left temporal lobectomy patients and that larger amounts of right temporal tissue resected were associated with greater degrees of impairment on the MFD.

Korman and Blumberg (1963) compared the MFD scores of 52 patients with those of 40 matched subjects (no mention is made of the 12 patients who were unmatched). The authors administered the Trials Test, the Spiral Aftereffect Test, the Bender–Gestalt, the MFD, and the Vocabulary subtest of the WAIS. They found that, when they used an optimum cutoff point (not the value reported in the MFD manual), they were able to achieve a 90% accuracy rate, which was the highest on all of the tests evaluated.

There is an important consideration in assessing the utility of these experimental results for clinical practice: Although some of these studies report reasonable hit rates, they do so with different cutoff points. Generally, when the cutoff points suggested by the manual are used, there are many misclassifications. However, manipulation of the cutoff points results in more accurate classifications, and each study reports a different optimum cutoff point. To be useful in clinical settings, there must be a standardized cutoff point with reasonable accuracy, or the MFD must remain a research instrument.

PAIRED ASSOCIATES

The use of paired associates in assessing learning and memory has a long history in laboratory research. David Wechsler included this procedure when he devised his Wechsler Memory Scales. The Randt Memory Test is another clinical instrument that uses a paired-associates procedure. This type of procedure has also been used in clinical research into memory deficits.

For example, Ottosson (1960) developed a memory test to evaluate the memory changes associated with electroconvulsive therapy (ECT). This test has three components, one of which is a paired-associates task. There are two alternate forms in the Swedish language. The Ottosson test uses both immediate recall of the pairs and a delayed recall. In a sample of 120 psychiatric subjects, Ottosson reported Kuder–Richardson (K–R) 20 values of .84 and .69 for the two forms in the immediate-recall condition and .87 and .82 in the delayed-recall condition. In a further evaluation of this instrument, Cronhorn and Ottosson (1963) administered the test to 112 psychiatric patients. They found K–R 20 values equivalent to the first study but also reported significant differences between the values obtained on the two forms by the same subjects. To assess the concurrent validity, they calculated point biserial correlations between values on the test and membership in a group that had received ECT or in a group with a similar diagnosis that had not received ECT. The resulting values were .89 and .62 for the two forms. Apparently, the two forms are not exactly equivalent. In a modification of the Fiske–Campbell multitrait–multimethod matrix methodology, Cronham and Ottosson reported higher correlations between the immediate recall condition of the paired associates and two other immediate-recall procedures and the relevant delayed-recall conditions of the same procedures. However, conclusions must be limited because of the modifications imposed on the method. Other types of reliability and validity must also be investigated. Sternberg and Jarvik (1976) translated the test into English and shortened it. These authors did not investigate the properties of the test, but they did find that performance on their modification of the test varied with the degree of depressive symptomatology.

The paired-associates procedure potentially gives the clinician information about the type of memory deficit manifested by a given client. Because the Wechsler version includes both pairs with high a priori associative value and pairs with low associative value, a difference in performance is possible. Using this idea and Tulving's concept (1972) of semantic versus episodic memory, Wilson, Bacon, Kaszniak, and Fox (1982) investigated memory in 39 senile dementia patients. They concluded that the pairs with low associative value draw on episodic memory alone, and that the pairs with high associative value draw on both episodic and semantic memory.

The construct validity of the paired-associates procedure needs to be carefully evaluated. Although this procedure is often used as a test of memory, it is important to keep in mind that it can also be conceptualized as a test of learning. Lambert (1970) found that scores on a paired-associates procedure could be used to predict scores on vocabulary achievement tests. When a stepwise multiple-regression methodology was used, the score on the paired-associates procedure was entered ahead of socioeconomic status and the other achievement variables. Rohwer and Lynch (1968) found that mentally retarded individuals performed more poorly on the test than normals, even when the mental age of the subjects was equated across the two groups. Finally, Schwenn and Postman (1967) found that prior exposure to the task improved performance even when different lists were used.

In conclusion, the paired-associates procedure has great potential as a clinical assessment device. However, a standardized form needs to be developed and evaluated in terms of the aforementioned considerations.

TRIGRAMS

The use of trigrams (nonsense "words" composed of three letters) has a long history in experimental settings. Because the three-letter combinations are largely without semantic meaning, they can be used in the evaluation of verbal stimuli without the influence of contextual meaning. Not all trigrams are without meaning because of the use in our culture of acronyms. Witmer (1935) provided estimates of the association value of various trigram combinations by asking normal subjects to rate the trigrams by the number of associations that could be made. The cultural substrate that provides meaning changes over time. Therefore, Constantini and Blackwood (1968) provided updated tables of associative value for 343 trigrams. For example, in 1935, few people could generate associations with the trigram JFK. After the 1960s, there was an increase in the number of people who made associations with this trigram.

Trigrams have been used in the assessment of immediate and delayed memory. They can be useful in the evaluation of memory decay. Peterson and Peterson (1959) reported that, in an experiment with normal college students, 72% of 48 sets of trigrams were retained after 3 seconds and only 38% were retained after 9 seconds. Paniak et al. (1997) presented normative information for the consonant trigrams procedure in a group of 714 children between the ages of 9 and 15 years.

Trigrams have also been used in the experimental investigation of unilateral neglect. Heilman, Watson, and Schulman (1974) presented consonant trigrams to either ear of eight subjects with unilateral neglect and concluded that unilateral neglect is the result of an arousal or alerting deficit. DeLuca, Cermak, and Butters (1975) used consonant trigrams and random shapes to investigate memory deficits in patients with Korsakoff's disease. In addition, Hannay and Malone (1976) used trigrams to assess differences in laterality associated with the sex of the subject.

There are no reliability studies for the trigram procedure, nor are there guides for the clinical interpretation of the results of an evaluation using trigrams. Milner (1972) stated that deficits in trigram performance are related to the extent of the involvement of the left hippocampus. Samuels, Butters, Fedio (1972) reported that there were no differences between left-temporal- and right-temporal-lesioned subjects when the trigrams were presented visually. However, when the trigrams were presented auditorally, the left-temporal-lesioned subjects performed significantly worse. Stuss et al. (1985) reported that consonant trigrams are sensitive to different levels of severity of closed head injury and the performance improves with recovery.

These studies indicate the potential utility of the trigram procedure in clinical settings. However, more information is needed before the procedure can be recommended.

WORD SPAN

Word-span procedures have been a popular means of assessing memory. They are very similar to digit span procedures. In the word-span procedure, a list of words is presented to the subject, and the subject is then asked to repeat the list back to the examiner. Although there is no standardized word-span procedure that stands independently, there are several memory tests that use word-span procedures. These include the Wechsler Memory Scale, the Randt Memory Test, and the Luria–Nebraska Neuropsychological Battery (LNNB). The LNNB has the added twist of asking the subject to predict how many of the seven words she or he expects to remember each time.

Although there are no standardized word-span procedures, there are data to suggest the utility of such a procedure in a neuropsychological evaluation. Basso, Spinnler, Vallar, and Zanobio (1982) suggested that the word-span procedure may be useful in the evaluation of individuals with left hemisphere damage. However, the data also suggest that a word-span procedure needs to be carefully constructed.

Although Talland (1965) found no differences in performance on word span across age in subjects who were grouped by decades (20s, 30s, 40s, 50s, and 60s), Kausler and Puckett (1979) found that there was a significant age effect on the length of the word span. Weingartner and Silberman (1982) found that the presence of clinical depression significantly affected performance on a word-span task. Schutz and Keisler (1972) found that there was an interaction between social class and the type of words used in the word-span procedure in children. Children of lower socioeconomic status performed significantly poorer than other children when the lists in the word span were composed of functors (prepositions and conjunctions), but not when the lists were composed of nouns or verbs. This result was replicated by the Laboratory of Comparative Human Cognition (1976).

Word-span procedures have also been used to investigate the memory deficits involved in certain disorders. Normal individuals remember the words at the beginning and the end of the list are better remembered because they are entered into long-term memory without proactive inhibition from earlier words. The words at the end of the list are better remembered because they are still in short-term memory when the recall occurs. However, the words in the middle of the list are affected by both retroactive and proactive inhibition. Miller (1971, 1973) used these ideas to investigate the memory deficits involved in Alzheimer's disease. He found that people with Alzheimer's disease remembered the words at the beginning of the list as poorly as the words in the middle of the list. He concluded that the memory deficit associated with Alzheimer's disease involves impairment in the transfer from short- to long-term storage. Oltmanns (1978) used a modified word-span procedure to study attention in schizophrenic and manic subjects and concluded that the attention problems demonstrated by schizophrenic subjects were associated with the thought disorder and not with the recognition and sensory-storage stages of processing.

Although the word-span procedure shows great promise as a clinical assessment technique, the lack of reliability and validity data on the freestanding procedure do not allow it to be recommended. However, when used in a procedure such as the Wechsler Memory Scale, the data regarding that particular instrument should be consulted.

THE REY AUDITORY–VERBAL LEARNING TEST

The Rey Auditory–Verbal Learning Test (RAVLT) is a short test of auditory memory that allows the examiner to evaluate immediate recall, repetitive learning, and the influence of interference by the use of two lists of 15 words each. The test was originally normed on French-speaking subjects, but it has become somewhat popular among English-speaking neuropsychologists. Rey (1964) presented normative data based on a sample of 25 manual laborers, 30 professionals, 47 students, 15 laborers over the age of 70, and 15 professionals over the age of 70. Especially because of the sample sizes, it is important to provide normative data based on English-speaking populations. Savage and Gouvier (1992) reported that gender did not have an effect on RAVLT performance, but the acquisition was affected by age. Interestingly, age did not seem to influence retention in comparisons of the last learning trial and the delayed recall trial. Selnes et al. (1991) presented normative observations for the RAVLT in a sample of 733 homosexual and bisexual men stratified by age and education. Mitrushina, Satz, Chervinsky, and D'Elia (1991) presented normative observations on 156 healthy elderly subjects divided into four age groups between 57 and 85 years old. Wiens, McMinn, and Crossen (1988) presented normative data for 222 adults. Anderson and Lajoie (1996) provided data on 376 normal children between the ages of 7 and 14 years. There is a Dutch version of the AVLT that has been normed on 225 children (van den Burg & Kingma, 1999). These same authors generated "parallel" forms using a rational strategy. Each child was tested twice over a 3-month interval with no significant differences in mean scores or distributions and with a reliability coefficient of .59 when corrected for age. The total number correct had the highest stability.

Lezak (1983) investigated the test–retest reliability of the RAVLT in a sample of 23 young male subjects and reported statistically significant practice effects over intervals that ranged from 6 months to 1 year. Delaney, Prevey, Cramer, Mattson, and the VA Epilepsy Cooperative Study No. 264 Research Group (1992) report good test–retest reliability in a small sample of normal control subjects. Additional information is needed to more fully evaluate the reliability of the AVLT. In particular, it will be important to evaluate the stability of the test results in a sample of chronically impaired subjects.

As noted in the section on the CVLT, use of the RAVLT may result in a smaller likelihood of conclusions of impairment than the CVLT (Stallings et al., 1995), perhaps owing to the high level of functioning of the subjects in the CVLT normative sample, but this point is in need of empirical examination. Crossen and Wiens (1994a) reported that the CVLT resulted in lower performance than the RAVLT in a small sample of healthy normal adults; however, they attributed this difference to the longer word list of the CVLT (by one word). (See also Crossen & Wiens, 1994b for erratum.)

Alternate forms of the RAVLT (Form A and Form C) have been proposed. For example, using the discrepancy between scores on the WAIS-R and the WMS, Ryan and Geisser (1986) divided a sample of VA patients into 41 subjects with intact memory and 32 subjects with impaired memory. Forms A and C of the RAVLT were administered in counterbalanced order with an interval of 2½ hours. Discriminant function analyses showed similar classification rates in the use of the two forms. Only the sum of scores from Trials I to V significantly contributed to the discriminant function. However, t-tests revealed significant differences between the two groups on three variables: the sum of Subtests I to V, the score on subtest VI, and the recognition score. Ryan, Geisser, Randall, and Georgemiller (1986) administered the two forms of the RAVLT to a sample of 85 VA patients. Once again, there was a counterbalanced order but with an interval of 140 minutes. The correlations between equivalent subtests ranged from .60 to .71. There were significant differences between the two forms on Trials IV and V, Form A having higher scores in both cases. List C is suggested as an alternative to either List A or B if either list is spoiled in its presentation. Uchimaya et al. (1995) reported reasonable equivalence between the two forms with the exception of intrusion errors. Fuller, Gouvier, and Savage (1997) reported that List B has different initial recall than does List C, possibly owing to the presence of lower frequency words on List B. More empirical work is needed before the equivalency of the two forms can be fully accepted or rejected.

Crawford, Stewart, and Moore (1989) developed an "alternate" alternate form and reported on the equivalency using a small sample of 30 subjects. Another alternate form was developed by Shapiro and Harrison (1990), but this included only initial learning and did not contain a delayed recall or recognition procedure. These researchers found no differences among the groups and correlations among the forms ranging from .67 to .90; however, the limited sample size may account for the lack of statistically significant differences that have been fairly reliably reported by other investigators. Geffen, Butterworth, and Geffen (1994) reported an alternate form, but based their conclusions of equivalence on a limited sample of 51 control subjects. It should be noted that the most highly reliable score (total words) correlated only .77 across the two forms. Majdan, Sziklas, and Jones-Gotman (1996) administered the C list, the Crawford et al. (1989) list, and a new list generated for the purposes of the study to groups of 38 subjects each. The learning trials, delayed recall, and recognition procedures all had basically equivalent scores in these college students. Although promising, the equivalency of each of these alternate forms should be considered hypothetical until additional data from later samples are obtained.

To evaluate the utility of the RAVLT, Mungas (1983) administered it to five groups of six subjects each: amnesiacs, head trauma victims, schizophrenics, nonpsychotic psychiatric subjects, and subjects with a diagnosis of attention deficit disorder. He found that although the delayed-recall score did not differentiate among the groups, the five-trial initial-word-list procedure did, especially as the number of trials increased. These results are intriguing but are in need of replication with a much larger sample. The delayed recall score may be the most sensitive index available from the Rey. For example, Roman et al. (1997) reported that the delayed recall score improved dramatically following cardiac transplant. Tierney et al. (1994) reported that healthy elderly subjects performed better than subjects with Parkinson's, who performed better than patients with moderate Alzheimer's, who performed better in turn than patients with severe Alzheimer's. Furthermore, the Alzheimer's patients showed greater recency than primacy effects and also had poor recognition scores. All of these differences were consistent with the theories involving the various disease processes. Powell, Cripe, and Dodrill (1992) reported that the RAVLT was better able to classify subjects as neurologically impaired or nonimpaired than was any single test of the Halstead–Reitan Neuropsychological Battery.

There is some evidence that the results of the RAVLT may overlap with the results of an intellectual evaluation. Query and Megran (1983) administered the RAVLT to 677 Caucasian male VA inpatients, including 23 subjects over the age of 70. There were moderately low correlations between results on the AVLT and level of education. However, the learning score correlated .82 in the subjects between the ages of 30 and 34, and .60 in the subjects between the ages of 50 and 54. An earlier study, by Query and Berger (1980), looked at this issue slightly more directly. The RAVLT and the WAIS were administered to 49 acutely neurologically impaired subjects (mainly victims of trauma and cardiovascular accidents), 40 chronically neurologically impaired subjects (mainly alcoholics), and 143 subjects with no evidence of neurological impairment. Multiple-regression methodology was used to partial out the influence of age, education, and WAIS Full Scale IQ (FSIQ). The adjusted group means indicated that the acutely neurologically impaired subjects performed more poorly than either the chronically impaired subjects or the nonimpaired subjects. However, no tests of statistical significance were reported, and the data in the report do not allow us to perform any tests. Bishop, Knights, and Stoddart (1990) reported moderate correlations between the RAVLT and IQ as measured by either the WPPSI or the WISC-R.

Rosenberg, Ryan, and Prifitera (1984) also evaluated VA inpatients using the AVLT. Their sample consisted of 92 psychologically and neurologically impaired subjects. These subjects were divided into groups of 45 memory-impaired and 47 non-memory-impaired subjects on the basis of WAIS and Wechsler Memory Scale results. A subject was classified as memory-impaired if his Wechsler Memory Scale MQ was at least 12 points below his WAIS FSIQ, or if his MQ was less than 85. The memory-impaired subjects scored significantly worse than the nonimpaired subjects.

As a test of the construct validity of the RAVLT, Ryan, Rosenberg, and Mittenberg (1984b) administered the Wechsler Memory Scale, the WAIS, and the RAVLT to 108 mixed psychiatric and neurological male VA inpatients. A principal-components factor analysis was performed using the scree test to determine the number of factors to be extracted and varimax rotation. The results indicated that the RAVLT scores loaded most heavily on the verbal factor. However, Moses (1986b) conducted a factor analysis on the RAVLT scores of VA inpatients and found that the RAVLT loaded highly on the same factor, as did the Benton Visual Retention Test, a finding indicating that the scores of the RAVLT may not be purely modality specific. When the RAVLT itself is subjected to a factor analysis, the results indicate that the scores are reflective of acquisition, storage, and retention (Vakil & Blachstein, 1993). Binder, Villanueva, Howieson, and Moore (1993) reported that the recognition trial of the RAVLT may be sensitive to different levels of motivation.

The RAVLT is sensitive to multiple physiological and neurological variables. For example, Valencia-Flores, Bliwise, Guilleminault, Cilveti, and Clerk (1996) reported that the delayed recall score of the RAVLT is associated with improvement in alertness for patients with sleep apnea who receive nocturnal positive airway pressure treatment. Because it is a verbal list learning task, performance on the RAVLT may be sensitive to language impairment as well as memory impairment. Records, Tomblin, and Buckwalter (1995) found that although individuals with a specific language impairment performed poorly on Trials 1 and 3 of List A and on List B, there were no differences on learning rate or retention in comparison to a control group. Therefore, improvement over time and retention may be more pure measures of memory on the RAVLT. In a sample of cardiac surgery patients, performance on the RAVLT was significantly related to duration of cardiac complaints and the presence of a preoperatively enlarged heart (Vingerhoets, van Nooten, & Jannes, 1997).

Talley (1986) administered the RAVLT and Digit Span to a sample of 153 children between the ages of 7 and 16 years. All of the children had been diagnosed as learning disabled. The AVLT did not predict the digits-forward scores and shared only 7% of the variance with digits backward. A principal-factors analysis with varimax rotation resulted in a three-factor solution that accounted for 71% of the total variance. The factors were interpreted as long-term memory, short-term memory, and short-term memory with control processes. Adult norms may be inappropriate in evaluating children, and Forrester and Geffen (1991) have provided normative information based on a sample of children between the ages of 7 and 15 years. Using the norms from Forrester and Geffen (1991), Kinsella et al. (1997) reported that performance on the RAVLT predicted placement in special education services 2 years following injury for children with mild to severe closed head injury.

Lezak (1979) administered the AVLT to 24 male head-trauma patients at 1, 2, and 3 years post-accident. There were eight left-hemisphere-damaged subjects, eight right-hemisphere-damaged subjects, and eight bilaterally damaged subjects. The AVLT scores tended to improve over time. However, these results must be considered in the light of Lezak's (1982) study which demonstrated significant practice effects.

Since the publication of the first edition of this book, there has been additional normative data on English-speaking subjects, reliability data, and validity studies using other than male VA inpatient samples. Callahan and Johnstone (1987) administered the RAVLT along with other neuropsychological instruments to a sample of outpatients who had experienced closed head injury. They focused on the meaning of Trial V of the RAVLT and found that it could be predicted by gender, WMS-R Delayed Memory Index, and Trail Making Test B, indicating it was related to global neuropsychological functioning as well as to specific memorial processes. Tuokko and Woodward (1996) presented a set of demographic corrections for age, gender, and education based on a sample of 2339 Canadian subjects.

In an examination of the ecological validity of the RAVLT, Millis et al. (1994) found that RAVLT and Trail Making Test B, administered to traumatic brain injury patients after emergence from posttraumatic amnesia, predicted scores on the Community Reintegration Questionnaire, a self-report instrument, 1 year later. Ross et al. (1997) reported that the RAVLT and the TMT also predicted reports of others regarding the psychosocial outcome of traumatic brain injury patients.

Ripich, Carpenter, and Ziol (1997) reported that although Caucasian subjects with Alzheimer's disease tended to score higher than African-American subjects, these differences were not significant and did not indicate the need for separate norms.

Vakil and Blachstein (1997) developed a Hebrew version of the RAVLT and administered it to 528 individuals between the ages of 21 and 91 years. Females tended to score higher than males. Age-related differences were minimal until 60 years, at which time age norms became more important. The delayed recall score showed the greatest sensitivity to age. Neyens and Aldenkamp (1997) developed a Dutch version of the RAVLT and reported acceptable test–retest reliability when 59 children were tested 3 times with a 6-month interval each time. There is also a German version of the RAVLT that has demonstrated construct validity related to short-term and long-term memory (Mueller, Hasse-Sander, Horn, Helmstaedter, & Elger, 1997). A Norwegian version was shown to be sensitive to the effects of whiplash injury (Gimse, Bjorgen, Tjell, Tyssedal, & Bo, 1997).

Detection of Response Bias

The RAVLT has received examination of two different strategies in the detection of less than optimal effort: investigation of patterns of performance and use of the recognition trial (Bernard, 1990, 1991; Bernard, Houston, and Natoli, 1993). Binder et al. (1993) examined scores on the recognition trial, dividing their subjects into those seeking compensation and those not seeking compensation. In addition, the subjects seeking compensation were divided on the basis of their performance on the PDRT. These researchers concluded that extremely poor performance on the recognition trial is indicative of motivation to exaggerate deficits, at least in subjects with mild head injury and negative neurological findings. King, Gfeller, and Davis (1998) criticized these studies for their failure to take into account estimated base rates of malingered performance in clinical settings. They found that the recognition trial could discriminate between analog malingerers and control subjects, but the discriminant function did not generalize well to a separate clinical sample.

A discriminant function derived on the clinical sample did separate the suspected malingerers well, indicating the sample specificity of derived formulae.

DIGIT SPAN

The use of strings of numbers presented in an auditory modality for the purposes of eliciting a repetition from the subject is common in many forms of evaluation. It is generally thought of as a measure of short-term memory, attention, and concentration. The most common form is exemplified in the Digit Span subtest of the Wechsler intelligence tests and in the Wechsler Memory Scale. Those scales have standardized lists and orders of digits and have been investigated in the contexts of their respective tests.

The use of this procedure can also be found in a heterogeneity of methods and lists. Often, a report in the literature will state that the numbers were chosen at random. This approach makes replication difficult. It also clouds the interpretation of studies in which different random lists are used as pre- and postintervention measures.

Blackburn and Benton (1957) suggested an alternate method to the customary one as exemplified by the Wechsler tests. In this procedure, the subject is given both series of each length, a procedure adopted in the development of the WAIS-R and the WISC-R. Other changes include terminating the administration when three consecutive failures have been recorded, rather than after two consecutive failures, and scoring 1 point for each series that is successfully repeated rather than using the length of the last successful series as the score. Blackburn and Benton (1957) concluded that these changes result in increases in reliability. Normative data for this set of procedures are presented in Hamsher et al. (1980). Norms for aged subjects are presented in Benton, Eslinger, and Damasio (1981).

Another variation is the supraspan procedure, in which a series of either eight or nine digits is repeated until the subject is successful in two consecutive attempts or until 12 trials have occurred. Bauer (1979) reported significant differences between the performance of seven learning disabled and seven normal children in a supraspan procedure. The description of how the learning disabled children were identified indicates that there were multiple sources of information that had not been standardized across subjects. The fact that differences were found shows the robustness of the procedure and supports efforts to further standardize the procedure. Hamsher, Benton, and Digre (1980) presented normative data on the supraspan procedure based on 500 subjects and reported that, in a comparison study, the supraspan procedure was more sensitive to neurological impairment than was the usual digit span procedure. Similarly, Drachman and Arbit (1966) and Drachman and Hughes (1971) reported that the supraspan procedure is more sensitive to neurological impairment than is the usual digit span procedure.

Hebb (in Milner, 1971) presented a potentially useful variation on the digit span method. He used nine digit series and repeated a certain series every third presentation. In that way, a learning curve was generated and longer term memory could also be evaluated with the same procedure.

Digit span procedures appear to be sensitive to both neurological impairment and age (Parkinson, 1980). Other research suggests that variability in digit span performance can be attributed to the time in the diurnal cycle: morning performance was superior to afternoon performance in the same subjects (Baddeley, Hatter, Scott, & Snashall, 1970). It will be important to partial out extraneous influences on digit span performance to specify its clinical meaning. Weinberg, Diller, Gerstman, and Schulman (1972) found that, although patients with left-hemisphere lesions performed more poorly than normals on digit span both forward and backward, subjects with right-hemisphere lesions performed more poorly only on the backward procedure. Black and Strub (1978) investigated the relationship of the quadrant of locus of lesion to digit span performance. They found that, for the forward procedure, right-anterior-, left-anterior-, and left-posterior-lesioned subjects performed more poorly than did normals. For the backward procedure, there were no significant differences between any of the groups.

In conclusion, there are procedures (the Wechsler tests, the Randt Memory Test, and the procedures proposed by Benton and Hebb) that have been standardized, and for which there is some knowledge of the psychometric properties. However, validation studies need to be conducted to show the clinical usefulness of the tests. In particular, research should be directed at partialing out extraneous influences, such as time of day and emotional state, and at specifying the physiological correlates.

PACED AUDITORY SERIAL ADDITION TEST (PASAT)

Technically, the PASAT is a test of attention and concentration. However, because it has sometimes been invoked as a measure of working memory and because assessment of attentional processes is frequently subsumed in a memory evaluation, the PASAT is considered in this chapter. The PASAT was originally developed on a somewhat limited standardization and normative sample (Gronwall, 1974). It has acquired a substantial normative base with the publication of information derived from a sample of 821 adult subjects stratified by age and intellectual status (Wiens, Fuller, & Crossen, 1997). The PASAT is very sensitive, even to mild cerebral dysfunction and injury. Gimse et al. (1997) reported that the PASAT discriminated between individuals with whiplash injury and those without such an injury. Cicerone (1997) reported that the PASAT was sensitive to the effects of minor closed head injury. In addition, patients with multiple sclerosis tend to perform poorly on the PASAT (Diamond, DeLuca, Kim, & Kelly, 1997).

The original version of the PASAT had 244 items. A revised version has 200 items (Levin, Benton, & Grossman, 1982). Diehr, Heaton, Miller, and Grant (1998) presented norms for the 200-item version in a sample of 566 adult subjects. These researchers found differences attributable to age, education, and ethnicity and provided regression formulas to correct for the influence of those variables. Sherman, Strauss, and Spellacy (1997) examined the relationships between a modified PASAT, using only the 2- and 1.6-second interval trials of the original form. These researchers found that although the PASAT correlated with other measures of attention in a sample of 441 adults with head injury, the PASAT also correlated with measures of arithmetic knowledge, verbal ability, academic achievement, visual memory, and visual–spatial ability. All correlations were in the low to moderate range. It may be that the PASAT measures some aspect of attention that is basic to several other skills, or that the PASAT does not specifically measure attention.

KIMURA'S RECURRING FIGURES TEST

Kimura's Recurring Figures Test is conceptualized as a measure of visual recognition. There is only one report of its reliability: Rixecker and Hartje (1980) administered the test to 427 German subjects. They reported a Kuder–Richardson reliability coefficient of .94.

They also reported that there were significant differences in level of performance attributable to college education. There are no other reports of any other form of reliability.

Depending on the scoring system used, right-temporal-lobectomy patients scored worse than or the same as left-temporal-lobectomy patients. Both left- and right-lobectomy patients scored worse than the 11 control subjects in this study (Kimura, 1963). In another small-sample experiment, head injury patients scored poorly long after the incidence of injury (Brooks, 1972). Brooks (1974) found that 34 head-injured patients scored more poorly than 34 orthopedic patients. The number of false-positive identifications by the head-injured subjects was about equal to the number emitted by the control subjects. The number of false-negative identifications by the head-injured subjects was greater than that by the control subjects.

As well as investigations of the reliability of this test, there need to be investigations of its construct, concurrent, and predictive validity.

KNOX'S CUBE TEST

Knox's Cube Test (KCT) was developed by Dr. H. Knox to aid him in detecting cognitive impairment in adult immigrants who did not speak English. The KCT has gone through several revisions since its initial formulation in 1914. The current version consists of four standardized blocks, which are glued to a baseboard in a straight line. The administrator uses a smaller fifth block to tap out a pattern on the four stimulus blocks, and the subject is to copy the tapping pattern. There are two forms available, a Junior and a Senior version. These forms differ only in that the Junior Form, for ages 2 to 8 years, starts with a smaller series of two taps and ends with a series of six taps, whereas the Senior Form, for ages 8 and over, starts with a series of three taps and concludes with a series of eight taps. The exact order of the tapping sequences is specified in the manual (Stone & Wright, 1980). Testing continues until five consecutive errors are made by the subject.

Scoring is conducted by assigning a value of 1 for each success and a value of 0 for each failure. The score for each item is then summed. Reliability values based on classical test theory are available for early versions of the KCT. The current version of the KCT was evaluated by use of the Rasch model, a set of statistical procedures that is sometimes known as item response theory. The test authors combined information from previous studies to estimate the reliability of each item. These studies covered a range of more than 60 years and were derived from all of the versions. Therefore, it may be necessary to update the norms by using the current version.

The use of the Rasch model allows the examiner to calculate the best estimate of the subject's ability level and to construct boundaries around this estimate. Failures below the boundaries or successes above the boundaries cast doubt on the validity of the results. Scores are then translated into values of the KCT variable. The use of the Rasch model also allows the examiner to separate estimates of the subject's ability from the difficulty level of the item. Finally, the use of the scoring procedures suggested in the manual results in an age equivalence score.

The use of the Rasch model to evaluate the KCT represents an advance in the evaluation of the instrument. However, the psychometric properties of the KCT have not been as well evaluated by use of the methodology of classical test theory. As the Rasch model is meant as an adjunct to classical test theory rather than as a substitute for it, it is desirable to evaluate the KCT under classical test theory as well.

Using subjects drawn from a population of medical, surgical, and nonpsychotic psychiatric inpatients, Sterne (1966) reported a test–retest reliability coefficient for the KCT of .64 for 56 adult male subjects with a reported interval of "not more than four days." Although Sterne did not report an evaluation of a test for the significance of differences between mean levels of performance, this evaluation was easy to perform, given the data regarding the means and the standard deviations. There were no significant differences. To investigate the possibilities of increasing the reliability values, Sterne then administered the KCT twice in the same day to a group of 50 male subjects drawn from the same sample as described previously. The test was readministered twice the following day. Averages were computed for each day's performance, and these averages were used as the data for the evaluation of the test's reliability. The correlation between the two averages was .82, and again, there were no significant differences. Because of the methodology of the second study, it is difficult to separate the effect of shortening the interval from the effect of averaging two test performances. However, the results indicate that the test–retest reliability may be beneficially affected by one or both of the manipulations used.

Although the KCT is thought to measure attention and short-term spatial memory, there has been little work to investigate the veracity of this assumption. There are studies of note that have attempted to evaluate the validity of the KCT.

Brooks (1976) administered the KCT to 55 Maori 4-year-olds and 55 Pakeha 4-year-olds in New Zealand. He reported that there were no significant differences attributable to socioeconomic status or to ethnic background. There were significant differences attributable to sex in the Maori sample, the females scoring higher than the males.

In an attempt to evaluate the discriminant validity of the KCT, Paletz and Hirshoren (1972) administered both the KCT and the Visual–Sequential Memory subtest of the Illinois Test of Psycholinguistic Ability. There were 96 subjects, 12 subjects in each of the six cells formed by crossing sex with school grade level in the kindergarten, second, fourth, and sixth grades. The resulting correlation coefficients ranged from .08 for the fourth-grade subjects to .57 for the kindergarten subjects. Paletz and Hirschoren concluded that the two tests measured different aspects of visual memory.

Horan, Ashton, and Minto (1980) compared the effects of bilateral and unilateral ECT on performance on the KCT by comparing the pre- and post-ECT performance of each subject. Performance improved significantly in the right-sided unilateral ECT subjects. Because the subjects used in this study numbered only 20, an attempt was made at replication. In the second study, there were ten matched controls who did not receive ECT, seven subjects who received bilateral ECT, and seven subjects who received unilateral right ECT. The unilateral ECT subjects manifested significant improvements in KCT performance, which were not demonstrated by either the control subjects or the bilateral ECT subjects.

None of the above studies were conducted with subjects with neuropsychological impairment. To remediate this deficiency (from the point of view of the clinical neuropsychologist), Bornstein (1983a) administered the KCT as well as the Halstead–Reitan Neuropsychological Battery, the WAIS, the Wechsler Memory Scale, and the Verbal Concept Attainment Test to 300 subjects who had been referred for neuropsychological evaluation. The subjects were divided into two equivalent samples. Identical statistical analyses were conducted on both samples, consisting of principal-factors analysis. In both analyses, the KCT loaded most heavily on factors that were interpreted as reflecting visual and auditory attention span. The results of this study indicate the potential utility of the KCT as a neuropsychological assessment instrument. However, more work needs to be done to specify the construct underlying the KCT, as well as the sensitivity of the KCT to particular forms of neurological impairment.

CORSI BLOCK TAPPING TEST

The Corsi Block Tapping Test may be seen as a spatial equivalent of the word and digit span tests that are sometimes used to measure aspects of memory. The test consists of nine uniformly small, white wooden blocks, which are distributed over a rectangular board. Numbers from 1 to 9 are printed on the sides of the blocks that face the examiner. The examiner taps the blocks in a pattern that is then copied by the subject. Five sequences are tapped for each series. A correct performance is scored when the subject is able to correctly copy three of the five sequences. When a correct response is given, the next sequence is given until a series of eight blocks is given or until the subject is unable to copy three of the five sequences. For a correct response to be scored, the subject must tap only one block at a time and must tap directly on the top of the block, not to the side. The pattern of taps is repeated for every third sequence; however, the intervening taps are not repeated. Normal subjects improve on the repeated stimuli, but not necessarily on the nonrepeated sequences.

The reliability of this instrument has not been investigated. However, some evidence has been presented in the literature that addresses the validity of the Corsi Block Tapping Test. Cantone, Orsini, Grossi, and De Michele (1978) investigated the performance of 85 subjects on the Corsi Block Tapping Test and the Digit Span subtest from the WAIS. The groups were constituted of the following subjects: 90 control subjects, 20 subjects with a diagnosis of Huntington's disease, 25 subjects with multiinfarct dementia, 15 subjects with cerebral atrophy, 21 subjects with a diagnosis of suspected Alzheimer's, subjects with senile dementia, 4 subjects with Pick's syndrome, and 2 subjects with normal-pressure hydrocephalus.

There were significant differences between the controls and the other groups on both the Digit Span and the Corsi Block Tapping Test, with the exception of the comparison between the controls and the multiinfarct dementia subjects. Cantone et al. (1978) also examined the ratio between the verbal span measure and the spatial span measure. Significant differences, in comparison with the control group, were found only for the senile dementia and the Alzheimer's groups. The authors concluded that verbal memory was more affected by dementia than was spatial memory.

Milner (1971) examined the performance of temporal lobectomy subjects on the Corsi Block Tapping Test. In this study, there were 12 subjects with right temporal lobectomy and minimal hippocampal removal, 13 subjects with right temporal lobectomy and radical hippocampal removal, 11 subjects with left temporal lobectomy and minimal hippocampal removal, 8 subjects with left temporal lobectomy and radical hippocampal removal, and 1 subject with bilateral temporal lobectomy and radical hippocampal removal. All of the subjects had roughly equivalent error rates on the nonrepeated sequences. But the subjects with right temporal lobectomy, radical hippocampal removal, and bilateral temporal lobectomy had roughly one half the rate of correct responses of the other groups. No statistical tests of significance were performed on the data. However, it appears that radical hippocampal removal in conjunction with right temporal lobectomy impairs performance.

De Renzi, Faglioni, and Previdi (1977) reported a study in which they examined the performance of left- and right-brain-damaged subjects with and without visual field defects. The presence and laterality of the brain damage had been determined by neurological exam, brain scan, EEG, and neuroradiological findings. There were 20 subjects in each of the four experimental groups, as well as 40 control subjects. Multiple comparisons were performed, but the only significant differences found were between the experimental groups with visual field defects and the controls. None of the other pairwise comparisons were significant. The authors then allowed the subjects to learn the sequences to criterion to a maximum of 50 trials. Only 65% of the right-hemisphere-damaged subjects with visual field defects were able to learn the sequences. The authors concluded that the right occipital region was implicated in the spatial memory task. It is apparent that left hemisphere lesions also impair performance, although to a lesser extent.

Because of its spatial components, the Corsi Block Tapping Test was originally hypothesized to be sensitive to damage to the right hemisphere. To test this hypothesis, De Renzi and Nichelli (1975) examined the performance of 30 control subjects and 125 neurologically impaired subjects. The neurologically impaired subjects included 39 left-hemisphere-injured subjects without visual field defects, 31 left-hemisphere subjects with visual field defects, 23 right-hemisphere subjects without visual field defects, and 32 right-hemisphere subjects with visual field defects. The authors found that visual field defects tended to lower performance on the Corsi Block Tapping Test regardless of the lateralization of the injury. Although the right-hemisphere subjects tended to score somewhat lower than the left-hemisphere subjects, the left-hemisphere subjects with visual field defects scored significantly lower than the controls. The authors concluded that the Corsi Block Tapping Test can be used to lateralize the site of damage only when it is used in conjunction with other tests such as the digit span, which has more specific lateralization and which can be used to rule out left-hemisphere involvement.

Orsini, Schiappa, and Grossi (1981) investigated the effects of sex and urban versus rural home environments on performance on the Corsi Block Tapping Test and on the Digits Forward subtest of the WISC-R. This study evaluated 1113 Italian children between the ages of 4 and 10 years. Four subgroups were formed by crossing the gender variable with the environment variable. Across all subjects, the Corsi Block Tapping Test correlated .53 with Digits Forward. Urban subjects performed significantly better than rural subjects on both tests. Boys performed better than girls only on the Corsi Block Tapping Test. Apparently, the Corsi Block Tapping Test is sensitive to variables other than cortical integrity, and separate norms may be necessary of accurate interpretation of the results of an evaluation using this instrument.

One variable of interest is the length and the spatial arrangement of the paths formed by the tapping. Milner (1971) and most other clinicians and researchers have used random paths. This procedure raises the possibility that performance on the Corsi Block Tapping Test is related to characteristics of the task; that is, one randomly chosen path may be more difficult than another path, and subjects given the first path may perform more poorly without actually having more organic impairment. To investigate this hypothesis, Smirni, Villardita, and Zappala (1983) varied path length and sequence in a group of 83 normal subjects. In addition, the administration of the Corsi Block Tapping Test varied from the usual in that all the subjects were given the maximum number of sequences. Fifty-eight percent of the subjects passed later sequences after failing earlier, shorter sequences. This result indicates that the complexity, as well as the length of the path, and possibly other characteristics are all important variables to consider in the use of this procedure. The authors then suggested a possible sequence of paths that could be used in a standardized fashion. The next step is the provision of norms for these standardized sequences. Hopefully, the authors of this study are engaged in that activity.

The Corsi Block Tapping Test would seem to be a useful addition to the armamentarium of neuropsychological assessment techniques. It has a unique set of task demands and appears to be sensitive to neurological impairment. However, as Smirni et al. (1983) pointed out, the usefulness is limited by a lack of standardized procedures. Berch, Kirkorian, and Huha (1998) reviewed several studies utilizing the Corsi Block Tapping Test in its various manifestations. Smirini et al. (1983) suggested standardized sequences go a long way toward remediating the existing shortcomings of this procedure. Additional research is needed to better specify the psychometric properties of the test, as well as to determine the utility of the new procedures. It is particularly important to investigate the construct validity of the instrument in light of the findings that poor performance is associated with visual field defects as much as with the location of the lesion (De Renzi et al., 1977) and that at least in patients with dementia, the forward digit span score is discriminable from the backward digit span and from both the forward and backward Corsi span, all three of which tended to covary (Carlesimo, Fadda, Lorusso, & Caltagirone, 1994; Sahgal, McKeith, Galloway, Tasker, & Steckler, 1995).

CONTINUOUS VISUAL MEMORY TEST

The Continuous Visual Memory Test (CVMT) is a test of recognition memory for recurring abstract designs. The manual (Trahan & Larrabee, 1988) specifies normative data stratified by age in four different age groups; 18 to 29 years old, 30 to 49 years old, 50 to 69 years old, and older than 70 years. The total standardization sample contains 310 individuals. There were only 30 individuals over the age of 70. Hall, Pinkston, Szalda-Petree, and Coronis (1996) reported that a substantial proportion of their older normal sample was classified as being impaired on the CVMT, indicating the need for better normative information at the upper ranges of the lifespan. Additional normative information is provided by Paolo, Troster, and Ryan (1998a), who reported data based on a sample of 177 healthy older individuals between the ages of 60 and 94 years. Children's norms were provided by Ullman, McKee, Campbell, Larrabee, and Trahan (1997) based on a sample of 138 children in grades 1 through 5. There do not appear to be gender-related differences on the CVMT (Trahan & Quintana, 1990).

Paolo, Troster, and Ryan (1998b) reported the test–retest reliability in a sample of healthy elderly tested over an interval of approximately 1 year. Both the Delayed Recognition score and the D-Prime score improved significantly across the two occasions. Furthermore, those two variables as well as the Total score had rather moderate correlations (.44 to .49). Because of the limited stability, the standard error of difference and 90% cutoff values for gains or decrements were calculated. As an antidote to the practice effects,

Trahan, Larrabee, Fritzche, and Curtiss (1996) presented an alternate form and examined the equivalency of the two forms in a sample of 40 normal subjects and 52 patients with mixed diagnoses. Using generalizability theory, these researchers were able to calculate generalizability coefficients of .66 for the Total score, .53 for the D-Prime score, and .57 for the Delayed Recognition score.

The CVMT would seem to be a fairly pure measure of nonverbal memory, but data suggest that it is sensitive to both left- and right-hemisphere dysfunction, at least in temporal lobe epilepsy patients (Snitz, Roman, & Beniak, 1996). Part of the lack of effect may be due to an inaccurate hypothesize regarding localization rather than laterality. Retzlaff and Morris (1996) reported greater event-related potentials over the frontal lobes during this task. In examining the construct validity of the CVMT using a factor analysis methodology, Larrabee, Trahan, and Curtiss (1992) found that while the acquisition score was related to verbal and nonverbal intelligence and attention, the delayed recall score appeared to be a relatively pure measure of visual memory. In a comparison of unilateral CVA patients, the right-hemisphere-lesioned patients performed more poorly than the left-hemisphere-lesioned patients, especially for the delayed recall measure (Trahan, Larrabee, & Quintana, 1990).

Because of the relative emphasis on visual functions and lack of explicit verbal representations for the test stimuli, it could be hypothesized that right temporal dysfunction might have a greater effect on CVMT performance than would left temporal dysfunction. This does not appear to be the case for seizure patients, in whom there were no significant group differences after IQ was partialed out (Snitz, Roman, & Beniak, 1996).

HOPKINS VERBAL LEARNING TEST

The Hopkins Verbal Learning Test or HVLT (Brandt, 1991) is a 12-word learning task with three recall trials and a recognition trial. A later incarnation of the HVLT includes a 20-minute delayed recall before the recognition. There are six alternate forms. The HVLT has been found to discriminate between patients with Alzheimer's and patients with Huntington's dementias (Brandt, Corwin, & Drafft, 1992). In comparing Alzheimer's patients with vascular dementia patients, the Alzheimer's patients tended to show a greater number of false-positive errors on the recognition task (Barr, Benedict, Tune, & Brandt, 1992). Rasmusen, Bylsma, and Brandt (1995) reported moderate stability using alternate forms over a 9-month interval in a sample of healthy elderly persons. Lacritz and Cullum (1998) compared the HVLT and CVLT and found differences in some of the scores available from both, such as the type of error and similarities in other scores such as recognition indices and the number correct across trials. The advice of these researchers to not interpret HVLT scores based on the literature on the CVLT seems sound when talking about any two tests. There is a revised version of the HVLT in which a 20-minute delayed free recall is administered prior to the recognition trial. Benedict, Schretlen, Groninger, and Brandt (1998) presented normative data based on a sample of 541 subjects between the ages of 17 and 88 years. In addition, these authors provided test–retest and alternate form reliability data. The revised form is probably preferable to the original form, owing to the inclusion of the delayed recall trial.

MEMORY ASSESSMENT SCALES

The Memory Assessment Scales, or MAS (Williams, 1991), are an attempt to blend cognitive neurosciences with clinical assessment. Zielinski (1993) provided a conceptual comparison of the MAS with the WMS-R and concluded that the MAS was better normed, more psychometrically sophisticated, and less verbally dependent. However, empirical evidence is necessary to complete this comparison. Golden, White, Combs, Morgan, and McLane (1999) administered the MAS and WMS-R to 51 clinical patients and found that no correlations between the two tests' scales exceeded .60, and when corrected for reliability none of the correlations exceeded .75. Although there was fair agreement among verbal subtests, the visual scales of the WMS-R tended to have equivalent correlations with both the verbal and the visual scales of the MAS. Furthermore, there was little agreement between the general composite memory scores of the two tests. It is likely that the WMS-R and MAS measure different aspects of memory, a conclusion further supported by similar findings by Hilsabeck et al. (1996). Patients with multiple sclerosis perform more poorly than control subjects on the MAS regardless of whether the patients are receiving interferon beta 1-B; even their scores are not within the impaired range (Selby, Ling, Williams, & Dawson, 1998). The MAS is sensitive to memory disturbance in subjects exposed to environmental neurotoxins; however, the presence of affective symptoms in the same subjects may have clouded the issue of etiology (Bowler, Hartney, & Ngo, 1998).

Evidence for concurrent validity is provided by Taylor, Musgrave, and Crimando (1996), who reported moderate correlations between the MAS and the Perceptual Memory Test in a rehabilitation sample. Again, there may be differences in the construct measured by the MAS and this criterion variable. Response bias on the MAS has been investigated by Betar and Williams (1995), who found agreement between the MAS and the Rey Dot Counting Test. The relevant measures on the MAS were related to the recognition items.

WARRINGTON RECOGNITION MEMORY TEST

The Warrington Recognition Memory Test or RMT (Warrington, 1984) is a test specifically designed to evaluate the ability of the patient to recognize printed words and photographs of faces after a single exposure. The recognition assessment involves forced choices among pairs of stimuli. Because both the words and the faces are presented visually there may be some overlap in the skills tapped by the two subtests. The standardization sample consisted of a group of 310 volunteer subjects who were receiving inpatient treatment for non-central nervous system disease.

The internal consistency of the RMT appears to be adequate (Malina, Bowers, Millis, & Uekert, 1998). The test–retest reliability is unknown.

Where the RMT was studied in a sample of patients with Alzheimer's disease, there was a relation between right hemisphere hippocampal and temporal volume and Faces Recognition, but a relationship between left hemisphere volume and Word Recognition was found only in female subjects (Cahn et al., 1998). The RMT was found to be a superior predictor of lateralization of seizure origin in comparison to the WMS-R, and both tests were inferior to the intracarotid amobarbitol procedure (Kneebone, Chelune, & Lueders, 1997). Baxendale (1997) found that the RMT showed laterality specific deficits in a sample of patients with temporal pathology following surgical treatment, a result also reported by Morris, Abrahams, and Polkey (1995). However, the relationship of the RMT to laterality of lesion is not unequivocal. Hermann, Connell, Barr, and Wyler (1995) reported that performance on the Words subtests but not the Faces subtest declined in epilepsy surgery patients regardless of the laterality of surgical lesions. Furthermore Bigler et al. (1996) found a stronger relationship of left than right hippocampal atrophy to poor performance on both the Words and the Faces subtests of the RMT when subjects were tested 90 days following traumatic brain injury. Rapcsak, Polster, Comer, and Rubens (1994) suggested that poor performance on the Faces subtests may be due to deficits in left hemisphere strategies involving feature analysis. When the RMT was factor analyzed along with the WMS, the resulting solution contained factors of verbal and visual memory associated with the WMS and a single recognition factor on which both subtests of the RMT loaded (Compton, Sherer, & Adams, 1992). In a separate factor analysis involving patients with chronic spinal cord injury, Dowler et al. (1997) found that rather than loading on a memory factor, the RMT-Faces loaded on the same factor as the Benton Facial Recognition Test. Therefore, at least for the Faces subtest, the RMT may be sensitive to factors other than memory.

The RMT may be useful in determining material specific deficits in recognition memory as distinct from recall memory, but these deficits may be differentially related to laterality in different etiologies and populations. Kelly, Johnson, and Govern (1996) reported that in a sample of head-injured individuals, both the RMT-Words and the RMT-Faces scores were correlated with the WMS scores and to a lesser extent with the WMS-R scores. Neither of the RMT scores were correlated with the Glasgow Coma Scale, but RMT-Words was correlated with the period of posttraumatic amnesia.

Because the forced choice method is used, there may be some utility of the RMT in the assessment of nonoptimal effort. Millis (1992) reported that individuals with minor traumatic brain injury and who were seeking compensation exhibited lower recognition scores than did individuals with severe traumatic brain injury. Iverson and Franzen (1994) found no false-positive classification for control subjects and patients with traumatic brain injury and 80% correct classification of experimental malingerers. Subsequent research indicated 100% correct classification and 97% on cross-validation (Iverson & Franzen, 1998).

BUSCHKE SELECTIVE REMINDING TEST

The Buschke Selective Reminding Test (Buschke, 1973) may be more frequently used in neurological than in other settings, but it is gaining increased use, especially in clinical trials of drugs intended to treat the memory impairment associated with the dementias. There are five trials to learn a list of 12 words and after each trial only the nonrecalled words from the prior trial are presented again. The Buschke allows scoring to index short-term recall, random long-term recall, and consistent long-term recall.

Tuokko and Woodward (1996) have presented data from more than 2000 normal control subjects with suggested corrections for age, gender, and education. The availability of this large set of data may further increase the use of the Buschke. The Buschke has been used more frequently in geriatric settings. Stricks, Pittman, Jacobs, Sano, and Stern (1998) presented normative data on community (northern Manhattan) dwelling elderly for 480 English-speaking and 416 Spanish-speaking individuals over the age of 65 years. The sample was stratified for age and education. Yet another set of normative data adjusted for age is represented by Ivnik et al. (1997). Sliwinski, Buschke, Stewart, Masur, and Lipton (1997) presented data related to age- and education-corrected norms for the Buschke and point out the difficulties in using these corrections in diagnostic determinations because age is a risk factor for dementia. They suggest using noncorrected cutoffs for diagnostic determinations. All of these sets of normative data are useful, but the Buschke is still in need of basic reliability data as well as validity data, especially with regard to diagnostic utility.

The construct validity of the Buschke has been examined in terms of the relationship of recalled words in early trials to delayed recall performance. In general, the predicted relationships were found through examination of conditional probabilities in a sample of 99 individuals diagnosed with multiple sclerosis (Beatty et al., 1996a). Examination of the relation to external variables would help bolster confidence in the construct validity of these indices. Beatty et al. (1996b) found that these same patients exhibited a range of memory impairment related to a mixture of learning and retrieval impairments and that these patients could be clustered into three groups using scores from the Buschke. Whether different patterns of performance may also characterize patients with different etiologies remains an empirical question.

Tests of Verbal Functions

OBJECT-NAMING TESTS

Object-naming tasks have been a popular form of evaluation of neurologically impaired individuals. Some form of object naming is included in many standardized procedures, including the Luria–Nebraska Neuropsychological Battery. The use of nonstandardized procedures is risky, as several variables can influence performance on this test, including the familiarity of the subject with the object, the use of an object itself as opposed to a picture of the object, and whether the object word can also be used as a verb (Barker & Lawson, 1968). To subvert these potential problems, Oldfield and Wingfield (1965) developed a set of pictures that can be used in a standardized fashion. Newcombe, Oldfield, Ratcliffe, and Wingfield (1971) found this task to be sensitive to brain injury. However, the reliability and the specific validities of this procedure still need to be evaluated. Lawson and Barker (1968) administered an object-naming test to 100 individuals with organic dementia and 40 volunteers from an elderly persons' social club. They scored a failure to respond as well as the latency of response and found that both variables discriminated between the two groups significantly. They also found that demonstration facilitated naming in the impaired subjects but not in the control subjects. This information points to the possible clinical utility of the procedure.

MULTILINGUAL APHASIA EXAM

In Chapter 10, we discussed many of the procedures developed by Arthur Benton. Most of those procedures were related to visual–spatial function. Yet another area of substantial contribution was in the assessment of verbal functions in the form of the Multilingual Aphasia Exam or MAE (Benton & Hamsher, 1989). There are relatively small age-related effects in performance. Schum and Sivan (1997) examined age-related effects in 61 community-dwelling adults between the ages of 70 and 90 years and found declines only in the Sentence Repetition subtest, which might be due to the memory demands of this test. In an investigation of concurrent validity, Axelrod, Ricker, and Cherry (1994) reported that the Visual Naming subtest of the MAE had good agreement with the Boston Naming Test and was relatively unrelated to perceptual skills and attention. Crosson, Cooper, Lincoln, Bauer, and Velozo (1993) reported that the Visual Naming and Token subtests of the MAE were correlated with performance on a verbal learning task (the California Verbal Learning Test) in patients who had experienced closed head injury.

Controlled Oral Word Association Test

Perhaps the most frequently used component of the MAE is the Controlled Oral Word Association Test (COWAT). Verbal fluency has been implicated in a wide variety of neurological and medical syndromes including cardiac surgery (Bruggemans, Van de Vijver, & Huysman, 1997). In addition, depression may serve to decrease scores and result in more variability (Veiel, 1997b). Stricks, Pittman, Jacobs, Sano, and Stern (1998) presented normative data related to both English- and Spanish-speaking elderly living in an urban setting. Performance on the COWAT among Spanish-speaking individuals may be related to socioeconomic status (Artiola I Fortuny, Heaton, & Hermosilla, 1998). The COWAT is frequently used in the evaluation of older subjects, necessitating the acquisition of data regarding normative performance in this group as provided by Ivnik, Male, Smith, Tangalos, and Petersen (1996). The COWAT has two forms, one using the letters C, F, and L and one using the letters P, R, and W. Ruff, Light, Parker, and Levin (1996) report updated normative information. The two forms had adequate test–retest/equivalent reliability across a 6-month interval. However, the means were higher than the original norms, perhaps due to differences in the sample characteristics (rural vs. urban) and to increases due to a cohort effect. In addition, a popular form of verbal fluency uses the letters F, A, and S. Lacy et al. (1996) provided evidence regarding the equivalence of the two forms (FAS and CFL) in a sample 287 patients with various diagnoses. Johnson-Selfridge, Zalewski, and Abroudarham (1998) reported significant differences due to ethnicity among white, black, and Hispanic veterans even when income and education were covaried. Therefore, different norms may be necessary for these groups. In general, the largest number of words are generated in the early stages of the task, with fewer words and less frequent words being generated in the second half of the time period (Crowe, 1998).

An interesting use of the COWAT is in conjunction with a category fluency procedure. For example, after being asked to generate as many words as possible beginning with the letters F, A, and S, the subjects will be asked to generate words that are names of animals in a 60-second interval. Subjects with Alzheimer's disease tend to show greater impairment on the animal naming task than on the FAS (Crossley, D'Arcy, & Rawson, 1997). Normal subjects and subjects with ischemic vascular dementia tend to generate more animal names than words on the COWAT, but patients with Alzheimer's disease tend to generate more words on the COWAT. Patients with ischemic vascular dementia tend to generate fewer words on the COWAT than patients with Alzheimer's dementia, but the same number of words on the category fluency task (Carew, Lamar, Cloud, Grossman, & Libon, 1997). Bolla, Gray, Resnick, Galante, and Kawas (1998) examined COWAT and categorical fluency (including animals) in older individuals and found significant effects for age, education, and gender. They reported mean values for performance in their $n = 478$ sample and stratified these means by age and gender, by education and gender, and by North American Adult Reading Test and gender. Generally speaking, these individuals could generate approximately four more animals than the average number of words generated across the three letters of the COWAT. Age- and education-adjusted norms for animal naming based on a sample of 412 subjects over the age of 55 years are provided in Lucas et al. (1998a); however, comparison to FAS performance is not reported. There are also differences in animal naming due to ethnicity when comparisons are made among individuals who are Chinese, Hispanic, or Vietnamese immigrants (Kempler, Teng, Dick, Taussig, & Davis, 1998).

Fama et al. (1998) reported that patients with Alzheimer's disease tend to perform more poorly than patients with Parkinson's disease on the FAS but not on animal naming. Individuals with Alzheimer's dementia, Huntington's disease, and vascular dementia all show greater impairment on animal naming than on COWAT, although both are impaired (Barr & Brandt, 1996). Perhaps the strongest effects of Alzheimer's on verbal fluency are found in comparison with normal control subjects. Kessler, Bley, Mielke, and Kalbe (1997) reported that patients with Alzheimer's were impaired on both the FAS and Animal Naming in comparison to healthy subjects and the biggest differences were found for the Animal Naming task. In addition, there appeared to be differences in strategy, as the patients with Alzheimer's tended to give nouns for the phonemic fluency task and to generate words for fewer categories than did the healthy subjects, who were twice as likely to generate adjectives and verbs.

Suhr and Jones (1998) used the FAS in comparison to a semantic fluency task (naming animals, fruits or vegetables, and tools or kitchen utensils) and found no differences in patterns of performance among patients with Huntington's disease, Parkinson's disease, Alzheimer's disease, and normal controls. The relative difference between phonemic and categorical fluency needs to be better explicated before a single clinical interpretation can be advanced. Category fluency may be more sensitive to the effects of aging than is phonemic fluency (Kozora & Cullum, 1995).

The differences in phonemic versus semantic fluency may be related to anatomical site of lesion. Stuss et al. (1998) reported that superior medial frontal lesions were associated with poorer performance on the COWAT but the relationship of lesion site to animal naming was less clear. The laterality of the two fluency tasks may not be different, as both left- and right-temporal lobectomy result in decreases on both tasks (Loring, Meador, & Lee, 1994). When the number of categories is increased, there appears to be a greater relationship to measures of executive function (Hanes, Andrewes, Smith, & Pantelis, 1996). The use of switching strategies in phonemic fluency may be the essential component related to frontal functioning (Troyer, Moscovitch, & Winocur, 1997). Although Moscovitch (1994) had proposed that phonemic fluency was related to frontal functioning and semantic fluency was related to temporal functioning, Baldo and Shimimura (1998) reported that their sample of frontally lesioned patients were impaired on both phonemic and semantic fluency tasks and suggested that the frontal lobes had a more general role in fluency overall. Although the COWAT specifically was not used, Condon, Montaldi, Wilson, and Hadley (1997) reported that functional MRI during letter fluency performance indicated activation of Brodmann areas 44 and 6 (premotor cortex).

The use of phonemic versus category fluency does not have universal support in the differentiation of Alzheimer's disease from other disorders. Sherman and Massman (1999) found that in their sample of 217 patients with Alzheimer's disease, only 145 patients showed the expected advantage of category fluency over phonemic fluency and 72 patients showed the opposite advantage. The two groups differed in Folstein MMSE scores wherein the patients with the unexpected advantage had significantly higher scores. However, these researchers warn against the clinical application of this putative diagnostic indicator.

Gladsjo et al. (1999) presented normative data on the combined COWAT and Animal Naming procedures derived from a sample of 768 normal control adult subjects. Multiple regression techniques were used to calculate demographically corrected standardized scores. Tombaugh, Kozak, and Rees (1999) presented normative data derived from a sample of 1300 community-dwelling subjects between the ages of 16 and 95 years. Instead of regression corrections, these researchers presented tables stratified by three age groups and three levels of education. They reported that the FAS is more sensitive to the effects of education than of age and that Animal Naming is more sensitive to the effects of aging than of education. In general, individuals could generate between six and eight more words in the Animal Naming than on the average across the three trials of the FAS.

Although the COWAT letters were not used as stimuli, Cohen, Morgan, Vaughn, Riccio, and Hall (1999) reported developmental trends in letter fluency. Furthermore, children with dyseidetic dyslexia tended to perform better than children with dysphonetic dyslexia. Individuals with mild closed head injury tend to produce fewer words on both the FAS and Animal Naming. In addition, they make more errors involving perseveration and out of category production (Raskin & Rearick, 1996).

THE TOKEN TEST

The Token Test has gone through many different incarnations. As a result, several versions are extant. De Renzi and Vignolo (1962) published what is probably the first version of the Token Test. In this version, there were no standard stimuli or instructions, although the authors did describe the stimuli and the types of instructions they had used. Needless to say, this unstandardized approach resulted in the different versions that can be found in the literature. Some of the changes have been seemingly minor. For example, Boller and Vignolo (1966) changed the commands from take to touch. Other changes were made to facilitate ruling out the influence of other impairments from the production of errors. The commands are said to increase in difficulty level; however, this claim has not been investigated empirically. In another version, the blue-colored tokens were changed to black so as not to penalize subjects who might be blue–green color-blind.

In general, reliability studies have not been a major focus of evaluations of the Token Test. Gallagher (1979) investigated test–retest reliability by administering the Token Test to 30 aphasic subjects on three occasions interspersed in an 8-day period. Although the Wilcoxin Matched Pairs Signed Ranks test was not significant, the Spearman rank-correlation coefficients were .98 for the comparison of the first administration with the second, .96 for the comparison of the second with the third, and .95 for the comparison of the first with the third administration.

McNeil and Prescott (1978) presented a Revised Token Test in which they addressed some of the traditional psychometric issues in aphasia evaluation. For example, they stated that, in their version, the intrascale homogeneity is controlled by the use of standard stimuli. Unfortunately, they did not empirically evaluate this assumption. Test–retest reliability was evaluated by administering the test twice to 10 brain-damaged subjects across a 2-week interval. The average subtest correlation was .90. Intrascorer reliability was evaluated by videotaping nine administrations of the Revised Token Test. Three judges scored three administrations twice each. The agreement of the judges with themselves was about .99

for the mean subtest scores. Interscorer reliability was evaluated by having three judges score the same three videotaped administrations. Agreement for the subtest means ranged from .98 to .97. Unfortunately, the authors did not say what the subject characteristics were. If the subjects used were normal subjects, this level of agreement is not surprising. Also, we would want to know what the agreement of diagnosis was across the judges. Norms are available for non-brain-damaged subjects, brain-damaged subjects, and aphasic subjects. Unfortunately, the manual states that the Revised Token Test discriminates between aphasic and nonaphasic brain-damaged subjects at only slightly better than chance levels (55% correct). Concurrent validity was evaluated by administering the Revised Token Test and the Porch Index of Communicative Ability to a sample of 23 aphasic subjects. The overall correlation was .67.

Another form of the Token Test involves the use of concrete objects rather than tokens. Martino, Pizzamiglio, and Razzano (1976) reported that, in a sample of 70 brain-damaged and 10 normal subjects, there was good agreement between the results of the traditional Token Test and the results of the Concrete Objects Token Test.

Orgass and Poeck (1966) attempted one of the first empirical validation studies using the Token Test. They administered the test to 66 subjects without brain damage, 49 subjects with brain damage but without aphasia, and 26 aphasics. The subjects ranged in age from 5 to over 60 years. The authors stated that the aphasics demonstrated clear signs of aphasia, but they did not describe what they meant by "clear signs." They found that performance was significantly related to age and that there were differences due to age. The influence of education was significant but was not judged to be important in clinical situations. Using a cutoff score of 11 errors, the authors were able to correctly classify 84% of the aphasics, 96% of the brain-damaged but not aphasic subjects, and 100% of the normals. There was no attempt at cross-validation in this report.

Because the cutoff scores were determined by an examination of the distributions against which the accuracy of classification was checked, it is especially important to attempt a cross-validation. This procedure can be seen in Hartje, Kerschensteiner, Poeck, and Orgass (1973), who found that changing the cutoff score to 23 errors resulted in an optimal correct classification rate for this sample. Apparently, although the Token Test may be sensitive to aphasic disorders, the use of a single cutoff point for diagnosis causes problems.

Lass and Golden (1975) investigated the concurrent validity of the Token Test by correlating the scores obtained by 20 normal subjects on the Token Test with their scores on the Peabody Picture Vocabulary Test (PPVT). These authors found a correlation of .71. Because the PPVT is a test of verbal intelligence, the moderately high correlation calls into question the interpretation of the Token Test as a measure of purely verbal language capacity.

Performance on the Token Test is associated with metabolism rates in the parieto-temporal region, at least in patients with mild cerebral artery infarcts (Karbe et al., 1989). This localization is consistent with the theoretical anatomic underpinnings of the language functions tested by the Token Test. Poor performance on the Token Test may be the result of perseverative tendencies in patients with Alzheimer's rather than specifically related to poor verbal comprehension (Swihart et al., 1989). In children with unilateral brain lesions, poor performance on the Revised Token Test may be related to memory dysfunction as much as to language dysfunction (Aram & Ekelman, 1987). Similarly, poor readers (children) may exhibit poor performance on the Token Test as the result of memory dysfunction (Smith, Mann, & Shankweiler, 1986). Intelligence does not appear to affect performance, at least in children (Kitson, Vance, & Blosser, 1985). Normal aging may also result in poor performance, pointing out the need for age-related norms (Emery, 1986).

Spellacy and Spreen (1969) investigated a short form of the Token Test by using two types of scoring procedures: a weighted score procedure, in which more sensitive items were given heavier weights, and a pass–fail score procedure, in which all items were given equal weight. They administered their short form to 37 nonaphasic brain-damaged subjects and 67 subjects who had been judged aphasic by medical diagnosis. The internal consistency reliability determined by use of the weighted scoring procedure was .79. The internal consistency reliability determined by use of the pass–fail scoring procedure was .92. Using an optimal cutoff developed on the same sample resulted in 89% correct classification of the aphasic subjects and 72% classification of the nonaphasic subjects. With the use of the pass–fail scoring procedure, 79% of the aphasic subjects and 86% of the nonaphasic subjects were correctly classified. Cross-validation is likely to result in even less accurate classification rates.

De Renzi and Faglioni (1978) gave a short form of the Token Test to 215 control subjects and 280 aphasic subjects. Using a regression correction for the amount of education, they found that an optimal cutoff score correctly classified 95% of the normal subjects and 93% of the aphasic subjects. For the same reasons discussed earlier, this optimal cutoff score is in need of cross-validation.

Cole and Fewell (1983) investigated the use of De Renzi and Faglioni's short version of the Token Test (1978) in a sample of 90 children aged 31 months to 103 months with a mean age of 66.4 months. They also administered the Preschool Language Scale (PLS) to the same subjects. The Token Test correlated .78 with the language age derived from the PLS, .74 with the Auditory Comprehension scale of the PLS, and .76 with the Verbal Ability scale of the PLS. By choosing a cutoff score that resulted in zero false negatives, these authors obtained 11 false positives compared to diagnosis determined by the PLS.

Age-related norms are essential, as demonstrated in a sample of older Danish individuals (Nielsen, Lolk, & Kragh-Sorensen, 1995).

In short, the Token Test, although often used in language disorder clinics, as well as in neuropsychological settings, is in need of standardization and basic reliability and validity research.

THE NEW WORD LEARNING TEST

The New Word Learning Test operates on the principle that organically impaired individuals will demonstrate lower levels of performance than will organically intact individuals on a task requiring them to learn the meanings of unfamiliar words. Walton and Black (1957) and Walton (1957) reported that New Word Learning Test scores do indeed discriminate organically impaired subjects from psychotic subjects and normal subjects. These studies also found that, although intelligence, age, and size of working vocabulary were related to scores on the New Word Learning Test, these variables did not have an appreciable effect on the classification of the subjects.

Walton, White, Black, and Young (1959) revised the scoring system of the New Word

Learning Test so that low scores represented poor performance and high scores represented good performance. They also penalized the subjects for each additional repetition required before adequate performance was demonstrated. They administered the test to a sample of 83 normal subjects, 66 neurotic subjects, 32 psychotic subjects, 45 mentally retarded subjects, and 78 organically impaired subjects. Using a cutoff score of 26 points resulted in perfect classification of the normal, neurotic, and psychotic subjects. Fifteen percent of the organically impaired subjects were misclassified, as were a large proportion of the mentally defective subjects. These misclassifications may have been due to the authors' inexplicable inclusion of the mentally retarded subjects in the normal classification. However, it is apparent that scores on the New Word Learning Test are affected by IQ.

White (1959) found that the New Word Learning Test classified 74% of 40 non-impaired children (including 18 psychiatric subjects), 8 retarded subjects, and 10 neurologically impaired subjects, all of whom were between the ages of 6 and 16. In a second study contained in the same report, there were no significant differences between 17 neurologically impaired children and 17 matched controls. Evidently, the New Word Learning Test is not equally sensitive to neurological impairment in all age groups. The limits of its applicability have yet to be defined. In addition, Teasdale and Beaumont (1971) found that the presence of depressed mood can affect scores so that subjects may be misclassified as neurologically impaired when they are not.

The New Word Learning Test is in need of research to assess both its reliability and its validity.

BOSTON NAMING TEST

There has been an explosion of interest in the Boston Naming Test (BNT) in recent years. With the exception perhaps of the Controlled Oral Word Association Test, there is no test of verbal function that has received as much scrutiny and utilization in neuropsychological contexts as has the Boston Naming Test. This is partly due to the social need for instruments to evaluate the cognitive effects of dementia and the fact that Alzheimer's disease has a correlated decrease in semantic relationships, which the BNT is well suited to evaluate. The BNT has been translated into various languages, which is essential in the application of language-based measures. The BNT was originally an 85-item version, but was subsequently shortened to 60 items. The 60-item form appears to be more sensitive than the original 85-item version, probably because of more stringent cutoffs (Thompson & Heaton, 1989).

The BNT is in almost the exact opposite psychometric condition of most neuropsychological instruments. Whereas most neuropsychological instruments have been evaluated in terms of their validity but not in terms of their reliability, the BNT was originally evaluated in terms of its reliability but not in terms of its validity. In the original study reported in the manual (Goodglass & Kaplan, 1983), Kuder–Richardson reliability coefficients were calculated on the basis of data provided by 34 aphasics. Unfortunately, in this case, as in all subsequent cases, the authors failed to describe by what means the subjects had been classified as aphasic or whether the subjects also exhibited other forms of neuropsychological impairment. Flanagan and Jackson (1997) report that the BNT has adequate temporal reliability when administered to older adults across a period of 7 to 17 days.

Although early reports did not demonstrate significant age-related differences (La-Barge, Edwards, & Knesevich, 1986), there is an age effect (Albert, Heller, & Milberg, 1988) that is more likely to be an aging effect than a cohort effect (Au et al., 1995). Normative data are available on a sample of 78 healthy, independently living adults aged 59 to 80 years (Van Gorp, Satz, Kiersch, & Henry, 1986). Ross and Lichtenberg (1997) found that age and education had significant effects on BNT performance in healthy older individuals. Ross and Lichtenberg (1998) later expanded this sample to include 233 intact individuals between the ages of 65 and 95 years and presented normative information stratified by age and education. Tombaugh and Hubley (1997) provided normative data that are age and education stratified as does Ross, Lichtenberg, and Christensen (1995) and Ivnik et al. (1996). The effect of education may be specifically related to reading vocabulary (Hawkins et al., 1993). Lichtenberg, Ross, and Christensen (1994) presented normative observations on a limited sample of older African-American individuals with lower education levels. This may help alleviate the problem of false positives that was identified by Lichtenberg, Vangel, Kimbarow, and Ross (1996). It is also important to pay attention to the interaction of age and education, as there is less of an age effect in more highly educated individuals (Welch, Doineau, Johnson, & King, 1996). On the other end of the age spectrum, Kirk (1992a) did not find gender-related differences for children aged 5 to 23 years, but did find significant age-related effects similar to reports by Kindlon and Garrison (1984); Guilford and Nawojczyk (1989); and Cohen, Town, and Buff (1988). Yeates (1994) concatenated childhood norms from different studies into a single continuum.

Normative data are also available on the Dutch version in a sample of 200 Belgian subjects aged 55 to 91 years (Marieen, Mapaey, Vervaet, Saerens, & DeDeyn, 1998) as well as normative data available on the Spanish version from a sample of 200 young bilingual adults (Kohnert, Henandez, & Bates, 1998). From the same sample, data are available for correct responses regardless of the language used. Allegri et al. (1997) reported normative information on the Spanish version of the BNT and also found that education had a significant effect on score. Ardila and Rosselli (1994) reported developmental trends using the Spanish version of the BNT in normal 5- to 12-year-old children in Columbia. Although they putatively share the same language as citizens of the United States, there are separate norms for older Australian subjects (Worrall, Yiu, Hickson, & Barnett, 1995).

The effect of demographic variables on BNT performance has been studied. Heaton, Grant, and Matthews (1991) presented data on the 85-item experimental version of the BNT with regression-based corrections made for gender, age, and education. Unfortunately, the cell sizes for each combination of age, education, and gender are very small. That fact, coupled with the fact that most clinicians use the 60-item clinical version of the BNT, limit the utility of these norms. Based on Thompson and Heaton (1989), Heaton, Matthews, Grant, and Avitable (1996) recommended prorating performance on the 60-item version to compare to the 85-item norms, but this suggestion involves a procedure that is too far removed from actual data. Fastenau (1999) reported that these norms resulted in large overcorrections for education in less well educated subjects. It would be preferable to rely on one of the other available sets of norms available for different levels of age and education.

Cultural variables, which can be very important in language measures, have also been studied. Ferraro and Bercier (1996) did not find differential effects on the performance on older Native Americans. Henderson, Frank, Pigatt, Abramson, and Houston (1998) reported that there were no effects for gender or race (African-American vs. Caucasian), although education had a significant effect. The social construct of race may not be as important as the extent of integration into the dominant culture. Manly et al. (1998b) found that performance on the BNT was related to degree of acculturation in healthy African-American subjects. This relation makes common sense, as degree of familiarity with the words is related to lexical speeded reaction time in naming (Ferraro, Blaine, Flaig, & Bradford, 1998). Ripich, Carpenter, and Ziol (1997) found that performance on the BNT had a greater relationship to the Folstein Mini-Mental State Exam than it did to race in a sample of patients with Alzheimer's disease; however, the small sample may have precluded finding significance, as there was differences in mean score observed for Caucasians and African-Americans. However, in a sample of urban elderly impaired and unimpaired subjects (as defined by functional independence scores and measures of activities of daily living), there was a much greater relationship to education than to race (Lichtenberg, Ross, Youngblade, & Vangel, 1998).

Poor performance on the BNT in clinical populations is usually interpreted as reflecting impaired access to the lexicon in naming functions (word retrieval). However, as Johnson, Paivio, and Clark (1996) pointed out, poor performance on object naming from visual input can be the result of multiple forms of cognitive or perceptual dysfunction. Although the BNT, like the Wechsler Intelligence Scales, carries an aura of assumed construct validity, it has been investigated in different neuropsychological populations. Therefore, we do know something about the diagnostic correlates of the instrument, especially its relationship to a diagnosis of Alzheimer's disease (Knesevich, LaBarge, & Edwards, 1986). For example, Lukatela, Malloy, Jenkins, and Cohen (1998) reported that patients with early Alzheimer's disease demonstrated greater levels of error than did patients with early vascular dementia or healthy individuals, a finding in agreement with the report of Barr et al. (1992) using the same populations. In addition, score on the BNT is related to severity of disease in patients with Alzheimer's disease (Chenery, Murdoch, & Ingram, 1996). Patients with Alzheimer's disease perform even more poorly than patients with cerebrovascular accident (CVA) (Margolin, Pate, Friedrich, & Elia, 1990). However, there may not be complete diagnostic specificity with the BNT, as Pachana et al. (1996) reported that there were not differences between patients with Alzheimer's and patients with frontotemporal dementia.

Children with severe closed head injury score lower on the BNT than healthy children but children with posterior fossa tumor or acute lymphoblastic leukemia do not (Jordan, Murdoch, Hudson-Tennent, & Boon, 1996). The poor performance on the BNT may extend into adulthood for those children (Jordan & Murdoch, 1994). Similarly, adults with closed head injury perform poorly on the BNT (Kerr, 1995). Left-hemisphere language dominant epilepsy patients who undergo left temporal resection exhibit deficient performance on the BNT even 1 year after surgery (Langfitt & Rausch, 1996). Subjects may exhibit poor performance on the BNT even in the preclinical stages of Alzheimer's disease (Jacobs et al., 1995).

The BNT is a somewhat lengthy procedure and may be onerous to individuals with significant expressive communication deficits. There is a discontinuation rule of six consecutive failures; however, it is important to attend to whether the use of a phonemic cue constitutes a correct response or not. A comparison of the two rules for failures resulted in changes in score for only 3% of 655 normal elderly subjects and changes in score in 31% of 140 patients with Alzheimer's disease (Ferman, Ivnik, & Lucas, 1998).

The BNT could be useful in serial examinations of the recovery of speech functions or in the documentation of decline. To enhance the utility of the BNT in these contexts, Huff, Collins, Corkin, and Rosen (1986) divided its 85 items into two subtests of 42 items each and administered them to 15 healthy adults, 24 subjects with senile dementia of the Alzheimer's type, and 17 subjects with diagnosed brain lesions. Form I had an alpha coefficient of .96, as did Form II. The two alternate forms had similar means and standard deviations, and the correlation between the two forms was .97. The more recently available 60-item clinical form of the BNT has also been subjected to short form development. Williams, Mack, & Henderson (1989) found that an empirically derived 30-item short form classified patients with Alzheimer's versus other dementias fairly well, although the total sample included only 40 subjects. Mack, Freed, Williams, and Henderson (1992) presented and evaluated five 15-item forms and three 30-item forms and recommended that empirically derived 30-item form. In a much larger ($n = 320$) and clinically diverse sample, Franzen, Haut, Rankin, and Keefover (1995) investigated and compared eight of the short forms of the BNT and recommended the 30-item forms over the 15-item forms because of the high degree of misclassification possible. Larrain and Cimino (1998) similarly reported poor agreement between the long form of the BNT and the 15-item CERAD (Consortium to Establish a Registry for Alzheimer's Disease) in evaluating a sample of 58 subjects with probable Alzheimer's disease. Lansing, Ivnik, Cullum, and Randolph (1999) reported that the previously developed short forms were all sensitive to gender and developed a gender-neutral form of 15-item version of the BNT. They reported equivalent discriminability to the full-length form in differentiating Alzheimer's patients from normal controls.

BOSTON DIAGNOSTIC APHASIA EXAM

The Boston Diagnostic Aphasia Exam (BDAE) is a multiple subtest instrument for investigating the various aspects of language impairment that might be possible in adults. It is primarily derived on samples of patients with CVAs and has its greatest utility there. It is very lengthy and would not be efficient unless communication impairment was suspected or demonstrated. However, in those cases, the BDAE offers a comprehensive look at language function from a neuropsychological perspective.

Goodglass and Kaplan (1983) reported the results of administering the BDAE to 242 aphasics, a remarkable feat that must have taken much patience and effort—even in just locating that many aphasics. These authors then performed multiple statistical operations on their data to examine the reliability and the factorial structure of the instrument. The analysis of internal consistency reliability resulted in values ranging from .96 for the Word Discrimination test to .68 for the Body Parts Identification test. This sample of 34 subjects was used to generate standardized z scores. This system was replaced by the calculation of percentiles based on the later sample of 242 aphasics.

A factor analysis conducted on this sample of 242 aphasics yielded a set of 10 factors that the authors suggested can be used for interpretation. However, there is no empirical evidence linking these factors to observable referents, so that their utility is limited in a clinical setting. The authors did not specify the number-of-factors rule that they used to decide when to terminate extraction. In addition, 44 variables were used in the factor analysis, which would require triple the number of subjects used to provide a stable solution. Another factor analysis conducted with the same subjects and a smaller number of variables (only the language variables) yielded a similar factor structure. This result may mean only that the language and nonlanguage variables are independent, but it also speaks to the issue of the stability of the derived language variables' structure. A third factor analysis with the same subjects, which deleted the rating scale variables, generated a similar factor structure. A fourth factor analysis used only the variables that were normally distributed and a sample of 41 aphasics from the original sample. What is needed is an attempt at cross-validation that uses a separate sample.

In another attempt to investigate the multivariate properties of the instrument, the authors performed a discriminant function analysis using 41 aphasics divided among the diagnostic groups of Broca's aphasics, Wernicke's aphasics, conduction aphasics, and anomie aphasics. Ten variables were selected to be included in the predictors on a theoretical basis. Even with this attempt to pare the number of potential predictors, the sample should have been four times the size to give any confidence in the generalizability of the solution. Another drawback is that the a priori classifications (diagnoses) were determined partly on the basis of the scores on the variables, which were then used as predictors.

Borod, Goodglass, and Kaplan (1980) reported normative data on the BDAE, the Parietal Lobe Battery, and the BNT. These data were based on an evaluation of 147 normal subjects, and they go a long way toward increasing the utility of these instruments in a clinical diagnostic setting. The authors recommended the BDAE on the basis of its content and its face validity, which are considerable. However, much basic validation work needs to be conducted.

Tests of Visual and Construction Functions

THE REY–OSTERRIETH COMPLEX FIGURE TEST

The Rey–Osterrieth Complex Figure Test involves the copying and recall of abstract line drawings. Among neuropsychological assessment instruments, the Rey–Osterrieth Complex is unusual for two reasons. First, there are more different administration and scoring systems for the Rey–Osterrieth than for any other instrument. The copy and then the recall conditions allow the Rey–Osterrieth to be related to the evaluation of both visual–spatial construction and memory. The complex nature of the stimulus allows evaluation of the strategy used, thereby assessing aspects of planning and executive functions. Some versions require a copy condition and then an immediate, unwarned recall condition, but one version utilizes a 3-minute delay before the "immediate" recall condition. The delayed recall condition, which is also unwarned, is given in some versions after 30 minutes and in some versions after 45 minutes.

There are scoring systems that have differing degrees of articulation of the criteria for the accuracy of the recall; one of the more specific is that of Loring, Martin, Meador, and Lee (1990). Another scoring system is presented in Meyers and Meyers (1995a,b) which has the added benefit of a standardized recognition trial. The normative base of the Meyers and Meyers (1995) system is composed of 601 subjects between the ages of 18 and 90 years in 5-year cohorts. Finally, there are scoring systems that evaluate the copy strategy. This chapter is confined to information about the copy condition. For information regarding the recall condition, please refer to the chapter on memory instruments. The copy strategy may be related to accuracy of the memory. Chiuli, Haaland, LaRue, and Garry (1995) reported that, unlike the recall scores, the copy strategy did not change with age in a sample of elderly.

A fair amount of information is available regarding the interrater and internal consistency reliability of the test but not of the temporal reliability. One study indicated that the Rey–Osterrieth had reasonable temporal reliability in a sample of elderly subjects (Berry, Allen, & Schmitt, 1991). Tuppler, Welsch, Asare-Aboagye, and Dawson (1995) found that the original scoring system suggested by Osterrieth had excellent interrater reliability even though reliability for individual items was quite variable. In an interesting design, Liberman, Stewart, Seines, and Gordon (1994) had two raters score the figures on two different occasions separated by a period of 2 years to avoid contamination by memory. In this way they were able to evaluate both interrater reliability and "intrarater" reliability and found them to be good, with intrarater reliability being excellent. The Meyers and Meyers

(1995a,b) scoring system has a reported median interrater reliability of .94, and a temporal reliability coefficient of .76 for Immediate Recall, .88 for Delayed Recall, and .87 for Recognition in a small sample of 12 normal subjects tested twice across an average interval of 184 days.

Bennett-Levy (1984) administered the test to a sample of 107 normals and found that females performed significantly better than males, which appears to be true or younger ages. Females perform better than males between the ages of 7 and 12 years (Vlachos & Karapetsas, 1994), and in addition, the scores were significantly correlated with age. Waber and Holmes (1985) examined children's copy performance across age and suggested a scoring system that was sensitive to developmental trends and qualitative aspects of performance. The developmental trends were also seen in a sample of Columbian children (Ardila & Rosselli, 1994). As well as there being accuracy differences, there are qualitative differences. Up to the age of 9 years, children tend to break up the figure into smaller and simpler components (Askshoomoff & Stiles, 1995a,b). The sex differences may disappear in the elderly (Boone, Lesser, Hill-Gutierrez, E., Berman, & D'Elia, 1993). These data suggest the need for separate norms for sexes and age groups, which have not been provided yet.

An effort in that direction has been made by Waber and Holmes (1986), who administered the Rey–Osterrieth to a sample of 454 children between the ages of 5 and 14. All of the subjects were students in a normal classroom, and there was no effort to screen the subjects for learning disability. Instructions for immediate reproduction were given to 57% of the subjects, and the rest of the subjects were asked to reproduce the design after a 20-minute delay. Relatively detailed scoring criteria were given. The interrater reliability between two judges was found to be .94 in a random sample of protocols; the interrater agreement on the clinical rating of the same protocol was 84%. There was no attempt to validate the results against an outside criterion. Karapetsas and Vlachos (1997) reported that when they studied children between the ages of 5 years and 12 years old, the copy accuracy improved until the age of 10½ years for both boys and girls and for both right- and left-handed subjects. Using this scoring system, Waber and Bernstein (1995) subsequently found that although groups of normal children showed age (and inferentially, developmental) changes, children with learning disabilities tended to remain at the normative 8-year-old level until age 14 years, at which time some further developmental trends began.

Binder (1982) compared the performance of 14 normal, 14 right-hemisphere-damaged, and 14 left-hemisphere-damaged subjects. He reported that the right-hemisphere subjects demonstrated more distortions and that the left-hemisphere subjects were more likely than the normals to break the configural units into segments. King (1981) compared the performance of 71 normals, 22 left-hemisphere, 45 right-hemisphere, and 47 diffusely damaged subjects. He found that the left-hemisphere subjects were more likely to make simplification errors, and that the right-hemisphere subjects were more likely to make distortion errors, but that there was no difference between the two groups on the number of errors they made. All three of the brain-damaged groups made significantly more errors than the normals. There were no differences due to type of injury: trauma, cerebrovascular problems, or degenerative disorders. As evidence of the construct validity of the test, King (1981) reported that the test correlated .28 with the Visual Recall subtest of the Wechsler Memory Scale when the influences of age and sex were partialed out. Meyers and Meyers (1995b) reported convergent and discriminant validity coefficients in a sample of 100 subjects with documented neurological impairment. Intercorrelations with WAIS-R subtests, the Benton Visual Form Discrimination Test, Visual Retention Test, Sentence Repetition Test, Judgment of Line Orientation Test, Hooper Visual Organization Test, Trail Making Test, the Token Test, and Rey Auditory Verbal Learning Test followed expected and predicted patterns. Principal-components factor analyses in both the normative sample and the clinical sample resulted in a five-factor solution supporting the scores recommended for interpretation in the manual. The scores were able to discriminate among three groups of brain-injured patients, normal controls, and psychiatric patients ($n = 30$ in each group).

Taylor (1969) investigated the construct validity of the Rey–Osterrieth by administering it and a similar abstract-form-copying task to a series of patients who had undergone temporal lobectomies. Thee were 50 subjects altogether; 23 had received left temporal lobectomies, and 27 had received right temporal lobectomies. At the presurgery assessment, the two groups exhibited similar test scores. At 2 weeks postsurgery, the left-hemisphere subjects' copying scores had improved somewhat, and the right-hemisphere subjects' copying scores had declined. The delayed-recall score of the left-hemisphere subjects had improved, and that of the right-hemisphere subjects had remained about the same. These data may be interpreted as evidence of the role of an intact right temporal lobe in the successful completion of the Rey–Osterrieth Complex Figure Test, although replication and further evidence are needed.

Silverstein, Osborn, and Palumbo (1998) found that although chronic schizophrenics tended to use more abnormal copy strategies than acute schizophrenics or patients with other forms of psychosis, there were no differences in copy scores. The chronic schizophrenic patients furthermore had poorer recall, but there was no relationship between copy strategy and recall score. There appears to be a relationship between the organizational strategy scoring system of Hamby, Wilkins, and Barry (1993) and self-reported impulsivity in incarcerated offenders (Cornell, Roberts, & Oram, 1997). Rapport, Dutra, Webster, Charter, and Morrill (1995) presented a scoring system that takes into account the hemifield of errors and found that these scores were associated with inpatients falls among patients with cerebrovascular accidents (CVAs). The complexity of the Rey–Osterrieth makes it more sensitive to subtle hemispatial impairment.

In an investigation of two scoring systems for the copy and immediate recall conditions of the Rey–Osterrieth, the Lezak (1995), and the Denman (1984) systems, Rapport, Charter, Dutrea, Farchione, and Kingsley (1997) found that the two systems were equivalent in terms of excellent interrater reliability and internal consistency. The Denman system had a greater normative base but the Lezak system required less time to apply. As mentioned earlier, there are different scoring systems for qualitative aspects of the copy condition. Troyer and Wishart (1997) compared 10 of these systems and found the systems of Bennett-Levy (1984) and Bylsma Bobholz, Schretlen, and Correa (1995) to have the most favorable characteristics in terms of range of possible scores, number of qualitative criteria considered, and attention to the structural framework of the stimulus. The Boston Qualitative Scoring System (Stern et al., 1994) may be helpful in identifying organizational deficits in children with ADHD (Cahn et al., 1996).

THE ISHIHARA COLOR BLIND TEST

The Ishihara Color Blind Test can be used to determine the presence of color blindness in subjects. The determination of color blindness is an important issue when other test stimuli may be colored. Particularly for males, in whom color blindness can be genetic rather than acquired, the integrity of color vision may need to be documented before the possibility of a deficit in color-naming skills can be evaluated.

The Ishihara Color Blindness Test (Ishihara, 1970) contains 14 color plates composed of different-sized dots. The dots are of different hues. Same-colored dots are arranged in recognizable designs, such as numbers, or in trails. In the first case, the subject is asked to name the number outlined by the same-colored dots. In the second case, the subject is asked to trace the trails formed by the same-colored dots.

Internal consistency reliability was computed by use of the Kuder–Richardson Formula 20 in a sample of 90 mentally retarded boys aged 8 to 16. The reliability coefficient for the Numbers plates was .901; for the Trails plates, the coefficient was .927; and for the overall test, the coefficient was .914.

De Renzi and Spinnler (1967) reported that, in a sample of 100 control subjects, 100 left-hemisphere-injured patients, and 73 right-hemisphere-injured patients, the right-hemisphere-injured patients were more likely to produce impaired performances on the Ishihara. It was found that left-hemisphere-injured patients performed at a level commensurate with that of the control subjects. Performance on the Ishihara is apparently insensitive to the effects of intelligence. Salvia and Ysseldyke (1972) found that, in a sample of 90 boys aged 8 to 16 with IQ scores between 40 and 75, there was little indication of impaired performance. These results were consistent with earlier reports by Wilson and Wolfensberger (1963) and Salvia (1969).

More information is needed regarding the other forms of reliability of this test, as well as regarding the validity of using the Ishihara in diagnosing right-hemisphere damage. The Ishihara may have utility in the diagnosis of color agnosia or color aphasia. However, empirical data are needed on these points.

MEANINGFUL PICTURES

The meaningful pictures procedure has not been extensively used in research settings. However, it is an interesting procedure that uses an original methodology. The one report of the use of meaningful pictures in the literature was given by Battersby, Bender, Pollack, and Kahn (1956). This report describes the procedure as using five pictures chosen from color magazine illustrations. These pictures were chosen for their quality of being symmetrical about the median plane. The pictures are presented to the subject one at a time for 10 seconds each. Following the presentation of each picture, the subject is asked to describe the details and to note their relative position in the picture. The pictures are then given to the subject again, and she or he is asked to describe the details while holding the pictures. The "omission, faulty recall (or description) of numerous details on one side only was taken as an index of asymmetric spatial perception" (Battersby et al., 1956, p. 74). The authors studied the performance on this task of 42 spinal cord patients, 85 patients with space-occupying lesions, and 37 patients with nonlocalizable lesions. The results indicated that poor performance on this task was not related to the location of the lesion, but that it was related to sensory impairment superimposed on a condition of cognitive impairment. No information is available regarding the reliability of this procedure or the general aspects of the validity of this procedure. The procedure would also benefit from a statement of more explicit rules for scoring the results.

STICK CONSTRUCTION

A stick construction test has been reported in a few studies. The test usually involves having the subject copy a drawing of a figurative or nonfigurative organization of sticks, although the test may also involve constructing letters or figures with sticks by command rather than from a model. There have been no reports of investigation of the reliability of this test. Although right-hemisphere-lesioned subjects are more likely to exhibit impaired performance on this test than are left-hemisphere subjects (Hecaen & Assal, 1970), subjects with lateralized lesions will show impairment regardless of whether they are right- or left-hemisphere-lesioned (Benton, 1967). More research is needed before this test can be recommended for clinical use.

THE MINNESOTA PAPER FORM BOARD

The Minnesota Paper Form Board Test is purported to be a test of perceptual organization. It is a paper-and-pencil test that requires the subject to select the correct alternative depicting a figure made from a combination of the parts shown in the stimulus. For example, the stimulus may show two separate triangles, and the alternatives may be a circle, a square joined to a triangle, and two triangles connected to form a diamond. The Likert and Quasha manual (1948) provides normative data separately by sex and by occupation. No information is available regarding the reliability of this test. The construct validity of the Minnesota Paper Form Board is also in question (Lezak, 1983). Dee (1970) concluded that it was actually a measure of perceptual ability associated with constructional ability. However, Dee did not use the original form of this test but rather a shorter version and increased the size of the stimuli and the allowable time limits. Gazzaniga and LeDoux (1978) demonstrated that the performance of a single patient may vary with the method of administration. Because of the variability in administration in published reports of this test, it is difficult to draw any definite conclusions regarding its reliability or validity.

FIGURE–GROUND TESTS

Neurological impairment has often been associated with a disruption in the ability to discriminate figure–ground relationships. Gottschaldt's Hidden Figures Test has been used in some neuropsychological settings. There have been no investigations of the reliability of this instrument, but there has been some research that points to its sensitivity to brain abnormalities. Impaired performance on the Hidden Figures Test has been associated with penetrating head wounds (Tueber, Battersby, & Bender, 1960; Weinstein, 1964). Russo and Vignolo (1967) reported that left-hemisphere patients without aphasia scored in the unimpaired range; however, Corkin (1979) reported that impairment results regardless of the laterality of the lesion. Poor performance on this test is also associated with Korsakoff's disease (Talland, 1965) and uremic disease (Beniak, 1977). Apparently, there are many types of brain injury that will cause impaired performance. As well as reliability investigations, validation studies are needed to specify the functional systems involved. The exact construct implicated in the successful performance of the test also needs to be specified.

The Embedded Figures Test was designed as a measure of field dependence–

independence. As such, it was originally conceptualized as a measure of cognitive style rather than of ability. However, more recent work (Widiger, Knudson, & Rorer, 1980) has indicated that, in fact, the Embedded Figures Test correlates more highly with tests of ability than with tests of cognitive style. This finding suggests its potential utility in the assessment of neurologically impaired individuals. Research with undergraduate students majoring in business (DeSantis & Dunikoski, 1983) indicated that the reliability, the score distributions, and the sex differences are relatively robust in samples different from undergraduate liberal arts students, on which the test was normed. However, research evaluating the characteristics of the test in neuropsychological populations, as well as the validity of the instrument in the same population, still needs to be conducted.

HOOPER VISUAL ORGANIZATION TEST

The Hooper Visual Organization Test has been used widely in psychiatric settings. The reliability and the validity of the test were not well evaluated in the studies reported in the manual (Hooper, 1958), although later research has been more encouraging. Of the two studies reported in the manual, one demonstrated acceptable accuracy in identifying normal subjects and reasonable (79%) accuracy in identifying organically impaired subjects. In the second study, the classification of the subjects into criterion groups was partly accomplished by reference to scores on the Hooper, hopelessly confounding the significant differences that were then found. There were no reports of reliability evaluation in the manual. Wetzel and Murphy (1991) developed a discontinue rule to shorten the administration time (five consecutive errors) with a change in impairment classification rate of 1%. Regardless of whether the original length or the shortened length was used, specificity was greater than sensitivity.

Lezak (1982) evaluated the test–retest reliability of the Hooper in a sample of 23 normal male subjects. The test was given on three occasions with approximate intervals of 6 months and 1 year. The report of this study is somewhat confusing, as not all subjects were given the test on each occasion, and information is not provided about which subjects took the test on which occasion. The report is further confused by the fact that, although the text refers to significant differences in level in the Hooper scores, the accompanying table presents values that are not significant. Be that as it may, the pairwise correlation coefficients ranged from .92 for the first and second occasions to .77 for the second and third occasions. Moreover, there was a significant difference in one of the comparisons of mean levels. This study represents the only attempt to investigate the reliability of the instrument.

Sterne (1973) evaluated the diagnostic validity of the Hooper in a sample of 75 VA inpatients, 25 of whom had been diagnosed as organically impaired, 25 as psychiatric, and 25 as indeterminate. As well as the Hooper, the WAIS, the Benton Visual Retention Test, the Porteus Mazes, and Trails A and B were administered. All of these variables were entered as predictors in a multiple-regression equation, with diagnosis as the criterion. Unfortunately, the diagnosis was determined by the results of the psychological testing and the result was a confound. Even when the results of the Hooper were used to diagnose subjects, the Hooper was unable to provide significant prediction beyond that afforded by the other variables, a finding that initially called into serious question the validity of this instrument.

In general, the results of early validation attempts were not encouraging. Pershad and Verma (1980) found that, although scores on the Hooper were sensitive to neurological impairment in an Indian sample, the use of the cutoff points suggested in the manual resulted in both false positives and false negatives. Love (1970) reported similar results in a sample of 115 New Zealand psychiatric patients. Tamkin and Kunce (1985) had reported greater than chance identification of neurological impairment in a sample of inpatients in a Veterans psychiatric hospital; however, the criterion used was the opinion of the ward physician regarding neurological impairment.

Wang (1977) evaluated the diagnostic accuracy of the Hooper in classifying neuro-surgery patients as neurologically impaired. The sample included 49 neurologically impaired subjects (15 left-hemisphere, 19 right-hemisphere, and 15 bilateral) and 17 nonneuro-logically impaired subjects (largely with peripheral nervous system disorders). Using the cutoff points suggested in the manual eventuated in a 43% misclassification. Raising the cutoff to over double that in the manual still resulted in a 17% false-negative rate, although it did not result in any false positives. There were no differences among the right, left, or bilaterally impaired subjects.

Jackson and Culbertson (1977) evaluated the use of the Hooper in classifying children as organically impaired. This study used 20 normal children and 20 neurologically impaired children, as determined by their status in classes for the learning impaired. There were no reports of how these children had been placed in the classes. There was overlap in the distributions of the scores in the two groups, and the cutoff points suggested in the manual resulted in many incorrect classifications. The authors then readjusted the cutoffs to maximize correct classifications. The readjustment resulted in no false positives, but it still produced a large number of false negatives. This is a problem with many screening devices. Because screening devices can usually assess the integrity of a single system, they may not be sensitive to focal impairment in other systems. Seidel (1994) presented normative information on the Hooper for children aged 5 to 21 years. In addition, he reported that age correlated with the Hooper and furthermore the Hooper was sensitive to visual–spatial impairment in pediatric patients. Kirk's (1992b) normative sample of 434 children indicated that adult level scores could be attained by boys about age 12, although girls needed to be of greater age to reach adult scores. Hilgert and Treolar (1985) had found differences due to age but not to sex in children, but this was a much more limited sample than the Kirk (1992b) study. Hilgert and Treolar (1985) also reported correlations with the Performance IQ, suggesting the role of perceptual skills in the Hooper.

Boyd (1981) described an attempt at validation using 40 neurologically impaired subjects and 40 nonimpaired psychiatric subjects. The cutoff points in the manual produced 97.5% correct classifications of the control subjects but only 15% correct classifications of the neurologically impaired subjects. Using cutoffs that maximized correct classification resulted in 67.5% accuracy of classification in the neurologically impaired subjects and 80.0% accuracy in the control subjects, for an overall rate of 73.8% accuracy. There were no significant differences due to site of lesion or acuteness of injury. Boyd also correlated the Hooper scores with Peabody Picture Vocabulary Test (PPVT), IQ scores, age, and education. He found only moderate correlations with these variables.

Boyd (1981) was subsequently criticized by Rathbun and Smith (1982) for using the PPVT and for using a system-specific test such as the Hooper as a screen. They then cited two unpublished studies that they said supported their points. Rathbun and Smith (1982) recommended using Smith's own test, the Symbol Digit Modalities Test, as a screen. Boyd (1982a) replied that the studies cited by Rathbun and Smith actually used the Benton Visual Retention Test (BVRT) and Raven's Progressive Matrices and did not even use the Hooper. Obviously, what is needed is a study that compares the utility of the BVRT with the Hooper when used as screening devices.

Woodward (1982) also criticized Boyd (1981) on the grounds that there were no work-ups of the controls to rule out impairment and that the even ratio of impaired and nonimpaired subjects was artificial and may have inflated the accuracy rates. Boyd (1982b) replied that his study had been meant to demonstrate the sensitivity of the Hooper to neurological impairment, not to evaluate its use in uncovering the incidence of neurological impairment in the general population. These responses are fine, but they do not address the fact that the use of the Hooper in the original study resulted in a misclassification of many of the subjects.

Further research regarding the Hooper has resulted in more positive findings, although only when modifications are made in the cutoffs or when additional information is considered. For example, Lewis et al. (1997) found that when a sample of 153 African-American patients with acute cerebral lesions was compared with control subjects, the patients scored significantly lower than the comparison group. However, contrary to the original theory behind the Hooper, namely that poor performance reflects right parietal impairment, the patients with right anterior lesions scored lower than the other patient localization groups. On the other hand, Fitz, Conrad, Hom, Sarff, and Majowski (1992) reported lower scores in the patients with right parietal lesions. Nadler, Grace, White, Butters, and Malloy (1996) reported that the Hooper scores of right hemisphere CVA patients were lower than the scores of left hemisphere CVA patients, even though the left hemisphere CVA patients also produced impaired scores. But the data have not been consistent. Wetzel and Murphy (1991) had earlier reported that although the Hooper correctly identified brain impairment, there were no differences between left- and right-hemisphere-lesioned subjects.

In an examination of the possible cultural and educational influences on the Hooper, Verma, Pershad, and Khanna (1993) compared patient and control Eastern Indian subjects in three different educational levels and found no significant relationships to Hooper performance.

Walsh, Lichtenberg, and Rowe (1997) found that the Hooper could discriminate among severely cognitively impaired, moderately impaired, and intact subjects in a sample of geriatric rehabilitation inpatients. When the Hooper was used in geriatric African-American patients, a modified cutoff of 15 points resulted in 81% sensitivity and 79% specificity (Nabors, Vangel, Lichtenberg, & Walsh, 1997). Following a principal-components factor analysis using conceptually similar and dissimilar neuropsychological assessment instruments, Johnstone and Wilhelm (1997) concluded that the Hooper is best interpreted as a measure of global visual–spatial intelligence. The Hooper does not appear to be influenced by object naming skills and may be considered a measure of perceptual organization (Paolo, Cluff, & Ryan, 1996; Ricker & Axelrod, 1995). This is consistent with Seidel (1994), who found that children's performance on the Hooper is correlated with visual–spatial skills but not with verbal skills. Tamkin and Hyer (1984) had found differences in Hooper scores associated with age in a psychiatric population and subsequently norms based on age organized by decade.

The Hooper has shown remarkable resiliency in the neuropsychological literature. It appears to be a viable screening instrument, especially for visual-spatially based impairment. Its relationship to laterality of lesion is still somewhat uncertain, and its specificity appears to be greater than its sensitivity; however, it is useful in assessment of the elderly and the existence of age-related norms has enhanced its utility in the assessment of children.

SATZ BLOCK ROTATION TEST

The Block Rotation Test (BRT) was developed by Paul Satz as his dissertation project. After graduation, Satz continued to provide validation information regarding the BRT (Satz, 1966). Although the actual number of publications evaluating the BRT is minimal, the quality of these publications is generally good. The BRT was developed to be sensitive to neurological impairment in general. However, this was done in the context of knowing the difficulty of determining the existence of neurological impairment when neurological impairment is not viewed as a unitary construct.

The BRT is an interactive test that takes about an hour to administer to normal subjects. Its administration to impaired subjects takes somewhat longer, depending on the nature and the severity of the impairment. The stimulus items consist of red and white colored blocks similar to those used in the Block Design subtest of the WAIS. The object of the test is for the subject to reproduce the designs formed by the examiner, but rotated 90 degrees, either to the left or to the right. This is accomplished by moving the blocks one at a time. The test is divided into two parts. In the first part, the stimuli are presented aligned with the horizontal and vertical axes. In the second part, the stimuli are presented at an angle to the axes. There are 15 designs in Part A and 7 designs in Part B. For both parts, there is an initial practice period in which the subject's understanding of the task requirements is assessed.

Six scores are obtained from the use of this instrument. Duplication errors consist of designs that merely replicate the design without the required 90-degree rotation. Angulation errors are those subject designs that, although rotated to some degree, deviate from the required rotation. Time errors are the result of a failure to complete the task within the 65-second time limit. Part A errors are the sum of the errors in Part A. Part B errors are the sum of the errors in Part B. Total errors are the total sum of errors over the entire test.

Reliability

Test–retest reliability was assessed in a sample of 18 subjects who were involved in the standardization of the instrument. The reported test–retest interval was "about four weeks." Pearson product–moment correlation coefficients between the scores obtained on the two test occasions ranged from .91 for total errors to .67 for time errors. No information has been reported regarding the assessment of change of level of scores with the use of analysis of variance. Therefore, no conclusions can be drawn regarding the existence of practice effects.

Lawriw and Sutker (1978) reported internal-consistency reliability values using data from 57 (40 male and 17 female) consecutive referrals to a neuropsychological assessment service. They reported an alpha coefficient of .94. These authors also performed various split-half analyses and reported Spearman–Brown corrected split-half reliabilities ranging from .94 for right- versus left-turning items on Part A to .77 for right- versus left-turning items on Part B.

Validity

The original standardized sample for the BRT consisted of 122 adult male subjects from VA hospitals. These subjects were divided into four groups: normals (psychiatric nursing assistants), neurotic patients, schizophrenic patients, and neurological patients (Satz, 1966). The diagnoses were obtained from case records and were performed by the respective attending physicians. A linear discriminant-function analysis was obtained from the six test scores, the performance IQ as measured by the WAIS, and the age of the subjects as predictors. The criterion was the dichotomous division of organic or not organic. All of the variables were forced into the discriminant function regardless of the amount of discrimination provided. This fact may account for some of the later shrinkage observed in the cross-validation. The standardized beta weights are not reported, so we cannot judge the relative amounts of independent variance accounted for by the individual predictors.

The cutoff points for the values obtained from the discriminant function were determined by computing the mean of the group average discriminant function scores. This is a reasonable strategy when the distributions are normal. However, to the extent that the distributions may have been skewed toward each other, this procedure may have resulted in a less than optimum cutoff point. For example, if the nonorganic group's distribution was skewed to the right, the proposed cutoff point may not have minimized the number of false positives, as seems to have been the case in the derivation and cross-validation studies. Nevertheless, the resultant procedure resulted in an 89% correct classification rate overall. When the results were analyzed for the effects of type and location of lesion, it was concluded that the test was sensitive to nonspecific effects of neurological impairment.

An important point needs to be raised here. This original study used only male subjects. This is unfortunate, as the construct most probably measured by the BRT (visual–spatial skills) has been found to be significantly and robustly different in the two sexes (Tapley & Bryden, 1977). Therefore, any generalization of these results to female subjects is a problem.

The first cross-validation study, also reported in Satz (1966), used 100 consecutive referrals to a neuropsychological assessment service. The sex of these subjects and of the subjects in the subsequent cross-validation studies is not specified. As noted previously, sex is an important variable, and this represents an unfortunate omission of information. There were 48 neurological patients, as diagnosed by history, neurological examination, EEG, brain scan (not defined, but probably not CT scan because of the date of the publication), skull films, and, in some cases, arteriogram, angiogram, or pneumoencephalogram. The comparison groups consisted of 52 psychiatric, normal, or medical patient subjects, as determined by negative history, neurological exam, and sometimes a negative EEG, a skull film, an angiogram, or a pneumoencephalogram. When the discriminant function derived in the first study was used, there was 75% correct classification overall; 71% of the nonorganic subjects were correctly classified, and 79% of the organically impaired individuals were correctly classified. The cross-validation subjects were then combined with the original sample, and a new discriminant function was derived by the same methodology. The result was an 82% correct-classification rate overall: 88% correct for the nonorganic subjects and 76% correct for the organic subjects.

This discriminant function was then cross-validated on the next 151 consecutive referrals to the neuropsychology service (61 organic and 90 nonorganic subjects). The result was a 79% correct-classification rate overall: 83% correct for the nonorganic and 72% correct for the organic subjects. These subjects were then combined with the concatenated sample, and the same methodology was used. This last sample was composed of 157 organically impaired subjects and 210 nonorganically impaired subjects. This final procedure resulted in an 81% overall correct classification rate: 90% correct for the nonorganic subjects and 70% for the organic subjects. There was no cross-validation.

Classification by subgroup was also examined, with the result that adequate classification rates were obtained for the psychiatric patients, the medical patients, the CVA patients, and the arteriosclerotic subjects, but only 50% correct classification of the epilepsy patients. The BRT may be ineffective in identifying impairment in subjects with seizure disorder. Furthermore, using Bayesian methodology, Satz (1966) demonstrated that when the base rate of organic impairment is low (e.g., mental health settings), the accuracy of the BRT may be only 44%, but in inpatient medical setting where the base rate of organic impairment is high, the accuracy may be 91%.

Satz, Fennell, and Reilly (1970) examined the relationship of the BRT and neurological test procedures such as EEG, brain scan, skull X-ray film, arteriogram, and pneumoencephalogram to the diagnosis of organic disease. Even though there was a confound of method of diagnoses with diagnosis, the Goodman–Kruskal test of strength of association indicated that only the EEG and the BRT had strong and significant predictive relationships with the criterion of diagnosis.

Other types of validity have not been well investigated. Lawriw and Sutker (1978) performed a factor analysis, but the relationship to construct validity was not examined. No quantitative methods of comparison of factor solutions were used, but examination of the obtained factor structure in comparison to the original solution (Satz, 1966) indicated that only the spatial factor was replicated. The instability of the two-factor solutions may be due to the small sizes used in the two studies.

There are several areas where more information is needed on the BRT. The reliability of the test needs to be more fully evaluated. The scoring is based on examiner judgment. Therefore the most important type of reliability information missing is interscorer reliability. In addition, a test–retest sample of 18 subjects is not adequate. The issue of the sex of the subjects in the last three cross-validation samples may obviate the issue of the sex differences in spatial abilities if it turns out that females were included. Lastly, the final derived discriminant function needs to be cross-validated.

THE MINNESOTA PERCEPTO-DIAGNOSTIC TEST

The Minnesota Percepto-Diagnostic Test (MPDT) was first described by Fuller and Laird (1963) in a monograph. The revised version was described in a subsequent monograph (Fuller, 1969). Thirteen years later, the manual was published (Fuller, 1982). Much of the information provided in the manual is available in the monograph's descriptions of identical studies, including exactly the same subject characteristics.

The MPDT consists of six Gestalt designs that are to be copied by the subject. These designs are scored on the basis of the three dimensions of rotation, separation of the components of the design, and distortion of the designs. The rotation score is obtained by use of a protractor, 25 degrees being the maximum score. The other scores are qualitative and are scored for presence or absence.

Fuller (1969) denoted four uses of the MPDT: to classify the etiology of reading and learning disorders in children; to classify behavior-problem children as having normal, emotionally disturbed, or schizophrenic perception; to assess the maturational level of normal and retarded children; and to classify adults as normal, brain-damaged, or emotionally disturbed.

The normative data on the MPDT were obtained from 4000 students between the ages of 5 and 20 years. The author of the test attempted to correct for age and IQ in the test. This correction was accomplished with a methodology first used by Fuller, Sharp, and Hawkins (1967). Each of the age groups was examined for differences in test score due to age, separately for children with IQ scores over 88 and under 87. There were no significant differences for ages over 14 in the IQ-over-88 group, so these groups were collapsed together. For the same reason, the children with IQ scores under 87 were collapsed into groups of 5 to 9 years, 10 to 15 years, and 16 years and older. Then IQ was correlated with the test scores separately for each of the collapsed age groups. The solved regression formulas were used to predict the median test score for each group in the normative sample. The difference between the predicted and the obtained median test scores was then used as the correction factor. Although this seems to be a reasonable methodology, it must be pointed out that the extent to which the suggested procedure actually corrects for the influence of age and IQ has not been empirically demonstrated.

Reliability

The MPDT has a suggested alternate form, which actually consists of the same items given in a different order. The relationship between these two forms was examined in a sample of 1128 normal schoolchildren, who received both forms in counterbalanced order. The same mean rotation scores were obtained for both forms, but the standard deviations were different for the 9- and 10-year-old children. Therefore, the raw scores obtained by use of the alternate form should not be interpreted in these age groups. The alternate-form reliability coefficients for the rotation scores ranged from .34 for the 8-year-old children to .88 for the 14-year-old children. When corrected for the restricted range of the score values, the coefficients ranged from .74 for the 7-year-olds to .98 for the children older than 14.

Test–retest reliability over a 1-year interval was evaluated for 165 children. The coefficients ranged from .37 for the 7-year-old children to .60 for the 11-year-old children. When 177 children aged 9 to 12 were tested with a 3-month interval, the coefficients ranged from .53 to .70. The MPDT has differential temporal stability across age groups. The interpretation of gains or losses obtained on retest occasions should therefore be tempered by consideration of the age-appropriate reliability coefficients.

Split-half reliability was evaluated by comparing the rotation scores for the circle–diamond stimuli with the scores for the dot stimuli. No information was given about the subjects in this study reported in the manual (Fuller, 1982). The coefficients ranged from .40 to .73. Split-half reliability was also examined by comparing the rotation scores of the first half of the items with the second half. It was reported that the coefficients ranged from .52 to .86. All of these studies used children as subjects. There are no published reports of the reliability of the MPDT in adult subjects.

Vance, Lester, and Thatcher (1983) examined the interscorer reliability of the MPDT when one of the scorers had expert status (the author of the test) and one scorer had novice status (a testing technician with 2 hours of instruction). The subject sample used was a group of 30 children (18 males and 12 females) who had been referred for evaluation. The authors found no significant differences between the two scorers on the Separation of Circle–Diamond and Distortion of Dot scores, but they did find significant differences on the Rotation scores and the Distortion of Circle–Diamond scores. These results indicate the sensitivity of the test results to the level of training of the scorer.

In all of the above reliability studies, the values of the coefficients were moderate at best. This fact has implications for the clinical utility of the MPDT. Without reliable scores, diagnosis conducted with the MPDT is likely to be of uncertain accuracy. Fuller (1969) argued that a more appropriate test of reliability would be to assess the stability of diagnostic decisions based on data from the MPDT. However, to date, no study has examined this facet of the instrument.

Validity

In the original description of the development of the MPDT (Fuller, 1969), the diagnostic validity of the test was evaluated on a sample of 5552 children divided among the categories of normal, emotionally disturbed, schizophrenic, reading disabled, brain-damaged, and good readers. The reading disabled children were identified by scores 2 or more years below their expected scores on either the Gates–MacGinitie Reading Tests or Gray's Oral Reading Test. Similarly, good readers were identified by scores on the same reading tests that were 1 or more years ahead of expected scores. Membership in the other groups was determined by decisions made by various professionals using unspecified criteria. By examining the distribution of scores, optimal cutoff points were determined that correctly classified 84% of the normal, 80% of the emotionally disturbed, and 81% of the brain-damaged children. These rates are likely to shrink in any attempt to apply the cutoff points to subjects who were not in the derivation sample. There is no report of an examination of the diagnostic accuracy of these cutoff points in a cross-validation sample.

An evaluation of the validity of an instrument includes an assessment of the extent to which it provides data that covary with conceptually similar information and the extent to which they do not covary with conceptually dissimilar information. Helmes, Holden, and Howe (1980) reported that the MPDT does not correlate with the Smith Symbol Digits Modality Test, a test that is also supposed to tap aspects of cortical integrity. Snow, Hynd, Hartlage, and Grant (1983) reported that the MPDT does not correlate well with any of the clinical scales of the Luria–Nebraska Neuropsychological Battery-Children's Revision (LNNB-C). These authors argued that this result was due to the MPDT's being sensitive to aspects of cortical functioning that are not tapped by the LNNB-C. However, this is unlikely for two reasons. First, the LNNB-C taps an extremely wide range of cortical functioning. Second, as mentioned previously, the MPDT has not been reported to correlate with other tests of cortical integrity.

Scores on the MPDT may be sensitive to other variables. For example, Fuller and

Friedrich (1979) reported that, in a sample of 60 black and 60 Caucasian children, with IQ as a covariate, scores on the MPDT were sensitive to both academic achievement and race. Lin and Rennick (1973) found that relationships between the rotation score of the MPDT and IQ were different by sex in a sample of 117 epileptic men and 60 epileptic women.

Many of the uses of the MPDT proposed in the manual are related to the detection of perceptual problems that would adversely affect academic achievement. A direct assessment of the validity of the instrument would involve an evaluation of the relationship of scores obtained from the instrument to other measures of perception. There are no published reports of such a study. A less direct assessment of the validity of the instrument would involve an evaluation of the relation between the MPDT and some measure of academic achievement. Fuller and Wallbrown (1983) reported that, in a sample of 69 first-grade children, the scores of the MPDT were related to academic achievement as measured by the California Achievement Test. However, the largest correlation coefficient had a value of $-.59$, explaining only 35% of the variance. Wallbrown, Wallbrown, and Engin (1977) examined the relationship of the MPDT to California Achievement Test scores in a sample of 153 third-grade students and found the highest correlation to be only $-.56$. Putman (1981) examined the relationship of the MPDT to reading achievement scores obtained from the Woodcock Reading Mastery Test. She used a sample of 102 remedial readers, and when the influence of mental age was partialed out, there was a correlation of $-.25$, which was not statistically significant. The modest correlations reported in these studies indicate the limited utility of the MPDT in this area.

A second proposed use of the MPDT involves the discrimination of brian-damaged and non-brain-damaged children. Fuller and Hawkins (1969) reported a hit rate of 85% in discriminating brain-damaged from non-brain-damaged adolescents. Fuller and Friedrich (1976) reported that Hillow (1971), in her unpublished master's thesis, had only a 45% hit rate using their actuarial system, but a 68% hit rate using a discriminant function analysis. Fuller and Friedrich (1976) reported a 63% hit rate using Hillow's discriminant function in a sample of 241 adolescents and a 79% hit rate using Fuller and Hawkin's actuarial formula (1969). Considering there were only two groups and almost a 50% chance of correct classification, none of these hit rates are very impressive.

Several studies have examined the ability of the MPDT to discriminate between brain-damaged, non-brain-damaged, and psychiatric adult subjects. Helmes et al. (1980) reported that the MPDT was not sensitive to the presence or absence of brain damage in 82 psychiatric subjects. Holland and Wadsworth (1974) found that the MPDT was unable to discriminate between 20 brain-damaged and 20 schizophrenic subjects when the influence of IQ was partialed out. Crookes and Coleman (1973) reported that, although rotation scores alone could not discriminate brain damage from psychiatric diagnoses, there was a significant difference between the overall scores (including qualitative scores) of brain-damaged and psychiatric subjects. George (1973) found that the MPDT was sensitive to all psychiatric disturbances, and that, the more severe the disturbance, the more similar to brain damage scores were the scores. Holland, Wadsworth, and Royer (1975b) reported that the MPDT could not discriminate between 20 brain-damaged and 20 schizophrenic subjects who were matched for age, educational level, and IQ. Crookes (1983) found that, overall, there was no significant difference between psychiatric and brain-damaged subjects on the MPDT, unless the subjects were matched for age.

This last point raises an important consideration. Although the manual (Fuller, 1982) recommends the use of the MPDT to discriminate adult brain-damaged subjects from psychiatric subjects, the scoring system is based on a normative sample whose oldest subject was 22 years old. The manual made a careful effort to partial out the effect of IQ and age in the scoring system, but only in subjects younger than 22. The inconclusiveness of the studies reviewed above may be partly the result of using an age-inappropriate scoring system.

Watson, Gasser, Schaefer, Buranen, and Wold (1981) attempted to improve the discriminative power of the MPDT by adding a background interference to the procedure. They used age-matched groups of married schizophrenics, unmarried schizophrenics, affective psychotics, alcoholics, subjects with neurotic personality disorders, and organically impaired individuals. There were 30 subjects in each group. Unfortunately, the basis for deciding whether or not a subject would be included in each group was not reported. The authors reported significant differences in the qualitative scores, but not in the rotation scores.

Fuller and Friedrich (1976) examined 112 subjects, 28 in each group of normal, personality disorder, psychotic, and organically impaired subjects. When age was covaried, the test scores were significantly affected by the group membership variable. However, because the authors did not report the group distributions, it is difficult to tell whether the MPDT would be useful for diagnostic purposes in the individual case.

Another reason for the inconclusive results of the validity studies may lie in the conceptual basis of the test. Wallbrown and Fuller (1984) stated that MDPT abnormal scores may be obtained as the result of either emotional or organic factors. The MDPT is said to measure accurate perception, which is sensitive to a wide range of factors. Because the test requires the subject to draw, it is also a measure of fine-motor control and of the reproduction of spatial relationships. The utility of the instrument would be enhanced if the scoring method allowed a means of separating these factors. Wallbrown and Fuller (1984) provided a five-step method of interpreting the MDPT but failed to provide adequate empirical evidence regarding the accuracy of this procedure. In addition, the five-step method does allow one to decompose the test results into the skill areas that are described in the manual.

Reliability information is lacking for adult populations and for special populations of children, such as retarded or brain-damaged children. There is no published research that examines the ability of the instrument to classify children's perceptions as normal, emotionally disturbed, schizophrenic, or brain-damaged. Also needed is research that demonstrates the relation between the diagnoses made by the five-step method and diagnostic decisions made from independent information. Another line of research would investigate the treatment implications of diagnoses made with the instrument. Treatments for different diagnoses are themselves different. Therefore, research is needed investigating the effectiveness of treatments prescribed on the basis of the information provided by the instrument. Wallbrown and Fuller (1984) described three different types of reading disabilities that can be identified by the MDPT, but more research is needed to evaluate the validity of the instrument in performing these diagnoses.

Tests of Higher Cognitive Function

THE PORTEUS MAZE

The Porteus Maze Test is a series of increasingly difficult mazes, which the manual states are designed to examine the ability to use "planning capacity, prudence, and mental alertness in a new situation of a concrete nature" (Golden, 1978b). The manual also asserts that performance on the test is affected by "impulsiveness, suggestibility, irresolution, and excitability" (p. 1). The user is told to expect practice effects, but not to worry about their presence because practice is built into the test. The Porteus has held fascination for clinical neuropsychologists for a long time. It has often been used as a dependent measure in experimental and clinical investigation, but its diagnostic utility is largely unknown.

Because of its hypothesized relationship to planning skills and impulsivity, the Porteus has been suggested as a useful measure in the assessment of attention deficit hyperactivity disorder (ADHD). Porteus (1965) reviewed developmental studies, but these had largely been completed in the first half of the twentieth century. Krikorian and Bartok (1998) subsequently published developmental data on the Porteus in 340 normal subjects aged 7 to 21 years. Socioeconomic status had a significant but weak relationship with Porteus score (age-corrected semipartial $r = -.15$) and a significant but weak relationship to IQ estimated by PPVT-R (age-corrected semipartial $r = .17$). Male subjects performed better than female subjects, but at a clinically insubstantial level. The other beneficial outcome of this study was an estimate of internal consistency reliability (Cronbach's coefficient alpha = .81).

Because of its reliance on successful planning, inhibition of impulsive behavior, and ability to change set, the Porteus has been used to document the behavioral effects of psychosurgery of the frontal regions. Smith and Kinder (1959) examined schizophrenics before surgery and 8 years postsurgery. Their study group consisted of 28 operated schizophrenics and 24 nonoperated schizophrenics. The subjects were further divided into young and old individuals, and the operated subjects were divided into orbital-topectomy subjects and superior-topectomy subjects. Both the pre- and post-evaluations were actually pairs of evaluations 1 month apart in each case. The means of each of these two evaluations were taken as the pre- and post-measures. At the 8-year follow-up, the operated schizophrenics demonstrated significantly worse performance than did the nonoperated subjects. There were no significant differences due to age or locus of surgery.

Smith (1960) also examined the impact of psychosurgery on Porteus Maze performance. With the same subjects as were evaluated by Smith and Kinder (1959), and with the addition of 16 more operated schizophrenic subjects, the analysis was conducted using only one each of the pre- and postsurgery Porteus measurements. In addition, Porteus scores taken shortly after surgery were included in the analysis. In this analysis, there was a significant age-by-site interaction; the postsurgery scores of the younger orbital-site subjects actually increased slightly. However, in general, the scores decreased both following surgery and at the 8-year follow-up. Smith interpreted the results in terms of the effects on the frontal lobe; namely, a dysfunctional frontal lobe results in decrements in certain psychological functions over time, as the brain no longer has its "executive" to direct learning. These results were at odds with earlier studies, which had reported that postoperative losses in Porteus scores were recovered over time. Riddle and Roberts (1978) reviewed several of these studies and concluded that most of the postoperative recovery was due to practice effects, which had gone unnoticed because of the lack of a control group in the design. The study reported by Smith (1960) had such a control group, which is why he was able to document the permanence of the effects.

Meier and Story (1967) studied subjects who had received subthalamotomy as a treatment for Parkinsonism. Twelve subjects had received left thalamotomy and 17 subjects had received right thalamotomy. The subjects were administered the Porteus, Trails A and B, and the Wechsler–Bellevue Intelligence Scale 1 week before surgery and between 5 and 15 months after surgery. There were no changes in the Trails or Wechsler–Bellevue scores; however, there was a statistically significant average decrease of 3 years in mental age score on the Porteus in the right-subthalamotomy subjects and a nonsignificant decrease of 1 year in mental age score in the left-subthalamotomy subjects. The authors hypothesized that the decrements occurred because the surgeries had been done on areas in the fields of Forel, which have abundant innervation to the frontal lobes.

Gow and Ward (1982) administered the Porteus to 90 subjects across a range of IQ values. They divided their subjects into three groups of 30 subjects each: a group with IQ scores between 135 and 116, a group with IQ scores between 115 and 86, and a group with IQ scores of less than 85. They found significant differences among the groups, indicating that the Porteus is sensitive to intelligence. However, it is likely that the Porteus measures a more narrowly defined skill than is usually thought of as intelligence, as might be construed from the Meier and Story (1967) study, in which there were effects for the Porteus but not for the measure of general intelligence. Research to partial out the particular constructs of the Porteus is now needed. This is particularly important, as Riddle and Roberts (1977) indicate that scores on the Porteus are partly affected by degree of impulsivity and the presence of delinquency in younger subjects.

The practice effects need to be documented clearly by test–retest reliability studies. In addition, other forms of reliability, particularly interscorer reliability, need to be investigated. Finally, the construct validity of the Porteus needs to be investigated.

ELITHORN'S PERCEPTUAL MAZE

Elithorn's Perceptual Maze Test (PMT) was designed to study the effects of psychosurgery (specifically prefrontal leukotomy) on intellectual functioning (Elithorn, 1955). Because at the time the Porteus Maze was considered the most sensitive measure of frontal damage, a maze procedure was used. The PMT consists of 30 patterns that have dots superimposed on a lattice background. The subject is required to connect the dots in a way that maximizes the number of dots transversed by the line. However, the subject can draw the line only forward and is not allowed to back up to connect additional dots. In the original version, the paper on which the pattern was drawn was pulled through a mask via a motor that standardized the speed of movement of the piece of paper. However, the time constraints seemed to intimidate some subjects, so this procedure was discontinued in favor of a flat sheet of paper on which the pattern was printed. Performance was then timed.

Elithorn, Mornington, and Stavrou (1982) stated that the intent of the test is to adhere to the experimental rather than the psychometric tradition. The test is therefore criterion- rather than norm-referenced, and little has been done to investigate the statistical and psychometric properties of the test.

In the procedure used in the original report (Elithorn, 1955), 30 patterns were used. There was one best solution for each pattern. If the subject did not solve the maze in 60 seconds, the solution was shown, and the next pattern was presented. Testing was discontinued when the subject failed to solve four consecutive mazes within the 30-second time limit for each maze. The score consists of 1 point for each successful solution and 1 bonus point for each solution within the 30-second limit.

Three groups of subjects were used (Elithorn, 1955). The first group consisted of 20 individuals who had psychosurgical procedures and who were tested pre- and postsurgery. Of the 15 subjects given a prefrontal leukotomy, 12 improved their scores on the PMT an average of 10 points. Of the five subjects with temporal lobectomies, all decreased their score on the PMT an average of 8 points. In the second group of subjects in this report, 22 individuals were given a full leukotomy, and 13 were given a partial leukotomy. No presurgery data are available for these subjects. The subjects who received partial leukoto- mies scored 5 points higher on the average; however, this difference was not statistically significant. The 85 subjects in the third group consisted of neurological and psychiatric inpatients who did not have psychosurgery. These individuals were administered the PMT and the Vocabulary subtest and Block Design subtest of the WAIS. There was a correlation of .46 with the Vocabulary subtest and .74 with the Block Design. The author concluded that the PMT was sensitive to frontal dysfunction and that the PMT tapped spatial skills (Elithorn, 1955).

There is also a group form available for the PMT. The group form consists of two parts: Part A, which has 30 patterns, and Part B, which has 20 patterns. An alternate form of these two parts consists of inverted copies of the patterns. The group form is timed, and there is no feedback regarding performance as there is in the individually administered form. Subjects are allowed 10 minutes to finish each part. Elithorn, Kerr, and Mott (1960) reported the results of an investigation of these forms of the PMT Some of the subjects in this study were administered the original form twice, and some of the subjects were administered first the original form and then the alternate form. With a 14-day test–retest interval, the correlation for the same form was .89. For the alternate form with the same interval, the correlation was .81. The difference between the two correlation values is not statistically significant. No data are available regarding alternate-form reliability when the order of administration is counterbalanced, or when no time interval separates the adminis- tration of the two forms. No test–retest reliability is available for the individually adminis- tered form.

There is also a computerized version of the PMT that can be individually administered. Elithorn, Mornington, and Stavrou (1982) stated that many more potential scores are available with the computerized form, such as reaction time and a record of the solution strategy. However, the characteristics of these scores have not been investigated.

There has been research investigating the validity of the PMT as a measure of spatial visual–perceptual skills and of planning. Lee (1967) reported that performance on the PMT was relatively independent of previously acquired skills and was sensitive to brain damage. Weinman and Cooper (1981) administered the PMT to a group of 817 first-year secondary school children in the United Kingdom, with an average age of 11.4 years. The authors found that the response characteristics were related to the overall level of perceptual-problem-solving skills.

Jahoda (1969) administered the PMT to 280 male students at the University of Ghana and found that the scores were normally distributed. Sixty-six of these subjects were also administered the Block Design subtest of the WAIS, the Embedded Figures Test, and a test of algebraic ability. There was a correlation of .52 with the Block Design Test, .46 with the Embedded Figures Test, and .40 with algebraic ability. The students who came from a literate family scored significantly better than the students from an illiterate family. These results indicate that the PMT is sensitive to more than just visual–perceptual skills, consistent with the conclusion of Elithorn et al. (1982) that performance on the PMT is sensitive to the personality variable of introversion–extroversion, as conceptualized by Eysenck (1952).

In order to investigate the organic substrate of performance on the PMT, Elithorn, Svancara, and Weinman (1971) administered the PMT to 14 pairs of monozygotic twins and 17 pairs of dizygotic twins. When the score used was the number of trials successfully completed and the influence of age was partialed out, there was a .28 correlation between monozygotic twins and of .41 between dizygotic twins. When the score used was the total number of dots connected, there was a correlation of .70 between the monozygotic twins and of .60 between the dizygotic twins. Apparently, the degree of genetic organic substrate underlying performance on the PMT depends partially on which score is used.

Colonna and Faglioni (1966) administered the PMT to 112 subjects with unilateral hemispheric lesions as diagnosed by X-ray films, EEGs, and a neurological exam. There were 53 subjects with right-hemisphere lesions and 59 subjects with left-hemisphere lesions. An analysis of covariance was performed, with age and education used as the covariates. The results of this analysis indicated that the right-hemisphere subjects performed significantly worse than the left-hemisphere subjects, that subjects with visual field defects performed significantly worse than subjects without defects, and that aphasics performed significantly worse than the nonaphasics.

Archibald (1978) administered the PMT to 29 left-hemisphere-lesioned subjects (18 of whom were aphasic), to 19 right-hemisphere-lesioned subjects, and to 30 normal control subjects. There were no significant differences among the groups in age or education. All of the lesions had been caused by cerebrovascular accidents (CVAs), and all subjects were tested at least 3 months post-CVA. When time limits were used, the normals scored significantly better than either the right- or left-hemisphere-lesioned subjects, and the left-hemisphere-lesioned subjects scored better than the right-hemisphere-lesioned subjects. There were no differences between the aphasic and the nonaphasic left-hemisphere-lesioned subjects. When the performance was measured without time limits, there were no differences between the left-hemisphere subjects and the normals, although the right-hemisphere subjects performed significantly worse than either.

Benton, Elithorn, Fogel, and Kerr (1963) examined performance on the PMT and on the 27 tests in Benton's assessment battery in 100 brain-damaged and 100 normal subjects. They found that the PMT was one of the most sensitive indicators of brain damage in the battery of 28 tests used. In addition, the PMT differentiated between the right- and left-hemisphere-lesioned subjects.

The PMT appears to be a sensitive indicator of frontal lobe damage, of right-hemisphere damage, and of brain damage in general. However, research can increase the usefulness of this procedure in a clinical setting. In light of the various forms and scores available, a standardized version would be useful in evaluating individual subjects. In particular, although the original intent of the test was not psychometric, that type of evaluation can provide needed information about the characteristics of the various scores that can be derived. The theoretical meaning of poor performance on the PMT needs to be delineated; such a delineation will help provide localization information as well as an elucidation of the functional significance of performance on the PMT.

VERBAL CONCEPT ATTAINMENT TEST

The Verbal Concept Attainment Test (VCAT) is a verbal problem-solving test that can be seen as a verbal analog of tests such as the Category Test or the Wisconsin Card Sorting Test. In the VCAT, the subject is presented with a list of 16 words arranged on a page in a 4-by-4 matrix. The subject is told that one word in each row has something in common with one word in each of the other three rows and is asked to underline those four words that form a concept. There are no reports of evaluations of any form of reliability of this test.

Bornstein (1982b) administered the VCAT and the Halstead–Reitan to 109 patients who had been referred for neuropsychological evaluation. He found that the VCAT correlated with all of the Halstead–Reitan measures except the Finger Tapping Test. The Wisconsin Card Sorting Test was administered to 92 of the subjects. There was a small but significant correlation (.31) between the VCAT and the Wisconsin Card Sorting Test. (The score from the Wisconsin Card Sorting Test was not reported, but most likely, it was the total error score.) The data were then submitted to an unspecified form of factor analysis with varimax rotation. The VCAT was found to load on the verbal reasoning factor and the nonverbal reasoning factor. Bornstein (1983a) found similar correlation patterns in a sample of 75 patients who had been referred for neuropsychological evaluation. A booklet form of this test was found to have a significant relation to the Impairment Index of the Halstead–Reitan in the same report. Bornstein and Leason (1985) administered the VCAT to 97 patients with unilateral lesions, 52 patients with right-hemisphere lesions, and 45 patients with left-hemisphere lesions. In addition, the patients were divided into frontal and nonfrontal lesions. An analysis of variance conducted on the data indicated that the left-hemisphere patients scored significantly worse than the right-hemisphere patients. The frontal lesion patients scored significantly worse than the nonfrontal lesion patients.

Bornstein (1986b) compared the Halstead Category Test, the Wisconsin Card Sorting Test, and the VCAT in their response to unilateral lesions in a sample of 53 patients who had been diagnosed with the aid of computed tomography (CT), EEG, and angiography. An analysis of variance (ANOVA) indicated that there were no significant effects of caudality or laterality on Halstead Category Test performance, and that there was an effect of caudality only on the Wisconsin Card Sorting Test perseverative score (frontal injuries were associated with worse performance). However, there was a significant interaction effect of caudality and laterality on VCAT performance (left-hemisphere injuries and anterior injuries were associated with worse performance). A discriminant function analysis resulted in 67.9% correct classification into the quadrant of lesion, with VCAT scores entered first into the stepwise equation. However, there was a low ratio of subjects to predictors, and the results are in need of cross-validation.

These results imply the promise of the instrument in clinical settings. However, the reliability of the instrument needs to be determined. In addition, cutoff points and interpretation guidelines need to be developed.

WEIGL COLOR-FORM SORTING TEST

The Weigl Color-Form Sorting Test was designed by Weigl (1941) as a test sensitive to structural brain lesions. In particular, Weigl was interested in the abstraction-skills deficits demonstrated by aphasics. The test has been revised and currently consists of three subtests. In the first subtest, the subject is given nine plastic figures of three shapes (a triangle, a square, and a circle) and three colors (red, blue, and yellow). The subject is asked to sort the plastic figures on the basis of the two categories of color and shape. In the second subtest, there are 18 figures: the original 9 and 9 additional figures, which are the same as the originals except that they are one half their size. In the third subtest, there are 36 figures: the figures from the second subtest plus their replicas constructed of cardboard. In each subtest, the variable of interest is the ability of the subject to shift categories while sorting. The reliability of the Weigl has not been investigated.

There is some intriguing information that suggests the clinical usefulness of the Weigl. In an investigation of the construct validity of the Weigl Test, Tamkin and Kunce (1982) reported small correlations with WAIS Verbal IQ scores ($r = .46$), the Similarities subtest of the WAIS ($r = .42$), Bender Gestalt recall scores ($r = .32$), and the Hooper Visual Organization Test ($r = .30$) in a sample of 38 male psychiatric inpatients. Further, there was a negative correlation with age ($r = -.33$). There was no significant correlation with education. In a stepwise multiple-regression application, there was a multiple R of .52 when the Verbal IQ (VIQ) and age were used to predict Weigl scores. An earlier study had demonstrated an effect of education on Weigl scores (Tamkin, 1980). Ward (1982) investigated the Weigl in a sample of 400 children aged 8 to 11 years and reported a significant relationship with age. There is apparently a relationship between Weigl scores and age and education that needs to be articulated before widespread clinical use of the instrument can be recommended.

The accuracy of the Weigl in diagnosis has been investigated. McFie and Piercy (1952) examined Weigl performance in 74 brain-damaged individuals. There was a wide variety of etiologies and of locations of lesions, so the results are difficult to interpret. The authors concluded that the Weigl is sensitive to left-hemisphere impairment and is not related to aphasia. In contrast, De Renzi, Faglioni, Savoiardo, and Vignolo (1966) examined Weigl performance in 40 control subjects, 40 right-hemisphere-impaired subjects, 22 nonaphasic left-hemisphere-impaired subjects, and 45 aphasic left-hemisphere-impaired subjects. These investigators covaried out the influence of age and education and found that only the aphasic subjects scored significantly worse that the control subjects. In addition, the aphasic left-hemisphere subjects scored significantly worse than the nonaphasic left-hemisphere subjects. There was no significant difference between the performance of the nonaphasic left-hemisphere subjects and the right-hemisphere subjects. The authors concluded that the Weigl was sensitive to aphasia and insensitive to neurological impairment in general. Although the more rigorous design of the De Renzi et al. study allows us to have more confidence in its results, more research is needed before definitive conclusions can be reached.

The Weigl is based on the assumption that it is more difficult to sort to shape than to sort to color (Grewal & Haward, 1984). Byrne, Bucks, and Ceurden (1998) subsequently developed a scoring system that codes for individuals who sort to shape and then fail to switch to color. In examining the performance of older subjects attending a memory disorders clinic, a preference for sorting to color was found, but the failure to switch set exhibited high specificity and low sensitivity.

WISCONSIN CARD SORTING TEST

The Wisconsin Card Sorting Test (WCST) is an old and well-known instrument in clinical neuropsychology. The test was originally designed by Berg (1948), but there have been several variations. Today, the most commonly used version is that by Heaton (1981). In the WCST, the subject is asked to sort a double stack of 64 cards each into categories identified by four stimulus cards. The cards can be sorted by color, form, or number. The subject is allowed to sort, and the examiner provides feedback regarding the accuracy of each sort. Unbeknownst to the subject, the correct principle changes each time the subject performs 10 consecutive correct sortings. The test is therefore an evaluation of the subject's ability to use abstraction skills as well as of his or her ability to change sets. Visual evoked potentials indicate activation of the prefrontal and right parieto-occipital regions in the first card following set change (Silberstein, Ciorciari, & Pipingas, 1995), implying a role of the frontal structures in WCST performance in normal subjects. The reliability of the WCST has not been extensively evaluated. Developmental norms for the WCST were derived from children between the ages of 6 and 12 years in a sample of 103 subjects (Chelune & Baer, 1986). Subsequent research indicated that level of intelligence may also need to be taken into consideration. For example, Arffa, Lovell, Podell, and Goldberg (1998) reported that children with IQ scores above 110 performed significantly better than the published norms (Chelune & Baer, 1986), to the extent that the mean score of the high IQ children was at the 90th percentile of the norms. Additional norms with corrections for age and education for the WCST can be found in Heaton, Chelune, Talley, Kay, and Curtiss (1993). Fastenau (1999) found that use of the education and age corrections resulted in overcorrections for age.

There is both a manually administered "card" version of the test and a computerized version. Artiola I Fortuny and Heaton (1996) reported that there are no differences in performance on the two across the two methods, at least for normal subjects. The same researchers found no differences due to ethnicity in comparing North American Caucasian subjects with natives of Spain.

It has been assumed that exposure to the test would invalidate future use because of a significant practice effect. Tate, Perdices, and Maggiotto (1998) examined this premise in a sample of individuals with traumatic brain injury (TBI) who were tested an average of 9 months apart along with a sample of control siblings of the patients. The control subjects demonstrated good stability without showing ceiling effects. The TBI patients demonstrated improvement across the two occasions. The reliability coefficients were used to calculate the magnitude of reliable change. Similar results were reported by Ferland, Ramsay, Engeland, and O'Hara (1998) using a 5-month interval in a sample of 85 TBI patients and 50 college students.

Heaton (1981) provided rules for determining several scores, but the scores that have generated the most interest are the perseverative-responses and the perseverative-errors scores. The rules for scoring perseveration are complex and are potentially susceptible to interscorer error. This fact has not been documented, most likely because it is extremely evident to anyone who has tried to teach another individual to score the WCST. Flashman, Horner, and Freides (1991) provided further explication of the scoring for perseverations and Berry (1996) provided a diagram to follow when scoring the WCST.

Osmon (1992) revised the WCST to require that subjects verbalize their sorting intention prior to sorting each card. This modification was intended to enhance the assessment of elderly subjects, but it may also have utility in further evaluating frontal lobe functions. Osmon and Suchy (1996) factor-analyzed the resulting new scores along with the number of categories completed in a sample of 71 geriatric, neurological, and orthopedic patients. They found three factors that they interpret as reflecting forming, maintaining, and switching sets. These factors, as well as the new scores themselves, are in need of further empirical validation. Nelson (1976) also modified the WCST to facilitate evaluation of elderly patients. This modification (MCST) uses only those 48 cards which can be sorted unambiguously. In comparing the two forms, van Gorp et al. (1997) found that the number of perseverative errors relative to categories achieved was comparable across the two forms, but that other indices were not comparable. Separate norms are therefore necessary for the clinical use of the MCST.

The WCST has been found to be sensitive to brain impairment. Both Parsons (1977) and Tarter and Parsons (1971) found that alcoholics demonstrated impaired performance on the WCST, mainly related to perseveration. Most of the interest in the WCST has been in its ability to diagnose frontal lobe impairment. Milner (1963) examined WCST performance in 71 subjects who had been given cortical excision as a treatment for intractable epilepsy. Eighteen of these patients had been afflicted in the dorsolateral frontal regions. The remaining 53 patients had involvement in other cerebral areas. Before the surgical intervention, the frontal subjects had more impaired scores on the total-errors and the perseverative-errors scores of the WCST. Following surgery, the frontal lobe subjects performed much worse, and the other subjects actually showed some improvement. Malmo (1974) used Milner's frontal subjects (1963) and compared their performance with that of 244 psychiatric patients divided into groups of schizophrenics, alcoholics, neurotics, and those with mixed diagnoses. The frontal lobe patients demonstrated statistically significantly more total errors than the other groups. Taylor (1979) found more perseverative errors associated with dorsolateral lesions of the frontal lobes; he also found that the left-frontal-lobe subjects tended to score worse than the right-frontal-lobe subjects. The effect of localization in WCST performance may be moderated by etiology. Patients with TBI do not differ on the WCST as a function of localization of lesion as indicated by magnetic resonance imaging (MRI), nor does score on the WCST vary with the size of the frontal lobe lesions in these same patients (Anderson, Bigler, & Blatter, 1995).

Drewe (1974) examined WCST performance in 22 left-frontal-lobe subjects, 21 right-frontal-lobe subjects, 24 left-nonfrontal subjects, and 24 right-nonfrontal subjects. He reported that left-frontal subjects performed significantly worse than the other subjects in total errors, in perseverative errors, and in the number of categories completed. In general, the combined frontal groups performed more poorly than the other subjects in perseverative errors and in the number of categories completed. The right-frontal subjects performed significantly better than the other subjects in nonperseverative errors. The patient groups and control subjects in the standardization sample were examined for classification using a discriminant function analysis. The patients groups were discriminable from the control subjects, but were not themselves accurately classified in terms of localization of lesion. Children with sickle-cell disease and subsequent frontal infarcts performed more poorly on the WCST than did children with sickle-cell disease but no infarcts and more poorly than sibling control subjects (Watkins et al., 1998). Horner, Flashman, Freides, Epstein, and Bakay (1996) reported that patients with temporal lobe epilepsy performed poorly on the WCST regardless of laterality of involvement. Hermann and Seidenberg (1995) concluded that poor performance on the WCST in temporal lobe patients was related to dysfunction of the extratemporal regions that are the substrate for executive function.

Robinson, Heaton, Lehman, and Stilson (1980) investigated the WCST in 123 normal control subjects and 107 subjects with structural lesions, 69 of whom had focal lesions. Following an analysis of covariance of age, education, and the Average Impairment Rating (AIR) of the Halstead–Reitan Neuropsychological Battery, these researchers found that the neurologically impaired subjects performed significantly worse than the control subjects, and that the frontal lobe subjects performed significantly worse than the non-frontal-lobe subjects. These authors then performed a discriminant-function analysis using the perseverative-errors score from the WCST, age, education, and the AIR as predictors of the presence of neurological impairment, with a 68% accuracy rate. When a discriminant-function analysis was performed using the perseverative-errors score of the WCST and the scores from the individual subtests of the Halstead–Reitan, there was an 85% correct classification rate.

Another way of looking at localization is to examine brain activity in normal subjects during performance on the task. Normal subjects tend to show inferior frontal and occipitotemporal increases in activation. Individuals who scored better also tended to show higher levels of activation of the dorsolateral and inferior regions (Raglund et al., 1997).

Because the Category test of the Halstead–Reitan is said to measure some of the same functions as the WCST, an important question is whether these two tests provide different information. King and Snow (1981) administered the WCST and the Category test to 89 neurologically impaired and 67 control subjects. The partial correlation between the number of categories completed in the WCST and the total-errors score of the Category test, when age and education were controlled for, was $-.55$. A second evaluation of these subjects was conducted from which those control subjects with a suggestion of neurological impairment were excluded. The number of control subjects decreased to 44. When the cutoff points suggested in the respective manuals were used, the Category Test correctly classified 85% of the neurologically impaired and 80% of the control subjects. The WCST correctly classified 68% of the neurologically impaired subjects and 89% of the control subjects. Apparently, the Category Test is more sensitive to neurological impairment in general.

In another attempt to determine the diagnostic utility of the WCST, Pendleton and Heaton (1982) administered the same two tests to 207 subjects with structural cerebral lesions (classified among frontal, nonfrontal, and diffuse lesions) and to 150 normal controls. The dependent measures were the total number of errors on the Category Test and the number of perseverative responses on the WCST. When the cutoff points from the manuals were used, the Category Test appeared to be more sensitive to neurological impairment. The two tests disagreed in 24% of the cases. In cases of disagreement, the WCST was more accurate for frontal injuries, and the Category test was more accurate for the subjects with nonfrontal and diffuse injuries.

It is important to remember that the utility of the WCST in localizing lesions is related to the concept of executive dysfunction. There are multiple etiologies beside frontal lesions that may cause executive dysfunction. Adolescents and young adults with ADHD perform poorly on the WCST (Seidman, Biederman, Faraone, Weber, & Ouelette, 1997), although it should be remembered that frontal immaturity is one of the theories regarding the etiology of ADHD. Striatal reduction, particularly in the left caudate and putamen, is associated with lowered performance on the WCST (Stratta et al., 1997). Furthermore, differential patterns of scores on the different indices available on the WCST may be related to the type of executive dysfunction. Degl'Innocenti, Agren, and Baeckman (1998) reported that depression may result in lower accuracy scores but not greater perseverative-error rates on the WCST, a finding corroborated by Channon (1996) in a sample of undergraduate students with dysphoria. The relationship of WCST performance to executive function is not certain. When patients with frontal lobe lesions were divided into two groups based on whether they exhibited dysexecutive syndrome or not, there were no differences on WCST scores between the two groups (Baddeley, Della Sala, Papagno, & Spinnler, 1997).

In addition, the WCST may be sensitive to chemical as well as structural changes in the brain. Volkow et al. (1998) reported that decreases in D2 (dopamine) receptors in the caudate and putamen associated with age were correlated with decreases in performance on the WCST. In contrast, patients with schizophrenia do not show the decrease in D2 receptors in the striatum, but at least one study has found decreased binding to D1 receptors in the prefrontal cortex, and these decreases are associated with poorer performance on the WCST (Okubu et al., 1997).

As with many neuropsychological tests, there are multiple other influences that may affect performance on the WCST. For example, Artiola I Fortuny, Heaton, and Hermosillo (1998) found that for Spanish-speaking residents of the border region between Texas and Mexico the amount of time spent living in the United States was correlated with WCST scores. These residents tended to perform more poorly than subjects living in Spain, although the differences between the two groups tended to disappear with higher levels of education. In studying the genetic component of performance on the WCST, Campana, Macciardi, Gambini, and Scarone (1996) found that monozygotic twins, dizygotic twins, and unrelated control pairs did not differ in intrapair correlation coefficients. This study used a very small sample, and it is possible that larger samples would uncover a modest association; however, it is noteworthy that environmental influences may play a role equivalent to that of genetic determinants. The WCST is associated with left frontal–

temporal activation which changes over the trials in normal subjects (Barcelo, Sanz, Molina, & Rubia, 1997). There is a secondary activation of temporal–parietal and medical temporal lobe structures during WCST performance by normals, suggesting the importance of working memory (Barcelo & Rubia, 1998). The role of working memory in WCST performance is not universally accepted. These two constructs may be differentiable, at least in schizophrenic subjects (Stratta et al., 1997). In a fascinating study of twins discordant for closed head injury, Kirby, van Horn, Ostrem, Weinberger, and Berman (1996) reported less activation (as measured by regional cerebral blood flow [rCBF]) during the WCST of the left inferior frontal lobe in the twin who had experienced the head injury. In general, in normal subjects the WCST tends to activate the frontal cortex as well as a complex set of other structures including the inferior parietal lobe (Berman et al., 1995).

The WCST may be useful in discriminating different diagnoses. For example, when matched for score on the Folstein Mini-Mental State Exam, age, and education, patients with multiple subcortical infarctions performed more poorly than patients with Alzheimer's dementia (Tei et al., 1997).

Construct Validity

MacInnes, Golden, McFadden, and Wilkening (1983) investigated the relationship between the WCST and the booklet form of the Category Test. They administered both tests in counterbalanced order to 30 neurologically impaired individuals and 31 normal control subjects. They calculated all 14 scores recommended in the WCST manual and found that age correlated significantly with 12 of these variables and that education correlated significantly with 10 of the variables. When the influence of age and education was partialed out, the largest correlation between the booklet form of the Category Test total-errors score and the WCST scores was −.52. With the use of a stepwise multiple-regression methodology, with age, education, and the 14 WCST scores as possible predictors, only the number of Categories completed was entered into the regression equation following age and education. Age and education accounted for 46% of the shared variance. When the various hit rates in diagnosis were compared (by use of the total number of errors score from the booklet form of the Category Test and the five scores that are given cutoff points in the WCST manual), the booklet form of the Category Test had a 59.0% hit rate overall. The WCST hit rates ranged from 59.0% to 70.5%. Significantly, the booklet form of the Category Test misclassified 11 of the 14 subjects over the age of 45. The authors concluded that, although the booklet form of the Category Test and the WCST have common properties, they provide distinctly different clinical information and should not be used interchangeably.

Bornstein (1986b) administered the Halstead Category test, the Wisconsin Card Sorting Test, and the Verbal Concept Attainment Test (VCAT) to a group of 53 patients with circumscribed lesions localized by the use of CT, EEG, and angiography. Although there were no effects of caudality or laterality on Category Test performance, there was a significant effect of caudality on the Wisconsin Card Sorting Test perseverative score, with the anterior- lesioned patient performing worse. Freedman, Black, Ebert, and Binns (1998) reported that six subjects with bilateral frontal lesions performed more poorly than control subjects on the WCST. It should be pointed out that all of these data are based on group studies. Heck and Bryer (1986) presented the case of an individual with 1.5 years of college education who had severe frontal atrophy and who performed in the superior range on the

Wisconsin Card Sorting Test. However, the performance of this individual may have been attributable to a high level of premorbid functioning. In a small sample of normal control subjects, performing the WCST resulted in activation of the left or bilateral dorsolateral prefrontal cortex as well as the inferior parietal lobes, the left superior occipital cortex, and the cerebellum. Multiple areas of the brain are most likely responsible for adequate performance. Functional MRI studies indicate activation of the mesial and dorsolateral prefrontal cortex in normal subjects administered the WCST (Mentzel et al., 1998).

It appears that increasing severity of brain injury and increasing volume of lesions in children with TBI was associated with poorer performance on the WCST (Levin et al., 1997) regardless of the site of maximum injury. Clearly, specific changes in the organic integrity of individuals across the life span will affect performance on the WCST. There are differences in WCST performance across the age span in normal subjects as well. Fristoe, Salthouse, and Woodard (1997) presented evidence to support the hypothesis that age-related changes in WCST scores are associated with changes in ability to utilize feedback as well as changes in working memory.

Factor Analyses

The WCST provides multiple index scores including number correct and number of errors, perseverative responses and errors, number of categories solved, failures to maintain set, and percent conceptual level responses. Some of these index scores are readily seen as related, such as the number of errors and the number correct. It is important to determine the relationships among all index scores as well. Greve, Brooks, Crouch, Williams, and Rice (1997) evaluated the factor structure in college students and in clinical subjects. They found two orthogonal factors, interpreted as executive function and attentional function. Subsequent research supported the interpretation of the second factor as measuring attentional processes (Greve, Williams, Haas, Littel, & Reinoso, 1996). In a sample of patients with schizophrenia, a factor analysis resulted in three factors interpreted as perseveration, errors, and inefficient sorting (Bell, Greig, Kaplan, & Bryson, 1997), a finding that was replicated fairly consistently in samples of patients with brain injury, stroke, dementia, and psychiatric diagnoses (Greve, Ingram, & Bianchini, 1998) and in a sample of 83 patients who had recently experienced a cerebrovascular accident (Greve, Bianchini, Hartley, & Adams, 1999). Koren et al. (1998) reported a three-factor solution (perseveration, failure to maintain set, and idiosyncratic sorting) in a sample of patients with schizophrenia. Paolo, Troster, Axelrod, and Koller (1995) reported a three-factor solution (accuracy, learning, and consistency of response) in their sample of normal control subjects, but reported that the nonperseverative errors variable loaded on the response consistency factor rather than the accuracy factor in their sample of patients with Parkinson's disease. The fact that different clinical diagnostic groups may have different factor structures was supported by the findings of Goldman et al. (1996), who reported a single-factor solution in a control sample and a two-factor solution in a mixed clinical sample.

All of the aforementioned studies used an orthogonal rotation method to allow greater interpretability of the solution. However, this may not be an accurate depiction of the relationship among the factors in an instrument where the various scores are not necessarily nonredundant. Weigner and Donders (1999) performed a factor analysis of the WCST using oblique rotation to account for the intercorrelation of obtained factors. These researchers further limited their sample to include only subjects with closed head injury. They found three factors: response accuracy, learning, and consistency of self-monitoring. A subsequent cluster analysis using the same subjects indicated that level of performance as related to education and length of coma could characterize the groups of subjects.

When the WCST is factor analyzed (using principal axes methods) along with other measures purported to measure prefrontal functioning (Stroop, Verbal Fluency, Digit Symbol) as well as variables not thought to be specifically related to prefrontal function (Rey–Osterrieth memory, WMS, and WAIS IQ score), the WCST variables tend to load together on the same factor interpreted as cognitive flexibility and the other prefrontal variables loaded on a speeded processing factor (Boone, Ponton, Gorsuch, Gonzalez, & Miller, 1998). In this particular study a mixed clinical sample was used.

Paolo, Troster, Axelrod, and Koller (1995) administered the WCST along with the Continuous Visual Memory Test, the California Verbal Learning Test, and the Digit Span to a group of 187 normal elderly and 181 elderly with Parkinson's disease. Two types of factor analyses were conducted, first using only the WCST variables, and second using the WCST and the other test variables. Three factors emerged from the WCST—only analyses for the normal subjects—conceptualization/problem-solving, failure to maintain set, and learning. The three factors obtained from the Parkinson's disease sample were similar, although initial conceptualization appeared to play a role in the second factor. In the analyses conducted using all of the test variables, the WCST did not load on any of the attention or memory measures, indicating that the WCST may measure problem-solving apart from memory.

A factor analysis of the WCST was performed in a sample of subjects with schizophrenia and a sample of control subjects. Following orthogonal rotation, three factors emerged, interpreted as perseveration, failure to maintain set, and idiosyncratic sorting (Koren et al., 1998). These factors were consistent across the two samples.

Ecological Validity

In an examination of ecological validity, Kibby, Schmitter-Edgecombe, and Long (1998) found that the WCST predicted occupational status in a group of 28 subjects who were 1 year to more than 5 years postsevere closed head injury. However, the WCST was not accurate in predicting job performance. The WCST was associated with the severity of drinking consequences in alcoholic subjects, indicating that executive dysfunction may mediate the effects of maladaptive behavior as well as be a cause of such behavior. Poor performance on the WCST is associated with violent acts committed by psychiatric inpatients while in the community (Krakowski et al., 1997). When dysexecutive impairment was defined behaviorally in patients with frontal lobe lesions, there were no differences on the WCST between those patients with dysexecutive impairment and those without (Baddeley, Della Sala, Papagano, & Spinnler, 1997). Although the WCST may have a fairly strong relationship to frontal lobe integrity, its relationship to executive functioning in the open environment needs to be better explicated. Lysaker, Bell, and Beam-Goulet (1995) reported that the WCST is a significant predictor of work performance in patients with schizophrenia.

Short Forms

Different short forms of the WCST have been suggested, including administering only the first deck of 64 cards and administering cards only until three categories are reached. Paolo, Axelrod, Troster, Blackwell, and Koller (1996) found that the 64-card version could discriminate among patients with Alzheimer's and patients with Parkinson's with dementia, in comparison to patients with Parkinson's without dementia and elderly control subjects. Another version is the WCST-3 version in which the cards are administered until three categories are reached. Robinson, Kester, Saykin, Kaplan, and Gur (1991) found that both the WCST-64 and the WCST-3 correlated well with full-length WCST and that both short forms accurately identified normal subjects, but that the WCST-64 was more accurate in identifying the clinical subjects. Axelrod, Henry, and Woodard (1992) compared the full-length WCST and WCST-64 in healthy elderly subjects and found good levels of agreement. Axelrod, Henry, and Woodard (1992); Haaland, Vranes, Goodwin, and Garry (1987); and Robinson et al. (1991) all provided information regarding mean scores and distributions of scores of the WCST-64, mainly related to older populations. The amount of normative information needs to be expanded, as Smith-Seemiller, Franzen, and Bowers (1997) point out the inaccuracies possible when transformed norms from the full-length version are applied to the 64-card version even though the two forms may correlate highly in most clinical populations, a point also raised by Axelrod, Paolo, and Abraham (1997) in their mixed sample of patients.

Detection of Response Bias

As with several other tests used in forensic evaluations, the WCST has been the subject of research to develop indices sensitive to response bias. Bernard, McGrath, and Houston (1996) used a set of simulating malingerers in comparison to control subjects and to patients with closed head injury or with other forms of central nervous system disease to derive discriminant functions. They then used the discriminant functions to predict group membership with overall accuracy of classification of 80% for the comparison with closed head injury patients and 91% for the comparison with patients with other forms of central nervous system disease. Both the classification formula for the closed head injury patients and that for the general central nervous system disease patients used the number of perseverative errors and the total number of categories solved as predictors. The sample size was limited and the prediction formulas, although promising, are in need of cross-validation in a separate sample.

TOWER OF LONDON

Cockburn (1995) found that the Tower of London did not discriminate between subjects with severe diffuse TBI and subjects with frontal lesions, nor did it discriminate between subjects with frontal lesions and subjects with nonfrontal lesions. Anderson, Anderson, and Lajoie (1996) demonstrated age-related trends in performance in a sample of 376 children ranging in age from 7 years to 13 years, 11 months. The greatest changes were between children 7 and 9 years old and between children 1 and 12 years old, consistent with developmental data from other executive tasks. Cullbertson and Zillmer (1998) reported age-related differences in children as well as differences between normal children and children with ADHD. Poor performance on the Tower of London was both sensitive and specific to ADHD. The Tower of London has been compared to the Tower of Hanoi, with the assumption that the two tasks may be comparable. The differences in methodology include aspects of the stimuli; namely the Tower of London involves three pegs of increasing length and three colored balls of equal size while the Tower of Hanoi involves three pegs of equal size and disks of increasing size. Humes, Welsh, Retzlaff, and Cookson (1997) found a small correlation between the two tasks which they attributed to low reliability of the Tower of London. More information is needed before either task can be confidently used in clinical applications.

Screening Devices

THE BENDER–GESTALT VISUAL–MOTOR INTEGRATION TEST

The Bender–Gestalt test has a long and varied history. It has four major scoring systems and has been used for several purposes, including the diagnosis of psychosis, the identification of learning disabilities in children, the description of personality, and the diagnosis of organicity. Because of this history of multiple usage, it is important to clarify which version of the Bender–Gestalt is under discussion at a given time. Unless otherwise noted, the discussion in this chapter is confined to the use of the Bender–Gestalt as an instrument for screening for organicity in adults [using the Hutt & Briskin (1960) scoring system] and its use to identify neurological and developmental disabilities in children [using the Koppitz (1960) scoring system].

The Bender–Gestalt is a relatively straightforward test to administer. The test materials consist of nine stimulus cards with designs printed on them. The subject is given a pencil and some plain white 8½″ × 11″ paper and is shown the stimulus cards one at a time. The subject is instructed to copy the designs as best she or he can. In the Hutt–Briskin scoring method, 12 errors can be made by the subject. These errors are different ways of distorting the designs. Each type of error can be scored only once per protocol. A score of five errors or more is representative of organic performance. The Koppitz scoring method consists of 30 characteristics of performance that are scored on the basis of absence or presence. These items are summed for possible scores ranging from 0 to 30 points.

There have been some suggested alterations in administration. There is a group administration method in which the subjects are simultaneously administered the test through the use of oversized cards. In another administration alteration, the subject is asked to reproduce the designs from memory. A third alteration presents the stimuli tachistoscopically, and a fourth version requires the subject to reproduce the design on paper on which is printed a background of interfering wavy lines.

Normative Data

Lacks (1984) presented normative data on the Hutt–Briskin method for 325 normals aged 17 to 59 years. Caucasian subjects, with a mean score of 1.58 errors, tended to perform better than black subjects, who had a mean score of 2.21 errors. Males, with a mean of 2.07 errors, tended to perform more poorly than females, who had a mean of 1.37. Normative data are also available on 334 normal adults over 60 years old. Although still scoring below the organicity cutoff of five errors, the older subjects tended to demonstrate more errors, with a mean of 3.45 errors, compared with the young-adult mean of 1.75 (Lacks & Storandt, 1982). Lubin and Sands (1992) provided a bibliography of the research related to the Bender–Gestalt. The book was revised (Lacks, 1999) with additional normative informa- tion and a more complete review of the research.

Normative data are available for the Koppitz scoring method for normal children between the ages of 5 years and 10 years, 11 months (Koppitz, 1960). Norms are also available for Puerto Rican and black children in a study in which 74 Puerto Rican and 47 African-American children were tested in the first grade and again in the third grade (Marmorale & Brown, 1977). Both the black and the Puerto Rican children performed more poorly than the Caucasian children. Extreme caution should be used in interpreting these norms because of the small sample size. Norms for adults with mental retardation were reported by Andert, Dinning, and Hustak (1976). The sample for this study was composed of 510 mentally retarded adults residing at a state school for the retarded. Norms are available for teenaged subjects only for the Pascal and Suttell scoring method (Grow, 1980).

Reliability

Lacks (1984) reviewed the reliability studies using the Bender–Gestalt. There is no alternate form for the Bender–Gestalt, and therefore, there is no estimate of alternate-form reliability. Lacks argued that, because of the nature of the test, there have been no split-half reliability studies. Given the Hutt–Briskin scoring system, it would be difficult to decide what split would be appropriate, as each of the items is different. Because categories of errors are counted only once for each protocol, it would be difficult to interpret any split- half coefficient even if it were obtained. A potential method of assessing split-half re- liability would be to score each half as if it were a whole, that is, to count each occurrence of an error in each half. Presumably, the organic deficit responsible for the error would be robust enough to cause more than one occurrence of that error. However, as noted previ- ously, the items are different and probably represent different stimulus values.

It is appropriate to evaluate test–retest reliability for the Bender–Gestalt. There are three indices on which to focus the evaluation of test–retest reliability: we can examine the stability of the total scores, the stability of the occurrence of each type of error, or the stability of the dichotomous decision of organic versus nonorganic subjects. In a study of 40 psychiatric patients (mixed inpatients and outpatients), Lacks (1984) reported a re- liability coefficient of .79 for total scores, a concordance rate of 86% for the occurrence of particular types of errors, and a 93% agreement rate for diagnosis of organicity. There was no attempt to correct for the low number of categories by the use of Cohen's kappa (Cohen, 1960) or some other method of assessing agreement in nominal data as discussed in Lawlis and Lu (1972) and Tinsley and Weiss (1975). This omission presents a minor problem with the test score data, which have 12 possible categories, but it is an especially important problem in the case of the dichotomous diagnosis of organicity. Here, the existence of only two categories means that there is a 50% concordance by chance alone. Another problem with this study is the failure of the author to take the base rate of diagnosis into account. As a result of these two deficiencies, the values reported are most likely inflated over their true values.

Lacks (1984) also reported the results of a test–retest reliability study using 25 individuals with a diagnosis of Alzheimer's disease and a test–retest interval of 12 months. The correlation coefficient relating the test scores was .66, the concordance of scores was 63%, and the agreement of diagnosis was 72%. The same problems discussed for the previous study—namely, failure to account for the number of categories in nominal data and failure to account for base rates—also apply to this study. There are additional problems, in that Alzheimer's disease is a progressively dementing disorder. Test–retest reliability is most accurately assessed when there is no intervening process that would change the true value of the obtained score. This study failed to provide adequate theoretical consideration of this fact. There are questions left unanswered. For example, would one expect more errors over time as a result of the progressive nature of the disorder, or would one expect more severe manifestations of the errors already present? The Hutt–Briskin scoring system would seem to be insufficient to document and account for changes associated with Alzheimer's disease.

Lacks and Newport (1980) examined the interscorer reliability of the Bender–Gestalt using four scoring methods and 12 scorers (3 using each method) at three levels of scorer expertise in a sample of 50 inpatient subjects. There were no differences between interscorer reliability coefficients among all of the methods except the Hain method. All of the scorers were able to distinguish the organic from the nonorganic patients in fair agreement with the discharge diagnosis. The Hutt–Briskin method was concluded to be the most accurate in diagnosis, with an 83% agreement with discharge diagnosis. Because of methodological flaws in the study, it is difficult to interpret the results. Once again, there was no attempt to correct for the number of categories in the nominal data or for the base rate of organicity in the sample. Diagnoses of organicity were determined by the attending psychiatrist and not by a neurologist, and the study included no examination of the variability engendered by having different psychiatrists perform the diagnoses or an indication of the level of experience of the psychiatrists. Lastly, the subjects who had diagnoses of chronic alcoholism were included in the nonorganic group, and this classification was justified on the basis of the Bender–Gestalt results of these subjects. This is a clear confound of the independent variable of Bender–Gestalt scores with the dependent variable of diagnosis.

Reliability has also been examined for the Koppitz scoring method. Test–retest and interscorer reliability were assessed in a sample of 30 second-grade, 24 fourth-grade, and 27 sixth-grade children (Ryckman, Rentfrow, Fargo, & McCartin, 1972). There was a 1-week interval between testing sessions. Two scorers were employed, one with an MA in psychology and the other with an Ed.D. The test–retest reliability coefficients for total obtained score were .67 for the first scorer and .64 for the second. The interscorer reliability coefficients were .85 for the first test and .83 for the retest. Because the Koppitz method results in scores with a range of 0 to 30 points, the problems of limited categories discussed earlier for the Hutt–Griskin method are not as applicable here.

Wallbrown, Wallbrown, and Engin (1976) investigated test–retest reliability in 144 first-grade children with a test–retest interval of from 9 to 14 days. The average time interval was not reported. The rest–retest reliability coefficient was .66. Engin and Wallbrown (1976) reported a test–retest coefficient of .63 in a sample of 157 second-grade students when the test interval ranged from 11 to 15 days. In neither of these studies were the children tested twice by the same examiner. Wallbrown et al. (1976) employed six examiners, and Engin and Wallbrown employed five examiners. Therefore, the test–retest coefficients reported in these studies also reflect interscorer variability.

Egeland, Rice, and Penny (1967) examined the interscorer reliability of the Koppitz scoring system in a sample of 80 retarded children with an average IQ of 78 as measured by either the Stanford–Binet or the WISC. The children were students in a university day-school program. Three doctoral students in a school psychology program served as the scorers. The mean correlation between total error scores for the three scorers was .90. The data were also submitted to an analysis of variance, which determined that there was a significant difference ($p < .01$) between the scores obtained by the three scorers. Although there was sufficient reliability of the relative position of the scores of each subject in the overall distribution, there was not sufficient reliability of the absolute level of scores. This result points out the necessity for caution when comparing absolute scores across scorers by the Koppitz method. Greater reliability of absolute scores is needed before an interpretation of the scores, including a comparison with cutoff points, can be accomplished.

Wallbrown and Fremont (1980) subsequently examined the test–retest reliability of Koppitz scores in a sample of 24 reading disabled children. The test–retest interval ranged from 12 to 24 days, but no average interval was reported. The protocols were scored by three licensed psychologists, and disagreements (the level of necessary agreement was not defined) regarding the scores were settled by discussion. The test–retest reliability coefficient was .83. This coefficient is somewhat larger than what might be expected in the usual testing situation. Because the scores were taken only when there was agreement, some of the error variability associated with an individual scorer across time may have been partialed out methodologically. This coefficient is therefore a more accurate estimate of the reliability of the test itself, separate from the reliability of the scorer. However, generalization of these results to an ordinary testing situation would cause problems.

In each of the studies investigating the test–retest reliability of the Koppitz scoring method, only the reliability of the total score was reported. There was no indication of an attempt to assess the concordance of agreement of type of error or the reliability of diagnoses based on the instrument. These issues remain to be addressed by future research.

Validity

Validity research involving the Bender–Gestalt is sadly deficient. There have been no investigations of the content validity of the test, nor of the construct validity. Lacks (1984) stated that investigations of the content validity of the Bender–Gestalt are inappropriate, but this argument begs the question of what the test is supposed to measure. The lack of such studies is very likely due to the paucity of a theoretical or rational substrate for the test. The closest description of a construct associated with the test is the notion of *organicity*. This concept has been discarded in the neuropsychological literature in favor of a multidimensional concept of *organic integrity* involving multiple, semi-independent skills. A case could be made for the construct of the test as involving visual–motor skills, as has been done in evaluations of children. But even here, no empirical investigations have been reported.

Investigation of the validity of the Bender–Gestalt has centered on the criterion-related validity of the instrument. The criterion usually used is a diagnosis of organicity.

The major shortcoming of this criterion lies in the nature of the concept of *organicity*. If we define the construct of organicity as the skills and behaviors for which brain integrity is responsible, several problems arise. The first is related to the content validity of the instrument. The Bender–Gestalt does not sample adequately from the realm of the skills that are mediated by the brain. The instrument is heavily loaded toward visual–perceptive and manual five-motor skills. Although the results of the test can be seen to be sensitive to receptive language skills, there is no systematic method of assessing the impact of such skills on the results of the test. The test is insensitive to organic deficits that give rise to specific behavioral deficits, such as deficits in reading comprehension, arithmetic ability, memory, attention, or expressive speech skills. It is possible for an individual to have deficits in these areas and still manifest a normal Bender–Gestalt score. With these points in mind, let us examine the research that has investigated the criterion-related validity of the Bender–Gestalt.

Lacks (1984) evaluated the data provided by three separate studies that she conducted over a period of 20 years. She collapsed the diagnostic information into three categories: schizophrenia, personality disorder, and organic impairment. The diagnoses were provided by a variety of clinicians, both neurologists and psychiatrists. Alcoholics were included in the personality disorder group because their Bender–Gestalt scores as a whole were not different from the scores of the nonorganic subjects. This procedure spuriously inflated the estimate of the diagnostic accuracy of the test. Decisions regarding the criterion should be made independently of the values of the independent variable. Because the diagnoses were conducted over a 20-year period, they represent at least two diagnostic systems (American Psychiatric Association, 1952, 1968). Only two diagnostic categories were used as the dependent measure: organically impaired or not organically impaired. Lacks found that 74% of the "nonorganic" psychiatric inpatients and 18% of the organic psychiatric inpatients had Bender–Gestalt scores in the impaired range. She stated that these results were different from what one would expect on the basis of chance or on the basis of base rates; however, she made no attempt to test this hypothesis statistically. It is therefore difficult to accept the conclusion that the Bender–Gestalt is an accurate diagnostic instrument.

Lacks et al. (1970) compared the diagnostic accuracy of the Bender–Gestalt to that of their own shortened form of the Halstead–Reitan Neuropsychological Battery. For an unexplained reason, these investigators did not administer the Trails A or B, Grip Strength, Finger Tip Writing, or Visual Field tests. To obtain an impairment index, they prorated the results of the tests that they did administer. The subjects were 64 Caucasian male inpatients from a VA hospital who were divided into the following groups: 19 organic, 27 schizophrenic, and 18 general medical. The modified impairment index correctly identified 84% of the organics and 62% of the nonorganics, and the Bender–Gestalt correctly identified 74% of the organics and 91% of the nonorganics. It is difficult to draw conclusions from this study because of the use of a modified version of the Halstead–Reitan battery. Because the Bender–Gestalt tended to underdiagnose "organicity" in relation to the modified Halstead–Reitan impairment index, these results may actually be seen as evidence of the relative insensitivity of the Bender–Gestalt to certain types of organic impairment.

Levine and Feirstein (1972) found significant differences between the scores of organics, medical patients, and schizophrenics but did not investigate the diagnostic accuracy of the instrument. Norton (1978) compared the diagnostic accuracy of the

Bender–Gestalt against both the results of a more thorough neuropsychological examination and the results of a neurological examination, an EEG, a pneumoencephalogram, an arteriogram, or a CT scan in a sample of 598 inpatients. The results indicated that 21% of the subjects classified as normal by the Bender–Gestalt were classified as impaired by the neuropsychological examination; 33% of the subjects classed as normal by the Bender–Gestalt had abnormal objective neurological findings.

Because of the poor performance of the Bender–Gestalt in discriminating between organically impaired individuals and schizophrenic patients, Canter (1966) suggested a background interference procedure. In this procedure, the subject is first asked to perform the Bender–Gestalt under standard administration procedures and then to perform the Bender–Gestalt by reproducing the designs on a sheet of paper that contains an array of wavy lines. Performance under the two conditions is compared, with the general idea that organically impaired individuals will show a greater decline in performance under the interference condition. Canter (1976) reported fairly good results with this procedure. However, Adams and Kenny (1982) were unable to obtain favorable diagnostic hit rates in a sample of children aged 6 to 16 years. The hit rate was 81% in the children aged 12 to 16 years but was only 60% in the children aged 6 to 11 years. Boake and Adams (1982) found a hit rate of 61% in a sample of adults and stated that the background interference procedure was not as accurate as standard neurodiagnostic techniques such as the EEG.

Part of the reason for the diagnostic inaccuracy may be that the Bender–Gestalt appears to be sensitive to variables other than organic integrity. Adams, Boake, and Crain (1982) reported that performance in the Bender–Gestalt background interference procedure is affected by age, education, race, and IQ to the extent that misdiagnosis can occur when these variables are not taken into account. The subjects in this study were 97 brain-damaged and 62 non-brain-damaged male inpatients. The results indicated that older, less educated, less intelligent, non-Caucasian subjects were more likely to be misdiagnosed as brain-damaged when the Bender–Gestalt was used. On the other hand, when age-, sex-, and education-matched Indian subjects were administered the Bender–Gestalt along with epileptic subjects, there were higher frequencies of errors among the epileptic subjects.

Lacks (1979, 1982) and Bigler and Ehrfurth (1980, 1981) have engaged in a disagreement regarding the clinical utility of the Bender–Gestalt. Lacks has argued that the test is short and accurate and can be administered by a technician with minimal training. Bigler and Ehrfurth, on the other hand, have argued the Bender–Gestalt is inaccurate and that the interpretation of the Bender–Gestalt results in information that is naively simplistic. They presented case material on subjects who had given normal Bender–Gestalt performances in spite of massive brain damage, as demonstrated by CT scans and a more rigorous neuropsychological evaluation (Bigler & Ehrfurth, 1980, 1981). Similar evidence from case material was presented by Russell (1976).

Although this case material is certainly impressive, the issue of the diagnostic accuracy of the Bender–Gestalt is more directly addressed by data obtained from many subjects analyzed in a group design. This question cannot be answered until a well-controlled and well-designed study is conducted. However, the issue of whether the Bender–Gestalt results in useful information can be debated without such a study. At the present time, the dichotomous question of whether or not the subject is organically impaired is on the verge of becoming an extinct concern. It is more likely that a neuropsychological evaluation would be sought to provide corroborative information detailing the nature of a subject's neurological disorder, or to define a subject's limitations and strengths for the purpose of treatment planning. In either of these cases, information provided by the Bender–Gestalt would be ineffectual.

Marsico and Wagner (1990) reported that the Bender–Gestalt is more effective than the WAIS IQ in discriminating between brain-damaged and non-brain-damaged subjects. Friedt and Gouvier (1989) report that the Bender–Gestalt was ineffectual at discriminating among brain damaged, schizophrenic, and unimpaired adult male patients in a state forensic hospital.

The clinical interpretation of the Bender–Gestalt by use of the Koppitz scoring system is similarly beset by problems. Although the Bender–Gestalt has been argued to be culture-fair because of its nonreliance on language skills, there is some evidence suggesting that it is, in fact, sensitive to characteristics of the subjects that are not related to neuropsychological ability.

Oakland and Feigenbaum (1979) investigated test bias on the Bender–Gestalt due to the age, sex, family size and structure, birth order, health, race, socioeconomic status, and urban versus rural residence of 436 elementary school children. They examined the effects of these subject variables on internal consistency, item difficulty indices, item total correlations, correlations with California Ability Test (CAT) scores, and factor structure when principal-components factor analysis was conducted using Bender scores in conjunction with WISC-R data. Mexican-American children had lower internal-consistency coefficients than their Caucasian and black counterparts. Correlations with the CAT were differentiated on the basis of socioeconomic status, family size, and sex. There were no effects on factor structure attributable to any of the subject variables.

Sattler and Gwynne (1982a) investigated the effects of race on Bender–Gestalt performance in children when the Koppitz scoring system was used. Their study evaluated 1938 Caucasian, black, and Puerto Rican children between the ages of 5 and 11 years. These authors found that the black children performed more poorly than the Caucasian children at all age levels and more poorly than the Puerto Rican children at all ages except 8 years. In addition, the Puerto Rican children performed more poorly than the Caucasian children at ages 5 and 8 years. Robin and Shea (1983) found that children from Papua New Guinea ($n = 245$) scored significantly worse than children from Australia ($n = 74$). In addition, the children from Papua New Guinea tended to lag 3 to 4 years behind the American sample on which the Koppitz scoring system was normed.

Validity of the Koppitz Scoring System

The concurrent validity of the Bender–Gestalt as a measure of cognitive ability has been evaluated by Wallbrown, Wallbrown, and Engin (1977). These authors found significant but modest correlations (ranging from $-.18$ to $-.27$) between the Bender–Gestalt and scores on the CAT. Giebink and Birch (1970) reported a correlation of $-.19$ between Bender–Gestalt scores and reading achievement as measured by the CAT. Schneider and Spivack (1979) found no differences in Bender–Gestalt performance between reading disabled and normal children.

Caskey and Larson (1980) correlated the scores derived from both a group and an individual administration of the Bender–Gestalt with IQ scores from the Otis–Lennon Test in a sample of 92 rural and 101 suburban kindergarten students. They found significant correlations for the rural children: $-.71$ for group administration and $-.68$ for individual administration. The corresponding correlations for the suburban children were of a lower magnitude ($-.49$ for group administration and $-.31$ for individual administration), indicating that the demographic variable may intervene in the relationship between the Bender–Gestalt and the measure of cognitive ability. Dixon (1998) failed to find support for Koppitz's revised Emotional Indicators score. Venkatesan (1991) reported that the Bender–Gestalt significantly underestimates cognitive skill on the basis of the Stanford–Binet or the Vineland Social Maturity Scale in mentally handicapped Indian individuals.

The Bender–Gestalt is often used to predict academic performance. Because the Bender–Gestalt is also considered a measure of general cognitive ability, a reasonable question is whether the Bender–Gestalt can predict academic performance beyond that associated with cognitive ability. Wright and DeMers (1982) correlated the Bender–Gestalt with Wide Range Achievement Test (WRAT) scores, partialing out the influence of WISC-R IQ values in a group of 86 elementary school students who had been referred for psychoeducational evaluation. These authors found that the partial correlations were modest (.13 to .22) and did not always attain statistical significance. The possibility remains that the Bender–Gestalt roughly measures intellectual functioning rather than a broader concept of organicity.

Tymchuk (1974) investigated the discriminative validity of the Bender–Gestalt in a sample of 16 epileptic, 27 mentally retarded, and 33 behavior problem children. He found significant differences among the three groups. However, using the recommended cutoff scores resulted in a 50% accurate classification rate. It was because of this sort of data that, in a review of the research investigating the validity of the Bender–Gestalt in screening for brain damage in school-aged children, Eno and Deichmann (1980) concluded that, although brain-damaged children as a group tend to perform more poorly on the Bender–Gestalt, these differences are not always significant. More important, interpretation on the level of the single case results in a high rate of false positives and false negatives. Aside from its use as a general screening instrument, the Bender–Gestalt might be used as a measure of developmental visual–spatial construction skills; however, the modified Bender–Gestalt correlated only .54 with the Developmental Test of Visual Motor Integration (Moose & Brannigan, 1997). The modified version of the Bender–Gestalt had been developed for use with young children (Brannigan & Brunner, 1993; Brannigan, Aabye, Baker, & Ryan, 1995) with apparently adequate interscorer reliability (Fuller & Vance, 1995).

In another attempt to investigate the use of the Bender–Gestalt as a measure of visual–motor skill, Shapiro and Simpson (1994) administered the Bender–Gestalt and the Developmental Test of Visual Motor Integration to a sample of 78 emotionally disturbed adolescents. Unlike the VMI, the Bender–Gestalt did not correlate with age, showing developmental insensitivity, and did not demonstrate relationships with other measures of cognitive functioning. Goldstein and Britt (1994) found that the Bender–Gestalt did not predict reading, writing, or mathematics performance when the variance associated with the VMI was partialed out. Fuller and Vance (1993) report that the Bender–Gestalt is inferior to the Minnesota Percepto-Diagnostic Test-Revised in predicting academic achievement at the first-, third-, and fifth-grade levels.

The Bender–Gestalt has different validity for different diagnostic groups. Armstrong and Knopf (1982) reported the correlations between the Bender–Gestalt and the Beery Developmental Test of Visual Motor Integration for a group of 40 learning disabled children and 40 normal children. The correlation coefficient for the learning disabled children was .74, and the correlation coefficient for the normal children was .36. Hartlage and Lucas (1976) reported different correlations between the Bender–Gestalt and the WISC-R for black and Caucasian children. Buckley (1978) reviewed the research related to the use of the Bender–Gestalt in school settings and concluded that there was little evidence or support for the instrument in predicting academic achievement, diagnosing neurological impairment, or uncovering emotional disturbance in children.

The continued popularity of the Bender–Gestalt as a measure of general cognitive skill is difficult to fathom, although it may be that it is much more popular among general clinical psychologists than among clinical neuropsychologists and continues to be recommended as part of a basic psychological evaluation for Social Security Disability evaluations. Sullivan and Bowden (1997) presented evidence that at least among Australian accredited neuropsychologists, the Bender–Gestalt does not enjoy much popularity. However, Lees-Haley (1992) reported that among forensic psychologists, the Bender–Gestalt is among the most frequently used instruments, a finding that also appears to hold for forensic psychologists operating in juvenile courts (Pinkerman, Haynes, & Keiser, 1993).

THE CLOCK DRAWING TEST

The Clock Drawing Test (Freedman et al., 1994) has become a frequently used screening procedure in the evaluation for dementia. The basic procedure involves asking the subject to draw the face of a clock with the hands showing the time ten after eleven. There are six basic scoring procedures focusing on either quantitative or qualitative features. Cahn and Kaplan (1997) found little difference in performance among subjects between the ages of 66 and greater than 85 years old. Generally speaking, although the quantitative scoring systems are successful in detecting dementia, the qualitative scoring systems may be more helpful in lateralizing strokes and in differentiating cortical and subcortical strokes (Suhr, Grace, Allen, Nadler, & McKenna, 1998). The Clock Drawing test was reported to have a sensitivity of 84% and a specificity of 72% in a sample of 42 individuals with Alzheimer's disease and 237 control subjects (Cahn et al., 1996). Libon, Malamut, Swenson, Sands, and Cloud (1996) developed a scale related to graphomotor function and executive function in addition to the original scale related to placement and accuracy and found that this scale helped make a differentiation between Alzheimer's dementia and vascular dementia.

CLINICAL TESTS OF THE SENSORIUM

The Clinical Tests of the Sensorium (CTS) are a collection of short procedures that have been recommended as a method of performing a mental status exam and as an instrument to aid in the discrimination between organic and psychiatric disorders. In particular, the CTS is purported to assess levels of mental efficiency. The CTS consists of the subtests Orientation, Days of the Week Reversed, Serial Sevens, Recall of Address and Telephone Number, Babcock Sentence, Logical Memory Test, General Information, Digit Span, and Story Recall. The CTS exists in three alternate forms.

Withers and Hinton (1971) examined the alternate-form reliability and the test–retest reliability of the CTS. They administered all three forms in randomized order to 24 inpatients (8 medical inpatients and 16 psychiatric inpatients). They conducted an ANOVA and reported that few significant differences were found. However, they did not report the F ratio values or the means or standard deviations, so it is difficult to evaluate the report. For the unidentified subtests that did demonstrate significant differences, modified versions were constructed and examined for significant differences in a further sample of 24 inpatients. No significant differences were found, but again, the report of results is incomplete.

Withers and Hinton (1971) then administered the three forms of the CTS to 108 consecutive-admission psychiatric inpatients. There were 57 males and 51 females, with a mean age of 36 years and a mean WAIS Full Scale IQ of 110. The order of administration of the tests was randomized. The first two administrations occurred in the first week of hospitalization, and the third occurred when the subjects were judged to be at their optimal level of functioning. The criterion by which this judgment was made was not specified.

The values obtained on the three administrations were then correlated. For some unspecified reason, differences in level among the three forms were tested only for a subgroup of 88 subjects who did not have a brain lesion. Significant differences were reported for the Serial Sevens subtest of Form C and the Immediate Recall of Address subtest of Form B. Unfortunately, the authors did not state what the other form was in these significant comparisons. The correlations between the scores ranged from .50 to .80, and all were significant at the .05 level. The correlations between the first and second administrations were slightly higher than the correlations between the first and second administrations, a finding indicating that the reliability tends to decline over time. An important aspect to remember about this study is that the subjects were young and had relatively high IQ scores for psychiatric patients.

Using the same number of subjects with the same mean IQs and ages (and apparently the same actual subjects) as Withers and Hinton (1971), Hinton and Withers (1971) examined the validity of the CTS. They reported significant correlations between the CTS scores and age and education. There were significant differences between the psychiatric patients and patients with brain lesions. There were also significant correlations between nurses' ratings of anxiety and depression and scores on the CTS. When the symptoms of anxious subjects remitted, their scores improved on the Orientation, the Serial Sevens, and the Logical Memory subtests. When the symptoms of the depressed patients remitted, their scores on the Serial Sevens, Logical Memory, and Story subtests improved. In addition, scores improved on repetition, a finding indicating the presence of practice effects.

Although the CTS is apparently sensitive to the presence of brain lesions, it is also affected by age, education, and the presence of anxious or depressed mood. More work is needed before this test can be recommended for clinical use. The work needed includes norming by age and education or the provision of corrections for these variables, larger and more complete examinations of reliability, and examinations of discriminant validity and predictive validity.

THE NEUROPSYCHOLOGICAL IMPAIRMENT SCREEN

The Neuropsychological Impairment Screen (O'Donnell, Reynolds, & De Soto, 1983) is a self-report questionnaire that is intended to provide an overview of the possible symptoms associated with neuropsychological impairment. There are 45 questions related to symptoms and 5 questions related to response style or, as the authors refer to it, "test-taking attitude." Eleven of the items are regarded by the authors as being pathognomic; that is, a positive response to any one of them is considered indicative of impairment. In addition to the test-taking attitude scale (LIE) and the pathognomic scale (PAT), the total raw score of the 45 symptom questions is called the *global measure of impairment* (GMI); the total number of items endorsed is the TIC scale, and the ratio of the GMI value to the TIC value is the symptom intensity measure, or SIM scale.

The original research manual (O'Donnell & Reynolds, 1983) reports normative data based on a sample of 1750 adults. The subjects in the normative sample came from groups of medical patients, neuropsychiatric patients, and normal subjects. Internal-consistency reliability values (coefficient alpha) are reported based on data from the normative sample. For the PAT scale, the value is .74; for the GEN scale, the value is .82. The manual does not report values for the other scales, but it does report reliability values of two scales, the V–L (verbal learning) and the FRU (frustration) scales, which are not referred to in the rest of the manual or in any of the research reports.

A principal-factor analysis with orthogonal varimax rotation was reported for the 1750 normative subjects. The results and a discussion of this analysis occupy only a few sentences, but it appears that there were four factors in the solution. No recommendations are made for interpretation or clinical use of the factors.

Test–retest reliability was assessed by administering the test twice to a sample of 25 inpatient neuropsychiatric subjects over an average interval of 46.76 days. The authors stated that the diagnoses of these subjects were determined by standard current nomenclature; however, they did not state specifically what diagnostic system was used. In addition, they did not provide a rationale for working with these particular subjects. In any evaluation of the temporal stability of test scores, the subjects should be presumed to have static conditions, a point that the authors addressed in the discussion section. Unfortunately, the researchers did not address that issue in their sample. There are doubts that the conditions of these subjects were indeed stable, for three of the subjects had neoplastic disease and three of the subjects carried a diagnosis of degenerative disorder. This fact makes is difficult to interpret the obtained correlation coefficients of .85 for the SIM, .52 for LIE, .84 for PAT, .84 for TIC, and .87 for SIM. A sample of 82 undergraduate subjects was administered the Neuropsychological Impairment Screen (NIS) on two occasions with an average interval of 12.21 days and with similar values in correlation coefficients. Other forms of reliability estimates have not been conducted.

The initial validation study (O'Donnell et al., 1983) looked at the concurrent validity of the NIS by comparing its diagnostic agreement with performance on Trails A and B and the Digit Symbol subtest of the WAIS in a sample of 22 normals, 21 psychiatric patients, and 14 neurological patients. The normals exhibited the best performance on the NIS and on the three screening measures. The psychiatric subjects performed next best, and the neurological patients performed worst. Unfortunately, the subjects differed in age and education in exactly the same order as their performance on the tests. Because neuro-psychological performance is known to vary with these two demographic variables, and because the authors did not attempt to control for these variables, we cannot be sure that the obtained differences were due to diagnosis. Although the NIS measures correlated with the screening tests, we cannot be sure that these correlations reflected the influence of the demographic variables.

A second validity investigation (O'Donnell, Reynolds, & De Soto, 1984a) also examined the concurrent validity of the NIS by correlating it with the Impairment Index, the Category Test score, the Localization score of the Tactual performance Test, and Trail B of the Halstead–Reitan in a sample of 40 patients with unspecified diagnoses. The obtained correlation coefficients were only moderate, ranging from .50 to .08.

Another study by the same researchers (O'Donnell, De Soto, & Reynolds, 1984b) investigated the sensitivity and specificity of the NIS in a sample of 41 patients. The diagnoses arrived at by the use of the NIS were compared to diagnoses arrived at by the attending physicians. It is not clear if the physicians had access to the test results. At any rate, when either the GMI or the SIM or the PAT or the TIC was used, there was a reported sensitivity rate of 91% and a reported specificity rate of 43%. Clearly, the NIS tends to overestimate the prevalence of pathology, at least in this sample. O'Donnell, DeSoto, and DeSoto (1994) reported that scores on the NIS were related to severity of alcoholism, duration of abstinence, education, and age.

The subsequent clinical manual (O'Donnell, DeSoto, DeSoto, & Reynolds, 1994) describes improvements over the original version including deleting three of the items and adding 48 new items. The new version was normed on 1000 nonclinical subjects. The items response form was expanded from a four-point scale to a five-point scale. Split-half reliability was .93 when corrected for attenuation. In addition, Cronbach's alpha was calculated for the scales. Test–retest reliability was calculated on four different samples including 25 college students, 25 outpatient rehabilitation patients, and 25 neurological patients with short time intervals (ranging from 7 days to just over 5 weeks) and also administered twice to 25 outpatient rehabilitation patients with a longer time interval of over 1 year. The temporal reliability values were reasonable (.72 to .98). The stability of the resulting profiles was also examined by administering the NIS three times to neurological patients and was found to be adequate. Validity was examined via factor analyses, scale intercorrelations, correlations with neuropsychological performance measures, and by examining the screening accuracy. In general, the validity appears to be adequate and acceptable. The revised version of the NIS has initial reports that indicate reasonable temporal reliability as well as concurrent validity with measures of the HRNB, the WAIS-R, and the WMS-R (O'Donnell, DeSoto, & DeSoto, 1993).

Screening instruments are much needed in neuropsychological assessment, as they can help identify subjects who need lengthier and more costly complete evaluations. If only for that reason, the NIS can be a useful instrument in clinical settings. The subsequent research reports indicate the promise of this instrument. Further research will help define its utility.

THE STROOP WORD–COLOR TEST

Like many neuropsychological tests, the Stroop Word–Color Test has a long and interesting history. Also, like many neuropsychological tests, the Stroop had its origins in laboratory procedures. Stroop (1935) was originally interested in a perceptual interference effect, namely, the effect of interfering perceptual information on behavior. The phenomenon of perceptual interference as measured by the Stroop has been used in cognitive, personality, psychopathology, and neuropsychology research. A recent study suggests that semantic interference and not response competition is the basis for the Stroop effect (Luo, 1999). Regardless, the scores obtained from use of the Stroop have demonstrated clinical utility for neuropsychology. Because of the heterogeneous body of literature associated with the Stroop, this section limits its discussion to neuropsychological topics. The Stroop has also been suggested as a measure of executive functioning; however, owing to its brevity and sensitivity, it may be more frequently used to screen for cognitive dysfunction. Although the Stroop has existed in several forms, unless stated otherwise we consider here only the most recent standardized form as published by the Stoelting Company (Golden, 1978b).

The Stroop is an easily administered and easily scored test. It takes less than 10 minutes to administer. The necessary materials consist of three sheets of 8½" × 11" paper. On the first sheet of paper are printed five columns of words, which are color names (*red, blue*, and *green*). The subject is asked to read aloud, in order, the words on the sheet. (In the group form, the subjects are asked to read the words silently.) The subjects are prompted to correct their incorrect responses. The score is the number of correct responses obtained in 45 seconds. The second part consists of a sheet of paper on which are printed columns of Xs in three different colors (red, blue, and green), and the subjects are asked to name the color. The administration and scoring are the same as in the first part. The third part consists of the same words as those in the first part; however, they are printed in colors different from the colors named by the words. For example, the word *red* is printed in blue ink. The subjects are asked to name the color, ignoring the word. The scoring is again based on the number of correct responses in 45 seconds.

The three raw scores are translated into standardized scores to permit comparisons across the three parts. These scores can then be transformed into ratios (C/W, COO/C) and linear combinations (C + W, CW − C). In addition, the manual suggests age corrections; however, there is insufficient information about the appropriateness (or the size) of the sample used in the derivation of these standardized scores or in the age corrections. It is clear that age corrections are needed as the interference effect shows age effects (Uttl & Graf, 1997). Ivnik, Malec, Smith, Tangalos, and Petersen (1996) provided normative information with education corrections for 750 individuals over the age of 65 years.

Reliability

Test–retest reliability has been evaluated for the three raw scores. Jensen (1965) stated that the test–retest reliability coefficient of the Word score is .79, that of the Color score is .88, and that of the Color–Word score is .71. Jensen also stated that 50 of the subjects had had a test–retest interval of a few minutes (the exact time interval was not reported), 50 subjects had had an interval of 1 day, and 336 subjects had had an interval of 1 week. However, no characteristics of the subjects are known. It should be noted that this study did not use the standardized form. Instead, tall cards similar to those used in eye exams were used at a distance of 4 feet. Also, the scores used were based on the time it took for 100 responses to be made.

Golden (1975) examined the test–retest reliability of both the group and the individual administrations. Thirty subjects were given the individual form twice, but the interval was not specified, nor were any characteristics of the subjects described. The reliability coefficients reported were .86 for the Word score, .82 for the Color score, and .73 for the Color–

Word score. The test–retest reliability was assessed for the group form. Once again, the interval and the characteristics of the subjects were not specified.

Franzen, Tishelman, Sharp, and Friedman (1987) investigated the test–retest reliability of the Stroop in a sample of 62 normal individuals. Two intervals were used: 1 week and 2 weeks. There were no significant differences between the reliability coefficients for the 1- and 2-week intervals so the data were collapsed. The coefficient values were .83 for the Word score, .738 for the Color score, and .671 for the Color–Word score. Split-plot analyses of variance indicated that there were significant increases in scores for both of the intervals. Subsequent research by Connor, Franzen, and Sharp (1988) indicated that these increases tended to become asymptotic after three administrations.

In a sense, the group and individual forms may be construed as alternate forms. Therefore, the alternate-forms reliability is a pertinent question. Golden (1975) administered both the group and the individual forms in counterbalanced order to 60 subjects whose characteristics were not described. For the Word score, the alternate-forms reliability coefficient was .85; for the Color score, the coefficient was .81; and for the Color–Word score, the coefficient was .69. The single card version has been most frequently used in clinical settings, but a single trial version where the dependent measure is response time has been used in experimental research settings and may be a more sensitive measure of selective attention in schizophrenic patients (Perlstein, Carter, Barch, & Baird, 1998).

Validity

Golden (1976b) examined the validity of the Stroop in discriminating neurologically impaired subjects from normal subjects. The neurologically impaired subjects consisted of 30 left-hemisphere-injury patients, 43 diffuse injury patients, and 31 right-hemisphere patients. All of the subjects were diagnosed by history, results on the Halstead–Reitan Neuropsychological Battery, and neurological examination. The nonneurologically impaired subjects consisted of 35 schizophrenics and 37 normals. When a discriminant-function analysis was used with the three basic scores as predictors, 88.9% of the controls and 84.6% of the neurologically impaired subjects were correctly classified, for an overall rate of 87%. A second discriminant-function analysis was performed to classify the neurologically impaired subjects into three groups that described the location of their injury. This procedure resulted in only a 56.7% accuracy-of-classification rate. None of these results have been replicated. The Golden manual (1978b) reports rules for the interpretation of scores, but none of these rules have been empirically validated. The Stroop has been shown to be sensitive to gender (Golden, 1974; Peritti, 1969, 1971), stress (Houston & Jones, 1967), and various personality measures (Golden, 1978b). Therefore, the discriminant validity of the Stroop with regard to the detection of neurological impairment needs to be addressed.

The Stroop can be used as a measure of specific or focused attention. It has been found to be sensitive to the effects of mild closed head injury (Batchelor, Harvey, & Bryant, 1995). Rojas and Bennett (1995) reported that the Stroop was able to identify subjects with and without mild brain injury, which is fairly impressive, given that the Stroop takes about 3 minutes to administer. The Stroop may have limited specificity in certain diagnostic decisions. Pachana, Boone, Miller, Cummings, and Berman (1996) reported no differences between patients with Alzheimer's versus frontotemporal dementia, although both groups of patients scored lower than normal control subjects. Although the Stroop appears to be a good measure of attention in general, it does not appear to be able to discriminate between adults with attention deficit hyperactivity disorder (ADHD) and adults with attentional problems secondary to depression (Katz, Wood, Goldstein, Auchenbach, & Geckle, 1998).

As well as being useful as a screening measure for general cognitive functioning, the Stroop can also be used as a brief measure of executive functioning. Hanes, Andrewes, Smith, and Pantelis (1996) reported that the Stroop can discriminate between normal control subjects and patients with schizophrenia, Huntington's disease, and Parkinson's disease. Furthermore, the Stroop correlated with other executive measures and not with nonexecutive measures in these subjects. Other evidence suggests that the Stroop is related to frontal circulation (Larue, Celsis, Bes, & Marc-Vergnes, 1994) and prefrontal function (Vendrell et al., 1995). Although the Stroop was correlated with other measures of executive functioning in a sample of patients with Parkinson's disease, Huntington's disease, schizophrenia, and controls, it did not separate the groups as well as the other measures, indicating some nonspecificity in relationship to etiology of impairment (Hanes et al., 1996). On the other hand, the Stroop was not related to measure of skills other than executive functioning in the same study.

The Stroop interference effect is reported to be greater in older subjects with a corresponding greater change in frontal activation as measured by EEG (West & Bell, 1997). However, there is not complete agreement as to the relationship of aging to the Stroop interference effect, as Uttl and Graf (1997) described evidence to suggest that the effect of aging may be due to generalized slowing rather than a specific prefrontal decline, a conclusion that finds additional support in a study using a different methodology (Klein, Ponds, Houx, & Jolles, 1997). The effect of aging has important clinical implications, and the Stroop has increasing rates of false-positive results in subjects over the age of 50 years (Palmer, Boone, Lesser, & Wohl, 1998). The Stroop should not be used in isolation but it can be very useful in conjunction with other measures of general cognitive efficiency and executive function. The Stroop interference effect may be dependent upon adequate reading skill, at least in children (Cox et al., 1997).

The exact construct measured by the Stroop may vary by population. Although, as noted above, the Stroop can reasonably be interpreted as reflecting executive functioning, there is also evidence to suggest that it is the aspect of cognitive speed that allows the Stroop to identify cognitive impairment (Spikman, van Zomeren, & Deelman, 1996). Generally, it is assumed that a portion of the Stroop interference effect may be due to proactive interference from the simpler early tasks to the complex third task. However, Taylor (1998) showed that when the order of tasks on the Stroop is varied, there is no difference in obtained scores, indicating that the third page of the Stroop may be used in isolation. Of course when this occurs, there can be no comparison between performance on the Color and on the Color–Word page. Henik (1996) points out the limits in logical inferences possible when comparisons are not made between the interference effect and the neutral condition.

Carl Dodrill (1978) has developed a form specifically for use in his epilepsy battery, but that has found utility in other settings. This particular form consists of a single sheet of color names printed in an inconsistent color where the colors include red, green, orange, and blue. Sacks, Clark, and Geffen (1991) developed five other alternate forms to this test and reported on the equivalency of the forms. When the six forms were administered to normal subjects in a single setting, there were single practice effects only between the first and second trials, with relatively equivalent scores otherwise. This is consistent with the research of Franzen et al. (1987) and Connor, Franzen, and Sharp (1988), who reported asymptotes to the practice effects after the second administration of the commercially available form of the Stroop.

Conclusions

The Stroop Word–Color Test is a very useful quick test of general cognitive impairment and can be helpful in the evaluation of executive function. Further examination of the effects of aging and more extensive normative information regarding older individuals and special populations would increase the utility of this simple but elegant measure. In addition, it would be useful to investigate the relationship of Stroop performance to reading ability in adults similar to that known about children. Although the original research did not indicate that separate gender-related norms were needed, recent research has indicated that at least for African-American subjects, women may be faster than men (Strickland, D'Elia, James, & Stein, 1997). When the single stimulus version was used in a very small sample, men were slower than women (Mekarski, Cutmore, & Suborski, 1996), but it is unclear whether this difference was large enough to have clinical implications.

THE NEUROBEHAVIORAL COGNITIVE STATUS EXAMINATION

The Neurobehavioral Cognitive Status Examination, or NCSE (Northern California Neurobehavioral Group, 1988) is a recently developed instrument for screening across a variety of cognitive functioning areas. Standardization data have been supplied using a sample of 119 healthy subjects between the ages of 20 and 92 years (Kiernan, Mueller, Langston, & Van Dyke, 1987). In each area a screening or "metric" item is administered. If the patient passes this item, the examiner moves on to the next area. If the item is not passed, the examiner administers a few more items tapping the same construct graduated across levels of difficulty. The areas of cognitive function tapped include Orientation, Attention, Memory, Language Repetition, Comprehension, and Naming, Visual Spatial Construction, Calculation, Abstraction, and Judgment. Raw score performance in each of these areas is translated to an impairment rating of Normal, Mild, Moderate, or Severe. Because of this increased sampling of cognitive areas, the NCSE has been suggested as an effective screening measure in psychiatric patients (Van Dyke, Mueller, & Kiernan, 1987) and in neurosurgical patients (Cammermeyer & Evans, 1988). The NCSE has been found to be useful in evaluating stroke patients in rehabilitation settings (Mysiw, Beegan, & Gatens, 1989). Osmon, Smet, Winegarden, and Gandhavadi (1992) reported that although the NCSE can discriminate between stroke patients and control subjects, it did not discriminate between left-hemisphere- and right-hemisphere-lesioned patients. Alternately, Mendez et al. (1996) found that the NCSE might be useful in discriminating between patients with Alzheimer's disease and patients with frontotemporal dementia.

Schwamm, Klein, Kiernan, Merrin, and Mueller (1987) reported that the NCSE is fairly sensitive to different forms of cognitive impairment. The NCSE appears to be more sensitive and specific than the Folstein Mini-Mental State Exam (Dey, Mahapatra, Misra, Padma, & Desai, 1997; Schwamm, Van Dyke, Kiernan, Merrin, & Mueller, 1987). However, subtest scores on the NCSE have little agreement with more extended neuropsychological measures and should therefore be considered a general screen for cognitive impairment rather than a domain-specific assessment instrument (Marcotte, van Gorp, Hinkin, & Osato, 1997).

Although the NCSE subtests theoretically sensitive to aging correlated with age in a sample of psychiatric patients, the intercorrelations among the subtests did not correspond to the construct groupings in the manual (Logue, Tupler, D'Amico, & Schmitt, 1993). The results of the NCSE when administered to a sample of patients with schizophrenia, and other major psychiatric disorders indicated that the theoretical areas of cognitive impairment in schizophrenia were reflected in relatively poorer performance in those areas for the schizophrenic patients (Mitrushina, Abara, & Blumenfeld, 1996). Although performance on the NCSE for patients with different forms of dementia was related to severity of dementia rather than type in a multisite study, there were differences in the comparisons with other forms of neurological disorder (Cammermeyer, 1997). The relation of the NCSE subtests to standardized neuropsychological tests may be moderated by population. Nabors, Millis, and Rosenthal (1997) reported that the relevant NCSE subtests correlated with the California Verbal Learning Test, the Logical Memory subtest of the WMS-R, the Token Test, the Block Design subtest of the WAIS-R, and Trails a in a sample of 45 individuals who had experienced traumatic brain injury. However, the Wisconsin Card Sorting Test did not correlate with the Reasoning subtest of the NCSE.

Meek, Clark, and Solana (1989) recommend the NCSE in the evaluation of substance abuse patients but this recommendation is not universally accepted. Fals-Stewart (1997) found that the NCSE had little agreement with the Neuropsychological Screening Battery in a sample of 51 detoxified patients with diagnoses of substance abuse.

Because the elderly may be more likely to have fatigue interfering with more lengthy evaluations and because there is an increased prevalence of cognitive impairment in elderly, it would seem that the NCSE would be very useful in this population. However, some data suggest that although there is sensitivity to cognitive impairment when using the NCSE with elderly, there may be low levels of specificity (Drane & Osato, 1998; Osato, Yang, & LaRue, 1993). Increasing the criterion from one scale in the impaired range to two scales in the impaired range resulted in an increase in specificity but lowered sensitivity in identifying cognitive impairment in the elderly (Roper, Bieliauskas, & Peterson, 1996). Use of the NCSE in a general adult population may be warranted. The provision of more extensive norms in the elderly may be helpful. Negative findings in the elderly can be interpreted with more confidence.

Karzmark (1997) examined the sensitivity and specificity of the NCSE using the results of a comprehensive neuropsychological evaluation as the criterion when four or more tests in the evaluation were determined to be in the impaired range. Subjects were 50 consecutive referrals to an outpatient clinic. The sensitivity of the NCSE was found to be .74 and its specificity was .86, but the sensitivity of the individual subtests was much lower. The specificity of the subtests was moderate and at times higher than that of the entire test (for the language skills domain).

MATTIS DEMENTIA RATING SCALE

The Mattis Dementia Rating Scale, or MDRS (Mattis, 1988) has experienced a great increase in clinical application in the recent past. It is a short collection of procedures for the assessment of cognitive dysfunction in content areas associated with dementias in the older individual. The MDRS assesses performance in the areas of Attention, Initiation/Perseveration, Construction, Conceptualization, and Memory. In addition, a Total Score can be used to determine the probable presence of a dementing condition. It should be noted that the MDRS has a relationship to age, and the use of a cutoff score can be increasingly inaccurate with advancing age (Marcopulos, McLain, & Guiliano, 1997).

Coblentz et al. (1973) reported a 1-week test–retest reliability of .97 for the Total score. Split-half reliability of the Total score is reported to be .90 (Gardner, Oliver-Munoz, Fisher, & Empting, 1981). Vitaliano et al. (1984a) reported internal consistency estimates (coefficient alpha) between .75 and .95 for the subtests.

The initial normative information is based on an extremely limited sample of 11 healthy older adults (Coblentz et al., 1973). Subsequently, Schmidt et al. (1994) published a data base on a sample of 1001 healthy Austrian adults, stratified by age (50 to 80 years old) and by education. Differences in the educational systems and other cultural factors may limit the generalizability of this data to a North American population. Despite this potential limitation, the MDRS appears to be sensitive to cognitive impairment associated with dementia. Shay et al. (1991) found that the MDRS was able to accurately classify all of their subjects with Alzheimer's dementia as having cognitive impairment, although there was some inaccuracy in identifying the level of impairment. There was a tendency to underestimate the level if impairment. Vangel and Lichtenberg (1995) reported a set of normative data based on a sample of 90 nonimpaired elderly. Their sample was drawn from an urban population where the majority of subjects were African-American. Although the MDRS Total score was correlated with both age and education, the relationship with education was largely mediated by age. Therefore, these researchers published the mean values based on age in two groups, 62 to 79 years and 80 to 95 years. These same researchers found that the Total score successfully classified 87% of the normative sample when combined with a group of 105 cognitively impaired elderly subjects. The cutoff score was 120 with a sensitivity of 74% and a specificity of 93%. Marson, Dymek, Duke, and Harrell (1997) found that the subscales of the MDRS correlated highly with conceptually related standard neuropsychological measures. However, interpretation of this study must be tempered by the fact that there was substantial overlap of method variance in the pairs of measures. For example, the Initiation/Perseveration subtest uses the same methodology as the neuropsychological measure chosen for comparison in this study, namely the Controlled Oral Word Association Test. Other normative samples include that reported by Lucas et al. (1998b), which is a large sample of relatively high functioning healthy elderly.

The Total score correlates with the Wechsler Memory Scale (Chase et al., 1984) and with the WAIS (Coblentz, et al., 1973). The MDRS can be useful in the detection of dementia. Its ability to determine severity of the impairment may be limited. In addition, although initial studies have provided moderate support for its ability to differentially diagnose between Alzheimer's disease and other dementing conditions, including Huntington's disease (Salmon, Kwo-on-Yuen, Heindel, Butters, & Thal, 1989), progressive supranuclear palsy (van der Hurk & Hodges, 1995), and Binswanger disease (Bernard et al.,

1994), none of these studies have been cross-validated. The utility of the MDRS in this regard is in need of greater empirical explication. When the total score of the MDRS is subjected to a principal-components factor analysis along with other neuropsychological measures in a sample of cognitively impaired individuals, a single factor emerges; however, a two-factor solution (general cognitive and memory factors) emerges in a sample of intact individuals (Lichtenberg, Ross, Youngblade, & Vangel, 1998). The MDRS total score appears to be an adequate measure of general cognitive functioning in the elderly.

Tests of Achievement and Aptitude

THE GENERAL APTITUDE TEST BATTERY

The General Aptitude Test Battery (GATB) is a group of tests that are used to measure nine aptitudes. Twelve tests comprise the GATB, and its composition was determined by a series of factor analyses that were conducted on a larger number of tests. Unfortunately, the factor analyses were conducted on anywhere from 9 to 27 of the tests, and at no time were all of the tests that eventually made up the GATB used in the same factor analysis. To remediate this shortcoming, Watts and Everitt (1980) conducted a maximum-likelihood factor analysis on the correlation matrix as published in the GATB manual (U.S. Employment Service, 1970). Watts and Everitt failed to replicate the original factor structure, a result that is not surprising because the correlation matrix indicates that some tests correlate more highly with tests that are not in the same aptitude factor than with tests that are in the same aptitude factor. Hammond (1984) found that the GAB measured four higher order abilities rather than the nine factors specified in the manual. The GATB has become an extremely popular instrument in employment training and is reported to be used in 35 countries with 12 different language translations (Droege, 1984).

The GATB apparently has a fair amount of utility in occupational counseling (Bemis, 1968), but its usefulness for a neuropsychologically impaired population is largely unknown. Kish (1970) reported that the General, Verbal, and Numerical aptitudes of the GATB had moderate correlations with Shipley IQ scores in a sample of 71 male inpatient alcoholics in a VA hospital. The values ranged from .71 to .12. Groff and Hubble (1981) administered the GATB and the Trail Making Test to 40 incarcerated female adult subjects who were not suspected of neurological impairment. These authors concluded that the complex cognitive functions measured by the Trail Making Test are largely unrelated to the GATB. The GATB may need to be interpreted separately for different cultural groups, at least based on information obtained from a study of the Dutch translation of the GATB and comparing immigrants to majority group Dutch native-born subjects (Nijenhuis & van der Flier, 1997). This finding is consistent with the report of Avolio and Waldman (1994), who found significant relationships of the GATB with race (Caucasian, African-American, Hispanic) even after the influence of education, experience, occupation, and age were controlled. However, the factor structure of the GATB appears to be consistent for American and Saudi Arabian subjects (Dagenais, 1990). It may be that although the scales show similar patterns of relation among themselves, the relationships to external criteria may be different. For example, in a meta-analysis of GATB studies, Rothstein and McDaniel (1993) found greater accuracy in predicting job performance in woman than in men. The relationships of test scores to external criteria do not vary simply as a function of skill level (Waldman & Avolio, 1989). Clemmons, Fraser, Dodrill, Trejo, and Freelove (1987) found that the GATB correlated moderately with the cognitive measures in the Dodrill Neuropsychological Battery for Epilepsy.

Davison, Gasser, and Ding (1996) used multidimensional scaling to obtain profile types of the GATB and suggested interpretative guidelines; however, these guidelines are in need of external validation. Because of its demonstrated validity in occupational counseling, the GATB may one day be useful for a cognitive rehabilitation. However, its reliability and validity in such a population need to be evaluated before its use can be recommended. A possibly negative indicator is that for severely handicapped subjects, the GATB scores did not predict job satisfaction as well as training ratings did (Bolton & Brookings, 1993).

THE MCCARTHY SCALES OF CHILDREN'S ABILITIES

The McCarthy Scales of Children's Abilities is a collection of 18 subtests that are grouped into six scales on a theoretical basis. The manual (McCarthy, 1972) states that the McCarthy scales are appropriate for children between the ages of 2½ and 8½. The normative sample consisted of 1032 children who were divided among 10 age groups, so that approximately 100 children were in each age group. The normative sample was stratified by sex, race, geography, father's occupation, and urban versus rural residence in accordance with census data.

The raw scores were weighted and summed to provide the scale scores. The weights were based on the author's judgment of the relative importance of the subtests and under the secondary principle that tests with larger standard deviations were given larger weights. No justification is stated for the strategy used. The McCarthy scales result in a Mental Age score as well as scores for the General Cognitive, Verbal, Perceptual Performance, Quantitative, Memory, and Motor scales.

In order to evaluate the test–retest reliability of the McCarthy scales, 125 children from the normative sample were administered the tests on two occasions, with approximately 1 month's interval. The children were fairly evenly divided into groups of 3 to 3.5 years, 5 to 5.5 years, and 7.5 to 8.5 years. The General Cognitive Index (GCI) demonstrated a reliability coefficient of .90 for all ages overall. The other subtests' reliability coefficients ranged from .75 to .89 for all ages combined. Split-half reliabilities were calculated on the same sample. The largest reliability coefficient was for the GCI an .93. The lowest values were for Memory and Motor at .79. The reliability of handedness was also assessed. Reliable hand preference was demonstrated for 61% of the 3- to 3.5-year-olds, 70% of the 5- to 5.5-year olds, and 76% of the 7.5- to 8.5-year-olds. Eye preference was demonstrated in 75% of all age groups combined. Because of our knowledge of developmental issues in laterality, this information cannot actually be used as an assessment of the reliability of the McCarthy scales.

Naglieri and Maxwell (1981) reported an evaluation of the interrater reliability of the Draw-a-Child task from the McCarthy scales. They administered the McCarthy scales to 20 mentally retarded children, 20 learning disabled children, and 20 normal children and scored the drawings independently. The overall reliability coefficient was .93, with values of .97 for the mentally retarded, .88 for the learning disabled, and .83 for the normal children. Analyses were conducted on the standard scores and produced no significant differences between scores assigned by the two authors.

The manual (McCarthy, 1972) also reported an attempt to evaluate the concurrent validity of the instrument in a small subsample of the normative group consisting of 35 children aged 6 years to 6 years, 7 months. The GCI correlated .81 with the IQ scores obtained on a Stanford–Binet. In the same group, the GCI correlated .62 with the WPPSI PIQ, .63 with the VIQ, and .71 with the FSIQ. Predictive validity was estimated by correlating the McCarthy scales with Metropolitan Achievement Test scores obtained after a 4-month interval. The values ranged from −.07 to .57. These are very disappointing correlations. The potential limits of the McCarthy scales in predicting achievement are illustrated by a correlation of .06 between the Verbal scale and the MAT Word Knowledge subtest. There have been other, more positive findings. Karr et al. (1993) found that the McCarthy and the WPPSI-R correlated moderately in a small sample of preschool and kindergarten children. Naglieri (1985) reported that the McCarthy correlated well with the PIAT in normal children aged 6 to 8 years old.

The McCarthy was able to separate 54 children with autism and other severe developmental disorders into eight subtypes (Fein, Waterhouse, Lucci, & Snyder, 1985), but the external correlates of these subtypes is in need of explication. Bickett, Reuter, and Stancin (1984) reported that although the Mental Age scores of the McCarthy correlated well with the Mental Age scores from the Stanford–Binet and the Minnesota Child Development Inventory, valid index scores for children with IQ scores in the moderately mentally retarded range could not be computed based on the tables available in the manual for the McCarthy. These researchers warn against using the McCarthy to measure intellectual level in these children.

Faust and Hollingsworth (1991) found that the McCarthy agreed well with the WPPSI-R and with the PPVT-R. In an important study for the use of this instrument in a neuropsychological population, Backman, Cornwall, Stewart, and Byrne (1989) reported that the McCarthy could predict WISC-R scores 2 years down the line in children referred for neuropsychological evaluation. Of note is the fact that the verbal measures seemed to agree least. Zucker and Copeland (1988) found that the McCarthy and the K-ABC correlated in a sample of 51 at-risk and 33 normal preschoolers. However, the K-ABC scores tended to be higher than the GCIs in the at-risk sample and tended to be lower than the GCIs in the normal sample. The McCarthy showed concurrent validity with the Reading and Mathematics subtests of the California Achievement Test as well as teacher ratings of learning ability (Sturner, Funk, & Green, 1984) and with the WPPSI in Mexican-American children enrolled in Head Start (Valencia & Rothwell, 1984). The McCarthy administered before school entry predicted California Achievement Test scores in kindergarten, first grade, and second grade (Funk, Sturner, & Green, 1986). Massoth (1985) conducted a follow-up study over a 5-year period and found that the McCarthy administered in kindergarten predicted course grades and Comprehensive Testing Program achievement test scores in the sixth grade, a truly impressive finding.

Naglieri and Maxwell (1981) compared the age equivalents obtained from the Draw-a-Child task of the McCarthy scales to WISC-R IQS and found that there were no significant differences between the two. The authors concluded that this task had adequate concurrent validity. Gomez-Benito and Forns-Santacana (1993) found moderate correlations and little difference in score level in a comparison of the McCarthy with the Columbia Mental Maturity Scale.

Tivnan and Pillemer (1978) administered the McCarthy scales to 30 female and 36 male preschool children aged 4 years, 7 months to 5 years, 7 months to evaluate the influence of gender on performance. The female subjects scored consistently higher on each of the subtests. The differences were significant only for the Motor scale, but the use of the binomial test resulted in a significantly different pattern of scores for the two sexes.

Several factor analyses have been conducted on the McCarthy scales. Hollenbeck (1972), Kaufman (1975b), Kaufman and DiCuio (1975), and Kaufman and Hollenbeck (1973) each used the normative sample as their data. Although they used slightly different techniques and groupings of the subjects (e.g., separating them by race or age), the resulting factor structures were very similar. Teeter (1984) replicated the Kaufman factor structure results in a sample of 105 kindergarten children. Keith and Bolen (1980) conducted a factor analysis on a separate sample of 300 children who had been referred for education evaluation. These authors used both principal-factor and principal-components factor analyses, employing the varimax rotation method each time. When they used Harman's coefficient of congruence, it appeared that only two of the factors reported in the normative sample had been replicated. This finding indicates that the factor structure of the McCarthy scales may depend, at least partly, on characteristics of the sample.

Because the McCarthy scales are more often used in evaluating children who evidence learning difficulties, analyses with these subjects are likely to provide more useful information than analyses of the factor structure in normal children. In a factor analysis of 141 first-grade students, the solution seemed to support verbal and perceptual-performance factors, but not quantitative and memory factors. When Gomez-Benito and Forns-Santacana (1996) factor analyzed the McCarthy scores from a sample of 128 Spanish children, they were unable to provide a match to previous factor solutions using Tucker's coefficient of congruence. Factor analysis of data from a sample of British children indicated support for the General Cognitive, Perceptual-Performance, Verbal, and Motor indices, but not the Memory index (Trueman, Lynch, & Branthwaite, 1984).

Just as with the Wechsler scales of intellectual functioning, short forms of the McCarthy have been suggested. Valencia (1984) found that the full-length GCI and the Kaufman short form predicted equally well the Comprehensive Test of Basic Skills-Level C, Form S scores in a sample of 31 English-speaking and 43 Spanish-speaking Mexican-American second-grade students. Harrington and Jennings (1986) investigated the relationship of short form (GCI) values to the long form values as well as computed the test–retest reliability estimates. The short form suggested by Kaufman provided the strongest relationship to the full-length GCI values and also provided the highest test–retest correlations. Furthermore, the Kaufman short form of the McCarthy correlates well with the Stanford–Binet IV (Karr, Carvajal, and Palmer, 1992).

In general, despite their widespread use, the McCarthy scales are in need of further evaluation for reliability and validity. They seem to be especially applicable in normal or mildly impaired populations and may have limited application in significantly impaired children. This is a significant drawback in neuropsychological practice. The most important consideration is the now aging normative and standardization sample on which the instrument is based.

THE PEABODY INDIVIDUAL ACHIEVEMENT TEST

The Peabody Individual Achievement Test (PIAT) is made up of five subtests that measure achievement in different areas related to school performance. Therefore, it is often used in the assessment of children who demonstrate problems in academic performance. The manual (Dunn & Markwardt, 1970) reports that the standardized sample consisted of approximately 200 children at each of 13 grade levels, for a total sample of 2884 subjects. The sample was stratified to reflect data from the 1967 U.S. Census.

The manual reports test–retest data for groups of between 50 and 75 children in kindergarten and Grades 1, 3, 5, 8, and 12. The retest interval was about 1 month. The reliability coefficients had a median value of .78, with a low value of .42 for the Spelling test in the kindergarten sample and a high of .94 for the Reading Recognition test in the Grade 3 sample.

Using a 6-month interval, Lamanna and Ysseldyke (1973) reported test–retest reliability coefficients ranging from .44 for the Mathematics test to .81 for the Reading Recognition test in a sample of 58 first-grade children. Naglieri and Pfeiffer (1983) investigated the test–retest reliability of the PIAT in a sample of 36 children who had been referred for evaluation. With a mean interval of 12 months and a standard deviation of 8.3 months, there were no significant differences between the standardized scores obtained, and the correlation values were comparable to those obtained in the normative sample.

Wilson and Spangler (1974) investigated the internal consistency reliability of the PIAT in a sample of 83 children who had been referred for evaluation. There was high reliability, with values ranging from .95 to .97. Dean (1977) investigated the PIAT's internal consistency reliability in a sample of 30 Mexican-American and 30 Anglo children. He found no significant differences between the two samples, and he found values that were not significantly different from the normative data.

Reynolds and Gutkin (1980) presented tables of values for determining the significance of differences between the individual scale scores and the mean of all other scale scores. These tables can be very helpful in evaluating the presence of relative strengths and weaknesses.

The manual (Dunn & Markwardt, 1970) further reported that the content validity of the initial pool of 300 items was sufficient, a value judgment at best. However, items were discarded for reasons of item difficulty and discrimination, as well as for reasons of low item-total correlation values. The resulting scales have not been evaluated for content validity or for the adequacy of their sampling of the domain of interest. Concurrent validity was measured by correlating the PIAT with Peabody Picture Vocabulary Test IQS. The correlation values ranged from a high of .68 for the General Information Test to a low of .40 for the Spelling Test.

Soethe (1972) evaluated the concurrent validity of the PIAT by comparing it with the Wide Range Achievement Test (WRAT) and the WISC. There were 40 subjects in this study: 26 males and 14 females, all of whom had been referred for evaluation. He divided the subjects into a group of 13 normal subjects (IQ ~ 86 and no difference of more than 10 points between WISC and WRAT scores), a group of 12 reading disabled subjects (IQ > 86 and at least a 10-point difference between WISC and WRAT Reading scores), and 15 retarded subjects (WISC < 85). The PIAT correlated more highly with the WISC than with the WRAT, and the highest correlation was only .71. The higher values were obtained in the normal sample; the retarded sample had correlation values in the .44 to .60 range. This study raises serious questions about the construct validity of the PIAT, as it correlated more with a test of IQ than with another achievement test. In addition, the PIAT has different sensitivity across different levels of intelligence, limiting its general applicability. These results are supported by the research of Simpson (1982), who concluded that the PIAT was not valid for use with retarded subjects.

In another attempt to investigate the concurrent validity of the PIAT, Sanner and McManis (1978) administered the PIAT and the Stanford Achievement tests to a sample of 21 third- and 22 sixth-grade children who were average achievers. The Spearman rank-order correlations for the two tests were in the range of .42 to .88, and there were significant differences in the grade equivalents on the two tests.

Wilson and Spangler (1974) correlated grade equivalence scores obtained from the PIAT with IQ scores obtained from the Stanford–Binet, the WISC, and the Peabody Picture Vocabulary Test (PPVT), after first partialing out the influence of age. Different subjects were evaluated in each of these analyses. For the WISC ($n = 63$), the correlation was .58; for the Stanford–Binet ($n = 17$), the correlation was .49; and for the PPVT ($n = 57$), the correlation was .48. These results are encouraging because of their moderate correlations, indicating that there is a relationship between the PIAT and IQ. The moderate size of the coefficients also indicates that the PIAT is not a measure of IQ. Further evidence is needed to demonstrate that it is a measure of achievement.

Even though intelligence tests and achievement tests are intended to measure different constructs, much of the research that attempts to investigate the concurrent validity of the PIAT compares it with the WISC. Naglieri and Pfeiffer (1983) correlated WISC-R IQ scores with scores on the PIAT subtests in a sample of 36 children who had been referred for evaluation. All of the correlations with the VIQ were significant and in the range of .57 to .69. The only significant correlation for the PIQ was with the PIAT Mathematics scale (.42). All of the PIAT subtests correlated significantly with the FSIQ, ranging from .46 to .64. Beck, Lindsey, and Facziende (1979) correlated the General Information subtest of the PIAT with the Information subtest of the WISC-R in a sample of 100 children who had been referred for evaluation. The overall correlation coefficient had a value of .76; however, the correlation for a subsample of 43 children with IQS under 69 was .43, a finding indicating that the relationship between the PIAT and measures of IQ may be different for different levels of ability.

Wickoff (1979) administered both the WISC-R and the PIAT to a sample of 123 male and 57 female children who had been referred for evaluation. However, instead of stopping after correlating the two tests, he conducted factor analyses to attempt to see if the PIAT offered information beyond that gained from the use of the WISC-R. In the first factor analysis, he used both the PIAT and the WISC-R subtest scores. In a principle-factor analysis with varimax rotation, he decided that the four-factor solution was most meaningful and interpreted the factor as the three traditional WISC-R factors plus a word recognition factor formed largely by the PIAT. A separate factor analysis of only the PIAT data by means of the same methodology resulted in a two-factor solution that Wickoff interpreted as word recognition and school-related knowledge.

Dean (1977) analyzed the PIAT and WISC-R data from 100 Mexican American and 100 Anglo children to investigate the factor structure of the PIAT. However, instead of factor analysis, Dean used canonical correlation. He found that 72% of the variability in the

PIAT was redundant with 45% of the variability in the WISC-R in the Anglo sample. In the Mexican-American sample, 63% of the variability in the PIAT was redundant, with 43% of the variability in the WISC-R. Dean concluded that there was a substantial amount of overlap between the two tests. Although not consistent with Wickoff's conclusions, these results are consistent with Wickoff's data, as the first two factors in his four-factor solution had heavy loadings from both of the tests. If the PIAT is highly related to tests of intelligence, then the construct validity of the test is questionable. More research is needed on more varied samples than are referred to researchers for evaluation. In addition, the concurrent validity of the test needs to be assessed by comparison with other measures of achievement rather than with tests of intelligence.

WOODCOCK–JOHNSON PSYCHOEDUCATIONAL BATTERY

The Woodcock–Johnson Psychoeducational Battery-Revised (Woodcock & Johnson, 1989, 1990) is a revision and extension of the original Woodcock–Johnson into a battery of Tests of Achievement (Woodcock & Mather, 1989, 1990) and a battery of Tests of Cognitive Ability (Woodcock & Mather, 1989, 1990). The Tests of Achievement assess academic skills including the molar areas of Humanities and Social Science as well as the component skills for Reading (Word Attack, Letter–Word Identification, Reading Comprehension) and Mathematics. The Tests of Cognitive Ability evaluate aspects of mental processing that are hypothesized to be independent of academic experience although necessary for success in an academic setting.

The normative base is extensive, consisting of 705 preschool subjects, 3245 subjects between kindergarten and 12th grade, 916 subjects in college, and 1493 adult subjects not in college (up to the age of 90 years). Subjects were sampled from the four basic census regions of the country as well as from different sizes of community and different socio-economic status levels. The manuals report high internal consistency reliabilities values. Later investigations of test–retest reliability indicated that this may be lower than desired for tests on which educational decisions are to be made (Breen, 1984).

The manual reports that concurrent validity was assessed via correlations with the Boehm, the Bracken, the Kaufman Assessment Battery for Children, and the PPVT-R for a group of children approximately 3 years old. Concurrent validity was assessed via correlations with the BASIS, the KABC, the Kaufman Test of Educational Achievement, the PIAT, and the WRAT-R for children approximately 9 years old. Finally, concurrent validity was assessed via the BASIS, the KTEA, the PIAT, and the WRAT-R for subjects approximately 17 years old. Construct validity was evaluated through an examination of the scales intercorrelation matrix. For an instrument that is so sophisticated in its design and standardization, the extent of information regarding reliability and validity data is disappointing. A basic study found that the Test of Cognitive Ability correlated well with the WISC-R in a sample of gifted students, but the Woodcock–Johnson subtest seemed to have fairly high relationships to verbal measures (Ingram & Hakari, 1985).

McGrew and Murphy (1995) examined the factor relationships in the standardization sample for the Cognitive Tests and concluded that they possess both sufficient factor loadings and sufficient unique information to allow clinical interpretation. The concurrent validity of the Woodcock–Johnson Tests of Cognitive Ability was examined by administering it to 30 normal children aged 3 to 5 years old. The children were also administered the WPPSI-R. Although the Woodcock–Johnson Broad Cognitive Ability score correlated with the WPPSI-R Full Scale IQ (FSIQ) and Verbal IQ (VIQ), the Woodcock–Johnson score was 4.5 standard scores lower than the FSIQ of the WPPSI-R. The Performance IQ (PIQ) of the WPPSI-R correlated with the Woodcock–Johnson Visual Processing cluster score (Harrington, Kimbrell, & Dai, 1992). Unlike the relationship to the WISC-R where the FSIQ is generally higher than the Broad Cognitive Ability score (Coleman & Harmer, 1985; Estabrook, 1984), Gregg and Hoy (1985) found little difference between the WAIS and the Tests of Cognitive Ability in a sample of learning disabled college students. College freshman with histories of learning disabilities scored more poorly than those without learning disability (Dalke, 1988). Arffa, Rider, and Cummings (1984) reported that there are no differences between the Woodcock–Johnson and Stanford–Binet IQ scores, at least for their sample of 60 African-American preschool children. Correlations with the WISC-R suggest that the Woodcock–Johnson is highly verbally loaded (Phelps, Rosso, & Falasco, 1984, 1985).

Using confirmatory factor analysis, Ysseldyke (1990) concluded that the Woodcock–Johnson had a good fit to the Horn–Cattell theory of crystallized and fluid intelligence. McGrew (1987) reported factor analyses conducted on the school-aged standardization subjects and reported factors similar to those originally identified by Woodcock. Later studies did not find the same consistency of support for the hypothesized factor structure. Kaufman and O'Neal (1988a,b) found that a two-factor solution was viable for preschool children and a three-factor solution was viable for grade school on up to adult subjects. These researchers did not find specific factors in support of the construct validity of the Woodcock–Johnson theoretical composition. When the Cognitive Battery alone was factor analyzed, a single factor sufficed for the preschool sample and three-factor solution was interpreted for the school-aged children and adults. The loadings of the subtests on the general intelligence factor (g) increased with age. Using a sample of 286 conduct disordered adolescents, Rosso and Phelps (1988) did not find the perceptual speed and memory factors reported in the manual. Telzrow and Harr (1987) reported that the hypothesized measures of nonverbal processes in the Woodcock–Johnson, namely the Reasoning cluster and the subtests that comprise it, have a fairly high relationship to language measures.

In a study that has particular relevance for neuropsychological evaluations, Tupper (1990) examined the Tests of Cognitive Ability in a sample of individuals who had experienced closed head injury. He found that coma duration was related to scores on the Perceptual Speed and Memory clusters. Furthermore, although the Halstead Category Test did not correlate with any of the cluster scores, the Trail Making Test did, providing limited support for the use of the Woodcock–Johnson in neuropsychological evaluations. Aram and Ekelman (1988) reported that children with either left-hemisphere or right-hemisphere lesions performed more poorly on the reasoning, perceptual speed, and memory clusters scores. When the children were examined in terms of site of lesion, the children with left-hemisphere lesions performed more poorly on the written language cluster and children with right-hemisphere lesions performed more poorly on the reading, math, and written language clusters.

Salthouse (1998) reported that the age-related changes in performance on the Woodcock–Johnson may be correlated, and that interpretation of individual skill level changes should be tempered in light of that information. Laurent (1997) found gender-related differences on the Visual Matching, Picture Vocabulary, and Cross Out subtests in a sample of 121 college students, but did not find significant gender differences for other subtests. Gender-related differences were not reported in the manual. If these college age differences are cross-validated and generalized to another age group, it may be necessary to develop norms separated by gender. Bolen, Kimball, Hall, and Webster (1997) reported the Woodcock–Johnson is significantly different from the Learning Efficiency Test-II in terms of visual processing scores, but not in terms of auditory processing scores. However, the two sets of auditory processing scores did not correlate. More information about the underlying constructs of both of these tests is necessary to interpret these findings. The Tests of Achievement appear to have more support for their use in neuropsychological populations, especially when used to evaluate aspects of academic skills once the determination of organic etiology has been made.

THE WIDE-RANGE ACHIEVEMENT TEST

The Wide Range Achievement Test (WRAT) was originally designed to provide an estimate of children's level of functioning in the academic areas of Reading, Spelling, and Arithmetic (Jastek & Jastek, 1978). The raw scores can be translated into grade-level ratings, standard T-scores, and percentiles. The manual states that, in norming the test, no attempt was made to provide national representation. The normative sample was composed of 1800 children and 200 adults. The small sample of adults was biased toward younger subjects, and Ivnik et al. (1996) have complemented this data with normative values of the WRAT-R Reading subtest with education corrections in a sample of 750 subjects over the age of 65 years.

The manual reports split-half reliability values of .94 (Arithmetic), .96 (Spelling), and .98 (Reading) for children between the ages of 5 and 11 years and comparable values for subjects between the ages of 12 and 24. The sample sizes are not described. The manual also reports an overall alternate-form reliability of .90. Unfortunately, not enough information is given in any of these studies to allow a consideration of their generalizability. The WRAT-R demonstrated adequate stability in adolescent psychiatric inpatients (Dura, Myers, & Freathy, 1989).

Few validity studies are reported in the manual. In one of these studies, there was a correlation of .78 between WRAT Reading scores and teachers' informal evaluations on a 9-point scale. In a sample of 74 children aged 5 to 15 years, the Reading scale correlated .81, the Spelling scale correlated .74, and the Arithmetic scale correlated .84 with the California Mental Maturity Scale.

Because of the paucity of reliability information, Woodward, Santa Barbara, and Roverts (1975) investigated the test–retest reliability in a sample of 106 children who were enrolled in special-education classes for the emotionally disturbed or for slow learners. These children were between the ages of 5 and 12 years. There were two test–retest intervals: 2 weeks (63 subjects) and 22 weeks (43 subjects). The correlation coefficients were reasonably high, ranging from .87 to .98. The tests for changes in absolute level of scores resulted in significant differences in Spelling scores for the 2-week period and for the Reading scores at 22 weeks. The results for the 22-week interval are problematic, as one would expect changes as a result of the special education intervention. Johnson, Fisher,

Rhodes, and Booth (1996a) reported good stability of the WRAT-R across 200 days in a set of drug abusing subjects. Wiese, Struer, Piersel, and Schwarting (1987) report good stability in mentally retarded children as well as independent variance from the WISC-R.

Silverstein (1980) evaluated the 1976 and 1978 norms presented in the manual, looking at both scaled grade equivalents and scaled raw scores. He found that the grade equivalents were not comparable across the two sets of norms, even though they were based on the same subjects, particularly for Grades 8 to 11. The standard score comparisons resulted in small but systematic differences. He therefore recommended that retest situations use the same sets of norms in comparing scores. These results were in agreement with those of Sattler and Feldman (1981). Naglieri and Parks (1980) found similar results in evaluating the scores of 115 Hopi Indian children. They also conducted a 1-year test–retest study with the same subjects and reported moderate correlation coefficients ranging from .60 to .70. The WRAT-R is significantly related to the highest level of school grade achieved (Morgan, Tidwell, & Takarae, 1996).

Because the WRAT can be enthusiastically recommended for use with neurologically impaired adults as an index of cortical function, reliability and validity studies need to be conducted on these populations. Initial information regarding the relationship between the WRAT-R and the achievement-oriented subtests of the Luria–Nebraska Neuropsychological Battery indicates strong correlations and good agreement in classification (Nagel, Harrell, & Gray, 1997). The WRAT and WAIS-R correlate highly in young adults (Spruill & Beck, 1986) and in patients with dementia (Margolis, Greenlief, & Taylor, 1985). Sullivan and Hawkins (1995) reported that the Spelling subtest of the WRAT-R could be shortened by half in a neuropsychological population and still provide equivalent classification. In a sample of children with learning disabilities, the WRAT-R Arithmetic but not the Spelling or Reading subtests correlated with the WISC-III IQ scores (Slate, Jones, Graham, & Bower, 1994).

Furthermore, the test appears to be useful in the process of estimating premorbid function (see section on premorbid estimates), although Johnstone and Wilhelm (1996) demonstrated greater utility in predicting premorbid function in individuals who show decline or stability in intellectual capacity than for subjects who demonstrate improvement.

THE WECHSLER INDIVIDUAL ACHIEVEMENT TEST

The Wechsler Individual Achievement Test, or WIAT, attempts to determine achievement in the areas of language skills and mathematics. It does not evaluate skill or knowledge in content areas such as the sciences or humanities. It is normed on individuals from 6 years old through adulthood. It was co-normed on a subsample of children who were administered the WISC-III. Additional norms are available in a subsample of the WAIS-III standardization sample. In this way, it is possible to make statistical comparisons to scores obtained in an intellectual evaluation. There is also a method for evaluating and rating test related behaviors. Initial studies indicate that the factor of the WIAT may be different for children with different levels of score on indices of attention, cooperation, and avoidance (Maller, Konold, & Glutting, 1998), but the empirical consequences for interpretation are not known.

Because of the controversy regarding cultural bias in the assessment of intelligence, it is important to investigate the possible presence of test bias in the WIAT. One study that evaluated this possibility determined that there was no differential predictability of WIAT scores from WISC-III FSIQ across Caucasian, Hispanic, and African-American children, nor was there bias in a comparison of male and female children (Weiss & Prifitera, 1995).

The temporal stability of the standardized scores from the WIAT was fairly high in a sample of 224 children with learning disability evaluated twice across a period of 3 years (Gaskill & Brantley, 1996).

A short form of the WIAT known as the WIAT Screener is available. The main determination that can be concluded from use of the WIAT is whether the full form should be administered; however, Anolik and Stevens (1998) reported that the verbal and math scores from the WIAT Screener, along with scores from the WISC-III, predicted success for adolescents in a behavior modification program in a group home.

The WIAT is an especially promising instrument because of its co-norming with the WISC-III, the WAIS-III, and the WMS-III. However, to date only research with child populations has been reported. Parallel and even more extensive empirical investigation is necessary to describe the utility of this instrument in adult populations and in neuropsychological samples.

Methods for Evaluating the Validity of Test Scores

There is another burgeoning area of assessment methods, namely the development and evaluation of methods to estimate the validity of inferences drawn from the test data. In essence, these are meta-methods to determine the validity of the test data themselves as well as to determine the validity of the inferences drawn from the test data. The estimation of premorbid functioning against which to evaluate change demonstrated by the present scores and the estimation of the level of effort exhibited by the subject are two areas that have attracted much recent attention. Because premorbid scores from a prior test session are rarely available, methods have been developed to estimate premorbid functioning. Because the interpretation of scores requires an assumption of optimal effort, methods have been developed to assess the level of effort and aid decisions regarding the possible presence of response bias.

Excellent previous reviews regarding premorbid estimates include Crawford (1992), who provided a good explication of the use of the National Adult Reading Test, especially in a British population, and Vanderploeg (1994), who provided an excellent discussion of the demographic methods and the use of WAIS-R subtest scores in the context of a discussion of the applicability of the WAIS-R to clinical neuropsychological assessment. A later review is that of Franzen, Burgess, and Smith-Seemiller (1997). Excellent reviews regarding the detection of response bias include Franzen, Iverson, and McCracken (1990) and Nies and Sweet (1994).

THE BEST PERFORMANCE METHOD

Muriel Lezak (1995) described the clinical method to examine scores obtained on a collection of tests based on the deficit measurement model. For many reasons, including the assumption of heterogeneity of skill level and the assumption of equally error-free measurement across different tests, this method is not recommended (Franzen, Burgess, & Smith-Seemiller, 1997). Another approach is based on the "hold–don't hold" method to estimate premorbid ability based on the individual's current performance on a measure that is considered to be relatively resistant to neurological impairment. Most such approaches can be grouped into two major types: those based on patterns of performance on the Wechsler Intelligence scales, and those based on word reading ability.

Wechsler (1958) described a Deterioration Quotient, obtained by subtracting age scale scores for "don't hold" subtests from the sum of scaled scores for the "hold" tests. The "hold" tests are Vocabulary, Information, Object Assembly, and Picture Completion. The "don't hold" tests are Block Design, Digit Symbol, Digit Span, and Similarities. Other variations on this approach have been described. The choice of hold tests should be based on the type of impairment under consideration. For example, although Picture Completion is included among the hold tests, lesions of the occipital or parietal lobes may result in relative decrements in score on this subtest. A related approach is to develop formulas based on hold versus no-hold tests to distinguish a specific neurological condition from healthy controls. An example of this is the Fuld profile, also referred to as the "cholinergic profile." As discussed in the chapter on the WAIS-R, this method has many drawbacks and cannot be enthusiastically recommended.

Like other methods of estimating premorbid level of functioning, these approaches are also vulnerable to criticism based on their assumption that an individual functioned at similar levels across all areas of brain–behavior functions. It has also been found that some of the traditional "hold" subtests (such as Vocabulary) are more sensitive to acquired cerebral dysfunction than had been commonly assumed (Larrabee, Largen, and Levin, 1985b).

DEMOGRAPHIC VARIABLE METHODS

Demographic variables such as social class and education are correlated with scores on intelligence tests, and may provide information on an individual's premorbid level of intellectual functioning (Crawford, 1992). Actuarial methods have been developed for predicting premorbid intellectual ability utilizing demographic information. More recently, methods have been described that utilize a combination of demographic information and performance on tests that are considered to be relatively insensitive to the effects of acquired brain injury (Kareken, Gur, & Saykin, 1995). The use of actuarial approaches utilizing demographic information for predicting premorbid intellectual ability is attractive for a number of reasons. A frequently cited reason is that actuarial approaches are superior to clinical judgment because of the actuarial methods' higher rates of interrater reliability (Barona, Reynolds, & Chastain, 1984). Also, while it can be argued that a patient's performance on putative "hold" tests or abilities can be affected by acquired brain injury, demographic background is unaffected.

Wilson et al. (1978) developed regression equations to predict premorbid Wechsler Adult Intelligence Scale IQ scores by using data on age, sex, race, education, and occupation from the 1955 WAIS standardization sample. The resulting squared multiple correlations were somewhat disappointingly low: .54, .53, and .42 for the WAIS Full Scale, Verbal, and Performance IQ scores, respectively. Wilson et al. (1978) also provided a method for correcting for differences between the educational levels of the standardization sample and educational levels that were more current at the time their formulae were developed.

Attempts to empirically evaluate the Wilson et al. (1978) formula have been reported with equivocal results. For example, Karzmark, Heaton, Grant, and Matthews (1985) used a sample of 491 normal control subjects and found that when a standard of matching the actual IQ scores within one standard error of estimate (SEE) was used, 70% accuracy was achieved. Klesges, Sanchez, and Stanton (1981) reported that although the Wilson predictions and obtained WAIS IQ scores correlated significantly in their samples of 60 psychiatric inpatients and 106 outpatients referred for Workman's Compensation evaluations, there were significant differences in the exact IQ values predicted. Using the educational correction factor suggested by Wilson et al. (1978) resulted in accurate predictions for the outpatient sample but overprediction for the inpatient sample.

Karzmark et al. (1985) found that there was 66% accuracy when using only education as a predictor, and they recommended using only the simpler formula. Wilson, Rosenbaum, and Brown (1979) compared the 1978 Wilson formula with the Wechsler deterioration index in predicting which subjects could be classified as impaired or normal using discriminant function analysis and reported that the Wechsler method resulted in 62% accuracy of classification and the 1978 Wilson formula resulted in 73% accuracy.

Because the revised WAIS-R IQ scores are not directly comparable to those obtained with the original WAIS, IQ estimates obtained using Wilson's method would be expected to have attenuated validity in predicting WAIS-R IQ scores. Therefore, Barona, Reynolds, and Chastain (1984) utilized a similar approach to develop regression equations for predicting IQ scores on the Wechsler Adult Intelligence Scale-Revised. Education, race, and occupation were found to be the most powerful predictors in each equation. The squared multiple correlations between the equations obtained and actual WAIS-R IQ scores were .38, .24, and .36 for the Verbal, Performance, and Full Scale IQ scores, respectively. These equations will tend to artificially lower or raise the estimated scores for individuals who fall outside of one standard deviation of the population mean IQ. They note that this is particularly likely to be problematic if premorbid IQ scores are above 120 or below 69. Hale, Dingemans, Wekking, and Cornelissen (1993) found that the Wilson formula underpredicted IQ in a sample of 27 depressed and 34 nondepressed Dutch subjects.

Because of the restriction of range inherent in the use of the Barona and Wilson estimates, most IQ predictions will cluster in the average to high average range (Sweet, Moberg, & Tovian, 1990). Sweet et al. (1990) found that neither the Barona nor the Wilson formulas performed any better than chance in classifying subjects into IQ ranges. Ryan and Prifitera (1990), in a study of the Barona estimates' accuracy in predicting short form IQ scores, found it to be fairly reliable in predicting IQ scores between 90 and 109. Eppinger, Craig, Adams, and Parsons (1987) did find a strong correlation between formula-estimated IQ and obtained WAIS-R IQ in a sample of neurologically normal patients. The percentage of subjects who were correctly classified (as indicated by an obtained IQ score that was within one standard error of estimate of their predicted IQ score) ranged from 69% to 75%. In a study addressing the clinical utility of the Wilson equations, Bolter, Gouvier, Veneklasen, and Long (1982) did find a significant correlation between IQ estimates and measured IQ scores, but also found the method's accuracy to be limited in terms of predicting groups of head-injured patients and controls. Bolter et al. (1982) argued against the use of the Wilson equations with head trauma patients. In an examination of premorbid estimates of Performance IQ (PIQ) and Verbal IQ (VIQ) in the same subjects Gouvier, Bolter, Veneklasen, and Long (1983) reported similar results.

Paolo, Ryan, Troster, and Hilmer (1996c) generated demographic formulae using the standardization sample of the WAIS-R and an additional sample of 130 normal individuals aged 75 to 96 years. The derived formulae in a subset of the sample predicted IQ scores well in the cross-validation sample. When the two standardization samples were combined, the formulae performed well in a sample of 247 individuals with acquired neurological impairment. The authors provided confidence intervals for individual subtests. The original demographic regression formulae were based on a United States sample. Crawford and Allan (1997) replicated this approach in a sample of individuals in the United Kingdom. They found that PIQ was least well predicted, similar to the U.S. results.

Application of Demographic Formulae to Children

The issue of estimating premorbid level of functioning in children has received much less attention and activity than has the counterpart issue in adult populations. Reynolds and Gutkin (1979) modeled an approach on the same methods used in the adult literature on the Wechsler Intelligence Scale for Children-Revised or WISC-R. Klesges and Sanchez (1981) failed to replicate these results in a sample of 76 neurologically impaired and 23 unimpaired children. Only 35% of the impaired subjects had IQ discrepancies consistent with Reynolds and Gutkin's (1979) suggestions, and 12% of the unimpaired children had similar discrepancies. Klesges (1982) reported similarly disappointing findings in a separate sample of 35 nonimpaired and 26 neurologically impaired children.

Application of Demographic Formulae to the Elderly

There are two Barona formulae, one based on a regression prediction of IQ using the entire WAIS-R standardization sample (Barona et al., 1984) and another based on a regression prediction using black and white subjects over the age of 19 years from the WAIS-R standardization sample (Barona and Chastain, 1986). Attempts to cross-validate the 1984 formula have generally found that IQ tends to be overestimated in normal subjects (Eppinger et al., 1987), especially when Full Scale IQ (FSIQ) is less than 89, although there may actually be a tendency to underestimate IQ when FSIQ is above 110 (Ryan & Prifitera, 1987). Paolo and Ryan (1992) found that the 1984 Barona formula significantly underestimated VIQ and FSIQ in elderly healthy subjects while the 1986 Barona formula significantly underestimated only VIQ. In subjects with neurological disease, both the 1984 and 1986 formulae resulted in significantly greater predicted IQ scores than obtained IQ scores, which is the desired direction of difference when some deterioration has taken place. Ryan, Paolo, and Dunn (1995b) reported on the relationship between demographic variables and performance on the WAIS-R in a sample of 130 healthy individuals over the age of 75 years. Although these authors did not develop regression equations to predict IQ values, they did provide a table of mean IQ scores by levels of gender, education, and preretirement occupation for their overall sample. The authors suggest that values in this table can be used as rough estimates of predicted IQ against which to compare obtained IQ in older individuals. No empirical evaluation of this strategy was provided.

Combining Demographic and Test Values

Krull, Scott, and Sherer (1995) used demographic information and performance on the Vocabulary and Picture Completion subtests of the WAIS-R to predict IQ values, by dividing the standardization sample for the WAIS-R in half. Age, race, education, occupation, and the two subtest scores were used to predict VIQ, PIQ, and FSIQ in the first half of the sample. The resulting formula were then cross-validated using the second half of the sample. Sixty-three percent of the cross-validation sample had predicted IQ values in the same Wechsler category (Average, Low Average, etc.) as their obtained IQ values. Furthermore, 91% of the subjects had predicted FSIQ values within a confidence interval calculated on the basis of the SEE, and the problems of restricted range seen with the pure demographic method were not encountered here.

Vanderploeg and Schinka (1995a) reported the results of an investigation regarding their BEST-3 method. This method combines demographic and WAIS-R subtest scores in a multiple regression formula to predict premorbid IQ. These researchers (Vanderploeg & Schinka, 1995) then applied the method to a sample of neurologically impaired individuals and matched control subjects drawn from the standardization sample for the WAIS-R. They reported that although the Barona and the BEST-3 methods both resulted in different values for IQ than were obtained when the WAIS-R was actually administered to the neurologically impaired individuals, the BEST-3 method had the greater relationship to group membership when discrepancy scores (predicted minus actual IQ) were calculated. Taken together, these two studies indicate the potential utility of using some combined prediction method. Axelrod, Vanderploeg, and Schinka (1999) examined and compared five different methods of estimating premorbid IQ, all of which involved some aspect of demographic regression equation or estimates based on WAIS-R subtest scores. These methods included the Barona, Reynolds, and Chastain (1984) demographic regression, and the combined demographic and performance methods of Vanderploeg and Schinka (1995); Vanderploeg, Schinka, and Axelrod (1996); Krull, Scott, and Sherer (1995); and Williamson, Krull, and Scott (1996). The methods used to compare these formulae included correlations with obtained IQ scores in a control sample, comparison of the magnitude of difference with obtained IQ scores in a clinical sample, comparison of differences between the predicted score for the clinical sample and the obtained IQ scores for a matched control group, and the ability of the difference scores to differentiate between the clinical and the control sample. No differences were found among the methods. It would be further interesting to compare current performance measures such as the NART with the regression formulae. Helmes (1996) calculated the Barona IQ estimates for a sample of 866 Canadian individuals over the age of 65 years and found an approximately normal distribution with a mean of 100, as expected. However, for subjects over the age of 85 years, Helmes suggested that a small correction factor be added.

Some methods, such as the Oklahoma Premorbid Intelligence Estimation (OPIE), involve a combination of current performance and demographic variables. Scott, Krull, Williamson, Adams, and Iverson (1997) found that the OPIE predicted IQ scores in the extreme ranges without the degree of underprediction or overprediction seen with both the WRAT-R and the Barona formula. The subjects used included patients with closed head injury, penetrating head injury, dementia, cerebrovascular accident (CVA), neoplasm, and epilepsy.

Yeates and Taylor (1997) attempted to develop a combination-demographic regression method that also used parental ratings of premorbid academic functioning as a predictor. The other three predictor variables were maternal ethnicity, socioeconomic status, and performance on the Word Identification subtest of the Woodcock–Johnson test of Achievement-Revised. After deriving the optimal formula weights from a sample of children with orthopedic injuries, the formulae were used to predict prorated WISC-III Performance IQ, score on the Beery Visual Motor Integration test, and total correct score from the Children's CVLT. Although the children who had the most severe traumatic brain injury (TBI) had the largest discrepancies between predicted and obtained scores, the amount of variance accounted for by these independent variables ranged from 13% to 45%. Clearly this method is not sufficient for clinical practice, although it does represent a positive beginning.

WORD READING TASKS

Sight reading irregularly spelled words is thought to be a reasonable estimate of premorbid intellectual function because this task correlates well with Verbal IQ in non-neurologically impaired subjects (Lastine-Sobecks, Jackson, & Paolo, 1998), and performance on the task is relatively stable over time, even with the acquisition of neurological impairment (for a review of the rationale and methods, see Franzen, Burges, & Smith-Seemiller, 1997). A Dutch version of the National Adult Reading Test or NART resulted in stable estimates in normal elderly over a 6-year period and declined only 3 IQ points in individuals who were normal at the first evaluation but suspected of dementia at the 6-year follow-up. Individuals who had moderate or severe dementia at the 6-year follow-up demonstrated a 15-point decline in estimated IQ, indicating the limits of using this procedure in cases of severe cognitive impairment.

Reading ability is more resistant to dementia than is the WAIS Vocabulary subtest, and the reading of irregular words is more resistant to cognitive decline than is reading of regular words; word reading taps previous knowledge while minimizing the demands on current cognitive capacity. The Schonell Graded Word Reading Test (GWRT) (Schonell, 1942) proved to be a reasonable predictor of premorbid intellect in adults with average intelligence. However, it was originally designed to assess children's reading ability, and a ceiling effect occurred when used with adults of above average intelligence (predicted IQ scores had a ceiling of 115) (Schonell, 1942).

Nelson and McKenna (1975) developed the National Adult Reading Test, or NART, a reading test for irregularly spelled words. Ruddle and Bradshaw (1982) attempted a replication of Nelson and McKenna's (1975) study with a sample of 78 healthy subjects and 75 patients with heterogeneous cortical diseases, and reported generally consistent findings. Nelson (1982) subsequently standardized the NART on an unrelated series of 120 inpatients, 20 to 70 years of age, all of whom were diagnosed as having an extracerebral disorder, finding that age and social status did not have a significant effect on word reading ability.

Nelson and O'Connell (1978) derived regression equations to predict IQ from NART scores. Applying the prediction formula to a sample of 40 patients with bilateral cortical atrophy resulted in values 10 to 14 points higher than the obtained prorated IQ scores. These results seem to indicate that word reading skill is relatively preserved in acquired neurological impairment, but the exact accuracy of the IQ estimates may be less optimal. The prediction equations had broad standard errors of estimate (SEE). The SEE values were 7.6 for VIQ, 9.4 for PIQ, and 7.6 for FSIQ.

Starr, Whalley, Inch, and Shering (1992) investigated NART IQ estimates, Folstein Mini-Mental State Exam (MMSE) scores, and age in a sample of 598 healthy, unmedicated community dwelling elderly. Subjects ranged in age from 70 to 88 years. There was no correlation between age and NART IQ estimates, even though MMSE scores correlated both with age and with NART IQ estimates. Apparently, the variances shared by the MMSE with age and by the MMSE with the NART are orthogonal to each other.

The sensitivity of the NART to a progressive dementing condition is another way of evaluating its utility as a premorbid estimate. There are two basic methods to evaluate this proposition. The first is to determine whether there is a relationship between dementia severity and NART score. The second and more convincing method is to test progressive dementia subjects longitudinally. In an example of the first method, O'Carroll and Gillead (1986) reported that no such relationship was found in a sample of 30 dementia patients with heterogeneous diagnoses. These same authors reported that the Mill Hill Vocabulary test was similarly not related to the degree of cognitive impairment. Nebes, Martin, and Horn (1984) reported that although the average score on the NART was higher for a sample of 20 healthy elderly than it was for a sample of 20 demented individuals, this difference was not significant. However, a more recent study using the North American version of the NART found that in comparing normal healthy aged to older individuals with very mild or mild dementia, there were significant differences in NART performance. Furthermore, performance on the NART was correlated with performance on measures of semantic memory (Storandt, Stone, & LaBarge, 1995). The seeming difference in study results may be partly attributable to the sample size used. There were a total of 213 subjects in the Storandt, Stone, and Labarge (1995) study; 40 subjects in the Nebes, Martin, and Horn (1984) study; and 30 subjects in the O'Carroll and Gillead (1986) study.

O'Connell, Baikie, and Whittick (1987) administered the NART twice over a year interval to a sample of 30 subjects diagnosed with dementia. NART scores declined modestly, but the difference was not significant. Hart, Smith, and Swash (1986) found that although the NART was better than either the WAIS Vocabulary subtest or the GWRT in predicting IQ in a sample of 20 patients with Alzheimer's disease and 15 healthy elderly subjects, there were significant differences in NART scores between the two groups. The NART might still be sensitive to acquired impairment.

Stebbins, Gilley, Wilson, Bernard, and Fox (1990) administered the NART to a sample of 199 patients with probable senile dementia of the Alzheimer's type (SDAT), multi-infarct dementia, or a mixture of the two and to a sample of 26 healthy elderly. These researchers found that NART scores covaried with dementia severity. Stebbins, Gilley, Wilson, Bernard, and Fox (1990) found that the NART covaried with language disturbance. Fromm, Holland, Nebes, and Oakley (1991) found that the NART scores declined over time with progressive dementia, although the decline was slight, especially in the early and middle stages of the disease process.

Although the use of the NART in the United States has been criticized because of the differences in British pronunciation, some studies have examined the NART in a North American population. Carswell, Graves, Snow, and Tierney (1997) attempted to predict performance on the WAIS-R based on scores on the NART administered after an interval of 5 years in a cross-validation of the regression formula reported by Paolo and Ryan (1992). They found that a decline of at least 16 points was necessary for the NART to detect declines. A second formula using both NART error scores and WAIS-R Vocabulary scores showed improved accuracy, but this method is in need of a separate cross-validation study.

As with much of the research using the NART in other populations, the research using older populations was initially conducted with subjects from Great Britain. Ryan and Paolo

(1992) found shrinkage in attempting to extend these findings to a North American population. Sharpe and O'Carroll (1991) administered the NART to 20 healthy Canadian elderly and 20 Canadian elderly with dementia. NART IQ predictions were significantly higher than the Vocabulary IQ predictions, which were significantly higher than the obtained IQs.

Blair and Spreen (1989) modified The NART for use on a North American population. This instrument, initially referred to as the National Adult Reading Test-Revised (NART-R; Blair and Spreen, 1989), eventually became referred to as the North American Adult Reading Test (NAART: Spreen and Strauss, 1998). There are actually three major versions of the NART available. The first is the original version as developed by Nelson (hereafter referred to as the NART). The second is the Blair and Spreen version, which will be referred to as the NAART. The third is the version of Grober and Sliwinski (1991), which will be discussed later and will be referred to as the AMNART.

Wiens, Bryan, and Crossen (1993) provided further utility of the NAART by predicting current WAIS-R FSIQ scores in a sample of 302 healthy job applicants for civil service positions in the Pacific Northwest of the United States. In an analysis between NAART estimated FSIQ and the individual WAIS-R Verbal subtest, the highest correlations were with the Vocabulary ($r = .54$) and Information ($r = .50$) subtests. Comparatively, the NAART estimated FSIQ and Performance subtests were greatest with Block Design ($r = .20$) and Object Assembly ($r = .17$). Similar to what is shown by other studies, the WAIS-R FSIQ and NAART estimated FSIQ was .46 ($p < .001$) (Wiens et al., 1993).

Blair and Spreen's (1989) modification of the NART consisted of adding words and then performing a series of item analyses that eventually resulted in finding the words that proved to be the best predictors of the WAIS-R FSIQ. Items with correlations higher than .2 were considered acceptable as suggested by Nunnally (1978). During subsequent analyses using the 61 words, the coefficient alpha estimate of internal consistency was .935. The correlation between the NAART and WAIS-R FSIQ was .75 ($r = .75$). O'Carroll (1987) had previously demonstrated that the original NART had a relatively high degree of inter-rater reliability. In this study, 10 clinicians rated 12 consecutive outpatients whose responses to the NART were audiotaped. Of the 45 resulting correlations, 44 were greater than $r = .90$. However, raters were asked to return only a total score of correct responses; an item analysis to see whether particular words led to a greater degree of interrater disagreement would have provided more useful information. Blair and Spreen's (1989) measure of interscorer reliability with the NAART, which was based on the performance of 20 Canadian subjects, was nearly perfect, $r = .99$. While this is another indication that previous experience with the NAART is not a prerequisite for reliable scoring, these authors failed to reveal the number of raters, the number of scores, and how the analysis was performed. Correlations of the NAART and the WAIS-R (using all of the WAIS-R subtests) VIQ, PIQ, and FSIQ were .83, .40, and .75, respectively. The NAART is relatively insensitive to level of dementia, especially in comparison to a method of estimating IQ using the Vocabulary and Block Design subtests of the WAIS-R (Maddrey, Cullum, Weiner, & Filley, 1996). Yet another version of the NART is the NART-Revised (Blair & Spreen, 1989), which was developed on a Canadian sample. Raguet, Campbell, Berry, Schmitt, and Smith (1996) found that the NART-R has acceptable reliability over a 1-year period. The NART-R and Barona formula are fairly equivalent in predicting FSIQ 1 year prior, but the average between the Barona and the NART-R appear to be superior to either alone.

Grober and Sliwinski (1991) administered the North American version of the NART (AMNART) to a sample of 230 healthy urban elderly. An abbreviated version of the WAIS-R consisting of the Information, Vocabulary, and Digit Span subtests was prorated to obtain VIQ estimates. After removing five words that had low item-total correlations, the 45-item score was used, along with education, to predict prorated VIQ in the two samples produced by halving the original sample. The predicted VIQs were correlated with prorated VIQs separately for each sample. The prediction equation from neither sample was superior, so the entire sample was used to develop a prediction equation that was then applied to a sample of 25 individuals with dementia. The predicted VIQs in this demented sample were lower than the prorated VIQs by a minimum of 10 points. In contrast, this same magnitude of difference was observed in only 105 of the healthy subjects.

Lastine-Sobecks, Jackson, and Paolo (1998) tested 34 healthy control subjects and found a partial correlation of $-.68$ between VIQ and AMNART performance in a multiple-choice format. Smith, Bohac, Ivnik, and Malec (1997a) examined 271 older individuals who had been tested twice using the WAIS-R across a period of an average of 3.7 years. If the WAIS-R VIQ was stable across the two sessions, the AMNART score from the second occasion was regressed against the VIQ (using MOANS transformations) from the first session. This formula was used to compare premorbid MOANS VIQ in a sample of 24 individuals who had demonstrated cognitive decline over a period of 5 years. The discrepancy between predicted and actual premorbid VIQ exceeded 5 points in only 19% of the sample. Gladsjo, Heaton, Palmer, Taylor, and Jests (1999a) reported that the AMNART provides predictions of WAIS-R FSIQ, VIQ, and CVLT Learning score beyond that provided by demographic formula, but did not offer incremental information related to recall of a short story paragraph narrative or of the HRNB AIR. Performance on the AMNART may decline with increasing cognitive impairment in progressive dementia, but correction based on score on the Folstein Mini-Mental State Exam may obviate these declines (Taylor et al., 1996b).

Thus far, although the NART has shown to have promise as an instrument that is specifically designed to provide premorbid estimates of IQ, there are limitations. First, the NART was standardized on a British population and the studies derived thus far have been conducted with British subjects. Secondarily, the NART was compared against the WAIS. Currently, the WAIS has been revised and the WAIS-R is used in research and practice. To date, there has been no revision of the British version of the NART.

Berry et al. (1994) also recognized that a small sample of Americans were used in studying the NAART and cross-validated this instrument with an older American sample who had a mean age of 68 years. NAART errors were used to estimate WAIS-R IQ scores, which were then compared to actual WAIS-R scores obtained an average of 3.5 years earlier. NAART estimated IQ scores correlated with WAIS-R IQ scores (FSIQ $r = .70$; VIQ $r = .68$; PIQ $r = .61$; all p values $< .05$) (Berry et al., 1994).

Beardsall and Brayne (1990) proposed a short form of the NART. They found that people who score lower than 12 points on the first 30 items of the NART are unlikely to improve their performance by completing the test. A formula is used to predict scores for people who score between 12 and 20 correct on the first 30 items. People who score more than 20 correct should be administered the entire test. The predicted and obtained scores correlated .95 in a sample of 20 subjects with dementia and correlated .93 in a sample of 52 depressed elderly.

PREMORBID ESTIMATES USING OTHER TESTS OF CURRENT ABILITY

Zachary, Crumpton, and Spiegel (1985) reported that the Shipley Institute of Living Scale can be used to predict WAIS-R IQ with good accuracy in the mid-range of IQ values, but with less accuracy for IQs in the above average to superior range. The estimates were based on current IQ values, and there has been no empirical evaluation of the application of this method to subjects with neurological impairment.

Yet another method involves the use of a test similar to the NART in that it also involves word reading, namely the Wide-Range Achievement Test-Revised Initial studies indicate that the WRAT-R may be less likely to overpredict IQ in the lower ranges than is the NART, although the WRAT-R is just as likely to underpredict IQ in the upper ranges (Wiens, Bryan, & Crossen, 1993). Kareken, Gur, and Saykin (1995) subsequently reported that the WRAT-R was fairly accurate in predicting WAIS-R IQ, and that the inclusion of parental education level and race increased the accuracy. However, the subjects in this study were all nonimpaired, and the application to a sample with decreased cognitive skill is still necessary.

The Wide-Range Achievement Test-Revised Reading subtest is correlated with IQ in normal subjects even when the influence of demographic variables is controlled statistically, indicating that the WRAT-R may offer information beyond that provided by the use of demographic formulae such as the Barona (Kareken et al., 1995). When subjects were administered either the WRAT-R or the WRAT-3 as well as the WAIS-R over an average interval of 28 months, subjects with decline in FSIQ did not show changes in WRAT-R/3, indicating the potential utility of this instrument. The WRAT-R appears to accurately predict premorbid FSIQ in cocaine abusing subjects with average to low average FSIQ (Ollo, Lindquist, Alim, & Deutsch, 1995). The WRAT-R Reading subtest did not change in subjects who demonstrated intellectual decline over a 2-year period and furthermore correlated with the WAIS-R IQ scores obtained at the time of the first administration (Johnstone & Wilhelm, 1996).

Johnstone, Hexum, and Ashkanazi (1995) used the WRAT-R Reading subtests as an estimate of premorbid intelligence and then compared the standard (z) scores obtained for measures of memory (WMS-R), intelligence (WAIS-R), and general cognitive function (Trail Making Test). By subtracting obtained z scores from estimated scores, the authors calculated the amount of decline in head injury patients.

PREMORBID ESTIMATES OF OTHER SKILL AREAS

In one of the few studies to investigate the use of demographic methods in predicting performance in areas other than intellectual functioning, Karzmark, Heaton, Grant, and Matthews (1985) reported on the development of a formula to predict score on the average impairment rating (AIR) of the Halstead–Reitan Neuropsychological Battery (HRNB). The formula was developed on a sample of 370 normal control subjects and cross-validated on a separate sample of 121 normal control subjects. Klesges and Troster (1987) later applied the formula to a sample of 141 neurologically impaired subjects and 83 nonimpaired subjects. Following the suggested guidelines of Karzmark et al. (1985), namely that an estimated–obtained difference of at least .45 in the AIR would be suggestive of neurological impairment, Klesges and Troster (1987) reported a 61% correct classification rate. Unfortunately, there have been no follow-up studies using this approach.

The estimation of premorbid IQ is certainly an important question in clinical practice; however, the information derived from this process may not always provide explicit information about premorbid estimates of other skill areas. As noted previously in the discussion of the limitations of using the best subtest performance to predict overall IQ, there might be significant variability among levels of skills in a single individual. Furthermore, the relationship between IQ and skill level in other content areas is not well explicated. One would need some form of objective algorithm for estimating level of memory performance from the results of estimates of intellectual function. Optimally, this method would also involve reliability estimates or confidence intervals applied around the predicted values. Regression formulae to predict performance on the Wechsler Memory Scale-Revised from performance on the WAIS-R can help provide estimates of premorbid function. However, a preferable method would be to develop prediction formulae based directly upon the relationship between some assessment device relatively insensitive to acquired neurological impairment and the memory instrument of interest.

Without a comparable relationship of memory to another skill, Schlosser and Ivison (1989) attempted to develop premorbid estimates of WMS performance based upon word reading skills using the NART and GWRT. They administered the three instruments to a sample of 65 healthy Australian individuals between the ages of 65 and 89 years. Total raw score on the WMS was calculated from a regression formula using age and NART scores as predictors and from another regression formula that used age, NART scores, and GWRT scores as predictors. When the formula was applied to a sample of 16 patients with SDAT, the discrepancy between predicted and obtained WMS score, only 12.5% of the subjects with dementia scored within the range of discrepancies exhibited by the healthy subjects. There did not seem to be a difference between the formula that used the NART and the formula that used both the NART and the GWRT in terms of correlation value or standard error of prediction. However, the combined formula had a wider range of possible predicted WMS MQs (70 to 129 for 69-year-olds) than did the formula that used only the NART (100 to 133 for 69-year-olds).

Many prediction methods actually estimate intelligence scores and use these in comparison to current performance on other measures. Although this basic premise can be criticized on the basis of diffractionation of skills, Tremont, Hoffman, Scott, and Adams (1998) found support for the premise in data that suggest that WAIS-R tends to correlate with HRNB performance even at above average levels. Graves, Carswell, and Snow (1999) reviewed 22 studies in which either a demographic regression formula or a present ability (sight reading) method was used to predict premorbid level of functioning. By calculating the standard error of estimate and applying it to the obtained–predicted differences reported in each study, these researchers found that to have a sensitivity of 80%, the observed–predicted values must exceed an average of 25 points for the demographic methods and 20 points for the sight reading methods. However, it should also be noted that specificity would be higher at these criteria.

Comparison of NAART and WRAT-R

Johnstone, Callahan, Kapila, and Bouman (1996) compared the NAART with the Reading subtest from the WRAT-R in a sample of 118 individuals with TBI, 37 individuals with dementia, and 77 individuals with varied neurological impairment. Both the WRAT-R and the NAART tended to underestimate IQ in the upper ranges (> 110) and both tended to overestimate IQ in the lower ranges (< 90). However, because the WAIS-R IQ scores were obtained concurrently with the NAART and WRAT-R, this study speaks more to the ability to estimate current IQ than to the ability to estimate premorbid IQ. The exception is in the finding that there is underprediction in the upper IQ ranges as having a premorbid estimate that is less than the postmorbid measurement, which is certainly problematic.

There may be differential utility of different methods for different neuropsychological domains. Johnstone et al. (1997) found that premorbid estimates using educational level provided greater estimates of impairment for the WAIS-R FIQ and for motor measures, but that use of the WRAT-R Reading subtests provided greater estimates of impairment for the Trail Making Test and a greater degree of differentiation among neuropsychological skill areas, allowing greater determination of relative strengths and weaknesses.

Intellectual Correlates Scale

The Intellectual Correlates Scale (ICS) is a self-report instrument that assesses attitudes, beliefs, and interests that have been found to correlate with level of intelligence. The basic rationale is that these variables would not change much with cognitive decline and would therefore provide an estimate of optimal premorbid level of intellectual functioning. Schlottman and Johnson (1991) found that the ICS correlated with the WAIS-R in control subjects and predicted higher than obtained values in individuals with acquired neurological impairment. The standard errors of estimate were approximately 10 IQ points. Perez, Schlottman, Holloway, and Ozolins (1996) administered the ICS and WAIS-R to four groups of 20 subjects each: control, right-hemisphere, left-hemisphere, and diffuse injury. In addition, the Barona formulae were used to estimate premorbid IQ scores. There were no differences between estimated and obtained IQ scores for the control group, but there were significant differences between predicted and obtained IQ scores in each of the clinical groups. A negative indicator for the ICS is that the 1-year temporal stability is low (Raguet, Campbell, Berry, Schmitt, & Smith, 1996).

Tests of vocabulary have sometimes been invoked as estimates of premorbid intellectual functioning. The Shipley Institute of Living Scale is discussed as an estimate of current intellectual functioning in the chapter on general measures of intelligence. The Shipley has also been used as an estimate of premorbid functioning. Yuspeh, Vanderploeg, and Kershaw (1998) provide normative data related to the Shipley and its corresponding WAIS-R Full Scale IQ scores derived from a sample of 383 community-dwelling normal control subjects between the ages of 60 and 94 years. There was no relationship between age and Shipley score. Zachary, Crumpton, and Spiegel (1985) developed a regression equation to provide estimates of WAIS-R IQ from Shipley Vocabulary scores. Although useful, the application of this information requires a demonstration that Shipley scores remain relatively intact in the presence of cognitive impairment.

Conclusions Regarding Premorbid Prediction

There are many difficulties in estimating premorbid functioning and on the development of instruments and methods to achieve this goal. Chief among them is the ephemerality of the construct itself. However, this is an extremely important component of clinical assessment, for the interpretation of the rest of the data hinges on this information. Currently, no one single method can be assumed to be superior to other methods. Future research may develop methods to predict premorbid function in skill-specific areas. For the meanwhile, it may be necessary to use multiple methods and check for agreement among them.

EVALUATING THE PRESENCE OF NEGATIVE RESPONSE BIAS

Perhaps in no other area of clinical neuropsychological assessment have we witnessed such phenomenal growth in assessment methods. Unfortunately, some of these methods do not receive cross-validation efforts or attempts to gain information regarding performance under varying conditions. This chapter considers only those methods that have received significant attention. Early reviews include Franzen, Iverson, & McCracken (1990). An excellent later review can be found in Nies & Sweet (1994) who recommended a multi-dimensional, multimethod approach.

Most malingering studies involve the production of symptoms of closed head injury, because that is the condition that is most likely to be involved in legal disputes; however, it is also possible that other clinical conditions could be dissimulated. There may not be much difference in presentation. Klimczak, Donovick, and Burright (1997) reported little difference between the performance of subjects malingering the effects of closed head injury and subjects malingering the effects of multiple sclerosis. One of the difficulties both in the research and in clinical practice is that frank malingering is probably much less common than exaggeration of deficit in the presence of actual impairment (Palmer, Boone, Allman, & Castro, 1995). Similarly, although tests of cognitive function have received the most attention in detection of malingering, several of the self-report instruments related to neurobehavioral impairment may also be sensitive to simulation of symptoms (Wong, Regennitter, & Barrios, 1994). An early set of studies by Faust and colleagues (Faust, Hart, & Guilmette, 1988a; Faust, Hart, Guilmette, & Arkes, 1988b) indicated large inaccuracies in the ability of neuropsychologists to identify simulated malingering. Subsequent research by Trueblood and Binder (1997) indicated improvement in the capacity of neuropsychologists to identify malingering in clinical cases of malingering; however, the inclusion of data from forced choice tests of malingering did not substantially increase accuracy. Clearly more research is needed to evaluate the incremental validity of these tests.

Tests of Malingering and Effort

The Letter Memory Test (LMT) is a computer administered test that relies upon manipulation of face difficulty. The tests takes 15 minutes for administration. There are two facets of difficulty for which different levels are provided: the number of letters to be remembered (3, 4, or 5) and the number of choices (2, 3, or 4) in the recognition procedure. The initial report (Inman, Vickery, Lamb, Edwards, & Smith, 1998) is favorable in terms of sensitivity and specificity.

Yet another computerized assessment method for the evaluation of less than optimal effort involves a word stem completion and priming task. Student analog malingerers could be differentiated from students performing optimally in the research report (Davis et al., 1997b). This method has promise particularly because it does not involve a memory task, but external validity and generalization need to be investigated. Another task also computerized and also developed by the same group of researchers involves category classification; however, the study investigating this instrument included 10 amnesiac patients as well as student analog malingerers (Davis, King, Bloodworth, Spring, & Klebe, 1997a).

The 48-Pictures Test

Chouinard and Rouleau (1997) evaluated the effectiveness of a recognition test for pictorial information which had been originally designed for clinical purposes. This procedure discriminated between suspected and analog malingerers and clinical patients with a 96% correct classification rate using discriminant function analysis with the 48-Pictures Test, the immediate recall of the Rey–Osterrieth Complex Figure, and the immediate recognition procedures of the Rey Auditory–Verbal Learning Test. Three simulators and one clinical patient were misidentified. Cross-validation is necessary at this point.

Schagen, Schmand, de Sterke, and Lindeboom (1997) examined a Dutch-language forced choice test of memory. By manipulating the typicality of the choices, the chance performance of the test (and therefore the cutoffs to identify malingered performance) is more difficult to determine. These researchers report 100% classification of memory impaired subjects and analog malingerers. This method shows promise, especially since there is evidence that it may be simple to avoid detection on some of the early detection devices.

Paced Auditory Serial Addition Test

Analog malingerers tend to perform more poorly than individuals with closed head injury, but only 55% of the subjects were accurately classified in a comparison with individuals with closed head injury. There was a false-positive rate of 36%. Adding an auditory reaction time task greatly increased the specificity (Strauss, Spellacy, Hunter, & Berry, 1994). The PASAT may provide some useful information in the evaluation of negative response bias, but the test alone is insufficient in identifying malingering subjects.

Cognitive Behavioral Driver's Inventory

The Cognitive Behavioral Driver's Inventory is a computerized instrument to evaluate neuropsychological aspects related to the operation of motor vehicles. Because it includes measures of response time and accuracy, it might be possible to develop indices to estimate the probability of malingered effort on this test. Initial research (Ray et al., 1997) indicates that in classifying subjects as malingering college students or as truly impaired patients, the CDBI has very high specificity (>98%) and high sensitivity (>90%). Further cross-validation and investigations of clinical malingerers is warranted in further examining this instrument.

Prigatano and Amin (1993) presented consistent data in a sample of five known malingerers. Prigatano, Smason, Lamb, and Bortz (1997) subsequently cross-validated the capacity of the DMT to differentiate those malingerers from a sample of individuals with moderate to severe closed head injury, aphasia, or frontal or temporal dysfunction. However, the DMT could not reliably discriminate the malingerers from individuals with Alzheimer's dementia, which may limit the clinical utility of this approach in an elderly population. Rosenfeld, Sweet, Chuang, Ellwanger, and Song (1996) modified the Hiscock DMT to include the concurrent recording of event-related potentials which appeared to have provided additional information, but the technology involved may not be readily available in most clinic settings.

Guilmette, Hart, and Guiliano (1993) and Guilmette, Hart, Guiliano, and Leininger (1993) suggested that a cutoff of less than 90% correctly classifies malingerers, but Back et al. (1996) indicated that 27% of their sample of schizophrenic patients were misclassified using that cutoff. Rather than malingering being the underlying construct tapped by this procedure, it may be the Hiscock and Hiscock procedure is sensitive to that poor effort or motivation. The clinical decision of malingering requires greater amounts of information.

Denney (1996) developed symptom validity testing applied to remote memory for events reported to be under amnesia. This method has limited applicability due to the individual nature of the remote autobiographical data.

21-Item Wordlist

The symptom validity approach has also been refined using word lists (Wiggins & Brandt, 1988). The 21-Item Test (Iverson, Franzen, & McCracken, 1991, 1994) consists of 21 words that are presented orally, following which the patient is instructed to freely recall as many words as possible. The patient is then instructed to identify the target words within a two-alternative forced-choice procedure. In analog studies, the rates of detecting experimental malingerers have ranged from 20% to 80% depending on which cutoff scores were used (Frederick, Sarafaty, Johnston, & Powel, 1994; Iverson et al., 1991, 1994; Iverson & Franzen, 1996). The 21-Item Test takes approximately 5 minutes to administer and score. This test can be used at the beginning of the evaluation as a rapid screen for biased effort. Arnett and Franzen (1997) report that the 21-Item Wordlist is fairly specific even in a sample of significantly memory impaired subjects.

Wechsler Adult Intelligence Scale-Revised

There may be characteristic profiles associated with incomplete effort on the WAIS-R. Mittenberg, Theroux-Fichera, Zielinski, Fichera, and Heilbronner (1995) found that a discriminant function could classify head injury patients and analogs malingerers. Furthermore, using a formula of age-corrected scale score on the Vocabulary subtest minus score on the Digit Span subtest, 75% of the analog malingerers and 79% of the patients were correctly classified. Millis, Ross, and Ricker (1998) attempted to replicate these findings in a sample of head injury patients and patients involved in litigation who were judged to have given incomplete effort on the basis of the Recognition Memory Test. Examining the receiver operating characteristic curve of the subtest difference score resulted in an optimal cutoff that correctly classified 90% of the subjects.

Hiscock and Hiscock's Digit Memory Test

Prigatano and Amin (1993) presented consistent data in a sample of five known malingerers. Prigatano, Smason, Lamb, and Bortz (1997) subsequently cross-validated the capacity of the DMT to differentiate those malingerers from a sample of individuals with moderate to severe closed head injury, aphasia, or frontal or temporal dysfunction. However, the DMT could not reliably discriminate the malingerers from individuals with Alzheimer's dementia, which may limit the clinical utility of this approach in an elderly population. Rosenfeld et al. (1996) modified the Hiscock DMT to include the concurrent recording of event-related potentials which appeared to have provided additional information, but the technology involved may not be readily available in most clinic settings.

Guilmette et al. (1993, 1994) suggested that a cutoff of less than 90% correctly classifies malingerers, but Back et al. (1996) indicate that 27% of their sample of schizophrenic patients were misclassified using that cutoff. Rather than malingering being the underlying construct tapped by this procedure, it may be that the Hiscock and Hiscock procedure is sensitive to that poor effort or motivation. The clinical decision of malingering requires greater amounts of information.

Portland Digit Recognition

Similar to the DMT, the PDRT shows a subject a list of numbers and then requires the subject to choose which of the numbers he or she had seen before. Rose, Hall, Szalda-Petree, and Bach (1998) computerized the procedure and reports fairly accurate identification when response latency as well as accuracy is included as a criterion measure. Binder and Kelly (1996) collected data from previous reports regarding the PDRT and provided information regarding the distributions of scores across samples of neurologically impaired subjects with and without financial incentive as well as a small sample of analog malingerers. Perhaps the most important aspect of this collection of data is the finding that the use of less than chance performance as a cutoff is not sensitive. This is an important point that derives support from other forced choice tests as well. Although early conceptualizations of interpretation of forced choice procedures suggested chance performance levels as the cutoff, each individual test needs to have its own empirically derived cutoffs.

The PDRT appears to be relatively less sensitive to the effects of coaching in comparison to the 21-Item Wordlist, the Nonverbal Forced Choice Test (actually the Test of Nonverbal Intelligence with norms for malingered performance), and Rey's Dot Counting Test. The PDRT was able to correctly identify 70% of the coached malingerers.

Denny (1996) developed symptom validity testing applied to remote memory for events reported to be under amnesia. This method has limited applicability due to the individual nature of the remote autobiographical data.

Rey 15-Item Test

Millis and Kler (1995) report that the Memorization of Fifteen Items Test may have adequate specificity, but poor sensitivity. Back et al. (1996) report that the Memorization of 15 Items Test misclassifies schizophrenic patients as malingerers (13% of their sample). Greiffenstein, Baker, and Gola (1996a) reported that the Rey Memory for 15 Items Test can separate probable malingerers from actually impaired subjects but with lower sensitivity (64% to 69% depending upon the scoring system) than specificity (72% to 77%). Arnett, Hammeke, and Schwartz (1995) reported a similar pattern of very low sensitivity and high specificity in comparing neurological patients to simulators even in a new set of quantitative and qualitative indices. The issue may be related to the sensitivity of the 15 Items test to actual memory impairment, although generally severely impaired memory performance is necessary to affect the score on the 15 Items test (Morgan, 1991).

The Dot Counting Test procedure which was also suggested by Rey has been evaluated by Paul, Franzen, Cohen, and Fremouw (1992), who examined the reliability and validity found that using all six possible indices from the DCT resulted in 100% identification of analog malingerers. Subsequent research by Binks, Gouvier, and Waters (1997) indicated that the DCT could discriminate between clinical patients and analog malingerers even when those malingerers were given general information regarding effective simulation techniques. However, in a sample of schizophrenic patients, 13% were classified as malingering on the basis of the DCT. It may be that malingering is not the construct underlying the DCT and 15-Item Test, but instead low motivation or poor effort. Further research in larger clinical populations is warranted, but current research supports the use of the DCT in a battery of other techniques.

The Test of Memory Malingering

The Test of Memory Malingering (TOMM) is a test involving recognition memory for pictorial stimuli. Initial data regarding normative samples indicates that the TOMM is not influenced by demographic variables (Tombaugh, 1997) and may be fairly sensitive and specific for malingered performance (Rees, Tombaugh, Gansler, & Moczynski, 1998). However, information regarding its relative accuracy and well as cross-validation information would be helpful.

Pattern Analysis

Although it is not technically a test, examination of the pattern of results may also be helpful in determining nonoptimal effort. Greiffenstein, Baker, and Gola (1996b) reported atypical patterns of performance on motor measures (grip strength < finger tapping < grooved pegboard) among patients with postconcussive syndrome as opposed to patients with documented closed head injury. Rapport, Farchione, Goleman, and Axelrod (1998) evaluated the performance of control subjects, naive subjects instructed to malinger, and subjects instructed to malinger who also received information regarding the typical effects of brain injury. However these researchers failed to find the same pattern in their sample of malingerers. This method (examination of pattern) has the benefit of not requiring generalization from a test specifically designed to evaluate to the tests of interest in the construct being examined.

Digit Span

The maximum span on digit span forward is relatively impervious to acquired neurological impairment. The effect of neurological impairment appears to be more highly related to the consistency of accuracy on this task. Greiffenstein, Baker, and Gola (1994) found that by adding the maximum span correct on both trials for forward and backward digit span and comparing this to a cutoff of 7 points, probable malingerers could be separated from persons assumed to be genuinely impaired. A subsequent comparison of persons with severe traumatic brain injury and patients with presumed negative response bias showed the same results (Greiffenstein, Gola, & Baker, 1995). Using performance on a forced choice memory task as criterion, Meyers and Volbrecht (1998b) reported a 78% specificity and 95% sensitivity for the Digit Span index.

Conclusions Regarding Response Bias

The evaluation of response bias is a relatively new area but it is also an extremely important area. All clinical evaluation should contain some aspect of evaluating level of effort rather than assuming it. Etcoff and Kampfer (1996) presented suggestions for incorporating tests of effort in clinical evaluations. Suffice it to say that although no single measure is totally accurate, the clinician who does not use some form, and optimally, multiple methods of evaluating level of effort, may be risking the integrity of the data obtained. Each individual test needs to have its own empirically derived set of cutoffs and not rely on comparison to chance performance levels. In addition, the performance of the test under varying degrees of prevalence needs to be specified with false-positive and false-negative rates described in the context of positive predictive validity and negative predictive validity.

The Assessment of Child Neuropsychological Function

One of the areas in which there has been significant development and activity is in the realm of child neuropsychological assessment. In the past, the assessment of children depended upon the availability of child norms for adult instruments. This approach was always decried as being inappropriate, but there was a lack of child instruments otherwise available. The exception was, of course, the Wechsler Intelligence Scale for Children which can be viewed as a downward extension of the Wechsler adult scales. The optimal situation would be for an instrument to be developed out of a consideration of the types of referral questions asked in child assessment cases, using age-appropriate stimuli, reflecting developmentally relevant domains and methods, and possessing adequate age-related norms. The ideal is always brighter than the real, but significant progress has been accomplished in recent years.

Some of the instruments used for child assessment have been discussed in the chapters on the WISC and on achievement tests. In addition, the children's forms of the Halstead–Reitan and Luria–Nebraska Neuropsychological Batteries were already discussed in that chapter. This discussion is related only to those instruments specifically developed for child neuropsychological assessment.

WIDE-RANGE ASSESSMENT OF MEMORY AND LEARNING

The Wide-Range Assessment of Memory and Learning (WRAML) is a multiple subtest instrument designed to measure both verbal auditory and visual aspects of memory in children (Sheslow & Adams, 1990). It was the first available instrument to differentiate among different aspects of learning and memory in younger subjects. It was originally standardized in a control sample and then validated in a sample of learning disabled children. Subsequent research investigated the WRAML in other neuropsychological populations. The manual details reliability data related to internal consistency. As a test of learning and memory, significant practice effects would impact temporal reliability. However, because repeat assessments are likely, empirical data related to temporal reliability and the magnitude of average practice effects would be a welcome addition to the literature on this instrument.

Williams and Haut (1995) reported that the Verbal Memory score obtained on the WRAML is significantly lower for children with epilepsy than for children with substance abuse diagnoses or psychiatric diagnoses. There is some question as to what the various subtests of the WRAML actually measure, as there appears to be substantial overlap with attentional processes on several of the tasks. Aylward, Gioia, Velhulst, and Bell (1995) reported that a factor analysis of the WRAML in a sample of 323 children referred because of academic difficulties resulted in a three-factor solution: visual content, short-term verbal memory, and verbal semantic/strategic factor. The factor solution was similar in both of the age groups used to derive normative information. Phelps (1995) reported a similar factor structure in 115 children also referred for academic difficulties. Williams and Dykman (1994) reported the results of factor analysis using subtests from the WRAML as well as performance subtests from the WISC-R, the Visual Form Discrimination Test, and the Beery Visual–Motor Integration Test. The subtests from the WRAML did not fall out as separate memory measures and instead loaded on general visual processing and attention. It should be noted that in one study, the WRAML exhibited the predicted pattern of impairment in a sample of children with a diagnosis of attention deficit hyperactivity disorder (ADHD) and did not conflate memory and attention (Cahn & Marcotte, 1995).

Some researchers feel the attention/concentration features predominate on the WRAML and that the model of index scores of Verbal Memory, Visual Memory, and Learning proposed in the manual does not reflect the relations among the subtests. Dewey, Kaplan, and Crawford (1997) report that in their sample of children with ADHD or reading disability, a factor analysis of the WRAML resulted in a three-factor solution. The factors extracted were interpreted as verbal memory, visual memory, and attention. Contrary to the index structure of the scoring system, there was no learning factor obtained, a finding that was also reported in a confirmatory factor analysis of the standardization sample (Burton, Donders, & Mittenberg, 1996) and in a hierarchical exploratory principal-factors analysis of the standardization sample (Gioia, 1998). As a result, Gioia (1998) suggested that interpretation of the WRAML be based primarily on a consideration of subtest scores rather than index scores.

The intercorrelations among the WRAML subtests may vary as a function of clinical status in interaction with the age of the child. Putzke, Williams, Adams, and Boll (1999a) examined the relationships among the four subtests contained in the WRAML screening index (Verbal Learning, Story Memory, Design, and Picture Memory). These researchers reported that the correlations among these subtests did not vary between a group of control subjects aged 5 to 9 years, and a group aged 10 to 14 years. However, in a mixed clinical sample of similarly aged children, the subtests were more highly intercorrelated in the older group. Therefore, factor analyses of the WRAML using normal subjects may not be readily generalizable to clinical subjects. Furthermore, interpretation of the indexes of the WRAML may need to be based on a consideration of the age of the child.

As with many longer neuropsychological tests, there is a short form of the WRAML known as the WRAML-Screening. The WRAML-Screening consists of the Picture Memory, Design Memory, Verbal Learning, and Story Memory subtests of the full instrument. Woodward and Donders (1998) reported the results of a factor analysis of the WRAML-Screening first in the standardization sample and second in a sample of 100 children with traumatic brain injury. The normal sample analysis resulted in a two-factor (verbal and nonverbal) solution, but the clinical sample produced a one-factor solution. The WRAML-

Screening index correlated $-.50$ with the length of coma. The WRAML-Screening index was significantly lower for children with severe head injury than for children with mild or moderate head injury. There may be some limitations in using the Memory Screening index to predict the General Memory index in that substantial overprediction is possible. Kennedy and Guilmette (1997) reported that 41 of the 51 subjects administered the WRAML evidenced overprediction an average of 5.3 points.

CHILDREN'S MEMORY SCALE

The Children's Memory Scale or CMS (Cohen, 1997) is actually a downward extension of the WMS-III. In fact some of the test stimuli (e.g., Family Pictures) are identical to that of the WMS-III. The CMS was normed on a sample of 1000 children in 10 age groups from 5 to 16 years old. The sample was stratified in terms of geographic region, parent education, and gender. The manual provides useful and detailed information regarding the reliability of the instrument. As to be expected, there are significant practice effects. Validity was evaluated via confirmatory factors analyses to determine the validity of the index scale components. In addition, correlations with WPPSI-R and WISC-III demonstrated relationships with cognitive measures. The manual also presents data related to the performance of selected clinical groups on the test. Research from independent laboratories can help address the questions of interpretation as well as the ultimate factor structure of the battery.

TEST OF MEMORY AND LEARNING

The Test of Memory and Learning or TOMAL (Reynolds & Bigler, 1994) is a battery of tests of memory function that has been standardized for use with children between the ages of 5 years and 19 years, 11 months. The standardization sample consists of 1342 subjects from 17 states, stratified on the basis of the U.S. Census. There are 10 subtests equally divided between verbal and nonverbal tasks. The subtests are translated to standard scores with a mean of 10 and a standard deviation of 15. The index scores (Verbal, Nonverbal and Composite Memory, and Delayed Recall) have a mean of 100 and a standard deviation of 15. Subsequent factor analyses of the standardization sample resulted in factor solutions that were stable across the age groups (Reynolds & Bigler, 1996). A four-factor solution was interpreted as being comprised of complex memory, sequential memory, backwards memory, and spatial memory. The use of the factor indexes for clinical purposes was explicated by Reynolds (1997). Reynolds and Bigler (1996) developed normative tables for the calculation of scores on these factors which they recommend for clinical interpretation of an individual subject's test results. The TOMAL does not combine the forward and backward digit span procedures or the forward and backward letter span procedures into a single index score, this decision being supported by factor analyses and theoretical considerations (Reynolds, 1997).

The manual reports high internal consistency reliability as estimated by Cronbach's coefficient alpha. Similar values are reported for a sample of 99 adolescents with learning disabilities (Reynolds, 1998).

NEPSY

The NEPSY (Korkman, Kirk, & Kemp, 1998) is designed to be used with children between the ages of 3 and 12 years. There are 27 subtests although not all of them are given to each child. The NEPSY was standardized on a sample of 1000 children with 100 children in each of 10 age groups. The sample was stratified on the basis of geographical area, parental education, race/ethnicity, and gender. The manual provides information regarding internal consistency, test–retest, or generalizability reliability estimates for each of the subtests. All of these reliabilities are reasonably high. Interrater reliability was evaluated for those subtests in which judgment plays a role in scoring. These values were .99 for Design Copying, .99 for Visuomotor Precision, and .97 for Repetition of Nonsense Words. Although relatively new, the NEPSY has been found to provide significantly more impaired scores in children with very low birth weight and asphyxia (Korkman, Liikanen, & Fellman, 1996).

THE BEERY–BUKTENICA DEVELOPMENTAL TEST OF VISUAL–MOTOR INTEGRATION

The Beery–Buktenica Developmental Test of Visual–Motor Integration (VMI) is a venerable procedure in the armamentarium of child clinical neuropsychologists. It was first published in 1967 and has gone through four revisions. The most recent incarnation (Beery, 1997) is a much improved instrument with extended norms from the age of 3 years to the age of 17 years, 11 months. There are now additional tests of visual perception and motor coordination. The VMI is a series of developmentally graded geometric forms which the child is to copy. The standardized scores are based on a sample of 2614 children stratified by socioeconomic status, gender, ethnicity, and geographical region.

The VMI has been found to discriminate between children with Tourette's syndrome and control children (Schultz et al., 1998). Visuoperceptual and fine motor control processes predicted VMI performance but did not fully account for the difference in diagnostic groups. Furthermore, children with very low birth weight and asphyxia performed less well than other children using Finnish norms for the VMI (Korkman, Liikanen, & Fellman, 1996). Although the VMI was originally designed to assess progressive developmental trends in children, it may also be helpful in assessing declines associated with aging. Hall, Pinkston, Szalda-Petree, and Coronis (1996) reported that trends exist in their sample of adults between the ages of 60 and 92; a normative sample would be helpful in establishing aspects of normal decline with aging.

THE BAYLEY SCALES OF INFANT DEVELOPMENT

The Bayley Scales of Infant Development provide an assessment of the cognitive skills of very young children, aged 2 to 30 months (Bayley, 1969). There is a second edition (Bayley, 1993). A Mental Development Index (MDI), similar to an IQ score, can be calculated from the results of administering the Bayley, which is now available in a revised second edition. In addition, a Mental Scale and a Motor Scale are calculated. Tasbihsazan,

Nettelbeck, and Kirby (1997) investigated the original version in comparison to the second edition and reported that MDI gains were apparent using the first edition and subsequently suggested the use of the revised version. Goldstein, Fogle, Wieber, and O'Shea (1995) found that the two versions of the Bayley correlated well in a sample of 490 premature infants. Using the Bayley to classify the infants as normal, borderline, or abnormal resulted in excellent agreement.

Temporal reliability was examined in a sample of 80 infants judged to be at risk for developmental delays. The subjects were tested at 6 months old and again at 12 months old. The stability of the Mental Scale was .71 and the stability was .69 for the Motor Scale (Cook, Holder-Brown, Johnson, & Kilgo, 1989).

In an interesting study of twins, the twin who had lower Apgar scores and greater utilization of neonatal respiratory oxygen support also demonstrated lower scores on the Mental Development Index of the Bayley (Raz, Shah, & Sander, 1996).

The Bayley faces unusual challenges that would not be especially relevant for assessment instruments in which the developmental features did not change so rapidly in the normative group. Because qualitative features of cognitive operations may change in the early years as the same task is performed by children of different ages, the construct underlying the task may also change. This appears to be the case, at least for the timed items of the Bayley. Gyurke, Lynch, Lagasse, and Lipsitt (1992) conducted a factor analysis of the Bayley with data obtained from infants aged 4, 12, and 18 months old. The timed items seemed to load on a five motor control factor in the 12-month-old children and seemed to load on both a five motor control and a speed of performance factor in the 18-month-old children. Burns, W. J., Burns, K. A., and Kabacoff (1992) reported that the Bayley factors changed from difficulty constructs to content constructs from the ages of 3 to 24 months.

The Bayley may have greater power to predict cognitive status in layer years than in early infancy, a finding that is not surprising given the extreme variability in very young infants and the imprecision implicit in measuring such infants. Crowe, Deitz, and Bennett (1987) found that the Bayley was more accurate in predicting motor and cognitive **what** in preschoolers when the Bayley was administered at age 2 years than when it was administered at age 4 months or 1 year. Lewis, Jaskir, and Enright (1986) reported that the Bayley predicted scores on the Stanford–Binet better when the Bayley was administered at 24 months than when it was administered at 3 months or 1 year.

Postscript—Future Directions

To predict the future is a daunting task. At the time of publication of the previous edition of this book I certainly would not have predicted the developments in or the effects of outside forces such as managed care on the field. Perhaps instead of future directions, we should talk of necessary improvements. In general, I think the field will see a greater degree of psychometric sophistication among clinicians and researchers. The increased use of Item Response Theory and Generalizability Theory to evaluate the precision of measurement would be a positive development. Along those lines, the evaluation and conceptualization of validity as a diffractionable entity rather than a monolith will help us to better understand and use the assessment techniques at our disposal. The general conceptualization of a test as a method-construct unit will also aid our understanding.

Among the forms of validity, ecological validity will see a much greater emphasis. As behavioral scientists, it is important that we concentrate on our specialty—behavior—and the relationship of behavior to the environment. The greater use of confirmatory factor analysis will also positively impact on assessment methods. Exploratory factor analysis still has a place, but the greater certainty of comparing different factor solutions will help resolve some standing questions.

The most obvious direction for future research is to conduct studies that will help elucidate the relationships between traditional neuropsychological assessment results and behaviors in the open environment. This would require the development of methods to evaluate the degree of success in performing the behaviors. Relevant sources of information include direct behavioral observation, self-report, and report by significant others. An example of self-report instruments is the Cognitive Failures Questionnaire (Broadbent et al., 1982). An example of report by significant others is the Cognitive Behaviors Rating Scale (Williams, 1987).

An ancillary area would be to identify those variables that most likely operate as moderating variables in the relationship between test data and free behavior. Some of these variables, such as speed of information processing, degree of executive control required, and extent of distractions, have already been discussed. Other variables include level of motivation, extent of anxiety, and affective status.

The development of assessment techniques may follow two potentially fruitful avenues. First, examination of the task requirements of free behaviors may indicate the direction for future assessment instrument development. An example of this can be found in the everyday memory instrument developed by Crook and Larrabee; the memory instru-

355

ment developed by Wilson, Cockburn, and Baddeley (1991); or the communication skills instrument developed by Holland (1980). Another direction for instrument development may be similar to the Loewenstein Direct Assessment of Functional Status (Loewenstein et al., 1989) where behavioral assessment techniques are used to evaluate the capacity of an individual to complete simple behaviors related to everyday functioning.

Among the methods used in assessment, the rise of methods to predict premorbid functioning will continue, as will the rise of methods to determine the presence of response bias. We will almost certainly see an explosive growth in the number of instruments available to test children. Furthermore, increased attention can be fruitfully turned to the development and evaluation of interview techniques. So much of our information is derived from the interview and yet there is so much variability possible, both within the same individual and across individuals. These methods need to be evaluated in terms of their reliability and validity, just as has been done in the area of psychiatric diagnosis.

Finally, the last step in assessment is the clinical decision-making that goes on when a diagnosis is reached or treatment is suggested. It would benefit the field to study these decision processes with the eventual aim of suggesting mental algorithms.

Will these predictions be met? Maybe not. Should they be addressed as suggestions? Definitely. If any students read this book without coming away with ideas for theses, dissertations, or career paths, maybe this Postscript will provide that impetus.

References

Abell, S.C., Heiberger, A.M., & Johnson, J.E. (1994). Cognitive evaluations of young adults by means of human figure drawings: An empirical comparison of two methods. *Journal of Clinical Psychology, 50*, 900–905.

Abell, S.C., Horkheimer, R., & Nguyen, S.E. (1998). Intellectual evaluations of adolescents via human figure drawings: An empirical comparison of two methods. *Journal of Clinical Psychology, 54*, 811–815.

Abell, S.C., Von Briesen, P.D., & Watz, L.S. (1996). Intellectual evaluations of adolescents via human figure drawings: An empirical comparison of two methods. *Journal of Clinical Psychology, 52*, 67–74.

Abidin, R.R., & Bryne, A.W. (1967). Quick Test validation and examination of interform equivalency. *Psychological Reports, 20*, 735–739.

Abraham, E., Axelrod, B.N., & Ricker, J.H. (1996). Application of the Oral Trail Making Test to a mixed clinical sample. *Archives of Clinical Neuropsychology, 11*, 697–701.

Abraham, E., Axelrod, B.N., & Paolo, A.M. (1997). Comparison of WAIS-R selected subtest short forms in a mixed clinical population. *Assessment, 4*, 409–417.

Acker, M.B., & Davis, J.R. (1989). Psychology test scores associated with late outcome in head injury. *Neuropsychology, 3*, 123–133.

Adams, J., & Kenny, T.J. (1982). Cross-validation of the Canter Background Interference Procedure in identifying children with cerebral dysfunction. *Journal of Consulting and Clinical Psychology, 50*, 306–309.

Adams, K.M. (1980a). In search of Luria's battery: A false start. *Journal of Consulting and Clinical Psychology, 48*, 511–516.

Adams, K.M. (1980b). An end of innocence for behavioral neurology? Adams replies. *Journal of Consulting and Clinical Psychology, 48*, 522–524.

Adams, K.M., Kvale, V.I., & Keegan, J.F. (1984). Relative accuracy of three automated systems for neuropsychological interpretation. *Journal of Clinical Neuropsychology, 6*, 413–434.

Adams, R.L., Boake, C., & Crain, C. (1982). Bias in a neuropsychological test classification related to education, age, and ethnicity. *Journal of Consulting and Clinical Psychology, 50*, 143–145.

Aikman, K.G., Belter, R.W., & Finch, A.J. (1992). Human figure drawings: Validity in assessing intellectual level and academic achievement. *Journal of Clinical Psychology, 48*, 114–120.

Aita, J.A., Reitan, R.M., & Ruth, J.M. (1947). Rorschach's test as a diagnostic aid in brain injury. *American Journal of Psychiatry, 103*, 770–779.

Akshoomoff, N.A., & Stiles, J. (1995a). Developmental trends in visuospatial analysis and planning: II. Memory for a complex figure. *Neuropsychology, 9*, 378–389.

Akshoomoff, N.A., & Stiles, J. (1995b). Developmental trends in visuospatial analysis and planning: I. Copying a complex figure. *Neuropsychology, 9*, 364–377.

Albert, M.S., Heller, H.S., & Milberg, W. (1988). Changes in naming ability with aging. *Psychology and Aging, 3*, 173–178.

Alekoumbides, A., Charter, R.A., Adkins, T.G., & Seacat, G.F. (1987). The diagnosis of brain damage by the WAIS, WMS, and Reitan Battery utilizing standardized scores corrected for age and education. *International Journal of Clinical Neuropsychology, 9*, 11–28.

Alfano, D.P., Paniak, C.E., & Finlayson, M.A.J. (1993). The MMPI and closed head injury: A neurocorrective approach. *Neuropsychiatry, Neuropsychology, and Behavioral Neurology, 6*, 111–116.

Allegri, R.F., Mangone, C.A., Villavicencio, A.F., Rymberg, S., Taragano, F.E., & Baumann, D. (1997). Spanish Boston Naming Test norms. *The Clinical Neuropsychologist, 11*, 416–420.

357

Allen, D.N., Huegel, S.G., Seaton, B.E., Goldstein, G., Gurklis, J.A., & van Kammen, D.P. (1998). Confirmatory factor analysis of the WAIS-R in patients with schizophrenia. *Schizophrenia Research, 34,* 87–94.

Allen, S.R., & Thorndike, R.M. (1995a). Stability of the WAIS-R and WISC-III factor structure using cross-validation of covariance structure models. *Journal of Clinical Psychology, 51,* 648–657.

Allen, S.R. & Thorndike, R.M. (1995b). Stability of the WPPSI-R and WISC-III factor structure using cross-validation of covariance structure models. *Journal of Psychoeducational Assessment, 13,* 3–20.

Allison, H.W., & Allison, S.G. (1954). Personality changes following transorbital lobotomy. *Journal of Abnormal and Social Psychology, 49,* 218–223.

Altepeter, T. (1985). Use of the PPVT-R for intellectual screening with a preschool pediatric sample. *Journal of Pediatric Psychology,* 195–198.

Altepeter, T., & Handal, P.J. (1985). A factor analytic investigation of the use of the PPVT-R as a measure of general achievement. *Journal of Clinical Psychology, 41,* 540–543.

Altepeter, T., & Handal, P.J. (1986). Use of the PPVT-R for intellectual screening with school-aged children: A caution. *Journal of Psychoeducational Assessment, 4,* 145–154.

Altepeter, T.S., & Johnson, K.A. (1989). Use of the PPVT-R for intellectual screening with adults: A caution. *Journal of Psychoeducational Assessment, 7,* 39–45.

Alterman, A.I., Zaballero, A.R., Lin, M.M., Siddiqui, N., Brown, L.S., Rutherford, M.J., & McDermott, P.A. (1995). Personality Assessment Inventory (PAI) scores of lower-socioeconomic African-American and Latino methadone maintenance patients. *Assessment, 2,* 91–100.

American Educational Research Association, American Psychological Association, & National Council on Measurement in Education. (1985). *Standards for educational and psychological testing.* Washington, DC: American Psychological Association.

American Psychiatric Association. (1952). *Diagnostic and statistical manual of mental disorders* (1st ed.). Washington, DC: Author.

American Psychiatric Association. (1968). *Diagnostic and statistical manual of mental disorders* (2nd ed.). Washington, DC: Author.

American Psychiatric Association. (1994). *Diagnostic and statistical manual of mental disorders* (4th ed.). Washington, DC: Author.

Ames, L. (1966). Changes in Rorschach responses throughout the human life span. *Genetic Psychology Monographs, 74,* 89–125.

Ames, L., Learned, J., Metraux, R.W., & Walker, R.N. (1954). *Rorschach responses in old age.* New York: Hoeber.

Ames, L., Metraux, R.W., & Walker, R.N. (1971). *Adolescent Rorschach responses: Developmental trends from ten to sixteen years* (2nd ed.). New York: Brunner/Mazel.

Ames, L., Metraux, R.W., Rodell, J.L., & Walker, R.N. (1973). *Rorschach responses in old age.* New York: Brunner/Mazel.

Ames, L., Metraux, R.W., Rodell, J.L., & Walker, R.N. (1974). *Child Rorschach responses: Developmental trends from two to ten years* (rev. ed.). New York: Brunner/Mazel.

Amir, T., & Bahri, T. (1994). Effect of substance abuse on visuographic function. *Perceptual and Motor Skills, 78,* 235–241.

Ammons, R.B., & Ammons, C.H. (1962). The Quick Test (QT): Provisional manual, *Psychological Reports, 11,* 111–161.

Ammons, R.B., & Ammons, C.H. (1979a). Use and evaluation of the Quick Test (QT): Partial summary through October, 1979: 1. Published papers. *Psychological Reports, 45,* 943–946.

Ammons, R.B., & Ammons, C.H. (1979b). Use and evaluation of the Quick Test (QT): Partial summary through October, 1979: 2. Reviews, unpublished reports, and papers. *Psychological Reports, 45,* 953–954.

Anastasi, A. (1982). *Psychological testing* (5th ed.). New York: Macmillan.

Anastopolous, A.D., Spisto, M.A., & Maher, M.C. (1994). The WISC-III Freedom from Distractibility factor: Its utility in identifying children with attention deficit hyperactivity disorder. *Psychological Assessment, 6,* 368–371.

Anderson, A., & Hanvik, L. (1950). The psychometric localization of brain lesions: The differential effect of frontal and parietal lesions on MMPI profiles. *Journal of Clinical Psychology, 6,* 177–180.

Anderson, A., Anderson, V., & Lajoie, G. (1996). The Tower of London Test: Validation and standardization for pediatric populations. *The Clinical Neuropsychologist, 10,* 54–65.

Anderson, C.V., Bigler, E.D., & Blatter, D.D. (1995). Frontal lobe lesions, diffuse damage, and neuropsychological functioning in traumatic brain-injured patients. *Journal of Clinical and Experimental Neuropsychology, 17,* 900–908.

Anderson, P.L., Cronin, M.E., & Kazmierski, S. (1989). WISC-R stability and re-evaluation of learning disabled students. *Journal of Clinical Psychology, 46,* 941–944.

Anderson, V.A., & Lajoie, G. (1996). Development of memory and learning skills in schoolaged children: A neuropsychological perspective. *Applied Neuropsychology, 3,* 128–139.

Andert, J.N., Dinning, W.D., & Hustak, T.L. (1976). Koppitz errors on the Bender–Gestalt for adult retardates: Normative data. *Perceptual and Motor Skills, 42,* 451–454.

Andrich, D. (1988). *Rasch models for measurement.* Beverly Hills, CA: Sage.

Anolik, S.A., & Stevens, R. (1998). Predictors of success within a behavior modification program among male adolescents. *Psychological Reports, 83,* 723–731.

Anthony, W.Z., Heaton, R.K., & Lehman, R.A. (1980). An attempt to cross-validate two actuarial systems for neuropsychological test interpretation. *Journal of Consulting and Clinical Psychology, 48,* 317–326.

Aram, D.M., & Ekelman, B.L. (1987). Unilateral brain lesions in childhood: Performance on the Revised Token Test. *Brain and Language, 32,* 137–158.

Aram, D.M., & Ekelman, B.L. (1988). Scholastic aptitude and achievement among children with unilateral brain lesions. *Neuropsychologia, 26,* 903–916.

Arbisi, P.A., & Ben-Porath, Y.S. (1997). Characteristics of the MMPI-2 F(p) scale as a function of diagnosis in an inpatient sample of veterans. *Psychological Assessment, 9,* 102–105.

Arbisi, P.A., & Ben-Porath, Y.S. (1998). The ability of Minnesota Multiphasic Personality Inventory-2 validity scales to detect fake-bad responses in psychiatric inpatients. *Psychological Assessment, 10,* 221–228.

Arbit, J., & Zagar, R. (1979). The effects of age and sex on the factor structure of the Wechsler Memory Scale. *The Journal of Psychology, 102,* 185–190.

Archer, R.P. (1987). *Using the MMPI with adolescents.* Hillsdale, NJ: Lawrence J. Erlbaum.

Archer, R.P. (1992). *MMPI-A: Assessing adolescent psychopathology.* Hillsdale, NJ: Lawrence J. Erlbaum.

Archer, R.P., & Krishnamurthy, R. (1993). Combining the Rorschach and the MMPI in the assessment of adolescents. *Journal of Personality Assessment, 60,* 132–140.

Archer, R.P., & Krishnamurthy, R. (1997). MMPI-A scale-level factor structure: Replication in a clinical sample. *Assessment, 4,* 337–349.

Archer, R.P., & Slesinger, D. (1999). MMPI-A patterns related to the endorsement of suicidal ideation. *Assessment, 6,* 51–59.

Archer, R.P., Belevich, J.K.S., & Elkins, D.E. (1994). Item-level and scale-level factor structures of the MMPI-A. *Journal of Personality Assessment, 62,* 332–345.

Archer, R.P., Elkins, D.E., Aiduk, R., & Griffin, R. (1997). The incremental validity of MMPI-2 supplementary scales. *Assessment, 4,* 193–205.

Archer, R.P., Fontaine, J., & McCrae, R.R. (1998). Effects of two MMPI-2 validity scales on basic scale relations to external criteria. *Journal of Personality Assessment, 70,* 87–102.

Archibald, Y.M. (1978). Time as a variable in the performance of hemisphere-damaged patients on the Elithorn Perceptual Maze Test, *Cortex, 14,* 22–31.

Archibald, Y.M., Wepman, J.M., & Jones, L.V. (1967). Performance on nonverbal cognitive tests following unilateral cortical injury to the right and left hemisphere. *The Journal of Nervous and Mental Disease, 145,* 25–36.

Ardila, A., & Rosselli, M. (1994). Development of language, memory, and visuospatial abilities in 5- to 12-year old children using a neuropsychological battery. *Developmental Neuropsychology, 10,* 97–120.

Arffa, S., Rider, L.H., & Cummings, J.A. (1984). A validity study of the Woodcock–Johnson Psycho-Educational Battery and the Stanford–Binet with Black preschool children. *Journal of Psychoeducational Assessment, 2,* 73–77.

Arffa, S., Lovell, M.R., Podell, K., & Goldberg, E. (1998). Wisconsin Card Sorting Test performance in above average and superior school children: Relationship to intelligence and age. *Archives of Clinical Neuropsychology, 13,* 713–720.

Argulewicz, E.N., & Abel, R.R. (1984). Internal evidence of bias in the PPVT-R for Anglo-American and Mexican American children. *Journal of School Psychology, 22,* 299–303.

Arita, A.A., & Baer, R.A. (1998). Validity of selected MMPI-A content scales. *Psychological Assessment, 10,* 59–63.

Armstrong, B.D., & Knopf, K.F. (1982). Comparison of the Bender–Gestalt and Revised Developmental Test of Visual Motor Integration. *Perceptual and Motor Skills, 55,* 164–166.

Arnett, P.A., & Franzen, M.D. (1997). Performance of substance abusers with memory deficits on measures of malingering. *Archives of Clinical Neuropsychology, 12,* 513–518.

Arnett, P.A., Hammeke, T.A., & Schwartz, L. (1995). Quantitative and qualitative performance on Rey's 15-Item test in neurological patients and dissimulators. *The Clinical Neuropsychologist, 9,* 17–26.

Arrigoni, G., & DeRenzi, E. (1964). Constructional apraxia and hemispheric locus of lesion. *Cortex, 1,* 170–197.

Arthur, G. (1949). The Arthur Adaptation of the Leiter International Performance Scale. *Journal of Clinical Psychology, 5,* 345–349.

Artiola I Fortuny, L., & Heaton, R.K. (1996). Standard versus computerized administration of the Wisconsin Card Sorting Test. *The Clinical Neuropsychologist, 10,* 419–424.

Artiola I Fortuny, L., Heaton, R.K., & Hermosillo, D. (1998). Neuropsychological comparisons of Spanish-speaking participants from the U.S.–Mexico border region versus Spain. *Journal of International Neuropsychological Society, 4,* 363–379.

Artzy, G. (1994). Correction factors for the MMPI-2 in head-injured men and women. Unpublished doctoral dissertation, University of Victoria, British Columbia, Canada.

Atkinson, L. (1986). The comparative validities of the Rorschach and MMPI: A meta-analysis. *Canadian Psychology, 27,* 238–247.

Atkinson, L. (1989). Three standard errors of measurement and the Stanford–Binet Intelligence Scale, Fourth Edition. *Psychological Assessment, 1,* 242–244.

Atkinson, L. (1991a). Mental retardation and WAIS-R difference scores. *Journal of Mental Deficiency Research, 35,* 537–542.

Atkinson, L. (1991b). On WAIS-R difference scores in the standardization sample. *Psychological Assessment, 9,* 292–294.

Atkinson, L. (1991c). Some tables for statistically based interpretation of WAIS-R factor scores. *Psychological Assessment, 3,* 288–291.

Atkinson, L. (1991d). Concurrent use of the Wechsler Memory Scale-Revised and the WAIS-R. *British Journal of Clinical Psychology, 30,* 87–90.

Atkinson, L. (1991e). Three standard errors of measurement and the Wechsler Memory Scale-Revised. *Psychological Assessment, 3,* 136–138.

Atkinson, L. (1992a). Mental retardation and WAIS-R scatter analysis. *Journal of Intellectual Disability Research, 36,* 443–448.

Atkinson, L. (1992b). "On WAIS-R difference scores in the standardization sample": Correction. *Psychological Assessment, 4,* 117.

Atkinson, L. (1992c). The Wechsler Memory Scale-Revised: Abnormality of selected index differences. *Canadian Journal of Behavioral Science, 24,* 537–539.

Atkinson, L., & Cyr, J.J. (1984). Factor analysis of the WAIS-R: Psychiatric and standardization samples. *Journal of Consulting and Clinical Psychology, 52,* 714–716.

Atkinson, R.C., & Schiffrin, R.M. (1968). Human memory: A proposed system and its control processes. In K.W. Spence & J.T. Spence (Eds.), *The psychology of learning and motivation: Advances in research and theory* (Vol. 2). New York: Academic Press.

Atkinson, L., Quarrington, B., Alp, I.E., & Cyr, J.J. (1986). Rorschach validity: An empirical approach to the literature. *Journal of Clinical Psychology, 42,* 360–362.

Atkinson, L., Bowman, T.G., Dickens, S.E., Blackwell, J., Vasarhelyi, J., Szep, P., Dunleavy, B., MacIntyre, R., & Bury, A. (1990). Stability of Wechsler Adult Intelligence Scale-Revised factor scores across time. *Psychological Assessment, 2,* 447–450.

Atkinson, L., Bvec, I., Dickens, S., & Blackwell, J. (1992). Concurrent validities of the Stanford–Binet (Fourth Edition), Leiter, and Vineland with developmentally delayed children. *Journal of School Psychology, 30,* 165–173.

Atkinson, L., Cyr, J.J., Doxey, N.C., & Vigna, C.M. (1989). Generalizability of WAIS-R factor structure within and between populations. *Journal of Clinical Psychology, 45,* 124–129.

Atlas, J.A., Fortunato, M., & Lavin, V. (1990). Stability and concurrent validity of the PPVT-R in hospitalized psychotic adolescents. *Psychological Reports, 67,* 554.

Au, R., Joung, P., Nicholas, M., Obler, L.K., Kass, R., & Albert, M.L. (1995). Naming ability across the adult life span. *Aging and Cognition, 2,* 300–311.

Avolio, B.J., & Waldman, D.A. (1994). Variations in cognitive, perceptual, and psychomotor abilities across the working life span: Examining the effects of race, sex, experience, education, and occupational type. *Psychology and Aging, 9,* 430–442.

Axelrod, B.N., & Naugle, R.I. (1998). Evaluation of two brief and reliable estimates of the WAIS-R. *International Journal of Neuroscience, 94,* 85–91.

Axelrod, B.N., & Paolo, A.M. (1998). Utility of WAIS-R seven-subtest short form as applied to the standardization sample. *Psychological Assessment, 10*, 33–37.

Axelrod, B.N., Henry, R.R., & Woodard, J.L. (1992). Analysis of an abbreviated form of the Wisconsin Card Sorting Test. *The Clinical Neuropsychologist, 6*, 27–31.

Axelrod, B.N., Jiron, C.C., & Henry, R.R. (1993). Performance of adults aged 20 to 90 on the abbreviated Wisconsin Card Sorting Test. *The Clinical Neuropsychologist, 7*, 205–209.

Axelrod, B.N., Ricker, J.H., & Cherry, S.A. (1994). Concurrent validity of the MAE Visual Naming test. *Archives of Clinical Neuropsychology, 9*, 317–321.

Axelrod, B.N., Goldman, R.S., Heaton, R.K., Curtiss, G., Thompson, L.L., Chelune, G.J., & Kay, G.G. (1996). Discriminability of the Wisconsin Card Sorting Test using the standardization sample. *Journal of Clinical and Experimental Neuropsychology, 18*, 338–342.

Axelrod, B.N., Putnam, S.H., Woodard, J.L., & Adams, K.M. (1996). Cross-validation of predicted Wechsler Memory Scale-Revised scores. *Psychological Assessment, 8*, 73–75.

Axelrod, B.N., Woodard, J.L., Schretlen, D., & Benedict, R.H.B. (1996). Corrected estimates of WAIS-R short form reliability and standard error of measurement. *Psychological Assessment, 8*, 222–223.

Axelrod, B.N., Brines, B., & Rapaport, L.J. (1997). Estimating full scale IQ while minimizing the effects of practice. *Assessment, 4*, 221–227.

Axelrod, B.N., Paolo, A.M., & Abraham, E. (1997). Do normative data from the full WCST extend to the abbreviated WCST? *Assessment, 4*, 41–46.

Axelrod, B.N., Vanderploeg, R.D., & Schinka, J.A. (1999). Comparing methods for estimating premorbid intellectual functioning. *Archives of Clinical Neuropsychology, 14*, 341–346.

Ayers, J., Templer, D.L., & Ruff, C.F. (1975). The MMPI in the differential diagnosis of organicity vs. schizophrenia: Empirical findings and a somewhat different perspective. *Journal of Clinical Psychology, 31*, 685–686.

Ayers, M.R., Abrams, D.I., Newell, T.G., & Friedrich, F. (1987). Performance of individuals with AIDS on the Luria–Nebraska Neuropsychological Battery. *International Journal of Clinical Neuropsychology, 9*, 101–105.

Aylward, G.P, Gioia, G., Velhulst, S.J., & Bell, S. (1995). Factor structure of the Wide Range Assessment of Memory and Learning in a clinical population. *Journal of Psychoeducational Assessment, 13*, 132–142.

Bach, P.J., Harowski, K., Kirby, K., Peterson, P., & Schulein, M. (1981). The interrater reliability of the Luria–Nebraska Neuropsychological Battery. *Clinical Neuropsychologist, 3*, 19–21.

Bachna, K., Sieggreen, M.A., Cermak, L., Penk, W., & O'Connor, M. (1998). MMPI/MMPI-2: Comparisons of amnesic patients. *Archives of Clinical Neuropsychology, 13*, 535–542.

Bachrach, H. (1971). Studies in the expanded Word Association Test: 1. Effects of cerebral dysfunction. *Journal of Personality Assessment, 35*, 148–158.

Bachrach, H., & Mintz, J. (1974). The Wechsler Memory Scale as a tool for the detection of mild cerebral dysfunction. *Journal of Clinical Psychology, 30*, 58–60.

Back, C., Boone, K.B., Edwards, C., Parks, C., Burgoyne, K., & Silver, B. (1996). The performance of schizophrenics on three cognitive tests of malingering. Rey 15-Item Memory Test, Rey Dot Counting, and Hiscock Forced-Choice method. *Assessment, 3*, 449–457.

Backman, J.E., Cornwall, A., Stewart, M.L., & Byrne, J.M. (1989). Stability of children's neuropsychological profiles: Comparison of McCarthy Scales and WISC-R. *The Clinical Neuropsychologist, 3*, 157–161.

Baddeley, A.D., & Warrington, E.K. (1970). Amnesia and the distinction between long- and short-term memory. *Journal of Verbal Learning and Verbal Behavior, 9*, 176–189.

Baddeley, A.D., Hatter, J.E., Scott, D., & Snashall, A. (1970). Memory and time of day. *Quarterly Journal of Experimental Psychology, 22*, 605–609.

Baddeley, A., Della Sala, S., Papagno, C., & Spinnler, H. (1997). Dual-task performance in dysexecutive and nondysexecutive patients with frontal lesions. *Neuropsychology, 11*, 187–194.

Baer, R.A., & Sekirnjak, G. (1997). Detection of underreporting on the MMPI-2 in a clinical population: Effects of information about validity scales. *Journal of Personality Assessment, 69*, 517–533.

Baer, R., & Wetter, M.W. (1997). Effects of information about validity scales on underreporting of symptoms on the Personality Assessment Inventory. *Journal of Personality Assessment, 68*, 402–413.

Baer, R., Ballenger, J., & Kroll, L.S. (1998). Detection of underreporting on the MMPI-A in clinical and community samples. *Journal of Personality Assessment, 71*, 98–113.

Bagby, R.M., Rogers, R., Nicholson, R.A., Seeman, M.V., & Rector, N. (1997a). Does clinical training facilitate feigning schizophrenia on the MMPI-2? *Psychological Assessment, 9*, 106–112.

Bagby, R.M., Rogers, R., Nicholson, R.A., Buis, T. Seeman, M.V., & Rector, N.A. (1997b). Effectiveness of the MMPI-2 validity indicators in the detection of defensive responding in clinical and nonclinical samples. *Psychological Assessment, 9,* 406–413.

Bagby, R.M., Nicholson, R., & Buis, T. (1998). Utility of the Deceptive-Subtle items in the detection of malingering. *Journal of Personality Assessment, 70,* 405–415.

Bak, J.S., & Greene, R.L. (1980). Changes in neuropsychological functioning in an aging population. *Journal of Consulting and Clinical Psychology, 48,* 395–399.

Baker, F.B. (1985). *The basics of item response theory.* Portsmouth, NH: Heinemann.

Baker, G. (1956). Diagnosis of organic brain damage in the adult. In B. Klopfer, M.D. Ainsworth, G. Klopfer, & R. Holt (Eds.), *Developments in the Rorschach technique* (Vol. 2): *Fields of application.* New York: World.

Baldo, J.V., & Shimimura, A.P. (1998). Letter and category fluency in patients with frontal lobe lesions. *Neuropsychology, 12,* 259–267.

Banken, J.A., & Banken, C.H. (1987). Investigation of Wechsler Adult Intelligence Scale-Revised short forms in a sample of vocational rehabilitation applicants. *Journal of Psychoeducational Assessment, 5,* 281–286.

Barcelo, F., & Rubia, F.J. (1998). Non-frontal P3b-like activity evoked by the Wisconsin Card Sorting Test. *Neuroreport, 9,* 747–751.

Barcelo, F., Sanz, M., Molina, V., & Rubia, F.J. (1997). The Wisconsin Card Sorting Test and the assessment of frontal function: A validation study with event-related potentials. *Neuropsychologia, 35,* 399–408.

Barker, M. (1977). A short form of the Category Test. *Psychological Reports, 40,* 1243–1246.

Barker, M.G., & Lawson, J.S. (1968). Nominal aphasia in dementia. *British Journal of Psychiatry, 114,* 1351–1356.

Barnes, G.W., & Lucas, G.J. (1974). Cerebral dysfunction vs. psychogenesis in Halstead–Reitan Tests. *The Journal of Nervous and Mental Disease, 58*(1), 50–60.

Barona, A., & Chastain, R. (1986). An improved estimate of premorbid IQ for blacks and whites on the WAIS-R. *International Journal of Clinical Neuropsychology, 8,* 169–173.

Barona, A., Reynolds, C., & Chastain, R. (1984). A demographically based index of premorbid intelligence for the WAIS-R. *Journal of Consulting and Clinical Psychology, 52,* 885–887.

Barr, W.B. (1997). Receiver operating characteristic curve analysis of Wechsler Memory Scale-Revised scores in epilepsy surgery candidates. *Psychological Assessment, 9,* 171–176.

Barr, A., & Brandt, J. (1996). Word-list generation deficits in dementia. *Journal of Clinical and Experimental Neuropsychology, 18,* 810–822.

Barr, A., Benedict, R., Tune, L., & Brandt, J. (1992). Neuropsychological differentiation of Alzheimer's disease from vascular dementia. *International Journal of Geriatric Psychiatry, 7,* 621–627.

Barr, W.B., Chelune, G.J., Hermann, B.P., Loring, D.W., Pereine, K., Strauss, E., Trenerry, M.R., & Westerveld, M. (1997). The use of figural reproduction tests as measures of nonverbal memory in epilepsy surgery candidates. *Journal of the International Neuropsychological Society, 3,* 435–443.

Bartel, N.R., Grill, J.J., & Bartel, H.W. (1973). The syntactic-paradigmatic shift in learning disabled and normal children. *Journal of Learning Disabilities, 7,* 59–64.

Barthlow, D.L., Graham, J.R., Ben-Porath, Y.S., & McNulty, J.S (1999). Incremental validity of the MMPI-2 content scales in an outpatient mental health setting. *Psychological Assessment, 11,* 39–47.

Bartz, W.R. (1968). Relationship of WAIS, Bets, and Shipley–Hartford scores. *Psychological Reports, 22,* 676.

Basso, A., DeRenzi, E., Faglioni, P., Scotti, G., & Spinnler, H. (1973). Neuropsychological evidence for the existence of cerebral areas critical to the performance of intelligence tasks. *Brain, 96,* 715–728.

Basso, A., Spinnler, H., Vallar, G., & Zanobio, M.E. (1982). Left hemisphere damage and selective impairment of auditory verbal short-term memory: A case study. *Neuropsychologia,* 263–274.

Batchelor, J., Harvey, A.G., & Bryant, R.A. (1995). Stroop Colour Word Test as a measure of attentional deficit following mild head injury. *The Clinical Neuropsychologist, 9,* 180–186.

Battersby, W.S., Bender, M.B., Pollack, M., & Kahn, R.L. (1956). Unilateral "spatial agnosia" (inattention). *Brain, 73,* 66–93.

Bauer, R.H. (1979). Recall after a short delay and acquisition in learning disabled and nondisabled children. *Journal of Learning Disabilities, 12,* 596–607.

Bawden, H.N., & Byrne, J.M. (1991). Use of the Hobby WISC-R short form with patients referred for neuro-psychological assessment. *Psychological Assessment, 3,* 660–666.

Baxendale, S.A. (1997). The role of the hippocampus in recognition memory. *Neuropsychologia, 35,* 591–598.

Bayley, N. (1969). *Bayley Scales of Infant Development.* New York: Psychological Corporation.

Bayley, N. (1993). *The Bayley II Manual.* San Antonio, TX: The Psychological Corporation.

Beardsall, L., & Brayne, C. (1990). Estimation of verbal intelligence in an elderly community: A prediction analysis using a shortened NART. *British Journal of Clinical Psychology, 29*, 83–90.

Beatty, W.W., Krull, K.R., Wilbanks, S.L., Blanco, C.R., Hames, K.A., & Paul, R.H. (1996a). Further validation of constructs from the selective reminding test. *Journal of Clinical and Experimental Neuropsychology, 18*, 52–55.

Beatty, W.W., Wilbanks, S.L., Blanco, C.R., Hames, K.A., Tivis, R., & Paul, R.H. (1996b). Memory disturbance in multiple sclerosis: Reconsideration of patterns of performance on the selective reminding test. *Journal of Clinical and Experimental Neuropsychology, 18*, 56–62.

Beck, F.W., & Black, F.L. (1986). Comparison of PPVT-R and WISC-R in a mild/moderate handicapped sample. *Perceptual and Motor Skills, 62*, 891–894.

Beck, S.J., Beck, A.G., Levitt, E.E., & Molish, H.B. (1961). *Rorschach's test* (Vol. 1): *Basic processes* (3rd ed.). New York: Grune & Stratton.

Beck, F.W., Lindsey, J.D., & Facziende, B. (1979). A comparison of the general information subtest of the Peabody Individual Achievement Test with the Information subtest of the Wechsler Intelligence Scale for Children-Revised. *Educational and Psychological Measurement, 39*, 1073–1077.

Beck, F.W., Black, F.L., & Doles, J. (1985). The concurrent validity of the Peabody Picture Vocabulary Test-Revised relative to the Comprehensive Tests of Basic Skills. *Educational and Psychological Measurement, 45*, 705–710.

Becker, J.T., Lopez, O.L., & Boller, F. (1995). Understanding impaired analysis of faces by patients with probable Alzheimer's disease. *Cortex, 31*, 129–137.

Beery, K.E. (1997). *VMI administration, scoring, and teaching manual.* Parsippany, NJ: Modern Curriculum Press.

Betar, J.T., & Williams, J.M. (1995). Malingering response styles on the Memory Assessment Scales and symptom validity. *Archives of Clinical Neuropsychology, 10*, 57–72.

Bejar, I.I. (1983). Introduction to item response models and their assumptions. In R.K. Hambleton (Ed.), *Applications of item response theory.* Vancouver: Educational Research Institute of British Columbia.

Bell, M.D., Greig, T.C., Kaplan, E., & Bryson, G. (1997). Wisconsin Card Sorting Test dimensions in schizophrenia: Factorial, predictive, and divergent validity. *Journal of Clinical and Experimental Neuropsychology, 19*, 933–941.

Bell-Pringl, V.J., Pate, J.L., & Brown, R.C. (1997). Assessment of borderline personality disorder using the MMPI-2 and the Personality Assessment Inventory. *Assessment, 4*, 131–139.

Bemis, S.E. (1968). Occupational validity of the General Aptitude Test Battery. *Journal of Applied Psychology, 52*, 240–244.

Benedict, R.H.B., Schretlen, D., Groninger, L., & Brandt, J. (1998). Hopkins Verbal Learning Test-Revised: Normative Data and analysis of inter-form and test–retest reliability. *The Clinical Neuropsychologist, 12*, 43–55.

Beniak, T.E. (1977). The assessment of cognitive deficits in uremia. Presented at the International Neuropsychological Society, Oxford, England.

Bennett-Levy, J. (1984). Determinants of performance on the Rey–Osterrieth Complex Figure Test: An analysis and a new technique for single case assessment. *British Journal of Clinical Psychology, 23*, 109–119.

Ben-Porath, Y.S., & Butcher, J.N. (1989). The comparability of MMPI and MMPI-2 scales and profiles. *Psychological Assessment, 1*, 345–347.

Bensberg, G.J., & Sloan, W. (1951). Performance of brain-injured defectives on the Arthur Adaptation of the Leiter. *Psychological Service Center Journal, 3*, 181–184.

Bentler, P.M., & Woodward, J.A. (1980). Inequalities among lower bounds to reliability: With applications to test construction and factor analysis. *Psychometrika, 45*, 249–267.

Benton, A.L. (1945). Rorschach performance of suspected malingerers. *Journal of Abnormal and Social Psychology, 40*, 94–96.

Benton, A.L. (1950). A multiple choice type version of the Visual Retention Test. *Archives of Neurology and Psychiatry, 64*, 699–707.

Benton, A.L. (1955a). Development of finger localization capacity in school children. *Child Development, 26*, 225–230.

Benton, A.L. (1955b). Right-left discrimination and finger localization in defective children. *Archives of Neurology and Psychiatry, 74*, 583–589.

Benton, A.L. (1959). *Right–left discrimination and finger localization in defective children.* New York: Hoeper-Harper.

Benton, A.L. (1967). Constructional apraxia and the minor hemisphere. *Confinia Neurologica, 29*, 1–16.

Benton, A.L. (1968). Differential behavioral effects in frontal lobe disease. *Neuropsychologia, 6*, 53–60.

Benton, A.L. (1973). Visuoconstruction disability in patients with cerebral disease in relations to side of lesion and aphasic disorder. *Documents in Ophthalmology, 33*, 67–76.

Benton, A.L. (1974). *Revised Visual Retention Test* (4th ed.). New York: Psychological Corporation.

Benton, A.L., & Hamsher, K. deS. (1989). *Multilingual aphasia examination manual of instructions* (2nd ed.). Iowa City, IA: AJA Associates.

Benton, A.L., & Spreen, O. (1961). Visual Memory Test: The simulation of mental incompetence. *Archives of General Psychiatry, 4*, 79–83.

Benton, A.L., Elithorn, A., Fogel, M.L., & Kerr, M. (1963). A perceptual maze test sensitive to brain damage. *Journal of Neurology, Neurosurgery, and Psychiatry, 26*, 540–544.

Benton, A.L., Garfield, J.C., & Chorini, J.C. (1964). Motor impersistence in mental defectives. Proceedings, the International Congress on the Scientific Study of Mental Retardation, pp. 746–750.

Benton, A.L., Spreen, O., Fangman, M., & Carr, D. (1967). Visual Retention Test, Administration C: Norms for children. *Journal of Special Education, 1*, 151–156.

Benton, A.L., Hamsher, K. deS., & Stone, F. (1977). *Visual Retention Test: Multiple Choice: Form 1.* Iowa City: Department of Neurology, University of Iowa Hospitals.

Benton, A.L., Varney, N.R., & Hamsher, K. (1978). Visuospatial judgement: A clinical test. *Archives of Neurology, 35*, 364–367.

Benton, A.L., Eslinger, P.J., & Damasio, A.R. (1981). Normative observations on neuropsychological test performance in old age. *Journal of Clinical Neuropsychology, 3*, 33–42.

Benton, A.L., Hamsher, K. deS., Varney, N.R., & Spreen, O. (1983). *Contributions to neuropsychological assessment: A clinical manual.* New York: Oxford University Press.

Benton, A.L., Sivan, A., Hamsher, K., Varney, N., & Spreen, O. (1994). *Contributions to neuropsychological assessment: A clinical manual* (2nd ed.). New York: Oxford University Press.

Berch, D.B., Kirkorian, R., & Huha, E.M. (1998). The Coris block tapping task: Methodological and theoretical considerations. *Brain and Cognition, 38*, 317–338.

Berg, E.A. (1948). A simple objective test for measuring flexibility in thinking. *Journal of General Psychology, 39*, 15–22.

Berg, R.A., & Golden, C.J. (1981). Identification of neuropsychological deficits in epilepsy using the Luria–Nebraska Neuropsychological Battery. *Journal of Consulting and Clinical Psychology, 49*, 745–747.

Berg, R.A., Bolter, J.F., Ch'ien, L.T., Williams, S.J., Lancaster, W., & Cummins, J. (1984). Comparative diagnostic accuracy of the Halstead–Reitan and Luria–Nebraska Neuropsychological Adult and Children's batteries. *International Journal of Clinical Neuropsychology, 6*, 200–204.

Berger, S. (1998). The WAIS-R factors: Usefulness and construct validity in neuropsychological assessments. *Applied Neuropsychology, 5*, 37–42.

Berk, R.A. (Ed.). (1982a). *Handbook of methods for detecting test bias.* Baltimore, MD: Johns Hopkins University Press.

Berk, R.A. (1982b). Verbal-performance IQ discrepancy score: A comment on reliability, abnormality, and validity. *Journal of Clinical Psychology, 38*, 638–641.

Berman, K.F., Ostrem, J.L., Randolph, C., Gold, J., Goldberg, C., Coppola, M., Carson, J.H., Hersecovitch, R.T., & Weinberger, N. (1995). Physiological activation of a cortical network during performance of the Wisconsin Card Sorting Test: A positron emission study. *Neuropsychologia, 33*, 1027–1046.

Bernard, B.A., Wilson, R.S., Gilley, D.W., Fleischman, D.A., Whalen, M.E., & Bennett, D.A. (1994). The dementia of Binswanger's disease and Alzheimer's disease: Cognitive, affective, and behavioral aspects. *Neuropsychiatry, Neuropsychology, and Behavioral Neurology, 7*, 30–35.

Bernard, L.C. (1990). Prospects for faking believable memory deficits on neuropsychological tests and the use of incentives in simulation research. *Journal of Clinical and Experimental Neuropsychology, 5*, 715–728.

Bernard, L.C. (1991). The detection of faked deficits on the Rey Auditory Verbal Learning Test: The effect of serial position. *Archives of Clinical Neuropsychology, 6*, 81–88.

Bernard, L.C., Houston, W., & Natoli, L. (1993). Malingering on neuropsychological memory tests: Potential objective indicators. *Journal of Clinical Psychology, 49*, 49–53.

Bernard, L.C., McGrath, M.J., & Houston, W. (1996). The differential effects of simulating malingering, closed head injury, and other CNS pathology on the Wisconsin Card Sorting Test: Support for the "pattern of performance" hypothesis. *Archives of Clinical Neuropsychology, 11*, 231–245.

Berry, D.T., & Carpenter, G.S. (1992). Effect of four different delay periods on recall of the Rey–Osterrieth Complex Figure by older persons. *The Clinical Neuropsychologist, 6*, 80–84.

Berry, D.T., Allen, R.S., & Schmitt, F.A. (1991). Rey–Osterrieth Complex Figure: Psychometric characteristics in a geriatric sample. *The Clinical Neuropsychologist, 5*, 143–153.

Berry, D.T.R., Carpenter, G.S., Campbell, D.A., Schmitt, F.A., Helton, K., & Lipke-Molby, T. (1994). The New Adult Reading Test-Revised: Accuracy in estimating WAIS-R score obtained 3.5 years earlier from normal older person. *Archives of Clinical Neuropsychology, 9*, 239–250.

Berry, D.T.R., Jr., Adams, J.J., Smith, G.T., Greene, R.L., Sekirnak, G.C., Wieland, G., & Tharpe, B. (1997). MMPI-2 clinical scales and 2-point code types: Impact of varying levels of omitted items. *Psychological Assessment, 9*, 158–160.

Berry, S. (1996). Diagrammatic procedure for scoring the Wisconsin Card Sorting Test. *The Clinical Neuropsychologist, 10*, 117–121.

Beverly, L., & Bensberg, G.J. (1952). A comparison of the Leiter, the Cornell–Coxe, and Stanford–Binet with mental defectives. *American Journal of Mental Deficiency, 57*, 89–91.

Bickett, L., Reuter, J., & Stancin, T. (1984). The use of the McCarthy Scales of Children's Abilities to assess moderately mentally retarded children. *Psychology in the Schools, 21*, 305–312.

Bigler, E.D., & Ehrfurth, J.W. (1980). Critical limitations of the Bender–Gestalt test in clinical neuropsychology: Response to Lacks. *International Journal of Clinical Neuropsychology, 2*, 88–90.

Bigler, E.D., & Ehrfurth, J.W. (1981). The continued inappropriate use of the Bender Visual Motor Gestalt test. *Professional Psychology, 12*, 582–589.

Bigler, E.D., Johnson, S.C., Anderson, C.V., Blatter, D.D., Gale, S.D., Russo, A.A., Ryser, D.K., MacNamara, S.E., & Abildskov, T.J. (1996). Traumatic brain injury and memory: The role of hippocampal atrophy. *Neuropsychology, 10*, 333–342.

Binder, L.M. (1982). Constructional strategies on complex figure drawings after unilateral brain damage. *Journal of Clinical Neuropsychology, 4*, 51–58.

Binder, L.M., & Kelly, M.P. (1996). Portland Digit Recognition Test performance by brain dysfunction patients without financial incentives. *Assessment, 3*, 403–409.

Binder, L.M., & Willis, S.C. (1991). Assessment of motivation after financially compensable minor head trauma. *Psychological Assessment, 3*, 175–181.

Binder, L.M., Villaneuva, M.R., Howieson, D., & Moore, R.T. (1993). The Rey AVLT recognition memory task measures motivational impairment after mild head trauma. *Archives of Clinical Neuropsychology, 8*, 137–147.

Bing, J.R., & Bing, S.B. (1985). Alternate-form reliability of the PPVT-R for Head Start preschoolers. *Psychological Reports, 54*, 235–238.

Bing, S.B., & Bing, J.R. (1985). Comparison of the K-ABC and PPVT-R with Head Start children. *Psychology in the Schools, 22*, 245–249.

Binks, P.G., Gouvier, W.D., & Waters, W.F. (1997). Malingering detection with the Dot Counting Test. *Archives of Clinical Neuropsychology, 12*, 41–46.

Birch, H.G., & Diller, L. (1959). Rorschach signs of "organicity": A physiological basis of perceptual disturbances. *Journal of Projective Techniques, 23*, 184–197.

Birch, J.R., Stuckless, E.R., & Birch, J.W. (1963). An eleven year study of predicting school achievement in young deaf children. *American Annals of the Deaf, 108*, 236–240.

Bishop, J., Knights, R.M., & Stoddart, C. (1990). Rey Auditory–Verbal Learning test: Performance of English and French children aged 5 to 16. *The Clinical Neuropsychologist, 4*, 133–140.

Black, F.W. (1973a). Use of the Leiter International Performance Scale with aphasic children. *Journal of Speech and Hearing Research, 16*, 530–533.

Black, F.W. (1973b). Cognitive and memory performance in subjects with brain damage secondary to penetrating missile wounds and closed head injury. *Journal of Clinical Psychology, 29*, 441–442.

Black, F.W. (1973c). Memory and paired associates learning of patients with unilateral brain lesions. *Psychological Reports, 33*, 919–922.

Black, F.W. (1974a). The cognitive sequelae of penetrating missile wounds of the brain. *Military Medicine, 139*, 815–817.

Black, F.W. (1974b). The utility of Memory for Designs Test with patients with penetrating missile wounds of the brain. *Journal of Clinical Psychology, 30*, 75–77.

Black, F.W. (1975). Unilateral brain lesions and MMPI performance: A preliminary study. *Perceptual and Motor Skills, 40*, 87–93.

Black, F.W. (1986). Digit repetition in brain-damaged adults: Clinical and theoretical implications. *Journal of Clinical Psychology, 42*, 770–782.

Black, F.W., & Strub, R.L. (1978). Digit repetition performance in patients with focal brain damage. *Cortex, 14*, 12–21.

Blackburn, H.L., & Benton, A.L. (1957). Revised administration and scoring of the digit span test. *Journal of Consulting Psychology, 21*, 139–143.

Blacker, D. (1992). Reliability, validity, and the effects of misclassification in psychiatric research. In M. Fava & J.F. Rosenbaum (Eds.), *Research designs and methods in psychiatry*. New York: Elsevier.

Blackerby, W. F., III (1985). A latent-trait investigation of the Luria–Nebraska Neuropsychological Battery. *Dissertation Abstracts International, 46*, 342B. (Universiety Microfilms, No. 85-05, 223)

Blaha, J., & Wallbrown, F.H. (1982). Hierarchical factor structure of the Wechsler Adult Intelligence Scale-Revised. *Journal of Consulting and Clinical Psychology, 50*, 652–660.

Blaha, J., & Wallbrown, F.H. (1991). Hierarchical factor structure of the Wechsler Preschool and Primary Scale of Intelligence-Revised. *Psychological Assessment, 3*, 455–463.

Blair, J., & Spreen, O. (1989). Predicting premorbid IQ: A revision of the National Adult Reading Test. *The Clinical Neuropsychologist, 3*, 129–136.

Blanton, P.D., & Gouvier, W.D. (1985). A systematic solution to the Benton Visual Retention Test: A caveat to examiners. *International Journal of Clinical Neuropsychology, 7*, 95–96.

Bloom, A.S., Klee, S.H., & Raskin, L.M. (1977). A comparison of the Stanford–Binet abbreviated and complete forms for developmentally disabled children. *Journal of Clinical Psychology, 33*, 447–480.

Boake, C., & Adams, R.L. (1982). Clinical utility of the Background Interference Procedure for the Bender–Gestalt Test. *Journal of Clinical Psychology, 38*, 627–631.

Bobic, J., Pavicevic, L., & Drenovac, M. (1997). Intellectual deterioration in alcoholics. *European Journal of Psychiatry, 11*, 21–26.

Bock, R.D. (1973). Word and image: Sources of the verbal and spatial factors in mental test scores. *Psychometrika, 38*, 437–457.

Bolen, L.M. (1998). WISC-III score changes for EMH students. *Psychology in the Schools, 35*, 327–332.

Bolen, L.M., Kimball, D.J., Hall, C.W., & Webster, R.E. (1997). A comparison of visual and auditory processing tests on the Woodcock–Johnson Tests of Cognitive Ability, Revised and the Learning Efficiency Test-II. *Psychology in the Schools, 34*, 321–328.

Bolin, B.J. (1955). A comparison of Raven's Progressive Matrices (1938) with the ACE Psychological Examination and the Otis Gamma Mental Ability Test. *Journal of Consulting Psychology, 19*, 400.

Boll, T.J. (1981). The Halstead–Reitan Neuropsychology Battery. In S.B. Filskov & T.J. Boll (Eds.), *Handbook of clinical neuropsychology*. New York: Wiley-Interscience.

Boll, T. (1993). *Children's Category Test Manual*. San Antonio, TX: Psychological Corporation.

Boll, T.J., Heaton, R., & Reitan, R.M. (1974). Neuropsychological and emotional correlates of Huntington's chorea. *Journal of Nervous and Mental Disease, 158*, 61–69.

Bolla, K.I., Gray, S., Resnick, S.M., Galante, R., & Kawas, C. (1998). Category and letter fluency in highly educated older adults. *The Clinical Neuropsychologist, 12*, 330–338.

Boller, F., & Vignolo, L.A. (1966). Latent sensory aphasia in hemisphere damaged patients: An experimental study with the Token Test. *Brain, 89*, 815–830.

Bolter, J., Gouvier, W., Venklasen, J., & Long, C.J. (1982). Using demographic unformation to predict premorbid IQ: A test of clinical validity with head injury trauma patients. *Clinical Neuropsychology, 4*, 171–174.

Bolton, B., & Brookings, J.B. (1993). Prediction of job satisfactoriness for workers with severe handicaps from aptitudes, personality, and training ratings. *Journal of Business & Psychology, 7*, 359–366.

Bondi, M.W., Monsch, A.U., Galaskos, D., Butters, N., Salmon, D.P., & Delis, D.C. (1994). Preclinical cognitive markers of dementia of the Alzheimer's type. *Neuropsychology, 8*, 374–384.

Bondi, M.W., Drake, A.I., & Grant, I. (1998). Verbal learning and memory in alcohol abusers and polysubstance abusers with concurrent alcohol abuse. *Journal of the International Neuropsychological Society, 4*, 319–328.

Bondy, A.S., Constantino, R., Norcross, J.C., & Sheslow, D. (1984). Comparison of Slosson and McCarthy Scales for exceptional preschool children. *Perceptual and Motor Skills, 59*, 657–658.

Bonfield, R. (1972). Stability of the Pictorial Test of Intelligence with retarded children. *American Journal of Mental Deficiency, 77*, 108–110.

Boone, D. (1998). Internal consistency reliability of the Personality Assessment Inventory with psychiatric inpatients. *Journal of Clinical Psychology, 54*, 839–843.

Boone, D.E. (1991). Item-reduction vs. subtest-reduction short forms on the WAIS-R with psychiatric inpatients. *Journal of Clinical Psychology, 47*, 271–276.

Boone, D.E. (1992a). Reliability of the WAIS-R with psychiatric inpatients. *Journal of Clinical Psychology, 48*, 72–76.

Boone, D.E. (1992b). Evaluation of Kaufman's short forms of the WAIS-R with psychiatric patients. *Journal of Clinical Psychology, 48*, 239–245.

Boone, D. (1994). Reliability of the MMPI-2 subtle and obvious scales with psychiatric inpatients. *Journal of Personality Assessment, 62*, 346–351.

Boone, D.E. (1998). Specificity of the WAIS-R subtests with psychiatric inpatients. *Assessment, 5*, 123–126.

Boone, K.B., Lesser, I.M., Hill-Gutierrez, E., Berman, N.G., & D'Elia, L.F. (1993). Rey–Osterrieth Complex Figure performance in healthy, older adults: Relationship to age, education, sex, and IQ. *The Clinical Neuropsychologist, 7*, 22–28.

Boone, K.B., Ponton, M.O., Gorsuch, R.L., Gonzalez, J.J., & Miller, B.L. (1998). Factor analysis of four measures of prefrontal functioning. *Archives of Clinical Neuropsychology, 13*, 585–595.

Bornstein, R.A. (1982a). Effects of unilateral lesions of the Wechsler Memory Scale. *Journal of Clinical Psychology, 38*, 839–392.

Bornstein, R.A. (1982b). A factor analytic study of the construct validity of the Verbal Concept Attainment Test. *Journal of Clinical Neuropsychology, 4*, 43–50.

Bornstein, R.A. (1983a). Verbal Concept Attainment Test: Cross validation and validation of a booklet form. *Journal of Clinical Psychology, 39*, 743–745.

Bornstein, R.A. (1983b). Verbal IQ-Performance IQ discrepancies on the Wechsler Adult Intelligence Scale-Revised in patients with unilateral or bilateral cerebral dysfunction. *Journal of Consulting and Clinical Psychology, 51*, 779–780.

Bornstein, R.A. (1984). Unilateral lesions and the Wechsler Adult Intelligence Scale-Revised: No sex differences. *Journal of Consulting and Clinical Psychology, 52*, 604–608.

Bornstein, R.A. (1986a). Classification rates obtained with "standard" cut-off scores on selected neuropsychological measures. *Journal of Clinical and Experimental Neuropsychology, 8*, 413–420.

Bornstein, R.A. (1986b). Contribution of various neuropsychological measures to detection of frontal lobe impairment. *International Journal of Clinical Neuropsychology, 8*, 18–22.

Bornstein, R.A. (1986c). Normative data on intermanual differences on three tests of motor performance. *Journal of Clinical and Experimental Neuropsychology, 8*, 12–20.

Bornstein, R.A., & Chelune, G.J. (1988). Factor structure of the Wechsler Memory Scale-Revised. *The Clinical Neuropsychologist, 2*, 107–115.

Bornstein, R.A., & Leason, M. (1985). Effects of localized lesions on the Verbal Concept Attainment Test. *Journal of Clinical and Experimental Neuropsychology, 7*, 421–429.

Bornstein, R.A., Baker, G.B., & Douglass, A.B. (1987). Short-term test–retest reliability of the Halstead–Reitan Battery in a normal sample. *Journal of Nervous and Mental Disorder, 175*, 229–232.

Bornstein, R.A., Palkanis, A., & Drake, M.E. (1988). Verbal and nonverbal memory and learning in patients with complex partial seizures of temporal lobe origin. *Journal of Epilepsy, 1*, 203–208.

Bornstein, R.A., Chelune, G.J., & Prifitera, A. (1989). IQ–Memory discrepancies in normal and clinical samples. *Psychological Assessment, 1*, 203–206.

Bornstein, R.F. (1996). Construct validity of the Rorschach oral dependency scale: 1967–1995. *Psychological Assessment, 8*, 200–205.

Bornstein, R.F., Rossner, S.C., & Hill, E.L. (1994). Retest reliability of scores on objective and projective measures of dependency: Relationship to life events and intertest interval. *Journal of Personality Assessment, 62*, 398–415.

Bornstein, R.F., Hill, E.L., Robinson, K.J., Calabrese, C., & Bowers, K.S. (1996). Internal reliability of Rorschach Oral Dependency Scale scores. *Educational and Psychological Measurement, 56*, 130–138.

Borod, J.C., Goodglass, H., & Kaplan, E. (1980). Normative data on the Boston Diagnostic Aphasia Examination, Parietal Lobe Battery, and the Boston Naming Test. *Journal of Clinical Neuropsychology, 2*, 209–215.

Bowden, S.C., & Bell, R.C (1992). Relative usefulness of the WMS and WMS-R: A comment on D'Elia et al. (1989). *Journal of Clinical and Experimental Neuropsychology, 14*, 341–346.

Bowden, S.C., Whelan, G., Long, C.M., & Clifford, C.C. (1995). Temporal stability of the WAIS-R and WMS-R in a heterogeneous sample of alcohol dependent clients. *Clinical Neuropsychologist, 9*, 194–197.

Bowden, S.C., Dodds, B., Whelan, G., Long, C., Dudgeon, P., Ritter, A., & Clifford, C. (1997). Confirmatory factor analysis of the Wechsler Memory Scale-Revised in a sample of clients with alcohol dependency. *Journal of Clinical and Experimental Neuropsychology, 19,* 755–762.

Bowden, S.C., Carstairs, J.R., & Shores, E.A. (1999). Confirmatory factor analysis of combined Wechsler Adult Intelligence Scale-Revised and Wechsler Memory Scale-Revised scores in a healthy community sample. *Psychological Assessment, 11,* 339–344.

Bowers, T.L., & Pantle, M.L. (1998). Shipley Institute for Living Scale and the Kaufman Brief Intelligence Test as screening instruments for intelligence. *Assessment, 5,* 187–195.

Bowler, R.M., Hartney, C., & Ngo, L.H. (1998). Amnestic disturbance and posttraumatic stress disorder in the aftermath of a chemical release. *Archives of Clinical Neuropsychology, 13,* 455–471.

Boyd, J.L. (1981). A validity study of the Hooper Visual Organization Test. *Journal of Consulting and Clinical Psychology, 49,* 15–19.

Boyd, J.L. (1982a). Reply to Rathbun and Smith: Who made the Hooper blooper? *Journal of Consulting and Clinical Psychology, 50,* 284–285.

Boyd, J.L. (1982b). Reply to Woodard. *Journal of Consulting and Clinical Psychology, 50,* 289–290.

Boyd, T.A., & Tramontana, M.G. (1986). Cross-validation of a psychometric system for screening for neuropsychological abnormalities in older children. *Archives of Clinical Neuropsychology, 1,* 387–391.

Boyle, G.J. (1986). Clinical neuropsychological assessment: Abbreviating the Halstead Category Test of brain dysfunction. *Journal of Clinical Neuropsychology, 42,* 615–625.

Boyle, G.J. (1996). Some psychometric problems with the Personality Assessment Inventory: A reply to Morey's (1995) rejoinder. *Journal of Psychopathology and Behavioral Assessment, 18,* 197–204.

Boyle, G.J., & Lennon, T.J. (1994). Examination of the reliability and validity of the Personality Assessment Inventory. *Journal of Psychopathology and Behavioral Assessment, 16,* 173–187.

Boyle, G.J., Ward, J., & Lennon, T.J. (1994). Personality Assessment Inventory: A confirmatory factor analysis. *Perceptual and Motor Skills, 79,* 1441–1442.

Bracken, B.A., & Murray, A.M. (1984). Stability and predictive validity of the PPVT-R over an eleven month interval. *Educational and Psychological Research, 4,* 41–44.

Bracken, B.A., & Prassee, D.P. (1981). Alternate form reliability of the PPVT-R for white and black educable mentally retarded students. *Educational and Psychological Research, 1,* 151–155.

Braden, J.P. (1989). The criterion-related validity of the WISC-R Performance Scale and other nonverbal IQ tests for deaf children. *American Annals of the Deaf, 134,* 329–330.

Bradford, D.T. (1992). *Interpretive reasoning and the Halstead–Reitan tests.* Brandon, VT: Clinical Psychology Publishing.

Bradley, F.O., Hanna, G.S., & Lucas, B.A. (1980). The reliability of scoring the WISC-R. *Journal of Consulting and Clinical Psychology, 48,* 530–531.

Brandt, J. (1991). The Hopkins Verbal Learning Test: Development of a new memory test with six alternate forms. *The Clinical Neuropsychologist, 5,* 125–142.

Brandt, J., Corwin, J., & Drafft, L. (1992). Is verbal recognition memory really different in Huntington's and Alzheimer's disease? *Journal of Clinical and Experimental Neuropsychology, 14,* 773–784.

Brannigan, G.G., & Ash, T. (1977). Cognitive tempo and WISC-R performance. *Journal of Clinical Psychology, 48,* 530–531.

Brannigan, G.G., & Brunner, N.A. (1993). Comparison of the qualitative and developmental scoring systems of the Modified Version of the Bender–Gestalt Test. *Journal of School Psychology, 31,* 327–330.

Brannigan, G.G., Aabye, S.M., Baker, L.A., & Ryan, G.T. (1995). Further validation of the qualitative scoring system for the modified Bender–Gestalt Test. *Psychology in the Schools, 32,* 24–26.

Brasfield, D.M. (1971). An investigation of the use of the Venton Visual Retention Test with pre-school children. Master's Thesis, University of Victoria, British Columbia.

Brayne, C., & Beardsall, L. (1990). Estimation of verbal intelligence in an elderly community: An epidemiological study using NART. *British Journal of Clinical Psychology, 29,* 217–223.

Breen, M.J. (1984). The temporal stability of the Woodcock–Johnson Tests of Cognitive Ability for elementary-aged learning-disabled children. *Journal of Psychoeducational Assessment, 2,* 257–261.

Breen, M.J. (1985). The Woodcock–Johnson tests of cognitive ability: A comparison of two methods of cluster analysis for three learning disability subtypes. *Journal of Psychoeducational Assessment, 3,* 167–171.

Breidt, R. (1970). Moglichkeiten des Benton–Tests in der Untersuchung psychoorgaischer Storungen nach Hirneverletzungen. *Archives Psychologishe, 122,* 314–326.

Breier, J.I., Plenger, P.M., Castillo, R., Fuchs, K., Wheless, J.W., Thomas, A.B., Brokkshire, B.L., Willmore, L.J.,

& Papanicolaou, A. (1996). Effects of temporal lobe epilepsy on spatial and figural aspects of memory for a complex geometric figure. *Journal of the International Neuropsychological Society, 2,* 535–540.

Brems, C., & Lloyd, P. (1995). Validation of the MMPI-2 Low Self-Esteem content scale. *Journal of Personality Assessment, 65,* 550–556.

Brinkman, S.D., Largen, J.W., Gerganoff, S., & Pomara, N. (1983). Russell's Revised Wechsler Memory Scale in the evaluation of dementia. *Journal of Clinical Psychology, 39,* 989–993.

Broadbent, D.E., Cooper, P.F., Fitzgerald, P., & Parkes, K.R. (1982). The Cognitive Failures Questionnaire (CFQ) and its correlates. *British Journal of Clinical Psychology, 21,* 1–16.

Bromley, D.B. (1953). Primitive forms of response to the Matrices Test. *Journal of Mental Science, 99,* 379–393.

Brooker, B.H., & Cyr, J.J. (1986). Tables for clinicians to use to convert WAIS-R short forms. *Journal of Clinical Psychology, 46,* 982–986,

Brooks, C.R. (1977). WISC, WISC-R, S-B L & M, WRAT: Relationships and trends among children six to ten referred for psychological evaluation. *Psychology in the Schools, 14,* 30–33.

Brooks, D.N. (1972). Memory and head injury. *Journal of Nervous and Mental Disease, 155,* 350–355.

Brooks, D.N. (1974). Recognition memory and head injury. *Journal of Neurology, Neurosurgery, and Psychiatry, 37,* 794–801.

Brooks, I.R. (1976). Cognitive ability assessment with two New Zealand ethnic groups. *Journal of Cross-Cultural Psychology, 7,* 347–356.

Brooks, P.H., & Baumeister, A.A. (1977). A plea for consideration of ecological validity in the experimental psychology of mental retardation: A guest editorial. *American Journal of Mental Deficiency, 81,* 407–416.

Brossard, M.D., Reynolds, C.R., & Gutkin, T.B. (1980). A regression analysis of test bias on the Stanford–Binet Intelligence Scale for black and white children referred for psychological services. *Journal of Child Clinical Psychology, 9,* 52–54.

Brotsky, S.J., & Linton, M.L. (1969). The test–retest reliability of free associations following successive associations. *Psychonomic Science, 16,* 98–99.

Brown, D.C. (1994). Subgroup norming: Legitimate testing practice or reverse discrimination? *American Psychologist, 49,* 927–928.

Brown, F.G. (1970). *Principles of educational and psychological testing.* Hinsdale, IL: Dryden Press.

Brown, L.F., & Rice, J.A. (1967). Form equivalence of the Benton Visual Retention Test in low IQ children. *Perceptual and Motor Skills, 24,* 737–738.

Brown, R.J., & McMullen, P. (1982). An unbiased response mode for assessing intellectual ability in normal and physically disabled children. *Clinical Neuropsychology, 4,* 51–56.

Brown, S.J., Rourke, B.P., & Chiccetti, D.V. (1989). Reliability of tests and measures used in the neuropsychological assessment of children. *The Clinical Neuropsychologist, 3,* 353–368.

Brown, T.L. & Morgan, S.B. (1991). Concurrent validity of the Stanford–Binet: Fourth Edition: Agreement with the WISC-R in classifying learning disabled children. *Psychological Assessment, 3,* 247–253.

Bruggemans, E.F., Van de Vijver, F.J.R., & Huysman, H.A. (1997). Assessment of cognitive deterioration in individual patients following cardiac surgery: Correcting for measurement error and practice effects. *Journal of Clinical and Experimental Neuropsychology, 19,* 543–559.

Brulot, M.M., Strauss, E., & Spellacy, F. (1997). Validity of the Minnesota Multiphasic Personality Inventory-2 correction factors for use with patients with suspected head injury. *The Clinical Neuropsychologist, 11,* 391–401.

Brunswick, E. (1955). Representative design and probabilistic theory in functional psychology. *Psychological Review, 62,* 193–217.

Buckhalt, J.A., Whang, P.A., & Fischman, M.G. (1998). Reaction time and movement time relationships with intelligence in three different simple tasks. *Personality and Individual Differences, 24,* 493–497.

Buckley, P.D. (1978). The Bender Gestalt Test: A review of reported research with school age subjects: 1966–1977. *Psychology in the Schools, 15,* 327–338.

Budescu, D.V. (1980). Some new measures of profile dissimilarity. *Applied Psychological Measurement, 4,* 261–272.

Burger, M.C., Botwinick, J., & Storandt, M. (1987). Aging, alcoholism, and performance on the Luria–Nebraska Neuropsychological Battery. *Journal of Gerontology, 42,* 69–72.

Burke, H.R., & Gingham, W.C. (1969). Raven's Progressive Matrices: More on construct validity. *Journal of Psychology, 72,* 247–251.

Burns, W.J., Burns, K.A., & Kabacoff, R.I. (1992). Item and factor analyses of the Bayley Scales of Infant Development. *Advances in Infant Research, 7,* 199–214.

Burton, D.B., Naugle, R.I., & Schuster, J.M. (1995). A structural equation analysis of the Kaufman Brief Intelligence Test and the Wechsler Adult Intelligence Scale-Revised. *Psychological Assessment, 7,* 538–540.

Burton, D.B., Donders, J., & Mittenberg, W. (1996). A structural equation analysis of the Wide Range Assessment of Memory and Learning in the standardization sample. *Child Neuropsychology, 2,* 39–47.

Buschke, H. (1973). Selective reminding for analysis of memory and learning. *Journal of Verbal Learning and Verbal Behavior, 12,* 543–550.

Butcher, J.N., Graham, J.R., Dahlstrom, W.G., & Bowman, E. (1990). The MMPI-2 with college students. *Journal of Personality Assessment, 54,* 1–15.

Butters, N., Sax, D., Montgomery, K., & Tarlow, S. (1978). Comparison of the neuropsychological deficits associated with early and advanced Huntington's disease. *Archives of Neurology, 35,* 585–589.

Butters, N., Salmon, D.P., Cullum, C.M., Cairns, P., Troster, A.I., Jacobs, D., Moss, M., & Cermak, L.S. (1988). Differentiation of amnesic and demented patients with the Wechsler Memory Scale-Revised. *The Clinical Neuropsychologist, 2,* 133–148.

Bylsma, F.W., Bobholz, J.H., Schretlen, D., & Correa, D.D. (1995). A brief, reliable approach to coding how subjects copy the Rey–Osterrieth Complex Figure. [Abstract]. *Journal of the International Neuropsychological Society, 1,* 125.

Byrd, P.B., & Ingram, C.F. (1988). A comparison study of the Intermediate Category Test with the Halstead Category Test using behaviorally disordered and normal subjects. *International Journal of Clinical Neuropsychology, 10,* 23–24.

Byrne, L.M.T., Bucks, R.S., & Cuerden, J.M. (1998). Validation of a new scoring system for the Weigl Color Form Sorting Test in a memory disorders clinic sample. *Journal of Clinical and Experimental Neuropsychology, 20,* 286–292.

Cahan, S., & Gejman, A. (1994). Stability of IQ scores among gifted children. *Megamot, 36,* 67–77.

Cahn, D.A., & Kaplan, E. (1997). Clock drawing in the oldest old. *The Clinical Neuropsychologist, 11,* 96–100.

Cahn, D.A., & Marcotte, A.C. (1995). Rates of forgetting in attention deficit hyperactivity disorder. *Child Neuropsychology, 1,* 158–163.

Cahn, D.A., Marcotte, A.C., Stern, R.A., Arruda, J.E., Akshoomoff, N.A., & Leshko, I.C. (1996a). The Boston Qualitative Scoring System for the Rey–Osterrieth Complex Figure: A study of children with attention deficit hyperactivity disorder. *The Clinical Neuropsychologist, 10,* 397–406.

Cahn, D.A., Salmon, D.P., Monsch, A.U., Butters, N., Wiederholt, W.C., & Corey-Bloom, J. (1996b). Screening for dementia of the Alzheimer type in the community: The utility of the Clock Drawing test. *Archives of Clinical Neuropsychology, 11,* 529–539.

Cahn, D.A., Sullivan, E.V., Shear, P.K., Marsh, L., Fama, R., Lim, K.O., Yeasavage, J.A., Tinklenberg, J.R., & Pfefferbaum, A. (1998). Structural MRI correlates of recognition memory in Alzheimer's disease. *Journal of the International Neuropsychological Society, 4,* 106–114.

Callahan, C.D., & Johnstone, B. (1997). The clinical utility of the Rey Auditory–Verbal Learning Test in medical rehabilitation. *Journal of Clinical Psychology in Medical Settings, 1,* 261–268.

Callahan, C.D., Schopp, L., & Johnstone, B. (1997). Clinical utility of a seven subtest WAIS-R short form in the neuropsychological assessment of traumatic brain injury. *Archives of Clinical Neuropsychology, 12,* 133–138.

Camilli, G., & Shepard, L.A. (1994). *Methods for identifying biased test items.* Thousand Oaks, CA: Sage.

Cammermeyer, M. (1997). Profiles of cognitive functioning in subjects with neurological disorders. *Journal of Neuroscience Nursing, 29,* 163–169.

Cammermeyer, M., & Evans, J.E. (1988). A brief neurobehavioral exam useful for early detection of postoperative complications in neurosurgical patients. *Journal of Neuroscience Nursing, 20,* 314–323.

Campana, A., Macciardi, F., Gambini, O., & Scarone, S. (1996). The Wisconsin Card Sorting Test (WCST) performance in normal subjects: A twin study. *Neuropsychobiology, 34,* 14–17.

Campbell, D.C., & Oxbury, J.M. (1976). Recovery from unilateral visuospatial neglect? *Cortex, 12,* 303–312.

Campbell, D.T., & Fiske, D.W. (1959). Convergent and discriminant validation by the multitrait–multimethod matrix. *Psychological Bulletin, 56,* 81–105.

Campbell, D.T., & Stanley, J.C. (1963). *Experimental and quasiexperimental designs for research.* Chicago: Rand McNally.

Campbell, K.A., Rohlman, D.S., Storzbach, D., Anger, W.K., Kovera, C.A., Davis, K.L. & Grossman, S.J. (1999). Test–retest reliability of psychological and neurobehavioral tests self-administered by computer. *Assessment, 6,* 21–23.

Campbell, J.M. (1998). Internal and external validity of seven Wechsler Intelligence Scale for Children-Third Edition short forms in a sample of psychiatric inpatients. *Psychological Assessment, 10,* 431–434.

Candler, A.C., Maddux, C.D., & Johnson, D.L. (1986). Relationship of scores on PPVT–R and WISC–R with special education children. *Perceptual and Motor Skills, 62,* 417–418.

Canivez, G.L. (1995). Validity of the Kaufman Brief Intelligence Test: Comparison with the Wechsler Intelligence Scale for Children-Third Edition. *Assessment, 2,* 101–111.

Canivez, G.L. (1996). Validity and diagnostic efficiency of the Kaufman Brief Intelligence Test in reevaluating students with learning disability. *Journal of Psychoeducational Assessment, 14,* 4–19.

Canivez, G.L., & Watkins, M.W. (1998). Long-term stability of the Wechsler Intelligence Scale for Children-Third Edition. *Psychological Assessment, 10,* 285–291.

Canter, A. (1966). A background interference procedure to increase sensitivity of the Bender–Gestalt test to organic brain disorders. *Journal of Consulting Psychology, 30,* 91–97.

Canter, A. (1976). *The Canter Interference Procedure for the Bender–Gestalt test: Manual for administration, scoring, and interpretation.* Nashville, TN: Counselor Recordings and Tests.

Cantone, G., Orsini, A., Grossi, D., & De Michele, G. (1978). Verbal and spatial memory in dementia. *Acta Neurologica, 33,* 175–183.

Carew, T.G., Lamar, M., Cloud, B.S., Grossman, M., & Libon, D.J. (1997). Impairment in category fluency in ischemic vascular dementia. *Neuropsychology, 11,* 400–412.

Carlesimo, G.A., Fadda, L., Lorusso, S., & Caltagirone, C. (1994). Verbal and spatial memory spans in Alzheimer's and multi-infarct dementias. *Acta Neurologica Scandinavica, 89,* 132–138.

Carmichael, J.A., & MacDonald, J.W. (1984). Developmental norms for the Sentence Repetition Test. *Journal of Consulting and Clinical Psychology, 52,* 476–477.

Carmines, E.G., & Zeller, R.A. (1979). *Reliability and reliability assessment.* Beverly Hills, CA: Sage.

Carr, M.A., Sweet, J.J., & Rossini, E. (1986). Diagnostic validity of the Luria–Nebraska Neuropsychological Battery-Children's Revision. *Journal of Clinical and Consulting Psychology, 54,* 354–358.

Carroll, J.B. (1961). The nature of the data, or how to choose a correlation coefficient. *Psychometrika, 26,* 347–372.

Carswell, L.M., Graves, R.E., Snow, W.G., & Tierney, M.C. (1997). Postdicting verbal IQ of elderly individuals. *Journal of Clinical and Experimental Neuropsychology, 19,* 914–921.

Cartan, S. (1971). Use of the Queensland Test in the subnormal population. *Australian Journal of Mental Retardation, 1,* 231–234.

Carter, C.L., & Dacey, C.M. (1996). Validity of the Beck Depression Inventory, MMPI, and Rorschach in assessing adolescent depression. *Journal of Adolescence, 19,* 223–231.

Carvajal, H., Gerber, J., Hewes, P., & Weaver, K.A. (1987). Correlations between scores on Stanford–Binet IV and Wechsler Adult Intelligence Scale-Revised. *Psychological Reports, 61,* 83–86.

Carvajal, H., Gerber, J., & Smith, P.D. (1987). Relationship between scores of young adults on Stanford–Binet IV and Peabody Picture Vocabulary Test-Revised. *Perceptual and Motor Skills, 65,* 721–722.

Carvajal, H.H., Parks, J.P., Bays, K.J., Logan, R.A., & Hayes, J.E. (1991) Relationships between scores on Wechsler Preschool and Primary Scale of Intelligence-Revised and Stanford–Binet IV. *Psychological Reports, 69,* 23–26.

Carvajal, H., Hayes, J.E., Miller, H.R., Wiebe, D.A., & Gerber, J. (1993). Comparisons of the vocabulary scores and IQS on the Wechsler Intelligence Scale for Children-III and the Peabody Picture Vocabulary Test-Revised. *Perceptual and Motor Skills, 76,* 28–30.

Carvajal, H., Schrader, M.S., & Holmes, C.B. (1996). Retest reliability of the Wechsler Adult Intelligence-Revised for 18- to 19-year-olds. *Psychological Reports, 78,* 211–214.

Cascio, W.F., Zedeck, S., Goldstein, I.L., & Outtz, J. (1995). Selective science or selective interpretation? *American Psychologist, 50,* 881–882.

Casey, V.A., & Fennell, E.B. (1981). Emotional consequences of brain injury: Effect of litigation, sex, and laterality of lesion. Presented at the ninth annual meeting of the International Neuropsychological Society, Atlanta.

Cashel, M.L., Rogers, R., Sewell, K., Martin-Cannici, C. (1996). The Personality Assessment Inventory (PAI) and the detection of defensiveness. *Assessment, 2,* 333–342.

Cashel, M.L., Rogers, R., Sewell, K., & Holliman, N.B. (1998). Preliminary validation of the MMPI-A for a male delinquent sample: An investigation of clinical correlates and discriminant validity. *Journal of Personality Assessment, 71,* 46–69.

Caskey, W.E., & Larson, G.L. (1980). Scores on group and individually administered Bender–Gestalt test and Otis–Lennon IQ's of kindergarten children. *Perceptual and Motor Skills, 50*, 387–390.

Caslyn, D.A., O'Leary, M.R., & Chaney, E.F. (1980). Shortening the Category test. *Journal of Consulting and Clinical Psychology, 48*, 788–789.

Cass, W.A., Jr., & McReynolds, P. (1951). A contribution to Rorschach norms. *Journal of Consulting Psychology, 15*, 178–184.

Castlebury, F.D., Hilsenroth, M.J., Handler, L., & Durham, T.W. (1997). Use of the MMPI-2 personality disorder scales in the assessment of DSM-IV antisocial, borderline, and narcissistic personality disorders. *Assessment, 4*, 155–168.

Catron, D.W., & Thompson, C.C. (1979). Test–retest gains in WAIS scores after four retest intervals. *Journal of Clinical Psychology, 35*, 352–357.

Cattell, R.B. (1949). A note on factor invariance and the identification of factors. *British Journal of Psychology, 2*, 134.

Cattell, R.B., Balcar, K.R., Horn, J.L., & Nesselroade, J.R. (1969). Factor matching procedures: An improvement of the s index; with tables. *Educational and Psychological Measurement, 29*, 781–792.

Cauthen, N.R. (1977). Extension of the Wechsler Memory Scale norms to older age groups. *Journal of Clinical Psychology, 33*, 208–211.

Cella, D.F., Jacobsen, P.B., & Hymowitz, P. (1985). A comparison of the intertest accuracy of two short forms of the WAIS-R. *Journal of Clinical Psychology, 41*, 544–546.

Cermak, L.S., & Butters, N. (1972). The role of interference and encoding in the short-term memory deficits of Korsakoff patients. *Neuropsychologia, 10*, 89–96.

Cermak, L.S., & Butters, N. (1973). Information processing deficits of alcoholic Korsakoff patients. *Quarterly Journal of Studies on Alcohol, 34*, 1110–1132.

Chaney, E.F., Erickson, R.C., & O'Leary, M.R. (1977). Brain damage and five MMPI items with alcoholic patients. *Journal of Clinical Psychology, 33*, 307–308.

Channon, S. (1996). Executive dysfunction in depression: the Wisconsin Card Sorting Test. *Journal of Affective Disorders, 39*, 107–114.

Chapman, L.F., & Wolff, H.G. (1959). The cerebral hemisphere and the highest integrative functions of man. *Archives of Neurology, 1*, 357–424.

Charter, R.A., & Dobbs, S.M. (1998). Long and short forms of the Speech–Sounds Perception test: Item analysis and age and education corrections. *The Clinical Neuropsychologist, 12*, 213–216.

Charter, R.A., & Webster, J.S. (1997). Psychometric structure of the Seashore Rhythm Test. *The Clinical Neuropsychologist, 11*, 167–173.

Charter, R.A., Adkins, T.G., Alekoumbides, A., & Seacat, G.F. (1987). Reliability of the WAIS WMS, and Reitan Battery: Raw scores and standardized scores corrected for age and education. *International Journal of Clinical Neuropsychology, 9*, 28–36.

Charter, R.A., Swift, K.M., & Blusewicz, M.W. (1997). Age- and education-corrected, standardized short form of the Category Test. *The Clinical Neuropsychologist, 11*, 142–145.

Charter, R.A., Walden, D.K., & Hoffman, C. (1998). Interscorer reliabilities for the memory and localization scores of the Tactual Performance test. *The Clinical Neuropsychologist, 12*, 245–247.

Chase, T.N., Foster, N.L., Fedio, P., Brooks, R., Mansi, L., & DiChiro, G. (1984). Regional cortical dysfunction in Alzheimer's disease as determined by positron emission tomography. *Annals of Neurology, 15*(suppl.), S170–S174.

Chelune, G. (1982). A reexamination of the relationship between the Luria–Nebraska and Halstead–Reitan Batteries: Overlap with the WAIS. *Journal of Consulting and Clinical Psychology, 50*, 578–580.

Chelune, G.J., & Baer, R.A. (1986). Developmental norms for the Wisconsin Card Sorting Test. *Journal of Experimental and Clinical Neuropsychology, 8*, 219–228.

Chelune, G.J., & Bornstein, R.A. (1988). WMS-R patterns among patients with unilateral brain lesions. *The Clinical Neuropsychologist, 2*, 121–132.

Chelune, G.J., Eversole, C., Kane, M., & Talbott, R. (1987). WAIS versus WAIS-R subtest patterns: A problem of generalization. *The Clinical Neuropsychologist, 1*, 235–242.

Chelune, G.J., Naugle, R.I., Lueders, H., Sedlak, J. & Awad, I. (1993). Individual change after epilepsy surgery: Practice effects and base-rate information. *Neuropsychology, 7*, 41–52.

Chenery, H.J., Murdoch, B.E., & Ingram, J.C.L. (1996). An investigation of confrontation naming performance in Alzheimer's dementia as a function of disease severity. *Aphasiology, 10*, 423–441.

Chervinsky, A.B., Mitrushina, M., & Satz, P. (1992). Comparison of four methods of scoring the Rey-Complex Figure Drawing Test on four groups of normal elderly. *Brain Dysfunction, 5,* 267–287.

Cheung, F.M., & Ho, R.M. (1997). Standardization of the Chinese MMPI-A in Hong Kong: A preliminary study. *Psychological Assessment, 9,* 499–502.

Childers, J.S., Durham, T.W., & Wilson, S. (1994). Relation of performance on the Kaufman Brief Intelligence Test with the Peabody Picture Vocabulary Test-Revised among preschool children. *Perceptual and Motor Skills, 79,* 1195–1199.

Chiuli, S.J., Haaland, K.Y., La Rue, A., & Garry, P.J. (1995). Impact of age on drawing the Rey–Osterrieth Figure. *The Clinical Neuropsychologist, 9,* 219–224.

Chmielewski, C., & Golden, C.J. (1980). Alcoholism and brain damage: An investigation using the Luria–Nebraska Neuropsychological Battery. *International Journal of Neuroscience, 10,* 99–105.

Choca, J.P., Laatsch, L., Wetzel, L., & Agresti, A. (1997). The Halstead Category Test: A fifty year perspective. *Neuropsychology Review, 7,* 61–75.

Chouinard, M-J., & Rouleau, I. (1997). The 58-Pictures Test: A two-alternative forced-choice recognition test for the detection of malingering. *Journal of the International Neuropsychological Society, 3,* 545–552.

Christensen, A.L. (1975). *Luria's neuropsychological investigation.* New York: Spectrum.

Christensen, A.L. (1979). *Luria's Neuropsychological Investigation* (2nd ed.) Copenhagen: Monksgaard.

Cicchetti, D.V. (1997). Do recognition-free recall discrepancies detect retrieval deficits in closed head injury? Demonstrating the inaccuracy of a reviewer's critique. *Journal of Clinical and Experimental Neuropsychology, 19,* 144–148.

Cicerone, K.D. (1997). Clinical sensitivity of four measures of attention to mild traumatic brain injury. *The Clinical Neuropsychologist, 11,* 266–272.

Ciula, B.A., & Cody, J.J. (1978). Comparative study of validity of the WAIS and Quick Test as predictors of functioning in a psychiatric facility. *Psychological Reports, 42,* 971–974.

Clare, L., McKenna, P.J., Mortimer, A.M., & Baddeley, A.D. (1993). Memory in schizophrenia: What is impaired and what is not preserved? *Neuropsychologia, 31,* 1225–1241.

Clark, P., McCallum, R.S., Edwards, R.P. & Hildman, L.K. (1987). Use of the Slosson Intelligence Test in screening of gifted children. *Journal of School Psychology, 25,* 189–192.

Clarke, R., & Scagliotti, J. (1989). Are the Slosson Intelligence Test and the Wechsler Intelligence Scale for Children-Revised interchangeable for identifying gifted students? *Psychology—A Quarterly Journal of Human Behavior, 26,* 33–38.

Clayton, G.A., Sapp, G.L., O'Sullivan, P., & Hall, L. (1986). Comparative validity of two WAIS-R short forms with vocational rehabilitation clients. *Perceptual and Motor Skills, 63,* 1303–1308.

Clement, P. (1966). Analyse de l'echelle de memoire de Wechsler. *Revue de Psychologie, 16,* 197–244.

Clemmons, D.C., Fraser, R.T., Dodrill, C.B., Trejo, W.R., & Freelove, C. (1988). Neuropsychological correlates of tested vocational aptitudes for adults with epilepsy in a rehabilitation setting. *Journal of Applied Rehabilitation Counseling, 18,* 29–32.

Coblentz, J.M., Mattis, S. Zingesser, L.H., Kasoff, S.S., Wisniewski, H.M., & Katzman, R. (1973). Presenile dementia. *Archives of Neurology, 29,* 299–308.

Cockburn, J. (1995). Performance on the Tower of London test after severe head injury. *Journal of the International Neuropsychological Society, 1,* 537–544.

Cohen, J. (1950). Wechsler memory Scale performance on psychoneurotic, organic, and schizophrenic groups. *Journal of Consulting and Clinical Psychology, 14,* 371–375.

Cohen, J. (1960). A coefficient of agreement for nominal scales. *Educational and Psychological Measurement, 20,* 37–46.

Cohen, J. (1968). Weighted kappa: Nominal scale agreement with provision for scaled disagreement or partial credit. *Psychological Bulletin, 70,* 213–220.

Cohen, M., Town, P., & Buff, A. (1988). Neurodevelopmental differences in confrontational naming in children. *Developmental Neuropsychology, 4,* 75–81.

Cohen, M.J. (1997). *Children's Memory Scale.* San Antonio, TX: The Psychological Corporation.

Cohen, M.J., Morgan, A.M., Vaughn, M., Riccio, C.A., & Hall, J. (1999). Verbal fluency in children: Developmental issues and differential validity in distinguishing children with attention-deficit hyperactivity disorder and two subtypes of dyslexia. *Archives of Clinical Neuropsychology, 14,* 433–443.

Cole, D.A. (1987). Utility of confirmatory factor analysis in test validation research. *Journal of Consulting and Clinical Psychology, 55,* 584–594.

Cole, D.A., Howard, G.S., & Maxwell, S.E. (1981). Effects of mono- versus multiple-operationalization in construct validation efforts. *Journal of Consulting and Clinical Psychology, 49*, 395–405.

Cole, K.N., & Fewell, R.R. (1983). A quick language screening test for young children: The Token Test. *Journal of Psychoeducational Assessment, 1*, 149–153.

Coleman, A.R., Moberg, P.J., Raglund, J.D., & Gur, R.C. (1997). Comparison of the Halstead–Reitan and infrared light beam finger tappers. *Assessment, 4*, 277–286.

Coleman, M.C., & Harmer, W.R. (1985). The WISC-R and Woodcock-Johnson Tests of Cognitive Ability: A comparative study. *Psychology in the Schools, 22*, 127–132.

Coleman, R.D., Rapport, L.J., Millis, S.R., Ricker, J.H., & Farchione, T.J. (1998). Effects of coaching on detection of malingering on the California Verbal Learning Test. *Journal of Clinical and Experimental Neuropsychology, 20*, 210–210.

Collingwood, L.M., & Harrell, E.H. (1999). Performance of psychotic and substance abuse patients with or without head injury on the Halstead–Reitan Battery. *Applied Neuropsychology, 6*, 88–95.

Colombo, A., DeRenzi, E., & Faglioni, P. (1976). The occurrence of visual neglect in patients with unilateral cerebral disease. *Cortex, 12*, 221–231.

Colonna, A., & Faglioni, P. (1966). The performance of hemisphere-damaged patients on spatial intelligence tests. *Cortex, 2*, 291–307.

Compton, J.M., Sherer, M., & Adams, R.L. (1992). Factor analysis of the Wechsler Memory Scale-Revised and the Warrington Recognition Memory Test. *Archives of Clinical Neuropsychology, 7*, 165–173.

Condon, B., Montaldi, D.M, Wilson, J.T.L., & Hadley, D. (1997). The relation between MRI neuroactivation changes and response rate on a word-fluency task. *Applied Neuropsychology, 4*, 201–207.

Conger, A.J. (1974). Estimating profile reliability and maximally reliable composites. *Multivariate Behavioral Research, 9*, 85–104.

Conger, A.J. (1980). Integration and generalization of kappas for multiple raters. *Psychological Bulletin, 88*, 322–328.

Conger, A.J., & Conger, J. (1996). Did too, did not!: Controversies in the construct validity of the PAI. *Journal of Psychopathology and Behavioral Assessment, 18*, 205–212.

Conger, A.J., & Lipshitz, R. (1973). Measures of reliability for profiles and test batteries. *Psychometrika, 38*, 411–427.

Conger, A.J., Conger, J.C., Farrell, A.D., & Ward, D. (1979). What can the WISC-R measure? *Applied Psychological Measurement, 3*, 421–436.

Connor, A., Franzen, M.D., & Sharp, B. (1988). Effects of practice and differential instructions on Stroop performance. *International Journal of Clinical Neuropsychology, 10*, 1–4.

Constantini, A.F., & Blackwood, R.O. (1968). CCC trigrams of low association value: A reevaluation. *Psychonomic Science, 12*, 67–68.

Cook, M.J., Holder-Brown, L., Johnson, L.J., & Kilgo, J.L. (1989). An examination of the stability of the Bayley Scales of Infant Development with high-risk infants. *Journal of Early Intervention, 13*, 45–49.

Cook, T.D., & Campbell, D.T. (1979). *Quasi-experimentation: Design and analysis issues for field settings.* Chicago: Rand McNally.

Coop, R.H., Eckel, E., & Stuck, G.B. (1975). An assessment of the Pictorial Test of Intelligence with young cerebral-palsied children. *Developmental Medicine and Child Neurology, 17*, 287–292.

Cooper, H., & Hedges, L.V. (Eds.). (1994). *The handbook of research synthesis.* New York: Russell Sage Foundation.

Corkin, S. (1979). Hidden-Figures-Test performance: Lasting effects of unilateral penetrating head injury and transient effects of bilateral cingulotomy. *Neuropsychologia, 17*, 585–605.

Cornell, D.G., Roberts, M., & Oram, G. (1997). The Rey–Osterrieth Complex Figure Test as a neuropsychological measure in criminal offenders. *Archives of Clinical Neuropsychology, 12*, 47–56.

Costa, L., & Rourke, B. (Eds.). (1985). Abstracts of symposia: Symposium 7. *Journal of Clinical and Experimental Neuropsychology, 7*(2), 178.

Costa, L.D. (1976). Interset variability on the Raven Colored Progressive Matrices as an indicator of specific deficit in brain lesioned patients. *Cortex, 12*, 31–40.

Costa, L.D., & Vaughan, H.G. (1962). Performance of patients with lateralized cerebral lesions: 1. Verbal and perceptual tests. *Journal of Nervous and Mental Disease, 132*, 162–168.

Cottle, W.C. (1950). Card versus booklet forms of the MMPI. *Journal of Applied Psychology, 34*, 255–259.

Covin, T.M. (1977). Comparison of SIT and WISC-R IQ's among special education candidates. *Psychology in the Schools, 15*, 19–23.

Cox, C.S., Chee, E., Chase, G.A., Baumgardner, T.L., Schuerholz, L.J., Reder, M.J., Mohr, J., & Denckla, M.B. (1997). Reading proficiency affects the construct validity of the Stroop Test interference score. *The Clinical Neuropsychologist, 11*, 105–110.

Craig, R.J., & Olson, R.E. (1988). Relationship between Wechsler Scales and Quick Test IQS among disability applicants. *Professional Psychology: Research and Practice, 19*, 26–30.

Crawford, J.R. (1992). Estimation of premorbid intelligence: A review of recent developments. In J.R. Crawford & D.M. Parker (Eds.), *Developments in clinical and experimental neuropsychology* (pp. 55–74). New York: Plenum.

Crawford, J.R., & Allan, K.M. (1994). The Mahalanobis Distance index of WAIS-R subtests scatter: Psychometric properties in a healthy U.K. sample. *British Journal of Clinical Psychology, 33*, 65–69.

Crawford, J.R., & Allan, K.M. (1997). Estimating premorbid WIS-R IQ with demographic variables: Regression equations derived from a UK sample. *The Clinical Neuropsychologist, 11*, 192–197.

Crawford, J.R., Stewart, L.E., & Moore, J.W. (1989). Demonstrations of savings on the AVLT and development of a parallel form. *Journal of Clinical and Experimental Neuropsychology, 16*, 190–194.

Crawford, J.R., Allan, K.M., & Jack, A.M. (1992). Short forms of the UK WAIS-R: Regression equations and their predictive validity in a general population sample. *British Journal of Clinical Psychology, 31*, 191–202.

Crawford, J.R., Mychalkiw, B., Johnson, D.A., & Moore, J.W. (1996). WAIS-R short forms: Criterion validity in healthy and clinical samples. *British Journal of Clinical Psychology, 35*, 638–640.

Cripe, L.I. (1996). The MMPI in neuropsychological assessment: A murky measure. *Applied Neuropsychology, 3*, 97–103.

Crockett, D.J. (1993). Cross-validation of WAIS-R prototypical patterns of intellectual functioning using neuro-psychological test scores. *Journal of Clinical and Experimental Neuropsychology, 15*, 903–920.

Crockett, B.K., Rardin, M.W., & Pasework, R.A. (1975). Relationship between WPPSI and Stanford–Binet IQ's and subsequent WISC IQ's in Head Start children. *Journal of Consulting and Clinical Psychology, 43*, 922.

Crockett, D.J., Clark, C., Labreche, T., Lacoste, D. & Klonoff, H. (1982). Shortening the Speech-Sounds Perception test. *Journal of Clinical Neuropsychology, 4*, 167–171.

Crockett, D.J., Clark, C., Browning, J., & MacDonald, J. (1983). An application of the background interference procedure to the Benton Visual Retention Test. *Journal of Clinical Neuropsychology, 5*, 181–185.

Cronbach, L.J. (1951). Coefficient alpha and the internal structure of tests. *Psychometrika, 16*, 297–334.

Cronbach, L.J. (1984). *Essentials of psychological testing.* New York: Harper & Row.

Cronbach, L.J. (1988). Internal consistency of tests: Analyses old and new. *Psychometrika, 53*, 63–70.

Cronbach, L.J., & Gleser, G.C. (1965). *Psychological tests and personal decisions.* Urbana: University of Illinois Press.

Cronbach, L.J., & Meehl, P.E. (1955). Construct validity in psychological tests. *Psychological Bulletin, 52*, 281–302.

Cronbach, L.J., Rajaratnam, N., & Gleser, G.C. (1963). Theory of generalizability: A liberalization of reliability theory. *The British Journal of Statistical Psychology, 16*(2), 137–163.

Cronbach, L.J., Gleser, G.C., Nanda, H., & Rajaratnam, N. (1972). *The dependability of behavioral measurement: Theory of generalizability theory for scores and profiles.* New York: John Wiley & Sons.

Cronholm, B., & Ottosson, J. (1963). Reliability and validity of a memory test battery. *Acta Psychiatrica Scandinavica, 39*, 218–234.

Cronholm, B., & Schalling, D. (1963). Intellectual deterioration after focal brain injury. *Archives of Surgery, 86*, 670–687.

Crook, T.H., Youngjohn, J.R., & Larrabee, G.J. (1990). The Misplaced Objects test: A measure of everyday visual memory. *Journal of Clinical and Experimental Neuropsychology, 12*, 819–833.

Crookes, T.G. (1983). The Minnesota Percepto-Diagnostic Test and presenile dementia. *Journal of Clinical Neuropsychology, 5*, 187–190.

Crookes, T.G., & Coleman, J.A. (1973). The Minnesota Percepto-Diagnostic Test (MPD) in adult psychiatric practice. *Journal of Clinical Psychology, 29*, 204–206.

Crossen, J.R., & Wiens, A.N. (1994a). Comparison of the Auditory Verbal learning test and the California Verbal Learning Test. *Journal of Clinical and Experimental Neuropsychology, 16*, 190–194.

Crossen, J.R., & Wiens, A.N. (1994b). Comparison of the Auditory Verbal learning test and the California Verbal Learning Test: Erratum. *Journal of Clinical and Experimental Neuropsychology, 16*, 649.

Crossen, J.R., & Wiens, A.N. (1988). Wechsler Memory Scale-Revised: Deficits in performance associated with neurotoxic solvent exposure. *The Clinical Neuropsychologist, 2*, 181–187.

Crossley, M., D'Arcy, C., & Rawson, N.S.B. (1997). Letter and category fluency in community-dwelling Canadian seniors: A comparison of normal participants to those with dementia of the Alzheimer's or vascular type. *Journal of Clinical and Experimental Neuropsychology, 19*, 52–62.

Crosson, B., & Trautt, G.M. (1981). Cortical functioning during recovery from brain stem infarctions: A case report. *Clinical Neuropsychology, 3*, 3–7.

Crosson, B., & Warren, L.A. (1982). Use of the Luria-Nebraska Neuropsychological Battery in aphasia: A conceptual critique. *Journal of Consulting and Clinical Neuropsychology, 50*, 22–31.

Crosson, B., Hughes, C.W., Roth, D.L., & Monkowski, P.G. (1984). Review of Russell's (1975) norms for the Logical Memory and Visual Reproduction subtests of the Wechsler Memory Scale. *Journal of Clinical Psychology, 52*, 635–641.

Crosson, B., Novack, T.A., Trenerry, M.R., & Craig, P.L. (1988). California Verbal Learning Test (CVLT) performance in severely head-injured and neurologically normal adult males. *Journal of Clinical and Experimental Neuropsychology, 10*, 754–768.

Crosson, B., Cooper, P.V., Lincoln, R.K., Bauer, R.M., & Velozo, C.A. (1993). Relationship between verbal memory and language performance after blunt head injury. *The Clinical Neuropsychologist, 7*, 250–267.

Crowe, S.F. (1998). Decrease in performance on the verbal fluency test as a function of time: Evaluation in a young healthy sample. *Journal of Clinical and Experimental Neuropsychology, 20*, 391–401.

Crowe, T.K., Deitz, J.C., & Bennett, F.C. (1987). The relationship between the Bayley Scales of Infant Development and preschool gross motor and cognitive performance. *American Journal of Occupational Therapy, 41*, 374–378.

Culbertson, W.C., & Zillmer, E.A. (1998). The Tower of London: A standardized approach to assessing executive functioning in children. *Archives of Clinical Neuropsychology, 13*, 285–301.

Cullum, C.M., Filley, C.M., & Kozora, E. (1995). Episodic memory function in advanced aging and early Alzheimer's disease. *Journal of the International Neuropsychological Society, 1*, 100–103.

Cyr, J.J., & Atkinson, L. (1992). Use of population-specific parameters in generating WAIS-R short forms. *Psychological Reports, 69*, 151–167.

Cyr, J.J., & Brooker, B.H. (1984). Use of appropriate formulas for selecting WAIS-R short forms. *Journal of Consulting and Clinical Psychology, 52*, 903–905.

Dagenais, F. (1990). General Aptitude Test Battery factor structures for Saudi Arabian and American samples: A comparison. *Psychology and Developing Societies, 2*, 217–240.

Dahlstrom, W., & Welsh, G. (1960). *An MMPI handbook—A guide to use in clinical practice and research.* Minneapolis: University of Minnesota Press.

Dahlstrom, W.G., Welsh, G.S., & Dahlstrom, L.E. (1975). *An MMPI Handbook* (Vol. 11): *Research applications.* Minneapolis: University of Minnesota Press.

Dalke, C. (1988). Woodcock–Johnson Psycho-Educational Test Battery profiles: A comparative study of college freshman with and without learning disabilities. *Journal of Learning Disabilities, 21*, 567–570.

Dalton, J.E., & Pederson, S.L. (1987). Estimating WAIS-R IQ from the Quick Test. *International Journal of Clinical Neuropsychology, 9*, 135–136.

D'Amato, R.C., Gray, J.W., & Dean, R.S. (1987). Concurrent validity of the PPVT-R with the K-ABC for learning problem children. *Psychology in the Schools, 24*, 35–39.

D'Amato, R.C., Gray, J.W., & Dean, R.S. (1988). Construct validity of the PPVT with neuropsychological, intellectual, and achievement measures. *Journal of Clinical Psychology, 44*, 934–939.

D'Amato, R.C., Lidiak, S.E., & Lassiter, K.S. (1994). Comparing verbal and nonverbal intellectual functioning with the TONI and WISC-R. *Perceptual and Motor Skills, 78*, 701–702.

Davis, D.E. (1973). Concurrent validity of the McCarthy Scales of Children's Abilities. *Measurement and Evaluation in Guidance, 8*, 101–104.

Davis, H.P., King, J.H., Bloodworth, M.R., Spring, A., & Klebe, K.J. (1997a). The detection of simulated malingering using a computerized category classification test. *Archives of Clinical Neuropsychology, 12*, 191–198.

Davis, H.P., King, J.H., Klebe, K.J., Bajszar, G., Jr., Bloodworth, M.R., & Wallick, S.L. (1997). The detection of simulated malingering using a computerized priming test. *Archives of Clinical Neuropsychology, 12*, 145–153.

Davis, L.J., & Swenson, W.M. (1970). Factor analysis of the Wechsler Memory Scale. *Journal of Consulting and Clinical Psychology, 35*, 430.

Davis, L., Foldi, N.S., Gardner, H., & Zurif, E.B. (1978). Repetition in the transcortical aphasias. *Brain and Language, 6*, 226–238.

Davis, R.D., Adams, R.E., Gates, D.O., & Cheramie, G.M. (1989). Screening for learning disabilities: A neuropsychological approach. *Journal of Clinical Psychology*, 45, 423–428.

Davis, S.E. & Kramer, J.J. (1985). Comparison of the PPVT-R and WISC-R: A validation study with second grade students. *Psychology in the Schools*, 22, 265–268.

Davison, M.L., Gasser, M., & Ding, S. (1996). Identifying major profile patterns in a population: An exploratory of WAIS and GATB patterns. *Psychological Assessment*, 8, 26–31.

Dean, R.S. (1977). Patterns of emotional disturbance of the WISC-R. *Journal of Clinical Psychology*, 33, 486–490.

DeCato, C.M., & Husband, S.D. (1984). Quick Test and Wechsler Adult Intelligence Scale-Revised in a prison clinical setting. *Psychological Reports*, 54, 939–942.

Dee, H.L. (1970). Visuoconstructive and visuoperceptive deficit in patients with unilateral cerebral lesions. *Neuropsychologia*, 8, 305–314.

DeFilippis, N.A. (1992). *Category Test: Computer version, Research edition*. Odessa, FL: Psychological Assessment Resources, Inc.

DeFilippis, N.A., & Fulmer, K. (1980). Effects of age and IQ level on the validity of one short intelligence test used for screening purposes. *Educational and Psychological Measurement*, 40, 543–545.

DeFilippis, N.A., McCampbell, E., & Rogers, P. (1979). Development of a booklet form of the Category test: Normative and validity data. *Journal of Clinical Neuropsychology*, 1, 339–342.

Degl'Innocenti, A., Agren, H., & Baeckman, L. (1998). Executive deficits in major depression. *Acta Psychiatrica Scandinavica*, 97, 182–188.

Deisinger, J.A. (1995). Exploring the factor structure of the Personality Assessment Inventory. *Assessment*, 2, 173–179.

Delaney, R.C., Rosen, A.J., Mattson, R.H., & Novelly, R.A. (1980). Memory function in focal epilepsy: A comparison of non-surgical, unilateral temporal lobe and frontal lobe samples. *Cortex*, 16, 103–117.

Delaney, R.C., Prevey, M.L., Cramer, J., Mattson, R.H. & the VA Epilepsy Cooperative Study No. 264 Research Group. (1992). Test–retest comparability and control subject data for the Rey–Auditory Verbal and Rey–Osterrieth/Taylor Complex Figures. *Archives of Clinical Neuropsychology*, 7, 523–528.

Delay, J., Pichot, P., Lemperier, J., & Perse, J. (1958). *The Rorschach and the epileptic personality*. New York: Logos Press.

D'Elia, L., & Satz, P. (1989). *Color Trails 1 and 2*. Odessa, FL: Psychological Assessment Resources.

D'Elia, L., Satz, P., & Schretlen, D. (1989). Wechsler Memory Scale-Revised: A critical appraisal of the normative studies. *Journal of Clinical and Experimental Neuropsychology*, 11, 551–568.

Delis, D., & Kaplan, E. (1982). Assessment of aphasia with the Luria–Nebraska Neuropsychological Battery: A case critique. *Journal of Consulting and Clinical Psychology*, 51, 32–39.

Delis, D.C., Kramer, J.H., Kaplan, E., & Ober, B.A. (1987). *The California Verbal Learning Test: Research Edition*. New York: The Psychological Corporation.

Delis, D.C., Cullum, C.M., Butters, N., & Cairns, P. (1988a). Wechsler Memory Scale-Revised and California Verbal Learning Test: Convergence and divergence. *The Clinical Neuropsychologist*, 2, 188–196.

Delis, D.C., Freeland, J., Kramer, J.H., & Kaplan, E. (1988b). Integrating clinical assessment with cognitive neuroscience: Construct validation of the California Verbal Learning Test. *Journal of Consulting and Clinical Psychology*, 56, 123–130.

Delis, D.C., Massman, P.J., Kaplan, E., McKee, R., Kramer, J.H., & Gettman, D. (1991). Alternate form of the California Verbal Learning Test: Development and reliability. *The Clinical Neuropsychologist*, 5, 154–162.

Delis, D.C., Kramer, J.H., Kaplan, E., & Ober, B.A. (1994). *California Verbal Learning Test: Children's Version*. San Antonio, TX: The Psychological Corporation.

DeLuca, D., Cermak, L.S., & Butters, N. (1975). An analysis of Korsakoff patients recall following varying types of distractor activity. *Neuropsychologia*, 13, 271–279.

Demsky, Y.Y., Gass, C.S., & Golden, C.J. (1997). Common short forms of the Spanish Wechsler Adult Intelligence Scale. *Perceptual and Motor Skills*, 85, 1121–1122.

Demsky, Y.I., Mittenberg, W., Quintar, B., Katell, A.D., & Golden, C.J. (1998). Bias in the use of standard American norms with Spanish translations of the Wechsler Memory Scale-Revised. *Assessment*, 5, 115–121.

Denes, F., Semenza, C., Stoppa, E., & Gradenigo, G. (1978). Selective improvement by unilateral brain damaged patients on Raven Coloured Progressive Matrices. *Neuropsychologia*, 16, 749–752.

Denman, S.B. (1984). *Manual for the Denman Memory Battery*. Charleston, S.C.: Author.

Denney, R.L. (1996). Symptom Validity Testing of remote memory in a criminal forensic setting. *Archives of Clinical Neuropsychology*, 11, 589–603.

De Renzi, E., & Faglioni, P. (1965). The comparative efficiency of intelligence and vigilance tests in detecting hemispheric cerebral damage. *Cortex, 1*, 410–433.

De Renzi, E., & Faglioni, P. (1978). Normative data and screening power of a shortened version of the Token Test. *Cortex, 14*, 41–49.

De Renzi, E., & Nichelli, P. (1975). Verbal and non-verbal short–term memory impairment following hemispheric damage. *Cortex, 11*, 341–354.

De Renzi, E., & Spinnler, H. (1967). Impaired performance on color tasks in patients with hemispheric damage. *Cortex, 3*, 194–217.

De Renzi, E., & Vignolo, L.A. (1962). The Token Test: A sensitive test to detect receptive disturbances in aphasics. *Brain, 85*, 665–678.

De Renzi, E., Faglioni, P., Savoiardo, M., & Vignolo, L.A. (1966). The influence of aphasia and of the hemispheric side of the cerebral lesion on abstract thinking. *Cortex, 2*, 399–420.

De Renzi, E., Pieczuro, A., & Vignolo, L.A. (1968). Ideational apraxia: A quantitative study. *Neuropsychologia, 6*, 41–52.

De Renzi, E., Faglioni, P., & Previdi, P. (1977). Spatial memory and hemispheric locus of lesion. *Cortex, 13*, 424–433.

Derry, P.A., Harnadek, M.C.S., McLachlan, R.S., & Sontrop, J. (1997). Influence of seizure content on interpreting psychopathology on the MMPI-2 in patients with epilepsy. *Journal of Clinical and Experimental Neuropsychology, 19*, 396–404.

Deshpande, S.A., Millis, S.R., Reeder, K.P., Fuerst, D., & Ricker, J.H. (1996). Verbal Learning subtypes in traumatic brain injury: A replication. *Journal of Clinical and Experimental Neuropsychology, 18*, 836–842.

DeSantis, G., & Dunikoski, R. (1983). Group Embedded Figures test: Psychometric data for a sample of business students. *Perceptual and Motor Skills, 56*, 707–710.

Des Rosiers, G., & Ivison, D. (1986). Paired associates learning: Normative data for differences between high and low associate word pairs. *Journal of Clinical and Experimental Neuropsychology, 8*, 637–642.

Des Rosiers, G., & Kavanaugh, D. (1987). Cognitive assessment in closed head injury: Stability, validity, and parallel forms for two neuropsychological measures of recovery. *International Journal of Clinical Neuropsychology, 9*, 162–173.

Deutsch, G., Bourbon, W.T., Papanicolaou, A.C., & Eisenberg, H.M. (1988). Visuospatial tasks compared via activation of regional cerebral blood flow. *Neuropsychologia, 26*, 445-452.

Dewey, D., Kaplan, B.J., & Crawford, S.G. (1997). Factor structure of the WRAML in children with ADHD or reading disabilities: Further evidence of an attention/concentration factor. *Developmental Neuropsychology, 13*, 501–506.

Dey, J., Mahapatra, A.K., Misra, A., Padma, M.V., & Desai, N.G. (1997). Cognitive function in younger Type II diabetics. *Diabetes Care, 20*, 32–35.

Diamant, J.J. (1981). Similarities and differences in the approach of R.M. Reitan and A.R. Luria. *Acta Psychiatrica Scandinavica, 63*, 441–443.

Diamond, B.J., DeLuca, J., Johnson, S.K., & Kelly, S.M. (1997a). Verbal learning in amnesic anterior communicating artery aneurysm patients and in patients with multiple sclerosis. *Applied Neuropsychology, 4*, 89–98.

Diamond, B.J., DeLuca, J., Kim, H., & Kelly, S.M. (1997b). The question of disproportianate impairments in visual and auditory information processing in multiple sclerosis. *Journal of Clinical and Experimental Neuropsychology, 19*, 34–42.

Diehr, M.C., Heaton, R.K., Miller, W., & Grant, I. (1998). The Paced Auditory Serial Addition Test (PASAT): Norms for age, education, and ethnicity. *Assessment, 5*, 375–387.

Dikmen, S., & Reitan, R.M. (1974a). Minnesota Multiphasic Personality Inventory correlates of dysphasic language disturbances. *Journal of Abnormal Psychology, 83*, 675–679.

Dikmen, S., & Reitan, R.M. (1974b). MMPI correlates of localized cerebral lesions. *Perceptual and Motor Skills, 39*, 831–840.

Dikmen, S., & Reitan, R.M. (1977). MMPI correlates of adaptive ability deficits in patients with brain lesions. *Journal of Nervous and Mental Disease, 165*, 247–254.

Dikmen, S.S., Heaton, R.K., Grant, I., & Temkin, N.R. (1999). Test–retest reliability and practice effects of Expanded Halstead–Reitan Neuropsychological Test Battery. *Journal of the International Neuropsychological Society, 5*, 346–356.

Dillon, R.F., Pohlmann, J.T., & Lohman, D.F. (1981). A factor analysis of Raven's advanced progressive matrices freed of difficulty factors. *Educational and Psychological Measurement, 41*, 1295–1302.

Dilworth, A., & French, J. (1990). Development of a cognitive ability test for 2-year-olds with motor or speech delays. *Journal of Psychoeducational Assessment*, *8*, 42–50.

Dixon, J.L. (1998). Concurrent validity of the Koppitz, Bender–Gestalt Emotional Indicators among women with mental retardation. *Perceptual and Motor Skills*, *86*, 195–197.

Dodge, G.R., & Kolstoe, R.H. (1971). The MMPI in differentiating early multiple sclerosis and conversion hysteria. *Psychological Reports*, *29*, 155–159.

Dodrill, C.B. (1978). A neuropsychological battery for epilepsy. *Epilepsia*, *19*, 611–623.

Dodrill, C.B. (1979). Sex differences on the Halstead–Reitan Neuropsychological Battery and on other neuropsychological measures. *Journal of Clinical Psychology*, *35*, 236–241.

Dodrill, C.B., & Clemmons, D. (1984). Use of neuropsychological tests to identify high school students with epilepsy who later demonstrate inadequate performances in life. *Journal of Consulting and Clinical Psychology*, *52*, 520–527.

Dodrill, C.B., & Troupin, A.S. (1975). Effects of repeated administrations of a comprehensive neuropsychological battery among chronic epileptics. *Journal of Nervous and Mental Disease*, *161*, 185–190.

Doehring, D., & Reitan, R.M. (1960). MMPI performances of aphasic and non-aphasic brain damaged patients. *Journal of Clinical Psychology*, *16*, 307–309.

Doehring, D.G., & Reitan, R.M. (1962). Concept attainment of human adults with lateralized cerebral lesions. *Perceptual and Motor Skills*, *14*, 27–33.

Dolke, A.M. (1976). Investigation into certain properties of Raven's Standard Progressive Matrices Test. *Indian Journal of Psychology*, *51*, 225–236.

Domrath, R.P. (1966). Motor impersistence in schizophrenia. *Cortex*, *2*, 474–483.

Donders, J. (1995). Validity of the Kaufman Brief Intelligence Test (K-BIT) in children with traumatic brain injury. *Assessment*, *2*, 219–224.

Donders, J. (1996). Validity of short forms of the intermediate Halstead Category Test in children with traumatic brain injury. *Archives of Clinical Neuropsychology*, *11*, 131–137.

Donders, J. (1997a). Sensitivity of the WISC-III to injury severity in children with traumatic head injury. *Assessment*, *4*, 107–109.

Donders, J. (1997b). A short form of the WISC-III for clinical use. *Psychological Assessment*, *9*, 15–20.

Donders, J. (1998). Performance discrepancies between the Children's Category Test (CCT) and the California Verbal Learning Test-Children's (CVLT-C) Version in the standardization sample. *Journal of the International Neuropsychological Society*, *4*, 242–246.

Donders, J., & Strom, D. (1995). Factor and cluster analysis of the Intermediate Halstead Category Test. *Child Neuropsychology*, *1*, 19–25.

Donders, J., & Warschausky, S. (1996a). A structural equations analysis of the WISC-III in children with traumatic head injury. *Child Neuropsychology*, *2*, 227–232.

Donders, J., & Warschausky, S. (1996b). WISC-III factor index score pattern after traumatic head injury in children. *Child Neuropsychology*, *3*, 71–78.

Donders, J., & Warschausky, S. (1996c). Validity of a short form of the WISC-III in children with traumatic head injury. *Child Neuropsychology*, *2*, 227–232.

Donias, S.H., Vassilopoulou, E.O., Golden, C.J., & Lovell, M.R. (1989). Reliability and clinical effectiveness of the standardized Greek version of the Luria–Nebraska Neuropsychological Battery. *International Journal of Clinical Neuropsychology*, *11*, 129–133.

Donovick, P.J., Burright, R.G., Burg, J.S., & Gronendyke, S.J. (1996). The K-BIT: A screen for IQ in six diverse populations. *Journal of Clinical Psychology in Medical Settings*, *3*, 131–140.

Dorken, H., & Kral, V.A. (1952). The psychological differentiation of organic brain lesions and their localization by means of the Rorschach test. *American Journal of Psychiatry*, *108*, 764–771.

Doss, G.H., Head, D.W., Blackburn, J.V., & Robertson, J.M. (1986). A quick measure of mental deficiency among adult offenders. *Federal Probation*, *50*, 57–59.

Dowler, R.N., Harrington, D.L., Haaland, K.Y., Swanda, R.M., Fee, F., & Fiedler, K. (1997). Profiles of cognitive functioning in chronic spinal cord injury and the role of moderating variables. *Journal of the International Neuropsychological Society*, *3*, 464–472.

Drachman, D.A., & Arbit, J. (1966). Memory and the hippocampal complex. *Archives of Neurology*, *15*, 52–61.

Drachman, D.A., & Hughes, J.R. (1971). Memory and the hippocampal complexes. *Neurology*, *21*, 1–14.

Drane, D.L., & Osato, S.S. (1998). Using the Neurobehavioral Cognitive Status Examination as a screening measure for older adults. *Archives of Clinical Neuropsychology*, *12*, 139–143.

Drewe, E.A. (1974). The effect of type and area of brain lesion of Wisconsin Card Sorting Test performance. *Cortex*, *10*, 159–170.

Droege, R.C. (1984). The General Aptitude Test Battery and its international use. *International Journal of Applied Psychology*, *33*, 413–416.

Drudge, J.P., Cyr, J.J., & Eccles, A.L. (1989). The relative accuracy of two WAIS-R short form approaches to IQ prediction. *Journal of Social Behavior and Personality*, *4*, 145–150.

Dudek, S.Z., Goldeberg, J.S., Lester, E.P., & Harris, B.R. (1969). The validity of cognitive, perceptual-motor, and personality variables for prediction of achievement in Grade 1 and Grade 2. *Journal of Clinical Psychology*, *25*, 165–170.

Dujovne, B.E., & Levy, B.I. (1971). The psychometric structure of the Wechsler Memory Scale. *Journal of Clinical Psychology*, *27*, 351–354.

Dumont, R., & Faro, C. (1993). A WISC-III short form for learning disabled students. *Psychology in the Schools*, *30*, 212–219.

Dumont, R., Cruse, C.L., Price, L., & Whelley, P. (1996). The relationship between the Differential Ability Scales (DAS) and the Wechsler Intelligence Scale for Children-Third Edition (WISC-III) for students with learning disabilities. *Psychology in the Schools*, *33*, 203–209.

Dumont, R., Farr, L.P., Willis, J.O., & Whelley, P. (1998). 30-second interval performance on the coding subtest of the WISC-III: Further evidence of WISC-III folklore? *Psychology in the Schools*, *35*, 111–117.

Dunn, J.A. (1967). Inter- and intra-scorer reliability of the New Goodenough–Harris Draw-A-Man Test. *Perceptual and Motor Skills*, *24*, 269–270.

Dunn, L.M., & Dunn, L.M. (1981). *Peabody Picture Vocabulary Test-Revised Manual*. Circle Pines, MN: American Guidance Service.

Dunn, L.M., & Markwardt, F.C. (1970). *Manual for the Peabody Individual Achievement Test*. Circle Pines, MN: American Guidance Service.

Dura, J.R., Myers, E.G., & Freathy, D.T. (1989). Stability of the Wide Range Achievement Test in an adolescent inpatient setting. *Educational and Psychological Measurement*, *49*, 253–256.

Durlak, J.A. (1995). Understanding meta-analysis. In L.G. Grimm & P.R. Yarnold (Eds.), *Reading and understanding multivariate statistics* (pp. 319–352). Washington, DC: American Psychological Association.

Dye, C. (1982). Factor structure of the Wechsler Memory Scale in an older population. *Journal of Clinical Psychology*, *38*, 163–166.

Dywan, J., Segalowitz, S.J., & Unsal, A. (1992). Speed of information processing, health, and cognitive performance in older adults. *Developmental Neuropsychology*, *8*, 473–490.

Eaves, R.C., Williams, P., Winshester, K., & Darch, C. (1994). Using teacher judgment and IQ to estimate reading and mathematics achievement in a remedial-reading program. *Psychology in the Schools*, *31*, 261–272.

Eckardt, M.J., & Matarazzo, J.D. (1981). Test–retest reliability of the Halstead impairment index in hospitalized alcoholic and non-alcoholic males with mild to moderate neuropsychological impairment. *Journal of Clinical Neuropsychology*, *3*, 257–269.

Eddy, D.M., Hasselblad, V., & Shachter, R. (1992). *Meta-analysis by the confidence profile method: The statistical synthesis of evidence*. Boston: Academic Press.

Egeland, B., Rice, J., & Penny, S. (1967). Interscorer reliability on the Bender Gestalt test and Revised Visual Retention Test. *American Journal of Mental Deficiency*, *72*, 96–99.

Ehrfurth, J.W., & Lezak, M. (1982). The battering of neuropsychology by the "hit rate": An appeal for peace and reason. Presented at the 10th annual meeting of the International Neuropsychological Society, Pittsburgh.

Eisenstein, N., & Engelhart, C.I. (1997). Comparison of the K-BIT with short forms of the WAIS-R in a neuropsychological population. *Psychological Assessment*, *9*, 57–62.

Elithorn, A. (1955). A preliminary report on a perceptual maze test sensitive to brain damage. *Journal of Neurology, Neurosurgery, and Psychiatry*, *18*, 287–292.

Elithorn, A., Kerr, M., & Mott, J. (1960). A group version of a perceptual maze test. *British Journal of Psychology*, *51*, 19–26.

Elithorn, A., Svancara, J., & Weinman, J. (1971). A twin study with the perceptual maze test. *Psychologia a Patopsychologia Dieteta*, *6*, 105–112.

Elithorn, A., Mornington, S., & Stavrou, A. (1982). Automated psychological testing: Some principles and practices. *International Journal of Man–Machine Studies*, *17*, 247–263.

Elliott, R.N. (1969). Comparative study of the Pictorial Test of Intelligence and the Peabody Picture Vocabulary Test. *Psychological Reports*, *25*, 528–530.

Elliott, S.N., & Bretzing, B.H. (1980). Using and updating local norms. *Psychology in the Schools, 17*, 196–201.

Ellis, D., & Zahn, B. (1985). Psychological functioning after severe closed head injury. *Journal of Personality Assessment, 49*, 125–128.

Elwood, R.W. (1991). The Wechsler Memory Scale-Revised: Psychometric characteristics and clinical applications. *Neuropsychology Review, 2*, 179–201.

Elwood, R.L. (1995). The California Verbal Learning Test: Psychometric characteristics and clinical application. *Neuropsychology Review, 5*, 173–201.

Emery, O.B. (1986). Linguistic decrement in normal aging. *Language and Communication, 6*, 47–64.

Engelsmann, F., Katz, J., Gharidian, A.M., & Schacter, D. (1988). Lithium and memory: A long term follow-up study. *Journal of Clinical Psychopharmacology, 8*, 207–212.

Engin, A.W., & Wallbrown, F.H. (1976). The stability of four kinds of perceptual errors on the Bender Gestalt. *Journal of Psychology, 84*, 123–126.

Eno, L., & Deichmann, J. (1980). A review of the Bender Gestalt test as a screening instrument for brain damage with school-aged children of normal intelligence since 1970. *The Journal of Special Education, 14*, 37–45.

Eppinger, M.G., Craig, P.L., Adams, R.L., & Parsons, O.A. (1987). The WAIS-R Index for estimating premorbid intelligence: Cross-validation and clinical utility. *Journal of Consulting and Clinical Psychology, 55*, 86–90.

Erlandson, G.L., Osmon, D.C., & Golden, C.J. (1981). Minnesota Multiphasic Personality Inventory correlates of the Luria–Nebraska Neuropsychological Battery in a psychiatric population. *International Journal of Neuroscience, 13*, 143–154.

Ernst, J., Warner, M.H., Morgan, A., Townes, B.D., Eiler, J., & Coppel, D.B. (1986). Factor analysis of the Wechsler Memory Scale: Is the Associate Learning subtest an unclear measure? *Archives of Clinical Neuropsychology, 8*, 637–642.

Estabrook, G.E. (1984). A canonical correlation analysis of the Wechsler Intelligence Scale for Children-Revised and the Woodcock–Johnson Tests of Cognitive Ability in a sample referred for suspected learning disability. *Journal of Educational Psychology, 76*, 1170–1177.

Etcoff, L.M., & Kampfer, K.M. (1996). Practical guidelines in the use of symptom validity and other psychological tests to measure malingering and symptom exaggeration in traumatic brain injury cases. *Neuropsychology Review, 6*, 171–201.

Ettlinger, G. (1970). Apraxia considered as a disorder of movements that are language-dependent: Evidence from cases of brain bisection. *Cortex, 5*, 285–289.

Evans, R.B., & Marmorston, J. (1963a). Improved mental functioning with Premarin therapy in atherosclerosis. *Proceedings of the Society for Experimental Biology and Medicine, 113*, 698–703.

Evans, R.B., & Marmorston, J. (1963b). Psychological test signs of brain damage in cerebral thrombosis. *Psychological Reports, 12*, 915–930.

Evans, R.B., & Marmorston, J. (1964). Rorschach signs of brain damage in cerebral thrombosis. *Perceptual and Motor Skills, 18*, 977–988.

Evans, R.B., & Marmorston, J. (1965). Mental functioning and Premarin therapy in cardiovascular and cerebrovascular disease. *Proceedings of the Society for Experimental Biology and Medicine, 118*, 529–533.

Exner, J.E. (1974). *The Rorschach: A comprehensive system*. New York: John Wiley & Sons.

Exner, J.E. (1978). *The Rorschach: A comprehensive system* (Vol. 2). New York: John Wiley & Sons.

Exner, J.E. (1982). *The Rorschach: A comprehensive system* (Vol. 3). New York: John Wiley & Sons.

Exner, J.E., Jr., Colligan, S.C., Boll, T.J., Stischer, B., & Hillman, L. (1996). Rorschach findings concerning closed head injury. *Assessment, 3*, 317–326.

Eysenck, H.J. (1952). *The scientific study of personality*. London: Routledge and Kegan Paul.

Fals-Stewart, W. (1996). The ability of individuals with psychoactive substance use disorders to dissimulate successfully on the Personality Assessment Inventory. *Psychological Assessment, 8*, 60–68.

Fals-Stewart, W. (1997). Detection of neuropsychological impairment among substance-abusing patients: Accuracy of the Neurobehavioral Cognitive Status Examination. *Experimental and Clinical Psychopharmacology, 5*, 269–276.

Fals-Stewart, W., & Lucente, S. (1997). Identifying positive dissimulation by substance-abusing individuals on the Personality Assessment Inventory. *Journal of Personality Assessment, 68*, 455–469.

Fama, R., Sullivan, E.V., Shear, P.K., Cahn-Weiner, D.A., Yesavage, J.A., Tinklenberg, J.R., & Pfefferbaum, A. (1998). Fluency patterns in Alzheimer's disease and Parkinson's disease. *The Clinical Neuropsychologist, 12*, 487–499.

Fantoni-Salvador, P., & Rogers, R. (1997). Spanish versions of the MMPI-2 and PAI: An investigation of concurrent validity with Hispanic patients. *Assessment, 4,* 29–39.

Farley, F.H. (1969). Further data on multiple choice versus open-ended estimates of vocabulary. *British Journal of Social and Clinical Psychology, 8,* 67–68.

Farmer, J.E., & Brazeal, T.J. (1998). Parent perceptions about the process and outcomes of child neuropsychological assessment. *Applied Neuropsychology, 5,* 194–210.

Fastenau, P.S. (1996). An elaborated administration of the Wechsler Memory Scale-Revised. *The Clinical Neuropsychologist, 10,* 425–434.

Fastenau, P.S. (1999). Validity of regression-based norms: An empirical test of the Comprehensive Norms with older adults. *Journal of Clinical and Experimental Neuropsychology, 20,* 906–916.

Fastenau, P.S., & Adams, K.M. (1996). Heaton, Grant, and Matthews' Comprehensive Norms: An overzealous attempt. *Journal of Clinical and Experimental Neuropsychology, 18,* 444–448.

Fastenau, P.S., Denburg, N.L., & Abeles, N. (1996). Age differences in retrieval: Further support for the resource-reduction hypothesis. *Psychology and Aging, 11,* 140–146.

Faust, D., Hart, K., & Guilmette, T.J. (1988a). Pediatric malingering: The capacity of children to fake believable deficits on neuropsychological testing. *Journal of Consulting and Clinical Psychology, 56,* 578–582.

Faust, D., Hart, K., Guilmette, T.J., & Arkes, H.R. (1988b). Neuropsychologists' capacity to detect adolescent malingerers. *Professional Psychology: Research and Practice, 19,* 508–515.

Faust, D.S., & Hollingsworth, J.O. (1991). Concurrent validity of the Wechsler Preschool and Primary Scale of Intelligence-Revised (WPPSI-R) with two criteria of cognitive abilities. *Journal of Psychoeducational Assessment, 9,* 224–229.

Fein, D., Waterhouse, L., Lucci, D., & Snyder, D. (1985). Cognitive subtypes in developmentally disabled children: A pilot study. *Journal of Autism and Developmental Disorders, 15,* 77–95.

Ferland, M.B., Ramsay, J., Engeland, C., & O'Hara, P. (1998). Comparison of the performance of normal individuals and survivors of traumatic brain injury on repeat administrations of the Wisconsin Card Sorting Test. *Journal of Clinical and Experimental Neuropsychology, 20,* 473–482.

Ferman, T.J., Ivnik, R.J., & Lucas, J.A. (1998). Boston Naming Test discontinuation rule: Rigorous vs. lenient interpretations. *Assessment, 5,* 13–18.

Ferraro, F.R., & Bercier, B. (1996). Boston Naming Test performance in a sample of Native American elderly adults. *Clinical Gerontologist, 17,* 58–60.

Ferraro, F.R., Blaine, T., Flaig, S., & Bradford, S. (1998). Familiarity norms for the Boston Naming Test stimuli. *Applied Neuropsychology, 5,* 43–47.

Field, M. (1987). Relation of language delayed preschooler's Leiter scores to later IQ. *Journal of Child Clinical Psychology, 16,* 111–115.

Fields, F.R. (1971). Relative effects of brain damage on Wechsler memory and intelligence quotients. *Diseases of the Nervous System, 32,* 673–675.

Filley, C.M., Kobayashi, J., & Heaton, R.K. (1987). Wechsler Intelligence Scale profiles, the cholinergic system, and Alzheimer's disease. *Journal of Clinical and Experimental Neuropsychology, 5,* 180–186.

Filskov, S.B., & Goldstein, S.G. (1974). Diagnostic validity of the Halstead–Reitan neuropsychological battery. *Journal of Consulting and Clinical Psychology, 42,* 382–388.

Filskov, S.B., & Leli, D. (1981). Assessment of the individual in neuropsychological practice. In S.B. Filskov & T.J. Boll (Eds.), *Handbook of clinical neuropsychology.* New York: Wiley-Interscience.

Finger, M.S., & Ones, D.S. (1999). Psychometric equivalence of the computer and booklet forms of the MMPI: A meta-analysis. *Psychological Assessment, 11,* 58–66.

Finger, S., & Stein, D.G. (1982). *Brain damage and recovery: Research and clinical perspectives.* New York: Academic Press.

Finlayson, M.A.J., Johnson, K.A., & Reitan, R.M. (1977). Relationship of level of education to neuropsychological measures in brain-damaged and non-brain-damaged adults. *Journal of Consulting and Clinical Psychology, 45,* 536–542.

Finton, M.J., Lucas, J.A., Graff-Radford, N.R., & Uitti, R.J. (1998). Analysis of visuospatial errors in patients with Alzheimer's disease or Parkinson's disease. *Journal of Clinical and Experimental Neuropsychology, 20,* 186–193.

Fish, J.M., & Sinkel, P. (1980). Correlation of scores on Wechsler Memory Scale and Wechsler Adult Intelligence Scale for chronic alcoholics and normals. *Psychological Reports, 47,* 940–942.

Fisher, J.S. (1988). Using the Wechsler Memory Scale-Revised to detect and characterize memory deficits in multiple sclerosis. *The Clinical Neuropsychologist, 2*, 149–172.

Fisher, J., Gonda, T., & Little, K.B. (1955). The Rorschach and central nervous system pathology. *American Journal of Psychiatry, 111*, 486–492.

Fiske, D.W. (1971). *Measuring the concepts of personality.* Chicago: Aldine.

Fiske, D.W. (1976). Can a personality construct have a singular validational pattern? Rejoinder to Huba and Hamilton. *Psychological Bulletin, 83*, 87.

Fiske, D.W. (1978). *Strategies for personality assessment.* San Francisco: Jossey-Bass.

Fitz, A.G., Conrad, P.M., Hom, D.L., Sarff, P.L., & Majovski, L.V. (1992). Hooper Visual Organization Test performance in lateralized brain injury. *Archives of Clinical Neuropsychology, 7*, 243–250.

Fitzhugh, K.B., Fitzhugh, L.C., & Reitan, R.M. (1961). Psychological deficits in relation to acuteness of brain dysfunction. *Journal of Consulting Psychology, 25*, 61–66.

Fitzhugh, K.B., Fitzhugh, L.C., & Reitan, R.M. (1964). Influence of age upon measures of problem solving and experimental background in subjects with longstanding cerebral dysfunction. *Journal of Gerontology, 19*, 132–134.

Flanagan, J.L. & Jackson, S.T. (1997). Test–retest reliability of three aphasia tests: Performance of non-brain-damaged older adults. *Journal of Communication Disorders, 30*, 33–43.

Flashman, L.A., Horner, M.D., & Freides, D. (1991a). Increasing interscorer reliability on the Wisconsin Card Sorting Test (WCST) using clarified scoring rules. (Abstract) *Journal of Clinical and Experimental Neuropsychology, 13*, 431.

Flashman, L.A., Horner, M.D., & Freides, D. (1991b). Note on scoring perseverations on the Wisconsin Card Sorting Test. *The Clinical Neuropsychologist, 5*, 190–194.

Flemmer, D.D., & Roid, G.H. (1997). Nonverbal intellectual assessment of Hispanic Speech impaired adolescents. *Psychological Reports, 80*, 1115–1122.

Flick, G.L., & Edwards, K.R. (1971). Prediction of organic brain dysfunction with the MMPI. *Newsletter for Research in Psychology, 13*, 18–19.

Flipsen, P. (1998). Assessing receptive vocabulary in small-town Canadian kindergarten children: Findings for the PPVT-R. *Journal of Speech-Language Pathology and Audiology, 22*, 88–93.

Flynn, J.R. (1984). The mean IQ of Americans: Massive gains 1932-1978. *Psychological Bulletin, 95*, 29–51.

Flynn, J.R. (1987). Massive IQ gains in 14 nations: What IQ tests really measures. *Psychological Bulletin, 101*, 171–191.

Flynn, J.R. (1990). Massive gains on the Scottish WISC. Evidence against Brand, et al.'s hypothesis. *Irish Journal of Psychology, 11*, 41–51.

Flynn, J.R. (1998). WAIS-III and WISC-III gains from 1972 to 1995: How to compensate for obsolete norms. *Perceptual and Motor Skills, 86*, 1231–1239.

Flynt, S.W., Warren, J.S., Morton, R.C., & Smith, F.H. (1997). Examining the question of gender bias in the Slosson Intelligence in relation to reading. *Reading Psychology, 18*, 237–248.

Forar, B.R., Farberow, N.L., Meyer, M.N., & Tolman, R.S. (1952). Consistency and agreement in the judgement of Rorschach signs. *Journal of Projective Techniques, 16*, 346–351.

Ford, M. (1946). The application of the Rorschach test to young children. *University of Minnesota Child Welfare Monograph*, No. 23.

Forrester, G., & Geffen, G. (1991). Performance measures of 7- to 15-year-old children on the Auditory Verbal Learning Test. *The Clinical Neuropsychologist, 5*, 345–359.

Fowler, P.C., Richards, H.C., Berent, S., & Boll, T.J. (1987). Epilepsy, neuropsychological deficits, and EEG lateralization. *Archives of Clinical Neuropsychology, 2*, 81–92.

Fowler, P.C., Zillmer, E., & Newman, A.C. (1988). A multifactor model of the Halstead–Reitan Neuropsychological Test Battery and its relationship to cognitive status and psychiatric diagnosis. *Journal of Clinical Psychology, 44*, 898–906.

Fraboni, M., & Saltstone, R. (1992). The WAIS-R number-of-factors quandary: A cluster analytic approach to construct validation. *Educational and Psychological Measurement, 52*, 603–613.

Frank, G. (1991). Research on the clinical usefulness of the Rorschach II: The assessment of cerebral dysfunction. *Perceptual and Motor Skills, 72*, 103–111.

Franzen, M.D., & Golden, C.J. (1984a). Multivariate techniques in neuropsychology: 2. Comparison of number of factors rules. *International Journal of Clinical Neuropsychology, 6*, 165–171.

Franzen, M.D., & Golden, C.J. (1984b). Multivariate techniques in neuropsychology: 3. Discriminant function analysis. *International Journal of Clinical Neuropsychology, 6,* 80–87.

Franzen, M.D., Tishelman, A.C., Sharp, B.H., & Friedman, A.G. (1987). Test–retest reliability of the Stroop Word Color Test across two intervals. *Archives of Clinical Neuropsychology, 2,* 265–272.

Franzen, M.D., Iverson, G.L., & McCracken, L.M. (1990). The detection of malingering in neuropsychological assessment. *Neuropsychology Review, 1,* 247–279.

Franzen, M.D., Haut, M.W., Rankin, E., & Keefover, R. (1995a). Empirical comparison of alternate forms of the Boston Naming Test. *The Clinical Neuropsychologist, 9,* 225–229.

Franzen, M.D., Wilhelm, K.L., & Haut, M.W. (1995b). The factor structure of the Wechsler Memory Scale-Revised and several brief neuropsychological screening instruments in recently detoxified substance abusers. *Archives of Clinical Neuropsychology, 10,* 193–294.

Franzen, M.D., Paul, D., & Iverson, G.L. (1996). Reliability of alternate forms of the Trail Making Test. *The Clinical Neuropsychologist, 10,* 125–129.

Franzen, M.D., Burgess, E.J., & Smith-Seemiller, L. (1997). Methods of estimating premorbid functioning. *Archives of Clinical Neuropsychology, 12,* 711–738.

Fraser, R.M., & Glass, I.B. (1980). Unilateral and bilateral ECT in elderly patients. *Acta Psychiatrica Scandinavica, 62,* 13–31.

Frederick, R.L., Sarafaty, S.D., Johnston, J.D., & Powel, J. (1994). Validation of a detector of response bias on a forced-choice test of noveral ability. *Neuropsychology, 8,* 118–125.

Freedman, M., Leach, L., Kaplan, E., Winocur, G., Shulman, K., & Delis, D. (1994). *Clock drawing: A neuropsychological analysis.* New York: Oxford University Press.

Freedman, M., Black, S., Ebert, S., & Binns, M. (1998). Orbitofrontal function, object alternation, and perseveration. *Cerebral Cortex, 8,* 18–27.

Freidt, L.R., & Gouvier, W.D. (1989). Bender–Gestalt screening for brain dysfunction in a forensic population. *Criminal Justice and Behavior, 16,* 455–464.

French, J.L. (1964). *Pictorial Test of Intelligence Manual.* Boston: Houghton Mifflin.

Freuh, B.C., & Kinder, B.N. (1994). The susceptibility of the Rorschach inkblot test to malingering of combat-related PTSD. *Journal of Personality Assessment, 62,* 280–298.

Frey, P.D. (1996). Comparison of visual-motor performance and nonverbal reasoning among children and adolescent patients in an urban psychiatric hospital. *Perceptual and Motor Skills, 82,* 179–184.

Friedman, S.H. (1950). Psychometric effects of frontal and parietal lobe brain damage. Unpublished doctoral dissertation, University of Minnesota.

Frisch, M.B., & Jessop, N.S. (1989). Improving WAIS-R estimates with the Shipley–Hartford and Wonderlic Personnel Tests: Need to control for reading ability. *Psychological Reports, 65,* 923–928.

Fristoe, N.M., Salthouse, T.A., & Woodard, J.L. (1997). Examination of age-related deficits on the Wisconsin Card Sorting Test. *Neuropsychology, 11,* 428–436.

Fromm, D., Holland, A.L., Nebes, R.D., & Oakley, M.A. (1991). A longitudinal study of word-reading ability in Alzheimer's disease: Evidence from the National Adult Reading Test. *Cortex, 27,* 367–376.

Fromm-Auch, D., & Yeudall, L.T. (1983). Normative data for the Halstead–Reitan Neuropsychological Tests. *Journal of Clinical and Experimental Neuropsychology, 9,* 221–238.

Fuerst, D.R. (1997). Some critical remarks regarding Veiel's comment on Wilde, et al. (1995). *Journal of Clinical and Experimental Neuropsychology, 19,* 149–152.

Fuld, P.A. (1983). Psychometric differentiation of the dementias: An overview. In B. Reisberg (Ed.), *Alzheimer's disease* (pp. 201–210). New York: Free Press.

Fuller, G.B. (1969). The Minnesota Percepto-Diagnostic Test (Revised). *Journal of Clinical Psychology* (Monograph Supplement), No. 28.

Fuller, G.B. (1982). *The Minnesota Percepto-Diagnostic Test (Revised) manual.* Brandon, VT: Clinical Psychology Publications.

Fuller, G.B., & Friedrich, D. (1976). Differential diagnosis of psychiatric patients with the Minnesota Percepto-Diagnostic Test. *Journal of Clinical Psychology, 32,* 335–337.

Fuller, G.B., & Friedrich, D. (1979). Visual-motor test performance: Race and achievement variables. *Journal of Clinical Psychology, 35,* 621–623.

Fuller, G.B., & Hawkins, W.F. (1969). Differentiation of organic from non-organic retarded children. *American Journal of Mental Deficiency, 74,* 104–110.

Fuller, G.B., & Laird, J. (1963). The Minnesota Percepto-Diagnostic Test. *Journal of Clinical Psychology* (Monograph Supplement), No. 16.

Fuller, G.B., & Vance, B. (1993). Comparison of the Minnesota Percepto-Diagnostic Test-Revised and Bender–Gestalt in predicting achievement. *Psychology in the Schools, 30,* 220–226.

Fuller, G.B., & Vance, B. (1995). Interscorer reliability of the Modified Version of the Bender–Gestalt Test for Preschool and Primary Children. *Psychology in the Schools, 32,* 264–266.

Fuller, G.B., & Wallbrown, F.H. (1983). Comparison of the Minnesota Percepto-Diagnostic Test and Bender Gestalt: Relationship with achievement criteria. *Journal of Clinical Psychology, 39,* 985–988.

Fuller, G.B., Sharp, H., & Hawkins, W.F. (1967). Minnesota Percepto-Diagnostic Test (MPD): Age norms and IQ adjustments. *Journal of Clinical Psychology, 23,* 456–461.

Fuller, K.H., Gouvier, W.D., & Savage, R.M. (1997). Comparison of list B and list C of the Rey Verbal Auditory Learning Test. *The Clinical Neuropsychologist, 11,* 201–204.

Funk, S.G., Sturner, R.A., & Green, J.A. (1986). Preschool prediction of early school performance: Relationship of McCarthy Scales of Children's Abilities prior to school entry to achievement in kindergarten, first, and second grades. *Journal of School Psychology, 24,* 181–194.

Gainotti, G., D'Erme, P., Villa, G., & Caltagirone, C. (1986). Focal brain lesions and intelligence: A study of a new version. *Journal of Clinical and Experimental Neuropsychology, 8,* 37–50.

Gale, S.D., Johnson, S.C., Bigler, E.D., & Blatter, D.D. (1994). Traumatic brain injury and temporal horn enlargement: Correlates with tests of intelligence and memory. *Neuropsychiatry, Neuropsychology, and Behavioral Neurology, 7,* 160–165.

Gale, S.D., Johnson, S.C., Bigler, E.D., & Blatter, D.D. (1995). Nonspecific white matter degeneration following traumatic brain injury. *Journal of the International Neuropsychological Society, 1,* 17–28.

Gallagher, A.J. (1979). Temporal reliability of aphasic performance on the Token Test. *Brain and Language, 7,* 34–41.

Gallen, R.T., & Berry, D.T.R. (1996). Detection of random responding in MMPI-2 protocols. *Assessment, 3,* 171–178.

Gallen, R.T., & Berry, D.T.R. (1997). Partially random MMPI-2 protocols: When are they interpretable? *Assessment, 4,* 61–68.

Gallucci, N.T. (1997). Correlates of MMPI-A substance abuse scales. *Assessment, 4,* 87–94.

Ganellen, R.J. (1994). Attempting to conceal psychological disturbance: MMPI defensive response sets and the Rorschach. *Journal of Personality Assessment, 63,* 423–437.

Ganellen, R.J. (1996). Exploring MMPI-Rorschach relationships. *Journal of Personality Assessment, 67,* 529–542.

Ganellen, R.J., Wasyliw, O.E., Haywood, T.W., & Grossman, L.S. (1996). Can psychosis be malingered on the Rorschach? An empirical study. *Journal of Personality Assessment, 66,* 65–80.

Garb, H.N., Florio, C.M., & Grove, W.M. (1998). The validity of the Rorschach and the Minnesota Multiphasic Personality Inventory. *Psychological Science, 9,* 402–404.

Garb, H.N., & Schramke, C.J. (1996). Judgement research and neuropsychological assessment: A narrative review and meta-analyses. *Psychological Bulletin, 120,* 140–153.

Gardner, R., Jr., Oliver-Munoz, S., Fisher, L., & Empting, L. (1981). Mattis Dementia Rating Scale: Internal reliability study using a diffusely impaired population. *Journal of Clinical Neuropsychology, 3,* 271–275.

Garfield, J.C. (1964). Motor impersistence in normal and brain-damaged children. *Neurology, 14,* 623–630.

Garfield, J.C., Benton, A.L., & McQueen, J.C. (1966). Motor impersistence in brain-damaged and cultural-familial defectives. *Journal of Nervous and Mental Disease, 142,* 434–440.

Garmoe, W.S., Schefft, B.K., & Moses, J.A., Jr. (1991). Evaluation of the diagnostic validity of the Luria–Nebraska Neuropsychological Battery-Form II. *International Journal of Neuroscience, 59,* 231–239.

Gass, C.S. (1991). MMPI-2 interpretation and closed-head trauma: A correction factor. *Psychological Assessment, 2,* 27–31.

Gass, C.S. (1992). MMPI-2 interpretation of patients with cerebrovascular disease: A correction factor. *Archives of Clinical Neuropsychology, 7,* 17–27.

Gass, C.S. (1995). A procedure for assessing storage and retrieval on the Wechsler Memory Scale-Revised. *Archives of Clinical Neuropsychology, 10,* 475–487.

Gass, C.S. (1996a). MMPI-2 interpretation and stroke: Cross-validation of a correction factor. *Journal of Clinical Psychology, 52,* 569–572.

Gass, C.S. (1996b). MMPI-2 variables in attention and memory test performance. *Psychological Assessment, 8*, 135–138.

Gass, C.S., & Ansley, J. (1994). MMPI correlates of poststroke neurobehavioral deficits. *Archives of Clinical Neuropsychology, 9*, 461–469.

Gass, C.S., & Apple, C. (1997). Cognitive complaints in closed-head injury: Relationship to memory test performance and emotional disturbance. *Journal of Clinical and Experimental Neuropsychology, 19*, 290–299.

Gass, C.S., & Lawhorn, L. (1991). Psychological adjustment to stroke: An MMPI study. *Psychological Assessment, 3*, 628–633.

Gass, C.S., & Russell, E.W. (1991). MMPI profiles of patients with closed-head trauma. Impact of neurologic complaints. *Journal of Clinical Psychology, 7*, 253–260.

Gass, C.S., & Wald, H.S. (1997). MMPI-2 interpretation and closed-head trauma: Cross-validation of a correction factor. *Archives of Clinical Neuropsychology, 12*, 199–205.

Gaskill, F.W., & Brantley, J. (1996). Changes in ability and achievement scores over time: Implications for children classified as learning disabled. *Journal of Psychoeducational Assessment, 14*, 220–228.

Gazzaniga, M.D., & LeDoux, J.E. (1978). *The integrated mind.* New York: Plenum Press.

Geffen, G., Butterworth, P., & Geffen, L. (1994). Test–retest reliability of a new form of the Auditory Verbal Learning Test (AVLT). *Archives of Clinical Neuropsychology, 9*, 303–316.

George, J. (1973). Differentiating clinical groups by means of the Minnesota Percepto-Diagnostic Test. *Journal of Clinical Psychology, 29*, 210–212.

Gerken, K.C., & Hodapp, A.F. (1992). Assessment of preschoolers at-risk with the WPPSI-R and the Stanford–Binet L-M. *Psychological Reports, 71*, 659–664.

Gfeller, J.D., Meldrum, D.L., & Jacobi, K.A. (1995). The impact of constructional impairment on the WMS-R Visual Reproduction subtests. *Journal of Clinical Psychology, 51*, 58–63.

Giambra, L.M., Arenberg, D., Zonderman, A.B., Kawas, C., & Costa, P.T., Jr. (1995). Adult life span changes in immediate visual memory and verbal intelligence. *Psychology and Aging, 10*, 123–139.

Giancola, P.R., Zeichner, A., Yarnell, J.E., & Dickson, K.E. (1996). Relation between executive dysfunctioning and the adverse consequences of alcohol use in social drinkers. *Alcoholism, Clinical and Experimental Research, 20*, 1094–1098.

Giebink, J.W., & Birch, R. (1970). The Bender Gestalt test as an ineffective predictor of reading achievement. *Journal of Clinical Psychology, 26*, 484–485.

Gilberstadt, H., & Farkas, E. (1961). Another look at MMPI profile types in multiple sclerosis. *Journal of Consulting Psychology, 25*, 440–444.

Gillen, R.W., Ginn, C., Strider, M.A., Kreuch, T.J., & Golden, C.J. (1983). The Luria–Nebraska Neuropsychological Battery and the Peabody Individual Achievement Test: A correlational analysis. *International Journal of Neuroscience, 21*, 51–62.

Gimse, R., Bjorgen, I.A., Tjell, C., Tyssedal, J.S., & Bo, K. (1997). Reduced cognitive functions in a group of whiplash patients with demonstrated disturbances in the posture control system. *Journal of Clinical and Experimental Neuropsychology, 19*, 838–849.

Gioia, G.A. (1998). Re-examining the factor structure of the Wide Range Assessment of Memory and Learning: Implications for clinical interpretation. *Assessment, 5*, 127–139.

Gladjso, J.A., Heaton, R.K., Palmer, B.W., Taylor, M.J., & Jests, D.V. (1999a). Use of oral reading to estimate premorbid intellectual and neuropsychological functioning. *Journal of the International Neuropsychological Society, 5*, 247–254.

Gladsjo, J.A., Schuman, C.C., Evans, J.D., Peavy, G.M., Miller, S.W., & Heaton, R.K. (1999b). Norms for letter and category fluency: Demographic corrections for age, education, and ethnicity. *Assessment, 6*, 147–178.

Glass, G.V., McGraw, B., & Smith, M.L. (1981). *Meta-analysis in social research.* Beverly Hills, CA: Sage.

Glaub, V.E., & Kamphaus, R.W. (1991). Construction of a nonverbal adaptation of the Stanford–Binet Fourth Edition. *Educational and Psychological Measurement, 51*, 231–241.

Glutting, J.J., Youngstrom, E.A., Ward, T., Ward, S., & Hale, R.L. (1997). Incremental efficacy of WISC-III factor scores in predicting achievement: What do they tell us? *Psychological Assessment, 9*, 295–301.

Godfrey, H.P.D., Partridge, F.M., Knight, R.G., & Bishara, S. (1993). Course of insight disorder and emotional dysfunction following closed head injury: A controlled cross-sectional follow-up study. *Journal of Clinical and Experimental Neuropsychology, 15*, 503–515.

Goebel, R.A. (1983). Detection of faking of the Halstead–Reitan Neuropsychological Test Battery. *Journal of Clinical Psychology, 39*, 731–742.

Gold, J.M., Randolph, C., Carpenter, C.J., Goldberg, T.E., & Weinberger, D.R. (1992). The performance of patients with schizophrenia on the Wechsler Memory Scale-Revised. *The Clinical Neuropsychologist, 6*, 367–373.

Golden, C.J. (1974). Sex differences in performance on the Stroop Color and Word Test. *Perceptual and Motor Skills, 39*, 1067–1070.

Golden, C.J. (1975). A group form of the Stroop Color and Word Test. *Journal of Personality Assessment, 39*, 386–388.

Golden, C.J. (1976a). The diagnosis of brain damage by the Stroop test. *Journal of Clinical Psychology, 32*, 652–658.

Golden, C.J. (1976b). The identification of brain damage by an abbreviated form of the Halstead–Reitan Neuropsychological Battery. *Journal of Clinical Psychology, 32*, 821–826.

Golden, C.J. (1977). Validity of the Halstead–Reitan Neuropsychological Battery in a mixed psychiatric and brain-injured population. *Journal of Consulting and Clinical Psychology, 45*, 1043–1051.

Golden, C.J. (1978a). *Diagnosis and rehabilitation in clinical neuropsychology.* Springfield, IL: Charles C Thomas.

Golden, C.J. (1978b). *Stroop Color and Word Test: A manual for clinical and experimental use.* Chicago: Stoelting.

Golden, C.J. (1980). In reply to Adams' "In search of Luria's battery: A false start." *Journal of Consulting and Clinical Psychology, 48*, 517–521.

Golden, C.J. (1989). Abbreviating administration of the LNNB in significantly impaired patients. *International Journal of Clinical Neuropsychology, 11*, 177–181.

Golden, C.J., & Maruish, M. (1986). The Luria–Nebraska Neuropsychological Battery. In T. Incagnoli, G. Goldstein, & C.J. Golden (Eds.), *Clinical application of neuropsychological test batteries* (pp. 193–234). New York: Plenum.

Golden, C.J., & Schlutter, L.C. (1978). The interaction of age and diagnosis in neuropsychological test results. *International Journal of Neurosciences, 8*, 61–63.

Golden, C.J., Hammeke, T.A., & Purisch, A.D. (1978). Diagnostic validity of a standardized neuropsychological battery derived from Luria's neuropsychological tests. *Journal of Consulting and Clinical Psychology, 46*, 1258–1265.

Golden, C.J., Sweet, J.J., & Osmon, D.C. (1979). The diagnosis of brain-damage by the MMPI: A comprehensive evaluation. *Journal of Personality Assessment, 2*, 138–142.

Golden, C.J., Graber, B., Moses, J.A., & Zatz, L.M. (1980a). Differentiation of chronic schizophrenics with and without ventricular enlargement by the Luria–Nebraska Neuropsychological Battery. *International Journal of Neuroscience, 11*, 131–138.

Golden, C.J., Hammeke, T.A., & Purisch, A.D. (1980b). *Luria–Nebraska Neuropsychological Battery manual.* Los Angeles: Western Psychological Services.

Golden, C.J., Kuperman, S.K., MacInnes, W.D., & Moses, J.A. (1980c). Cross-validation of an abbreviated form of the Halstead Category Test. *Journal of Consulting and Clinical Psychology, 49*, 606–607.

Golden, C.J., Fross, K.H., & Graber, B. (1981a). Split-half reliability of the Luria–Nebraska Neuropsychological Battery. *Journal of Consulting and Clinical Psychology, 49*, 304–305.

Golden, C.J., Kane, R.K., Sweet, J., Moses, J.A., Cardellino, J.P., Templeton, R., Vicente, P., & Graber, B. (1981b). Relationship of the Halstead–Reitan Neuropsychological Battery to the Luria–Nebraska Neuropsychological Battery. *Journal of Consulting and Clinical Psychology, 49*, 410–411.

Golden, C.J., Moses, J.A., Fishburne, F.J., Engum, E., Lewis, G.P., Wisniewsh, A.M., Conley, F.K., Berg, R.A., & Graber, B. (1981c). Cross-validation of the Luria–Nebraska Neuropsychological Battery of the presence, lateralization, and localization of brain damage. *Journal of Consulting and Clinical Psychology, 49*, 491–507.

Golden, C.J., Ariel, R.J., Wilkening, G.N., McKay, S.E., & MacInnes, W.D. (1982a). Analytic techniques in the interpretation of the Luria–Nebraska Neuropsychological Battery. *Journal of Consulting and Clinical Psychology, 50*, 40–48.

Golden, C.J., Berg, R.A., & Graber, B. (1982b). Test–retest reliability of the Luria–Nebraska Neuropsychological Battery in stable, chronically impaired patients. *Journal of Consulting and Clinical Psychology, 50*, 452–454.

Golden, C.J., Gustavson, J.L., & Ariel, R. (1982c). Correlations between the Luria–Nebraska and Halstead–Reitan batteries: Effects of partialling out education and post-morbid I.Q. *Journal of Consulting and Clinical Psychology, 50*, 770–771.

Golden, C.J., Hammeke, T.A., Purisch, A.D., Berg, R.A., Moses, J.A., Newlin, D.B., Wilkening, G.N., & Puente, A.E. (1982d). *Item interpretation of the Luria–Nebraska Neuropsychological Battery*. Lincoln: University of Nebraska Press.

Golden, C.J., MacInnes, W.D., Ariel, R.N., Ruedrich, S.L., Chu, C., Coffman, J.A., Graber, B., & Bloch, S. (1982e). Cross-validation of the Luria–Nebraska Neuropsychological Battery to discriminate chronic schizophrenics with and without ventricular enlargement. *Journal of Consulting and Clinical Psychology*, *50*, 87–95.

Golden, C.J., Purish, A.D., & Hammeke, T.A. (1985). *Luria–Nebraska Neuropsychological Battery: Forms I and II*. Los Angeles: Western Psychological Services.

Golden, C.J., White, L., Combs, T., Morgan, M., & McLane, D. (1999). WMS-R and MAS correlations in a neuropsychological population. *Archives of Clinical Neuropsychology*, *14*, 265–271.

Goldfried, M.R., Stricker, G., & Weiner, I.B. (1971). *Rorschach handbook of clinical and research applications*. Englewood Cliffs, NJ: Prentice-Hall.

Goldman, R.S., Axelrod, B.N., Giordani, B.J., Foster, N., & Berent, S. (1992). Longitudinal sensitivity of the Fuld cholinergic profile to Alzheimer's disease. *Journal of Clinical and Experimental Neuropsychology*, *14*, 566–574.

Goldman, R.S., Axelrod, B.N., Heaton, R.K., Chelune, G.J., Curtiss, G., Kay, G.G., & Thompson, L.L. (1996). Latent structure of the WCST with the standardization samples. *Assessment*, *3*, 73–78.

Goldstein, D.J., & Britt, T.W. (1994). Visual–motor coordination and intelligence as predictors of reading, mathematics, and written language ability. *Perceptual and Motor Skills*, *78*, 819–823.

Goldstein, D.J., Fogle, E.E., Wieber, E.E., & O'Shea, T.M. (1995). Comparison of the Bayley Scales of Infant Development Second Edition and the Bayley Scales of Infant Development with premature infants. *Journal of Psychoeducational Assessment*, *13*, 391–396.

Goldstein, G., & Shelly, C. (1973). Univariate vs. multivariate analysis in neuropsychological test assessment: A critical review. *Clinical Neuropsychology*, *2*, 49–51.

Goldstein, G., & Shelly, C. (1982). A further attempt to cross-validate the Russell, Neuringer, & Goldstein neuropsychological keys. *Journal of Consulting and Clinical Psychology*, *50*, 721–726.

Goldstein, G., & Shelly, C. (1984). Discriminative validity of various intelligence and neuropsychological tests. *Journal of Consulting and Clinical Psychology*, *52*, 383–389.

Goldstein, G., Shelly, C., McCue, M., & Kane, R.L. (1987). Classification with the Luria–Nebraska Neuropsychological Battery: An application of cluster and ipsative profile analysis. *Archives of Clinical Neuropsychology*, *2*, 215–235.

Goldstein, G., & Shemansky, W.J. (1997). Patterns of performance by neuropsychiatric patients on the Halstead Category Test: Evidence for conceptual learning in schizophrenic patients. *Archives of Clinical Neuropsychology*, *12*, 251–255.

Goldstein, G., Shemansky, W.J., Beers, S.R., George, T., & Roberts, K. (1996). A clarification of the Russell, Neuringer, and Goldstein Process Key: Implications for outcome. *Archives of Clinical Neuropsychology*, *11*, 581–587.

Goldstein, S.G., Deysach, R.E., & Kleinknecht, R.A. (1973). Effects of experience and amount of information on identification of cerebral impairment. *Journal of Consulting and Clinical Psychology*, *41*, 30–34.

Gomez-Benito, J., & Forns-Santacana, M. (1990). Factor structure of the McCarthy scales. *Psychology in the Schools*, *27*, 111–115.

Gomez-Benito, J., & Forns-Santacana, M. (1993). Concurrent validity between the Columbia Mental Maturity Scale and the McCarthy scales. *Perceptual and Motor Skills*, *76*, 1177–1178.

Gomez-Benito, J., & Forns-Santacana, M. (1996). Factor structure of the McCarthy Scales in 7-year-old Spanish children. *Psychology in the Schools*, *33*, 231–238.

Goodglass, H., & Kaplan, E. (1983). *The assessment of aphasia and related disorders*. Philadelphia: Lea & Febiger.

Gorsuch, R.L. (1974). *Factor analysis*. Philadelphia: W.B. Saunders.

Gottfredson, L.S. (1994). The science and politics of race-norming. *American Psychologist*, *49*, 955–963.

Gouvier, W.D., Bolter, J.F., Veneklasen, J.A., & Long, C.J. (1983). Predicting verbal and performance IQ from demographic data: Further findings with head trauma patients. *Clinical Neuropsychology*, *5*, 119–121.

Gow, L., & Ward, J. (1982). The Porteus Maze Test in the measurement of reflection/impulsivity. *Perceptual and Motor Skills*, *54*, 1043–1053.

Graham, F.K., & Kendall, B.S. (1960). Memory for Designs Test: Revised general manual. *Perceptual and Motor Skills, 11,* 147–188.

Graham, J.R., Smith, R.L., & Schwartz, G.F. (1986). Stability of MMPI configurations for psychiatric inpatients. *Journal of Consulting and Clinical Psychology, 54,* 375–380.

Grauer, D. (1953). Prognosis in paranoid schizophrenia on the basis of the Rorschach. *Journal of Consulting Psychology, 17,* 199–205.

Graves, R.E., Carswell, L.M., & Snow, W.G. (1999). An evaluation of the sensitivity of premorbid IQ estimators for detecting cognitive decline. *Psychological Assessment, 11,* 29–38.

Gravitz, M.A., & Gerton, M.I. (1976). An empirical study of internal consistency in the MMPI. *Journal of Clinical Psychology, 32,* 567–568.

Greene, R.L. (1990). Stability of MMPI scale scores within four codetypes across forty years. *Journal of Personality Assessment, 55,* 1–6.

Greene, R.L. (1991). *The MMPI-2/MMPI: An Interpretive Manual.* Boston: Allyn & Bacon.

Greene, V., & Carmines, E. (1980). Assessing the reliability of linear composites. In K.F. Schuessler (Ed.), *Sociological methodology 1980.* San Francisco: Jossey-Bass.

Gregg, N., & Hoy, C. (1985). A comparison of the WAIS-R and the Woodcock–Johnson Tests of Cognitive Ability with learning-disabled college students. *Journal of Psychoeducational Assessment, 3,* 267–274.

Gregory, R.J., Paul, J.J., & Morrison, M.W. (1979). A short form of the Category test for adults. *Journal of Clinical Psychology, 35,* 795–798.

Greiffenstein, M.F., Baker, W.J., & Gola, T. (1994). Validation of malingered amnesia measures with a large clinical sample. *Psychological Assessment, 6,* 218–224.

Greiffenstein, M.F., Gola, T., & Baker, W.J. (1995). MMPI-2 validity scales versus domain specific measures in detection of factitious traumatic brain injury. *The Clinical Neuropsychologist, 9,* 230–240.

Greiffenstein, M.F., Baker, W.J., & Gola, T. (1996a). Comparison of multiple scoring methods for Rey's malingered amnesia measures. *Archives of Clinical Neuropsychology, 11,* 283–293.

Greiffenstein, M.F., Baker, W.J., & Gola, T. (1996b). Motor dysfunction profiles in traumatic brain injury and post-concussive syndrome. *Journal of the International Neuropsychological Society, 2,* 477–485.

Greve, K.W., Williams, M.C., Haas, W.G., Littel, R.R., & Reinoso, C. (1996). The role of attention in Wisconsin Card Sorting Test performance. *Archives of Clinical Neuropsychology, 11,* 215–222.

Greve, K.W., Brooks, J., Crouch, J.A., Williams, M.C., & Rice, W.J. (1997). Factorial structure of the Wisconsin Card Sorting Test. *British Journal of Clinical Psychology, 36,* 283–285.

Greve, K.W., Ingram, F., & Bianchini, K.J. (1998). Latent structure of the Wisconsin Card Sorting Test in a clinical sample. *Archives of Clinical Neuropsychology, 13,* 597–609.

Greve, K.W., Bianchini, K.J., Hartley, S.M., & Adams, D. (1999). The Wisconsin Card Sorting Test: Factor structure and relationship to outcome. *Archives of Clinical Neuropsychology, 14,* 497–509.

Grewal, B.S., & Haward, L.R.C. (1984). Validation of a new Weigl scoring system in neurological diagnosis. *Medical Science, 12,* 602–603.

Grober, E., & Sliwinski, M. (1991) Development and validation of a model for estimating premorbid verbal intelligence in the elderly. *Journal of Clinical and Experimental Neuropsychology, 13,* 933–949.

Groff, M.G., & Hubble, I.M. (1981). A factor analytic investigation of the Trail Making Test. *Clinical Neuro-psychology, 3,* 11–13.

Groff, M., & Hubble, L. (1982). WISC-R factor structures of younger and older youths with low IQs. *Journal of Consulting and Clinical Psychology, 50,* 148–149.

Gronwall, D.M. (1974). Paced auditory serial addition test: A measure of recovery from concussion. *Perceptual and Motor Skills, 44,* 367–373.

Grossman, F.M. (1983). Percentage of WAIS-R standardization sample obtaining verbal–performance discrepancies. *Journal of Consulting and Clinical Psychology, 50,* 641–642.

Grossman, F.M., & Johnson, K.M. (1982). WISC-R factor scores as predictors of WRAT performance: A multivariate analysis. *Psychology in the Schools, 19,* 465–468.

Grow, R.T. (1980). Junior high norms for the Bender Gestalt. *Journal of School Psychology, 18,* 395–398.

Grundvig, J.L., Needham, W.E., & Ajax, E.T. (1970). Comparison of different scoring and administration procedures for the Memory for Designs Test. *Journal of Clinical Psychology, 26,* 353–367.

Guilford, A.M., & Nawojczyk, D.C. (1988). Standardization of the Boston Naming Test at the kindergarten and elementary school levels. *Language, Speech, and Hearing Services in the Schools, 19,* 395–400.

Guilmette, T.J., & Faust, D. (1991). Characteristics of neuropsychologists who prefer the Halstead–Reitan or the Luria–Nebraska Neuropsychological Battery. *Professional Psychology—Research and Practice, 22,* 80–83.

Guilmette, T.J., & Rasile, D. (1995). Sensitivity, specificity, and diagnostic accuracy of three verbal memory measures in the assessment of mild brain injury. *Neuropsychology, 9,* 338–344.

Guilmette, T.J., Faust, D., Hart, K., & Arkes, H.R. (1990). A national survey of psychologists who offer neuropsychological services. *Archives of Clinical Neuropsychology, 5,* 373–392.

Guilmette, T.J., Hart, K.J., & Guiliano, A.J. (1993). Malingering detection: The use of a forced-choice method in identifying organic versus simulated memory impairment. *The Clinical Neuropsychologist, 7,* 59–69.

Guilmette, T.J., Hart, K.J., Guiliano, A.J., & Leininger, B.E. (1994). Detecting simulated memory impairment: Comparison of the Rey Fifteen Item Test and the Hiscock Forced-Choice Method. *The Clinical Neuropsychologist, 7,* 59–69.

Guilmette, T.J., Dabrowski, J., Kennedy, M.L., & Gnys, J. (1999). A comparison of nine WAIS-R short forms in individuals with mild to severe traumatic brain injury. *Assessment, 6,* 33–41.

Gulliksen, H. (1987). *Theory of mental test.* Hillsdale, NJ: Lawrence J. Erlbaum.

Gutkin, T.B. (1978). Some useful statistics for the interpretation of the WISC-R. *Journal of Consulting and Clinical Psychology, 46,* 1561–1563.

Gutkin, T.B. (1979). The WISC-R Verbal Comprehension, Perceptual Organization, and Freedom from Distractibility deviation quotients: Data for practitioners. *Psychology in the Schools, 16,* 359–360.

Gyurke, J.S., Stone, B.J., & Beyer, M. (1990). A confirmatory factor analysis of the WPPSI-R. *Journal of Psychoeducational Assessment, 8,* 15–21.

Gyurke, J.S., Prifitera, A., & Sharp, S.A. (1991). Frequency of verbal and performance IQ discrepancies on the WPPSI-R at various levels of ability. *Journal of Psychoeducational Assessment, 9,* 230–239.

Gyurke, J.S., Lynch, S.J., Lagasse, L., & Lipsitt, L.P. (1992). Speeded items: What do they tell us about an infant's performance? *Advances in Infancy Research, 7,* 215–225.

Haaland, K., Linn, R.T., Hunt, W.C., & Goodwin, J.S. (1983). A normative study of Russell's variant of the Wechsler Memory Scale in a healthy elderly population. *Journal of Consulting and Clinical Psychology, 51,* 878–881.

Haaland, K.Y., Vranes, L.F., Goodwin, J.S., & Garry, P.J. (1987). Wisconsin Card Sorting Test performance in a healthy elderly population. *Journal of Gerontology, 42,* 345–346.

Haddad, F.A. (1987). Concurrent validity of the Test of Nonverbal Intelligence with learning disabled children. *Psychology in the Schools, 23,* 361–364.

Hale, R.L. (1978). The WISC-R as a predictor of WRAT performance. *Psychology in the Schools, 15,* 172–175.

Hale, W.W., Dingemans, P., Wekking, E., & Cornelissen, E. (1993). Depression and assessment of intellectual functioning. *Journal of Clinical Psychology, 49,* 773–776.

Hall, G.C.N., Bansal, A., & Lopez, I.R. (1999). Ethnicity and psychopathology: A meta-analytic review of 31 years of comparative MMPI/MMPI-2 research. *Psychological Assessment, 11,* 186–197.

Hall, J.C. (1957). Correlation of a modified form of Raven's Progressive Matrices (1938) with the Wechsler Adult Intelligence Test. *Journal of Consulting Psychology, 21,* 23–26.

Hall, J.C., & Toal, R. (1957). Reliability (internal consistency) of the Wechsler Memory Scale and correlation with the Wechsler–Bellevue Intelligence Scale. *Journal of Consulting Psychology, 21,* 131–135.

Hall, M.M., Hall, G.C., & Lavoie, P. (1968). Ideation in patients with unilateral or bilateral midline brain lesions. *Journal of Abnormal Psychology, 73,* 526–531.

Hall, S., Pinkston, S.L., Szalda-Petree, A.C., & Coronis, A.R. (1996). The performance of healthy older adults on the Continuous Visual Memory Test and the Visual Motor Integration Test: Preliminary findings. *Journal of Clinical Psychology, 52,* 449–454.

Halperin, J.M., Healey, J.M., Zeitchik, E., Ludman, W.L., & Weinstein, L. (1989). Developmental aspects of linguistic and mnestic abilities in normal children. *Journal of Clinical and Experimental Neuropsychology, 11,* 518–528.

Halperin, K.M., Neuringer, C., Davies, P.S., & Goldstein, G. (1977). Validation of the schizophrenia-organicity scale with brain-damaged and non-brain-damaged schizophrenics. *Journal of Consulting and Clinical Psychology, 45,* 949–950.

Halstead, W.C. (1947). *Brain and intelligence: A quantitative study of the frontal lobes.* Chicago: University of Chicago Press.

Haltiner, A.M., Temkin, N.R., Winn, H.R., & Dikmen, S.S. (1996). The impact of traumatic seizures on 1-year neuropsychological and psychological outcome of head injury. *Journal of the International Neuropsychological Society, 2,* 494–504.

Hambleton, R.K. (Ed.). (1983). *Applications of item response theory*. Vancouver: Educational Research Institute of British Columbia.

Hambleton, R.K., & Cook, L.L. (1977). Latent trait models and their use in the analysis of educational test data. *Journal of Educational Measurement, 14*, 75–95.

Hambleton, R.K., Swaminathan, H., & Rogers, H.J. (1991). *Fundamentals of item response theory*. Newbury Park, CA: Sage.

Hammond, S.M. (1984). An investigation into the factor structure of the General Aptitude Test Battery. *Journal of Occupational Psychology, 57*, 43–48.

Hamby, S.L., Wilkins, J.W., & Barry, N.S. (1993). Organizational quality on the Rey–Osterrieth and Taylor Complex Figure Tests: A new scoring system. *Psychological Assessment, 5*, 27–33.

Hamsher, K., Levin, H.S., & Benton, A.L. (1979). Facial recognition in patients with focal brain lesions. *Archives of Neurology, 36*, 837–839.

Hamsher, K., Benton, A.L., & Digre, K. (1980). Serial Digit Learning: Normative and clinical aspects. *Journal of Clinical Neuropsychology, 2*, 39–50.

Handel, R.W., Ben-Porath, Y.S., & Watt, M. (1999). Computerized adaptive assessment with the MMPI-2 in a clinical setting. *Psychological Assessment, 11*, 369–380.

Hanes, K.R., Andrewes, D.G., Smith, D.J., & Pantelis, C. (1996). A brief assessment of executive control dysfunction: Discriminant validity and homogeneity of planning, set shift, and fluency measures. *Archives of Clinical Neuropsychology, 11*, 185–191.

Hannay, J.H., Falgout, J.C., Leli, D.A., & Katholi, C.R. (1987). Focal right temporo-occipital blood flow changes associated with Judgment of Line Orientation. *Neuropsychologia, 25*, 755–763.

Hannay, H.J., & Malone, D.R. (1976). Visual field effects and short-term memory for verbal material. *Neuropsychologia, 14*, 203–209.

Harley, J.P., Leuthold, C.A., Matthews, C.G., & Bergs, L. (1980). *Wisconsin Neuropsychological Test Battery T-score norms for older Veterans Administration Medical Center patients*. Madison, WI: C.G. Matthews.

Harper, D.C., & Tanners, H. (1972). The French Pictorial Test of Intelligence and the Stanford–Binet, L-M: A concurrent validity study with physically impaired children. *Journal of Clinical Psychology, 28*, 178–181.

Harrington, R.G., & Jennings, V. (1986). A comparison of three short forms of the McCarthy Scales of Children's Abilities. *Contemporary Educational Psychology, 11*, 109–116.

Harrington, R.G., Kimbrell, J., & Dai, X. (1992). The relationship between the Woodcock–Johnson Psycho-Educational Battery-Revised (Early Development) and the Wechsler Preschool and Primary Scale of Intelligence-Revised. *Psychology in the Schools, 29*, 116–125.

Harris, D.B. (1963). *Children's drawings as measures of intellectual maturity*. New York: Harcourt Brace Jovanovich.

Harrison, K.A., & Wiebe, M.J. (1977). Correlation study of McCarthy, WISC, and Stanford–Binet Scales. *Perceptual and Motor Skills, 14*, 10–14.

Hart, S., Smith, C.M., & Swash, M. (1986). Assessing intellectual deterioration. *British Jouranl of Clinical Psychology, 25*, 119–124.

Hart, T., & Hayden, M.E. (1986). The ecological validity of neuropsychological assessment and remediation. In B.P. Uzzell & Y. Gross (Eds.), *The clinical neuropsychology of intervention*. Boston: Martinus Nijhoff Publishing.

Hartje, W., Kerschensteiner, M., Poeck, K., & Orgass, B. (1973). A cross-validation study on the Token Test. *Neuropsychologia, 11*, 119–121.

Hartlage, L.C., & Lucas, T.L. (1976). Differential correlation of Bender–Gestalt and Beery Visual-Motor Integration test for Black and for White children. *Journal of Clinical Psychology, 34*, 1039–1042.

Hartlage, L.C., & Steele, C.T. (1977). WISC and WISC-R correlates of academic achievement. *Psychology in the Schools, 14*, 15–18.

Hartman, M., & Potter, G. (1998). Sources of age differences on the Rey–Osterrieth Complex Figure Test. *The Clinical Neuropsychologist, 12*, 513–524.

Hasselblad, V., & Hedges, L.V. (1995). Meta-analysis of screening and diagnostic tests. *Psychological Bulletin, 117*, 167–178.

Hathaway, S.R., & McKinley, J.C. (1942). A multiphasic personality schedule (Minnesota): 3. The measurement of symptomatic depression. *Journal of Psychology, 14*, 73–84.

Hathaway, S.R., & Meehl, P.E. (1951). *An atlas for the clinical use of the MMPI*. Minneapolis: University of Minnesota Press.

Hattori, K., & Lynn, R. (1997). Male–female differences on the Japanese WAIS-R. *Personality and Individual Differences, 23*, 531–533.

Haut, M.W., & Shutty, M.S. (1992). Patterns of verbal learning after closed head injury. *Neuropsychology, 6*, 51–58.

Haut, M.W., Weber, A.M., Wilhelm, K.L., Keefover, R.W., & Rankin, E.D. (1994). The visual reproduction subtest as a measure of perceptual/constructional functioning in dementia of the Alzheimer's type. *Clinical Neuropsychologist, 8*, 187–192.

Haut, M.W., Weber, A.M., Demarest, D., Keefover, R.W., & Rankin, E.D. (1996). Controlling for constructional dysfunction with the visual reproduction subtest of the Wechsler Memory Scale-Revised in Alzheimer's disease. *The Clinical Neuropsychologist, 10*, 309–312.

Havlicek, L.L., & Peterson, N.L. (1977). Effect of the violation of assumptions upon significance levels of the Pearson. *Psychological Bulletin, 84*, 373–377.

Hawkins, K.A., & Sayward, H.K. (1994). Examiner judgment and actual stability of psychiatric inpatient intelligence. *The Clinical Neuropsychologist, 8*, 394–404.

Hawkins, K.A., Sledge, W.H., Orleans, J.F., Quinlan, D.M., Rakfeldt, J., & Hoffman, R.E. (1993). Normative implications of the relationship between reading vocabulary and Boston Naming Test. *Archives of Clinical Neuropsychology, 8*, 525–537.

Hawkins, K.A., Sullivan, T.E., & Choi, E.J. (1997). Memory deficits in schizophrenia: Inadequate assimilation or true amnesia? Findings from the Wechsler Memory Scale-Revised. *Journal of Psychiatry and Neuroscience, 22*, 169–179.

Hawkins, R.P. (1988). Selection of target behaviors. In R.O. Nelson & S.C. Hayes (Eds.), *Conceptual foundations of behavioral assessment* (pp. 331–385). New York: The Guilford Press.

Hayden, D.C., Furlong, M.J., & Linnemeyer, S. (1988). A comparison of the Kaufman Assessment Battery for Children and the Stanford–Binet IV for the assessment of gifted children. *Psychology in the Schools, 25*, 239–243.

Hays, W.L. (1973). *Statistics for the social sciences*. New York: Holt, Rinehart, & Winston.

Heaton, R.K. (1981). *A manual for the Wisconsin Card Sorting Test*. Odessa, FL: Psychological Assessment Resources.

Heaton, R.K., Smith, H.H., Jr., Lehman, R.A., & Vogt, A.T. (1978). Prospects for faking believable deficits on neuropsychological testing. *Journal of Consulting and Clinical Psychology, 46*, 892–900.

Heaton, R.K., Grant, L., Anthony, W.Z., & Lehman, R.A.W. (1981). A comparison of clinical and automated interpretation of the Halstead–Reitan Battery. *Journal of Consulting and Clinical Psychology, 3*, 121–141.

Heaton, R.K., Chelune, G.J., Talley, J.L., Kay, G.G., & Curtiss, G. (1993). *Wisconsin Card Sorting Test manual: Revised and expanded*. Odessa, FL: Psychological Assessment Resources.

Heaton, R.K., Grant, I., & Matthews, C.G. (1991). *Comprehensive norms for an expanded Halstead–Reitan Battery*. Odessa, FL: Psychological Assessment Resources.

Heaton, R.K., Matthews, C.G., Grant, I., & Avitable, N. (1996). Demographic corrections with comprehensive norms: An overzealous attempt or a good start? *Journal of Clinical and Experimental Neuropsychology, 18*, 449–458.

Hecaen, H., & Assal, G. (1970). A comparison of constructive deficits following right and left hemisphere lesions. *Neuropsychologia, 8*, 289–303.

Heck, E.T., & Bryer, J.B. (1986). Superior sorting and categorizing ability in a case of bilateral frontal atrophy: An exception to the rule. *Journal of Clinical and Experimental Neuropsychology, 8*, 313–316.

Hedges, L.V., & Olkin, I. (1985). *Statistical methods for meta-analysis*. Orlando, FL: Academic Press.

Heilman, K.M., Watson, R.T., & Schulman, H.M. (1974). A unilateral memory defect. *Journal of Neurology, Neurosurgery, and Psychiatry, 37*, 790–793.

Heinemann, A.W., Harper, R.G., Friedman, L.C., & Whitney, J. (1985). The relative utility of the Shipley Institute of Living Scale: Prediction of WAIS-R IQ. *Journal of Clinical Psychology, 41*, 547–551.

Heinrichs, R.W. (1989). Neuropsychological test performance and employment status in patients referred for assessment. *Perceptual and Motor Skills, 69*, 899–902.

Heinrichs, R.W., & Celinski, M.J. (1987). Frequency of occurrence of a WAIS dementia profile in male head trauma patients. *Journal of Clinical and Experimental Neuropsychology, 9*, 187–190.

Heise, D.R. (1969). Separating reliability and stability in test–retest correlation. *American Sociology Review, 34*, 93–101.

Helmes, E. (1996). Use of the Barona method to predict premorbid intelligence in the elderly. *The Clinical Neuropsychologist, 10*, 255–261.

Helmes, E., Holden, R.R., & Howe, M.G. (1980). An attempt at validation of the Minnesota Percepto-Diagnostic Test in a psychiatric setting. *Journal of Clinical Neuropsychology, 2,* 231–236.

Henderson, L.W., Frank, E.M., Pigatt, T., Abramson, R.K., & Houston, M. (1998). Race, gender, and educational level effects on Boston Naming Test scores. *Aphasiology, 12,* 901–911.

Henik, A. (1996). Paying attention to the Stroop effect. *Journal of the International Neuropsychological Society, 2,* 467–470.

Herkov, M.J., & Myers, W.C. (1996). MMPI profiles of depressed adolescents with and without conduct disorder. *Journal of Clinical Psychology, 52,* 705–710.

Herman, D.S., Weathers, F.W., Litz, B.T., & Keane, T.M. (1996). Psychometric properties of the embedded and stand-alone versions of the MMPI-2 Keane PTSD scale. *Assessment, 3,* 437–442.

Hermann, B.P., & Melyn, M. (1985). Identification of neuropsychological deficits in epilepsy using the Luria–Nebraska Neuropsychological Battery: A replication attempt. *Journal of Clinical and Experiment Neuro-psychology, 7,* 305–313.

Hermann, B., & Seidenberg, M. (1995). Executive system dysfunction in temporal lobe epilepsy: Effects of nociferous cortex versus hippocampal pathology. *Journal of Clinical and Experimental Neuropsychology, 17,* 809–819.

Hermann, B.P., Connell, B., Barr, W.B., & Wyler, A.R. (1996). The utility of the Warrington Recognition Memory Test for temporal lobe epilepsy: Pre- and post-operative results. *Journal of Epilepsy, 8,* 139–145.

Herrera-Graf, M., Dipert, Z.J., & Hinton, R.N. (1996). Exploring the effective use of the Vocabulary/Block Design short form with a special school population. *Educational and Psychological Measurement, 56,* 522–528.

Hertz, M.R. (1934). The reliability of the Rorschach ink-blot test. *Journal of Applied Psychology, 18,* 461–477.

Hertz, M.R., & Loehrke, L.M. (1954). The application of the Piotrowski and Hughes signs of organic defect to a group of patients suffering from post-traumatic encephalopathy. *Journal of Genetic Psychology, 62,* 189–215.

Hevern, V.W. (1980). Recent validity studies of the Halstead–Reitan approach to clinical neuropsychological assessment of lateralized brain damage. *Cortex, 9,* 204–216.

Hilgert, L.D., & Treolar, J.H. (1985). The relationship of the Hooper Visual Organization Test to sex, age, and intelligence of elementary school children. *Measurement and Evaluation in Counseling and Development, 17,* 203–206.

Hiller, J.B., Rosenthal, R., Bornstein, R.F., Berry, D.T.R., & Brunell-Neulieb, S. (1999). A comparative meta-analysis of Rorschach and MMPI validity. *Psychological Assessment, 11,* 278–296.

Hillow, P. (1971). Comparison of brain-damaged and non-brain-damaged retarded children on two visual-motor tasks. Unpublished master's thesis, North Carolina State University.

Hilsabeck, R.C., Dunn, J.T., & Less-Haley, P.R. (1996). An empirical comparison of the Wechsler Memory Scale-Revised and the Memory Assessment Scales in measuring four memory constructs. *Assessment, 3,* 417–422.

Hinshaw, S.P., Carte, E.T., & Morrison, D.C. (1986). Concurrent prediction of academic achievement in reading disabled children: The role of neuropsychological and intellectual measures at different ages. *International Journal of Clinical Neuropsychology, 8,* 3–8.

Hinton, J., & Withers, E. (1971). The usefulness of the Clinical Tests of the Sensorium. *British Journal of Psychiatry, 119,* 9–18.

Hirshoren, A., Kavale, K., Harley, O., & Hunt, J.T. (1977). Intercorrelations among tests of general mental ability and achievement for black and white deaf children. *Perceptual and Motor Skills, 46,* 1107–1113.

Hoffman, R.G., & Nelson, K.S. (1988). Cross-validation of six short forms of the WAIS-R in a healthy geriatric sample. *Journal of Clinical Psychology, 44,* 952–957.

Hoffman, R.G., Scott, J.G., Tremont, G., Adams, R.L., & Oommen, K.J. (1997a). Cross-validation of a method for predicting Wechsler Memory Scale-Revised index scores. *The Clinical Neuropsychologist, 11,* 402–406.

Hoffman, R.G., Tremont, G., Scott, J.G., Adams, R.L., & Mittenberg, W. (1997b). Cross-validation of predicted Wechsler Memory Scale-Revised scores in a normative sample of 25–34-year-old patients. *Archives of Clinical Neuropsychology, 12,* 677–682.

Holland, A.L. (1980). *Communicative Abilities in Daily Living. A test of functional communication for aphasic adults.* Austin, TX: Pro-Ed.

Holland, P.W., & Thayer, D.T. (1988). Differential item performance and the Mantel–Haenszel procedure. In H. Wainer & H.I. Braun (Eds.), *Test validity* (pp. 129–145). Hillsdale, NJ: Lawrence J. Erlbaum.

Holland, T.R., & Wadsworth, H.M. (1974). Incidence vs. degree of rotation on the Minnesota Percepto-Diagnostic Test in brain damaged and schizophrenic patients. *Perceptual and Motor Skills, 38,* 131–134.

Holland, T.R., Lowenfeld, J., & Wadsworth, H.M. (1975a). MMPI indices in the discrimination of brain-damaged and schizophrenic groups. *Journal of Consulting and Clinical Psychology, 43*, 426.

Holland, T.R., Wadsworth, H.M., & Royer, F.L. (1975b). The performance of brain-damaged and schizophrenic patients on the Minnesota Percepto-Diagnostic test under standard and BIP conditions of administration. *Journal of Clinical Psychology, 31*, 21–25.

Hollenbeck, G.P. (1972). A comparison of analyses using the first and second generation Little Jiffy's. *Educational and Psychological Measurement, 32*, 45–51.

Hollinger, C.L., & Sarvis, P.H. (1984). Interpretation of the PPVT-R: A pure measure of verbal comprehension? *Psychology in the Schools, 21*, 34–41.

Holzberg, J.D., & Alessi, S. (1949). Reliability of the shortened MMPI. *Journal of Consulting Psychology, 13*, 288–292.

Holzberg, J.D., & Wexler, M. (1950). The predictability of schizophrenic performance on the Rorschach test. *Journal of Consulting Psychology, 14*, 395–399.

Hom, J., Haley, R.W., & Kurt, T.L. (1997) Neuropsychological correlates of Gulf War Syndrome. *Archives of Clinical Neuropsychology, 12*, 531–544.

Hooper, H.E. (1958). *The Hooper Visual Organization Test: Manual*. Los Angeles: Western Psychological Services.

Hopkins, C.D., & Antes, R.L. (1978). *Classroom measurement and evaluation*. Itasca, IL: F.E. Peacock.

Hopp, G.A, Dixon, R.A., Grut, M., & Bacekman, L. (1997). Longitudinal and psychometric profiles of two cognitive status tests in very old adults. *Journal of Clinical Psychology, 53*, 673–686.

Horan, M., Ashton, R., & Minto, J. (1980). Using ECT to study hemispheric specialization for sequential processes. *British Journal of Psychology, 137*, 119–125.

Horan, W.P., Pogge, D.L., Borgaro, S.R., Stokes, J.M., & Harvey, P.D. (1997). Learning and memory in adolescent psychiatric inpatients with major depression: A normative study of the California Verbal Learning Test. *Archives of Clinical Neuropsychology, 12*, 575–584.

Horn, G.J., & Kelly, M.P. (1996). Strengths and limitations of the Short Category Test in neuropsychological examination following acute traumatic brain injury. *Applied Neuropsychology, 3*, 58–64.

Horn, J.L., Wanberg, K.W., & Appel, M. (1973). On the internal structure of the MMPI. *Multivariate Behavioral Research, 8*, 131–171.

Horner, M.D., Flashman, L.A., Freides, D., Epstein, C.M., & Bakay, R.A. (1996). Temporal lobe epilepsy and performance on the Wisconsin Card Sorting Test. *Journal of Clinical and Experimental Neuropsychology, 18*, 310–313.

Horton, A.M., Jr. (1995a). The alterative impairment index: A measure of neuropsychological deficit. *Perceptual and Motor Skills, 80*, 336–338.

Horton, A.M., Jr. (1995b). Cross-validation of the alternative impairment index. *Perceptual and Motor Skills, 81*, 1153–1154.

Horton, A.M., Jr. (1996). Revised children's version of the alternative impairment index. *Applied Neuropsychology, 3*, 178–180.

Horton, A.M., Jr. (1997). Alternate Impairment Index-Revised: A measure of neuropsychological deficit. *Applied Neuropsychology, 4*, 176–179.

Horton, A.M., Jr. (1998). Development of a Short-Form Screening Index for severity of brain damage in older children. *Applied Neuropsychology, 5*, 48–50.

Horton, A.M., Anilane, J., Puente, A.E., & Berg, R.A. (1988). Diagnostic parameters of an odd-even short-form of the Luria–Nebraska Neuropsychological Battery. *Archives of Clinical Neuropsychology, 3*, 375–381.

House, B.J. (1977). Scientific explanation and ecological validity: A reply to Brooks and Baumeister. *American Journal of Mental Deficiency, 81*, 534–542.

Houston, B.K., & Jones, T.H. (1967). Distraction and Stroop color word performance. *Journal of Experimental Psychology, 74*, 54–56.

Hovey, H.B. (1964). Brain lesions and five MMPI items. *Journal of Consulting Psychology, 28*, 78–79.

Howard, A., & Shoemaker, D.J. (1954). An evaluation of the Memory for Designs Test. *Journal of Consulting Psychology, 18*, 266.

Huba, G.J., & Hamilton, D.L. (1976). On the generality of trait relationships: Some analyses based on Fiske's paper. *Psychological Bulletin, 83*, 868–876.

Huff, F.J., Collins, C., Corkin, S., & Rosen, T.J. (1986). Equivalent forms of the Boston Naming Test. *Journal of Clinical and Experimental Neuropsychology, 8*, 556–562.

Hughes, R.M. (1948). Rorschach signs for the diagnosis of organic pathology. *Rorschach Research Exchange and Journal of Projective Techniques, 12*, 165–167.

Humes, G.E., Welsh, M.C., Retzlaff, P., & Cookson, N. (1997). Towers of Hanoi and London: Reliability and validity of two executive function tasks. *Assessment, 4*, 249–257.

Humphries, T., & Bone, J. (1993). Validity of IQ–achievement discrepancy criteria for identifying learning disabilities. *Canadian Journal of School Psychology, 9*, 181–191.

Hunsley, J., Hanson, R.K., & Parker, K.C. (1988). A summary of the reliability and stability of MMPI scales. *Journal of Clinical Psychology, 44*, 44–46.

Hunter, J.E., & Schmidt, F.L. (1990). *Methods of meta-analysis: Correcting error and bias in research findings.* Newbury Park, CA: Sage.

Hunter, J.E., Schmidt, F.L., & Jackson, G.B. (1982). *Meta-analysis: Cumulating research findings across studies.* Beverly Hills, CA: Sage.

Husband, S.D., & DeCato, D.M. (1982). The Quick Test compared with the Wechsler Adult Intelligence Scale-Revised. *Psychological Reports, 40*, 523–526.

Hutchinson, G.L. (1984). The Luria–Nebraska controversy: A reply to Spiers. *Journal of Consulting and Clinical Psychology, 52*, 539–545.

Hutt, M.L., & Briskin, G.J. (1960). *The clinical use of the revised Bender–Gestalt test.* New York: Grune & Stratton.

Imhof, E.A., & Archer, R.P. (1997). Correlates of the MMPI-A Immaturity (IMM) scale in an adolescent psychiatric sample. *Assessment, 4*, 169–179.

Incagnoli, T., Goldstein, G., & Golden, C. (Eds.). (1986). *Clinical application of neuropsychological test batteries.* New York: Plenum.

Inglis, J., & Lawson, J. (1981). Sex differences in the effects of unilateral brain damage on intelligence. *Science, 212*, 693–695.

Ingram, F., Caroselli, J., Robinson, H., Hetzel, R.D., Reed, K., & Masel, B.E. (1998). The PPVT-R as a quick screen of intelligence in a post-acute rehabilitation setting for brain-injured adults. *Journal of Clinical Psychology, 54*, 877–884.

Ingram, G.F., & Hakari, L.J. (1985). Validity of the Woodcock–Johnson Tests of Cognitive Ability for gifted children: A comparison study. *Journal for Education of the Gifted, 9*, 11–23.

Inman, T.H., Vickery, C.D., Lamb, D.G., Edwards, C.L., & Smith, G.T. (1998). Development and initial validation of a new procedure for evaluating adequacy of effort given during neuropsychological testing: The Letter Memory Test. *Psychological Assessment, 10*, 128–139.

Innes, J.M. (1972). The relationship of word-association commonality response set to cognitive and personality variables. *British Journal of Psychology, 83*, 421–428.

Ironson, G.H. (1983). Using item response theory to measure item bias. In R.K. Hambleton (Ed.), *Applications of item response theory* (pp. 155–174). Vancouver, BC: Educational Research Institute of British Columbia.

Ishihara, S. (1970). *Ishihara Color Blind Test book.* Tokyo: Kanehara Shuppan.

Iversen, G.R. (1984). *Bayesian statistical inference.* Beverly Hills, CA: Sage.

Iverson, G.L. (1995). Qualitative aspects of malingering. *Brain Injury, 9*, 35–40.

Iverson, G.L., & Franzen, M.D. (1994). The recognition memory test, digit span, and Knox cube test as markers of malingered memory impairment. *Assessment, 1*, 323–334.

Iverson, G.L., & Franzen, M.D. (1996). Using multiple objective memory procedures to detect simulated malingering. *Journal of Clinical and Experimental Neuropsychology, 18*, 38–51.

Iverson, G.L., & Franzen, M.D. (1998). Detecting malingered memory deficits with the Recognition Memory Test. *Brain Injury, 12*, 275–282.

Iverson, G.L., Franzen, M.D., & McCracken, L.M. (1991). Evaluation of an objective assessment technique for the detection of malingered memory deficits. *Law and Human Behavior, 15*, 667–676.

Iverson, G.L., Franzen, M.D., & McCracken, L.M. (1994). Application of a forced-choice memory procedure designed to detect experimental-malingering. *Archives of Clinical Neuropsychology, 9*, 437–450.

Iverson, G.L., Myers, B., Bengston, M.L., & Adams, R.L. (1996). Concurrent validity of a WAIS-R seven-subtest short form in patients with brain impairment. *Psychological Assessment, 8*, 319–323.

Iverson, G.L., Myers, B., & Adams, R.L. (1997). Comparison of two computational formulas for a WAIS-R. *Journal of Clinical Psychology, 53*, 465–470.

Iverson, G.L., Sherman, E.M.S., & Smith-Seemiller, L. (1997a). Evaluation of a short form of the Visual Form Discrimination Test for assessing cognitive decline associated with dementia. *Journal of Cognitive Rehabilitation, 15*, 20–21.

Iverson, G.L., Slick, D., & Smith-Seemiller, L. (1997b). Screening for visual–perceptual deficits following closed head injury: A short form of the Visual Form Discrimination Test. *Brain Injury, 11*, 125–128.

Iverson, G.L., Guirguis, M., & Green, P. (1998). Assessing intellectual functioning in persons with schizophrenia spectrum disorders using a seven subtest short form of the WAIS-R. *Schizophrenia Research, 30*, 165–168.

Ivinskis, A., Allen, S., & Shaw, E. (1971). An extension of Wechsler Memory Scale norms to lower age groups. *Journal of Clinical Psychology, 27*, 354–357.

Ivison, D.J. (1977). The Wechsler Memory Scale: Preliminary findings toward an Australian standardisation. *Australian Psychologist, 12*, 303–312.

Ivnik, R.J., Smith, G.E., Malec, J.F., Petersen, R.C., & Tangalos, E.G. (1995). Long-term stability and intercorrelations of cognitive abilities in older persons. *Psychological Assessment, 7*, 155–161.

Ivnik, R.J., Malec, J.F., Smith, G.E., Tangalos, E.G., & Petersen, R.C. (1996). Neuropsychological tests' norms above age 55: COWAT, BNT, MAE Token, WRAT-R Reading, AMNART, STROOP, TMT, and JLO. *The Clinical Neuropsychologist, 10*, 262–278.

Ivnik, R.J., Smith, G.E., Lucas, J.A., Tangalos, E.G., Kokmen, E., & Petersen, R.C. (1997). Free and cues recall selective reminding test: MOANS norms. *Journal of Clinical and Experimental Neuropsychology, 19*, 676–691.

Jackson, B. (1978). The effects of unilateral and bilateral ECT on verbal and visual spatial memory. *Journal of Clinical Psychology, 34*, 4–13.

Jackson, D.N. (1969). Multimethod factor analysis in the evaluation of convergent and discriminant validity. *Psychological Bulletin, 72*, 30–49.

Jackson, D.N., Fraboni, M., & Helmes, E. (1997). MMPI-2 content scales: How much content do they measure? *Assessment, 4*, 111–117.

Jackson, R.E., & Culbertson, W.C. (1977). The Elizur Test of Psycho-Organicity and the Hooper Visual Organization Test as measures of childhood neurological impairment. *Journal of Clinical Psychology, 33*, 213–214.

Jacob, H. (1984). *Using published data: Errors and remedies.* Beverly Hills, CA: Sage.

Jacobs, D.M., Sano, M., Dooneief, G., Marder, K., Bell, K.L., & Stern, Y. (1995). Neuropsychological detection and characterization of preclinical Alzheimer's disease. *Neurology, 45*, 957–962.

Jacobson, N.S., & Truax, P. (1991). Clinical significance: A statistical approach to defining meaningful change in psychotherapy research. *Journal of Consulting and Clinical Psychology, 59*, 12–19.

Jaffe, K.M., Fay, G.C., Polissar, N.L., Martin, K.M., Shurtleff, H.A., Rivara, J.B., & Winn, H.R. (1993). Severity of pediatric traumatic brain injury and neurobehavioral recovery at one year: A cohort study. *Archives of Physical Medicine and Rehabilitation, 74*, 587–595.

Jahoda, G. (1969). Cross-cultural use of the perceptual maze test. *British Journal of Educational Psychology, 39*, 82–86.

Janus, M-D., de Groot, C., & Toepfer, S.M. (1998). The MMPI-A and 13 year-old inpatients: How young is too young? *Assessment, 5*, 321–332.

Jarvis, P.E., & Barth, J.T. (1994). *Halstead–Reitan test battery: An interpretative guide* (2nd ed.). Odessa, FL: Psychological Assessment Resources.

Jastek, J.F., & Jastek, S. (1978). *Wide Range Achievement Test manual.* Wilmington, DE: Jastek.

Jenkins, M., Cohen, R., Malloy, P., Salloway, S., Johnson, E.G., Penn, J., & Marcotte, A. (1998). Neuropsychological measures which discriminate among adults with residual symptoms of attention deficit disorder and other attentional complaints. *The Clinical Neuropsychologist, 12*, 74–83.

Jensen, A. (1965). Scoring the Stroop test. *Acta Psychologica, 24*, 398–408.

Joesting, J. (1975). Correlations among different forms of the Quick Test. *Psychological Reports, 37*, 285–286.

Joesting, J., & Joesting, R. (1972). Children's Quick Test. Picture Interpretation, and Goodenough Draw-A-Person scores. *Psychological Reports, 30*, 941–942.

Johnson, C.J., Paivio, A., & Clark, J.M. (1996). Cognitive components of picture naming. *Psychological Bulletin, 120*, 113–139.

Johnson, D.L., & Johnson, C.A. (1971). Comparison of four intelligence tests commonly used with culturally disadvantaged children. *Psychological Reports, 28*, 209–210.

Johnson, J.E., & Oziel, L.J. (1970). An item analysis of the Raven Colored Progressive Matrices Test for paranoid and nonparanoid schizophrenic patients. *Journal of Clinical Psychology, 26*, 357–359.

Johnson, J.H., Klingler, D.E., & Williams, T.A. (1977). An external criterion study of the MMPI validity indices. *Journal of Clinical Psychology, 33*, 154–156.

Johnson, M.E., & Fisher, D.G. (1996). Evaluating three reading tests for use with alcohol and other drugs-abusing populations. *Alcoholism, Clinical and Experimental Research, 20*, 11125–1129.

Johnson, M.E., Fisher, D.G., Rhodes, F., & Booth, R. (1996a). Test–retest stability and concurrent validity of two reading tests with a drug-abusing population. *Assessment, 3,* 111–114.

Johnson, M.E., Jones, G., & Brems, C. (1996b). Concurrent validity of the MMPI-2 feminine gender role (GF) and masculine gender role (GM) scales. *Journal of Personality Assessment, 66,* 153–168.

Johnson-Selfridge, M.T., Zalewski, C., & Abroudarham, J.-F. (1998). The relationship between ethnicity and word fluency. *Archives of Clinical Neuropsychology, 13,* 319–325.

Johnstone, B., & Wilhelm, K.L. (1996). The longitudinal stability of the WRAT-R Reading subtest: Is it an appropriate estimate of premorbid intelligence? *Journal of International Neuropsychological Society, 2,* 282–285.

Johnstone, B., & Wilhelm, K.L. (1997). The construct validity of the Hooper Visual Organization Test. *Assessment, 4,* 243–248.

Johnstone, B., Erdal, K., & Stadler, M.A. (1995a). The relationship between the Wechsler Memory Scale-Revised (WMS-R) Attention index and putative measures of attention. *Journal of Clinical Psychology in Medical Settings, 2,* 195–204.

Johnstone, B., Hexum, C.L., & Ashkanazi, G. (1995b). Extent of cognitive decline in traumatic brain injury based on estimates of premorbid intelligence. *Brain Injury, 9,* 377–384.

Johnstone, B., Callahan, C.D., Kapila, C.J., & Bouman, D.E. (1996). The comparability of the WRAT-R Reading test and the NAART as estimates of premorbid intelligence in neurologically impaired patients. *Archives of Clinical Neuropsychology, 11,* 513–519.

Johnstone, B., Slaughter, J., Schopp, L., McAllister, J.A., Schwake, C., & Leubbering, A. (1997). Determining neuropsychological impairment using estimates of premorbid intelligence: Comparing methods based on level of education versus reading scores. *Archives of Clinical Neuropsychology, 12,* 591–601.

Jones, J., & Shea, J. (1974). Some problems in the comparison of divergent thinking scores across cultures. *Australian Psychologist, 9,* 47–51.

Jones-Gotman, M. (1986). Memory for designs: The hippocampal contribution. *Neuropsychologia, 24,* 193–203.

Jordan, F.M., & Murdoch, B.E. (1994). Severe closed-head injury in childhood: Linguistic outcomes into adulthood. *Brain Injury, 8,* 501–508.

Jordan, F.M., Murdoch, B.E., Hudson-Tennent, L.J., & Boon, D.L. (1996). Naming performance of brain-injured children. *Aphasiology, 10,* 755–766.

Jortner, S. (1965). A test of Hovey's MMPI scale for CNS disorder. *Journal of Clinical Psychology, 21,* 285–287.

Jurden, F.H., Franzen, M.D., Callahan, T., & Ledbetter, M. (1996). Factorial equivalence of the Wechsler Memory Scale-Revised across standardization and clinical samples. *Applied Neuropsychology, 3,* 65–74.

Kalechstein, A.D., & van Gorp, W.G. (1998). Outcomes research for forensic neuropsychology: Recommendations and considerations. *Applied Neuropsychology, 5,* 202–208.

Kalechstein, A.D., van Gorp, W., & Rapport, L.J. (1998). Variability in clinical classification of raw test scores across normative data sets. *The Clinical Neuropsychologist, 12,* 339–347.

Kane, R.L., Sweet, J.J., Golden, C.J., Parsons, O.A., & Moses, J.A. (1981). Comparative diagnostic accuracy of the Halstead–Reitan and standardized Luria–Nebraska Neuropsychological Batteries in a mixed psychiatric and brain-damaged population. *Journal of Consulting and Clinical Psychology, 49,* 484–485.

Kane, R.L., Parsons, O.A., & Goldstein, G. (1985). Statistical relationships and discrimination accuracy of the Halstead–Reitan, Luria–Nebraska, and Wechsler IQ scores in the identification of brain damage. *Journal of Clinical and Experimental Neuropsychology, 7,* 211–223.

Kaplan, C.H. (1992). Ceiling effects in assessing high-IQ children with the WPPSI-R. *Journal of Clinical Child Psychology, 21,* 403–406.

Kaplan, C.E. (1993). Predicting first-grade achievement from pre-kindergarten WPPSI-R scores. *Journal of Psychoeducational Assessment, 11,* 133–138.

Kaplan, C.E. (1996). Predictive validity of the WPPSI-R: A four year follow-up study. *Psychology in the Schools, 33,* 211–220.

Kaplan, C.H., Fox, L.M., & Paxton, L. (1991). Bright children and the revised WPPSI: Concurrent validity. *Journal of Psychoeducational Assessment, 9,* 240–246.

Kaplan, E. (1983). Achievement and process revisited. In S. Wapner & B. Kaplan (Eds.), *Toward a holistic developmental psychology.* Hillsdale, NJ: Lawrence J. Erlbaum.

Karapetsas, A.B., & Vlachos, F.M. (1997). Sex and handedness in development of visuomotor skills. *Perceptual and Motor Skills, 85,* 131–140.

Karbe, H., Herholz, K., Szelies, B., Pawlik, G., Weinhard, K., & Heiss, W.D. (1989). Regional metabolic correlates of Token Test results in cortical and subcortical left hemisphere infarction. *Neurology, 39,* 1083–1088.

Kareken, D.A., Gur, R.C., & Saykin, A.J. (1995). Reading on the Wide Range Achievement Test-Revised and parental education as predictors of IQ: Comparison with the Barona formula. *Archives of Clinical Neuropsychology, 10*, 147–157.

Kareken, D.A., Moberg, P.J., & Gur, R.C. (1996). Proactive inhibition and semantic organization: Relationship with verbal memory in patients with schizophrenia. *Journal of the International Neuropsychological Society, 2*, 486–493.

Karnes, F.A., & Oehler, J. (1986). Comparison of the renormed Slosson Intelligence Test with the WISC-R for gifted children. *Educational and Psychological Research, 6*, 207–211.

Karr, S.K., Carvajal, H.H., & Palmer, B.L. (1992). Comparison of Kaufman's short forms of the McCarthy Scales of Children's Abilities and the Stanford–Binet Intelligence Scales-Fourth Edition. *Perceptual and Motor Skills, 74*, 1120–1122.

Karr, S.K., Carvajal, H.H., Elser, D., Bays, K., Logan, R.A., & Page, G.L. (1993). Concurrent validity of the WPPSI-R and the McCarthy Scales of Children's Abilities. *Psychological Reports, 72*, 940–942.

Karras, D., Newlin, B.B., Franzen, M.D., Golden, C.J., Wilkening, G.N., Rothermel, R.D., Jr., & Tramontana, M.J. (1987). Development of factor scales for the Luria–Nebraska Neuropsychological Battery-Children's Revision. *Journal of Clinical Child Psychology, 16*, 19–28.

Karzmark, P. (1997). Operating characteristics of the Neurobehavioral Cognitive Status Exam using neuropsychological assessment as the criterion. *Assessment, 4*, 1–8.

Karzmark, P., Heaton, R.K., Grant, I., & Matthews, C.G. (1984). Use of demographic variables to predict overall level of performance on the Halstead–Reitan Battery. *Journal of Consulting and Clinical Psychology, 52*, 663–665.

Karzmark, P., Heaton, R.K., Grant, I., & Matthews, C.G. (1985). Use of demographic variables to predict Full Scale IQ: A replication and extension. *Journal of Clinical and Experimental Neuropsychology, 7*, 412–420.

Kashden, J. (1994). An interrater reliability study of the qualitative and quantitative scoring systems in the Luria–Nebraska Neuropsychological Battery Form-II. Doctoral Dissertation, West Virginia University.

Kaskie, B., & Storandt, M. (1995). Visuospatial deficit in dementia of the Alzheimer's type. *Archives of Neurology, 52*, 422–425.

Katz, L., & Goldstein, G. (1993). The Luria–Nebraska Neuropsychological Battery and the WAIS-R in assessment of adults with specific learning disabilities. *Rehabilitation Counseling Bulletin, 36*, 190–198.

Katz, L., Wood, D.S., Goldstein, G., Auchenbach, R.C., & Geckle, M. (1998). The utility of neuropsychological tests in evaluation of attention-deficit/hyperactivity disorder (ADHD) versus depression in adults. *Assessment, 5*, 45–51.

Kaufman, A.S. (1975a). Factor analysis of the WISC-R at 11 age levels between 6½ and 16½ years. *Journal of Consulting and Clinical Psychology, 43*, 135–147.

Kaufman, A.S. (1975b). Factor structure of the McCarthy Scales at five age levels between 2½ and 8½. *Educational and Psychological Measurement, 35*, 641–656.

Kaufman, A.S. (1979). *Intelligence testing with the WISC-R.* New York: John Wiley & Sons.

Kaufman, A.S., & DiCuio, R.F. (1975). Separate factor analyses for groups of black and white children. *Journal of School Psychology, 13*, 11–18.

Kaufman, A.S., & Hollenbeck, G.P. (1973). Factor analysis of the standardization edition of the McCarthy Scales. *Journal of Clinical Psychology, 29*, 519–532.

Kaufman, A.S., & Horn, J.L. (1996). Age changes on tests of fluid and crystallized ability for women and men on the Kaufman Adolescent and Adult Intelligence Test (KAIT) at ages 17–94 years. *Archives of Clinical Neuropsychology, 11*, 97–121.

Kaufman, A.S., & Kaufman, N.L. (1990). *Manual for the Kaufman Adolescent and Adult Intelligence Test (KAIT).* Circle Pines, MN: American Guidance Services.

Kaufman, A.S., & O'Neal, M.R. (1988a). Factor structure of the Woodcock–Johnson cognitive subtests from preschool to adulthood. *Journal of Psychoeducational Assessment, 6*, 35–48.

Kaufman, A.S., & O'Neal, M.R. (1988b). Analysis of the cognitive, achievement, and general factors underlying the Woodcock–Johnson Psycho-Educational Battery. *Journal of Child Clinical Psychology, 17*, 143–151.

Kaufman, A.S., & Van Hagen, J. (1977). Investigation of the WISC-R for use with retarded children: Correlation with the 1972 Stanford–Binet and comparison of WISC and WISC-R profiles. *Psychology in the Schools, 14*, 10–14.

Kaufman, A.S., & Wang, J. (1992). Gender, race, and education differences on the K-BIT at ages 4 to 90 years. *Journal of Psychoeducational Assessment, 10*, 219–229.

Kaufman, A.S., Ishikuma, T., & Kaufman-Packer, J.L. (1991). Amazingly short forms of the WAIS-R. *Journal of Psychoeducational Assessment, 9,* 4–15.

Kaufman, A.S., Kaufman, J.C., Balgopal, R., & McLean, J.E. (1996). Comparison of three WISC-III short forms: Weighing psychometric, clinical, and practical factors. *Journal of Clinical Child Psychology, 25,* 97–105.

Kausler, D.H., & Puckett, J.M. (1979). Effects of word frequency on adult age differences in word memory span. *Experimental Aging Research, 5,* 161–169.

Kear-Colwell, J.J. (1973). The structure of the Wechsler Memory Scale and its relationship to brain damage. *British Journal of Social and Clinical Psychology, 12,* 384–392.

Kear-Colwell, J.J. (1977). The structure of the Wechsler Memory Scale: A replication. *Journal of Clinical Psychology, 33,* 483–485.

Kear-Colwell, J.J., & Heller, M. (1978). A normative study of the Wechsler Memory Scale. *Journal of Clinical Psychology, 34,* 437–442.

Kear-Colwell, J.J., & Heller, M. (1980). The Wechsler Memory Scale and closed head injury. *Journal of Clinical Psychology, 36,* 782–787.

Keenan, P.A., Ricker, J.H., Lindamer, L.A., Jiron, C.C., & Jacobson, M.W. (1996). Relationship between WAIS-R Vocabulary and performance on the California Verbal Learning Test. *The Clinical Neuropsychologist, 10,* 455–458.

Keesler, T.Y., Schultz, E.E., Sciara, A.D., & Friedenberg, L. (1984). Equivalence of alternate subtests for the Russell revision of the Wechsler Memory Scale. *Journal of Clinical Neuropsychology, 6,* 215–219.

Keith, T.Z., & Bolen, L.M. (1980). Factor structure of the McCarthy scales for children experiencing problems in school. *Psychology in the Schools, 17,* 320–328.

Keller, W.K. (1971). A comparison of two procedures for assessing constructional praxis in patients with unilateral cerebral disease. Ph.D. dissertation, University of Iowa.

Kelley, D.M., Margulies, H., & Barrera, S.E. (1941). The stability of the Rorschach method as demonstrated in electric convulsive therapy cases. *Rorschach Research Exchange, 5,* 35–43.

Kelly, M.D., & Braden, J.P. (1990). Criterion-related validity of the WISC-R Performance scale with the Stanford Achievement Test-Hearing Impaired Edition. *Journal of School Psychology, 28,* 147–151.

Kelly, M.P. (1996). Recognition memory test: Validity in diffuse traumatic brain injury. *Applied Neuropsychology, 3,* 147–154.

Kelly, M.P., Johnson, C.T., & Govern, J.M. (1996). Recognition Memory Test: Validity in diffuse traumatic brain injury. *Applied Neuropsychology, 3,* 147–154.

Kemali, D., Maj, M., Galderisi, S., Salvati, A., Starace, F., Valente, A., & Pirozzi, R. (1986). Clinical, biological, and neuropsychological features associated with lateral ventricular enlargement in DSM-III schizophrenic disorder. *Psychiatry Research, 21,* 137–149.

Kempen, J.H., Kritchevsky, M., & Feldman, S.T. (1994). Effect of visual impairment on neuropsychological test performance. *Journal of Clinical and Experimental Neuropsychology, 16,* 223–231.

Kempler, D., Teng, E.L., Dick, M., Taussig, I.M., & Davis, D.S. (1998). The effects of age, education, and ethnicity on verbal fluency. *Journal of the International Neuropsychological Society, 4,* 532–538.

Kennedey, M.H., & Hiltonsmith, R.W. (1988). Relation ship among the K-ABC Nonverbal Scale, the Pictorial test of Intelligence, and the Hiskey–Nebraska Test of Learning Aptitude for speech- and language-disabled preschool children. *Journal of Psychoeducational Assessment, 6,* 49–54.

Kennedy, M.L., & Guilmette, T.J. (1997). The relationship between the WRAML memory screening and general memory indices in a clinical population. *Assessment, 4,* 69–72.

Kerr, C. (1995). Dysnomia following traumatic brain injury: An information-processing approach to assessment. *Brain Injury, 9,* 777–796.

Kerr, M. (1936). Temperamental differences in twins. *British Journal of Psychology, 27,* 51–59.

Kessler, J., Bley, M., Mielke, R., & Kalbe, E. (1997). Strategies and structures in verbal fluency tasks in patients with Alzheimer's disease. *Behavioural Neurology, 10,* 133–135.

Kibby, M.Y., Schmitter-Edgecombe, M., & Long, C.J. (1998). Ecological validity of neuropsychological tests: Focus on the California Verbal Learning Test and the Wisconsin Card Sorting Test. *Archives of Clinical Neuropsychology, 13,* 523–534.

Kiernan, R.J., Mueller, J., Langston, J.W., & Van Dyke, C. (1987). The Neurobehavioral Cognitive Status Examination: A brief but differentiated approach to cognitive assessment. *Annals of Internal Medicine, 107,* 481–485.

Kimura, D. (1963). Right temporal lobe damage. *Archives of Neurology, 8,* 264–271.

Kindlon, D.J., & Garrison, W. (1984). The Boston Naming Test: Norm data and cue utilization in a sample of 6- and 7-year-old children. *Brain and Language, 21*, 255–259.

King, D.A., Cox, C., Lyness, J.M., Conwell, Y., & Caines, E.D. (1998). Quantitative and qualitative differences in the verbal learning performance of elderly depressives and healthy controls. *Journal of the International Neuropsychological Society, 4*, 115–126.

King, G.D., Hannay, H.J., Masek, B.J., & Burns, J.W. (1978). Effects of anxiety and sex on neuropsychological tests. *Journal of Consulting and Clinical Psychology, 46*, 375–376.

King, J.H., Gfeller, J.D., & Davis, H.P. (1998). Detecting simulated memory impairment with the Rey Auditory Verbal Learning Test: Implications of base rates and study generalizability. *Journal of Clinical and Experimental Neuropsychology, 20*, 603–612.

King, M.C. (1981). Effects of non-focal brain dysfunction on visual memory. *Journal of Clinical Psychology, 37*, 638–643.

King, M.C., & Snow, W.G. (1981). Problem-solving task performance in brain damaged subjects. *Journal of Clinical Psychology, 37*, 400–404.

Kinsella, G.J., Prior, M., Sawyer, M., Ong, B, Murtagh, D., Eienmajer, R., Bryan, D., Anderson, V., & Klug, G. (1997). Predictors and indicators of academic outcome in children 2 years following traumatic brain injury. *Journal of the International Neuropsychological Society, 3*, 608–616.

Kirk, U. (1992a). Confrontation naming in normally developing children: Word retrieval or word knowledge? *The Clinical Neuropsychologist, 6*, 156–170.

Kirk, U. (1992b). Evidence for early acquisition of visual organization ability: A developmental study. *Clinical Neuropsychology, 6*, 171–177.

Kirkby, B.S., van Horn, J.D., Ostrem, J.L., Weinberger, D.R., & Berman, S. (1996). Cognitive activation during PET: A case study of monozygotic twins discordant for closed head injury. *Neuropsychologia, 34*, 689–697.

Kirkcaldy, B. (1987). Personality correlates of Benton's Visual Retention Test. *Personality and Individual Differences, 8*, 141–143.

Kish, G.B. (1970). Alcoholics' GATB and Shipley profiles and their interrelationships. *Journal of Clinical Psychology, 26*, 482–483.

Kitson, D.L., Vance, B. & Blosser, J. (1985). Comparison of the Token Test of Language Development and the Wechsler Intelligence Scale for Children-Revised. *Performance and Motor Skills, 61*, 532–534.

Klebanoff, S.G., Singer, J.L., & Wilensky, H. (1954). Psychological consequences of brain lesions and ablations. *Psychological Bulletin, 51*, 1–41.

Klein, S. (1993). Misuse of Luria–Nebraska localization scales: Commentary on a criminal case study. *The Clinical Neuropsychologist, 7*, 297–299.

Klein, M., Ponds, R.W.H.M., Houx, P.J., & Jolles, J. (1997). Effect of test duration on age-related differences in Stroop interference. *Journal of Clinical and Experimental Neuropsychology, 19*, 77–82.

Klesges, R.C. (1982). Establishing premorbid levels of intellecual functioning in children: An empirical investigation. *Clinical Neuropsychology, 4*, 15–17.

Klesges, R.C., & Sanchez, V.C. (1981). Cross-validation of an index of premorbid functioning in children. *Journal of Consulting and Clinical Psychology, 49*, 141.

Klesges, R.C., Sanchez, V.C., & Stanton, A.L. (1981). Cross-validation of an adult premorbid functioning index. *Clinical Neuropsychology, 3*, 13–15.

Klesges, R.C., & Troster, A.I. (1987). A review of premorbid indices of intellectual and neuropsychological functioning: What have we learned in the past five years? *International Journal of Clinical Neuropsychology, 9*, 1–11.

Klesges, R.C., Fisher, L., Pheley, A., Boschee, P., & Vasey, M. (1984). A major validation study of the Halstead–Reitan in the prediction of CAT-Scan assessed brain damage in adults. *International Journal of Clinical Neuropsychology, 6*, 29–34.

Klett, W.G., Watson, C.G., & Hoffman, P.T. (1986). The Henmon–Nelson and Slosson tests as predictors of WAIS-R IQ. *Journal of Clinical Psychology, 42*, 343–347.

Klimczak, N.J., Donovick, P.J., & Burright, R. (1997). The malingering of multiple sclerosis and mild traumatic brain injury. *Brain Injury, 11*, 343–352.

Kline, R.B., Snyder, J., Guilmette, S., & Castellanos, M. (1992). Relative usefulness of elevation, variability, and shape information from WISC-R, K-ABC, and Fourth Edition Stanford–Binet profiles in predicting achievement. *Psychological Assessment, 4*, 426–432.

Kljajic, I. (1975). Wechsler Memory Scale indices of brain pathology. *Journal of Clinical Psychology, 31*, 698–701.

Kljajic, I. (1976). The MFD and brain pathology. *Journal of Clinical Psychology, 32*, 91–93.

Klonoff, H., Fibiger, C.H., & Hutton, G. (1970). Neuropsychological patterns in chronic schizophrenia. *The Journal of Nervous and Mental Disease, 150*, 291–300.

Klopfer, B., & Davidson, H. (1962). *The Rorschach technique: An introductory manual.* New York: Harcourt.

Klove, H. (1959). Relationship of differential electroencephalographic patterns to distributions of Wechsler–Bellevue scores. *Neurology, 9*, 871–876.

Klove, H. (1963). Clinical neuropsychology. In F.M. Forster (Ed.), *The medical clinics of North America.* New York: W.B. Saunders.

Klove, H. (1974). Validation studies in adult clinical neuropsychology. In R.M. Reitan & L.A. Davison (Eds.), *Clinical neuropsychology: Current status and applications.* Washington, DC: Winston.

Klove, H., & Doehring, D.G. (1962). MMPI in epileptic groups with differential etiology. *Journal of Clinical Psychology, 18*, 149–153.

Kneebone, A.C., Chelune, G.J., & Lueders, H.O. (1997). Individual patient predictors of seizure lateralization in temporal lobe epilepsy: A comparison between neuropsychological memory measures and the Intracarotid Amobarbitol Procedure. *Journal of the International Neuropsychological Society, 3*, 159–168.

Kowalski, J.M., & Rossini, E.D. (1990). Reliability of the WAIS-R factors. *Psychological Reports, 66*, 111–114.

Knesevich, J.W., LaBarge, E., & Edwards, D. (1986). Predictive value of the Boston Naming Test in mild senile dementia of the Alzheimer type. *Psychiatry Research, 19*, 155–162.

Knight, R.G. (1983). On interpreting the several standard errors of the WAIS-R: Some further tables. *Journal of Consulting and Clinical Psychology, 51*, 671–673.

Knight, R.G. (1997). The Wechsler Adult Intelligence Scale-Revised in clinical neuropsychology practice. *New England Journal of Psychology, 26*, 2–19.

Kohnert, K.J., Hernandez, A.E., & Bates, E. (1998). Bilingual performance on the Boston Naming Test: Preliminary norms in Spanish and English. *Brain and Language, 65*, 422–440.

Koltai, D.C., Bowler, R.M., & Shore, M.D. (1996). The Rivermead Behavioural Memory Test and Wechsler Memory Scale-Revised: Relationship to everyday memory impairment. *Assessment, 3*, 443–448.

Konald, T.R., Kush, J.C., & Canivez, G.L. (1997). Factor replication of the WISC-III in three independent samples of children receiving special education. *Journal of Psychoeducational Assessment, 15*, 123–137.

Koppitz, E. (1960). The Bender–Gestalt test for children: A normative study. *Journal of Clinical Psychology, 16*, 432–435.

Koren, D., Seidman, L.J., Harrion, R.H., Lyons, M.J., Kremen, W.S., Caplan, B., Goldstein, J.M., Faraone, S.V., & Tsuang, M.T. (1998). Factor structure of the Wisconsin Card Sorting Test: Dimensions of deficit in schizophrenia. *Neuropsychology, 12*, 289–302.

Korkman, M., Liikanen, A., & Fellman, V. (1996). Neuropsychological consequences of very low birth weight and asphyxia at term: Follow-up until school age. *Journal of Clinical and Experimental Neuropsychology, 18*, 220–233.

Korkman, M., Kirk, U., & Kemp, S. (1998). *NEPSY Manual.* San Antonio, TX: The Psychological Corporation.

Korman, M., & Blumberg, S. (1963). Comparative efficiency of some tests of cerebral damage. *Journal of Consulting Psychology, 27*, 303–304.

Kowall, M.A., Watson, G.M., & Madak, P.R. (1990). Concurrent validity of the Test of Nonverbal Intelligence with referred suburban and Canadian native children. *Journal of Clinical Psychology, 46*, 632–636.

Kozel, J.J., & Meyers, J.E. (1998). A cross-validation of the Victoria Revision of the Category Test. *Archives of Clinical Neuropsychology, 13*, 327–332.

Kozora, A.K., & Cullum, C.M. (1995). Generative naming in normal aging: Total output and qualitative changes using phonemic and semantic constraints. *The Clinical Neuropsychologist, 9*, 313–320.

Krakowski, M., Czobor, P., Carpenter, M.D., Libiger, J., Kunz, M., Papezova, H., Parker, B.B., Schmader, L., & Abad, T. (1997). Community violence and inpatient assaults: Neurobiological deficits. *Journal of Neuropsychiatry and Clinical Neurosciences, 9*, 549–555.

Kramer, J.H., Delis, D.C., Kaplan, E., O'Donnell, L., & Prifitera, A. (1997). Developmental sex differences in verbal learning. *Neuropsychology, 11*, 577–584.

Krikorian, R., & Bartok, J.A. (1998). Developmental data for the Porteus Maze test. *The Clinical Neuropsychologist, 12*, 305–310.

Krishnamurthy, R., Archer, R.P., & House, J.J. (1996). The MMPI-A and Rorschach: A failure to establish convergent validity. *Assessment, 3*, 179–191.

Kristianson, P. (1974). A comparison between the personality changes in certain forms of psychomotor and grand mal epilepsy. *British Journal of Psychiatry, 125*, 34–35.

Kroger, R.O., & Turnbull, W. (1975). Invalidity of validity scales: The case of the MMPI. *Journal of Consulting and Clinical Psychology, 43*, 48–55.

Kronfol, Z., Hamsher, K., Digre, K., & Waziri, R. (1978). Depression and hemispheric functions: Changes associated with ECT. *British Journal of Psychiatry, 132*, 580–587.

Krull, K.R., Scott, J.G., & Sherer, M. (1995). Estimation of premorbid intelligence from combined performance and demographic variables. *The Clinical Neuropsychologist, 9*, 83–88.

Kuder, G.F., & Richardson, M.W. (1937). The theory of estimation of test reliabilities. *Psychometrika, 2*, 151–160.

Kuehn, S.M., & Snow, W.G. (1992). Are the Rey and Taylor figures equivalent? *Archives of Clinical Psychology, 7*, 445–448.

Kunen, S., Overstreet, S., & Salles, C. (1996). Concurrent validity study of the Slosson Intelligence-Revised in mental retardation testing. *Mental Retardation, 34*, 380–386.

Kush, J.C. (1996). Factor structure of the WISC-III for students with learning disabilities. *Journal of Psychoeducational Assessment, 14*, 32–40.

Kush, J.C., & Watkins, M.W. (1997). Construct validity of the WISC-III Verbal and Performance factors for Black special education students. *Assessment, 4*, 297–304.

LaBarge, E., Edwards, D., & Knesevich, J.W. (1986). Performance of normal elderly on the Boston Naming Test. *Brain and Language, 27*, 380–384.

Laboratory of Comparative Human Cognition. (1976). Memory span for nouns, verbs, and function words in low SES children: A replication and critique of Schutz and Keisler. *Journal of Verbal Learning and Verbal Behavior, 15*, 431–435.

Labreche, T.M. (1983). The Victoria Revision of the Halstead Category Test. Doctoral dissertation, University of British Columbia, Canada.

Lacey, M.A., Gore, P.A. Jr., Pliskin, N.H., Henry, G.K., Heilbronner, R.L., & Hamer, D.P. (1996). Verbal fluency task equivalency. *The Clinical Neuropsychologist, 10*, 305–308.

Lacks, P. (1982). Continued clinical popularity of the Bender–Gestalt test: Response to Bigler and Ehrfurth. *Professional Psychology, 13*, 677–680.

Lacks, P. (1984). *Bender Gestalt screening for brain dysfunction*. New York: John Wiley & Sons.

Lacks, P. (1999). *Bender Gestalt screening for brain impairment* (2nd ed.). New York: John Wiley & Sons.

Lacks, P., & Storandt, M. (1982). Bender Gestalt performance of normal older adults. *Journal of Clinical Psychology, 38*, 624–627.

Lacks, P.B. (1979). The use of the Bender Gestalt test in clinical neuropsychology. *Clinical Neuropsychology, 1*, 29–34.

Lacks, P.B., & Newport, K. (1980). A comparison of scoring systems and level of scorer experience on the Bender–Gestalt test. *Journal of Personality Assessment, 44*, 351–357.

Lacks, P.B., Colbert, J., Harrow, M., & Levine, J. (1970). Further evidence concerning the diagnostic accuracy of the Halstead organic test battery. *Journal of Clinical Psychology, 26*, 480–481.

Lacritz, L.H., & Cullum, C.M. (1998). The Hopkins Verbal Learning Test and CVLT: A preliminary comparison. *Archives of Clinical Neuropsychology, 13*, 623–628.

Ladd, J.S. (1998). The F(p) Infrequency-Psychopathology scale with chemically dependent inpatients. *Journal of Clinical Psychology, 54*, 665–671.

Lamanna, J.A., & Ysseldyke, J.E. (1973). Reliability of the Peabody Individual Achievement Test with first grade children. *Psychology in the Schools, 10*, 473–479.

Lambert, N.M. (1970). Paired associates learning, social status, and tests of logical concrete behavior as univariate and multivariate predictors of first grade reading achievement. *American Educational Research Journal, 7*, 511–528.

Lamp, R.E., & Barclay, A. (1967). The Quick Test as a screening device for intellectually subnormal children. *Psychological Reports, 20*, 763–766.

Landy, F.J. (1986). Stamp collecting versus science. *American Psychologist, 41*, 1183–1192.

Langfitt, J.T., & Rausch, R. (1996). Word-finding deficits persist after left anterotemporal lobectomy. *Archives of Neurology, 53*, 72–76.

Lansing, A.E., Ivnik, R.J., Cullum, C.M., & Randolph, C. (1999). An empirically derived short form of the Boston Naming Test. *Archives of Clinical Neuropsychology, 14*, 481–487.

Larrabee, G.J. (1998). Somatic malingering on the MMPI and MMPI-2 in personal injury litigants. *The Clinical Neuropsychologist, 12*, 179–188.

Larrabee, G.J., & Curtiss, G. (1995). Construct validity of various verbal and visual memory measures. *Journal of Clinical and Experimental Neuropsychology, 17*, 536–547.

Larrabee, G.J., Kane, R.L., & Schuck, J.R. (1983). Factor analysis of the WAIS and Wechsler Memory Scale: An analysis of the construct validity of the Wechsler Memory Scale. *Journal of Clinical Psychology, 5*, 159–168.

Larrabee, G.J., Kane, R.L., Shuck, J.R., & Francis, D.J. (1985a). Construct validity of various memory testing procedures. *Journal of Clinical and Experimental Neuropsychology, 7*, 239–250.

Larrabee, G.J., Largen, J.W., & Levin, H.S. (1985b). Sensitivity of age-decline resistant ("hold") WAIS subtests to Alzheimer's disease. *Journal of Clinical and Experimental Neuropsychology, 7*, 497–504.

Larrabee, G.J., Trahan, D.E., & Curtiss, G. (1992). Construct validity of the Continuous Visual Memory Test. *Archives of Clinical Neuropsychology, 7*, 395–405.

Larrain, C.M., & Cimino, C.R. (1998). Alternate forms of the Boston Naming Test in Alzheimer's disease. *The Clinical Neuropsychologist, 12*, 525–530.

Larue, V., Celsis, P., Bes, A., & Marc-Vergnes, J.P. (1994). The functional anatomy of attention in humans: Cerebral blood flow changes induced by reading, naming, and the Stroop effect. *Journal of Cerebral Blood Flow Metabolism, 14*, 958–962.

Lass, N.J., & Golden, S.S. (1975). A comparative study of children's performance on three tasks for receptive language abilities. *Journal of Auditory Research, 15*, 177–182.

Lassiter, K.S., & Bardos, A.N. (1992). A comparison of learning-disabled children's performance on the Test of Nonverbal Intelligence, K-ABC, and WISC-R. *Journal of Psychoeducational Assessment, 10*, 133–140.

Lassiter, K.S., & Bardos, A.N. (1995). The relationship between young children's academic achievement and measures of intelligence. *Psychology in the Schools, 32*, 170–177.

Lastine-Sobecks, J.L., Jackson, S.T., & Paolo, A.M. (1998). Identifying the pronunciation of irregularly spelled words: Relation to verbal IQ. *The Clinical Neuropsychologist, 12*, 189–192.

Laughlin, T. (1995). The school readiness composite of the Bracken Basic Concept scales as an intellectual screening instrument. *Journal of Psychoeducational Assessment, 13*, 294–302.

Laurent, J. (1997). Characteristics of the standard and supplemental batteries of the Woodcock–Johnson Tests of Cognitive Ability-Revised with a college sample. *Journal of School Psychology, 35*, 403–416.

Laurent, J., Swerdlik, M., & Ryburn, M. (1992). Review of validity research on the Stanford–Binet Intelligence Scale: Fourth Edition. *Psychological Assessment, 4*, 102–112.

Lavin, C. (1996). The Wechsler Intelligence Scale for Children-Third Edition and the Stanford–Binet Intelligence Scale-Fourth Edition: A preliminary study of validity. *Psychological Reports, 78*, 491–496.

Law, J.G., Price, D.R., & Herbert, D.A. (1981). Study of Quick Test, WAIS, and premorbid estimates of intelligence for neuropsychiatric patients. *Psychological Reports, 52*, 919–922.

Lawlis, G.F., & Lu, E. (1972). Judgement of counseling process: Reliability, agreement, and error. *Psychological Bulletin, 78*, 17–20.

Lawriw, I., & Sutker, L.W. (1978). A further analysis of the Block Rotation Test. *Journal of Clinical Psychology, 34*, 930–934.

Lawson, J.S., & Barker, M.G. (1968). The assessment of nominal aphasia in dementia: The use of reaction-time measures. *British Journal of Medical Psychology, 41*, 411–414.

Lawson, J.S., Inglis, J., & Stroud, T.W.F. (1983). A laterality index of cognitive impairment derived from a principal components analysis of the WAIS-R. *Journal of Consulting and Clinical Psychology, 51*, 841–847.

Lawson, T.T., & Evans, L.D. (1996). Stanford–Binet: Fourth edition short forms with underachieving and learning disabled students. *Psychological Reports, 79*, 47–50.

Lee, D. (1967). Graph-theoretical properties of Elithorn's Maze. *Journal of Mathematical Psychology, 4*, 341–347.

Lees-Haley, P.R. (1992). Efficacy of MMPI-2 validity scales I–II modifier scales for detecting spurious PTSD claims: F, F-K, Fake Bad Scale, Ego Strength, Subtle-Obvious Scales, Dis, and Deb. *Journal of Clinical Psychology, 48*, 681–689.

Lees-Haley, P.R., English, L.T., & Glenn, W.J. (1991). A fake bad scale on the MMPI-2 for personal injury claimants. *Psychological Reports, 68*, 203–210.

Lees-Haley, P.R., Smith, H.H., Williams, C.W., & Dunn, J.T. (1996). Forensic neuropsychological test usage: An empirical survey. *Archives of Clinical Neuropsychology, 11*, 45–51.

Leonard, F.C. (1994). Using Wechsler data to predict success from learning disabled college students. *Learning Disabilities Research and Practice, 6*, 17–24.

Lerner, H.L., & Lerner, P.M. (1986). Rorschach inkblot test. In D.J. Keyser & R.C. Sweetland (Eds.), *Test critiques* (Vol. 4). Kansas City: Test Corporation of America.

Levenson, R.L., & Lasher-Adelman, V. (1988). Stability of the Peabody Picture Vocabulary Test-Revised for emotionally handicapped middle-school-aged children. *Perceptual and Motor Skills, 67*, 392–394.

Levin, H. (1973). Motor impersistence in patients with unilateral cerebral disease: A cross-validational study. *Journal of Consulting and Clinical Psychology, 41,* 287–290.

Levin, H.S., & Benton, A.L. (1977). Facial recognition in "pseudoneurological" patients. *Journal of Nervous and Mental Disease, 164,* 135–138.

Levin, H.S., Grossman, R.G., & Kelly, P.J. (1977). Impairment of facial recognition after closed head injuries of varying severity. *Cortex, 13,* 119–130.

Levin, H.S., Benton, A.L., & Grossman, R.G. (1982). Neurobehavioral consequences of closed head injury. *The Lancet, 2,* 605–609.

Levin, H.S., Song, J., Scheibel, R.S., Fletcher, J.M., Harward, H., Lilly, M., & Goldstein, F. (1997). Concept formation and problem-solving following closed head injury in children. *Journal of the International Neuropsychological Society, 3,* 598–607.

Levine, J., & Feirstein, A. (1972). Differences in test performances between brain damaged, schizophrenic, and medical patients. *Journal of Consulting and Clinical Psychology, 39,* 508–511.

Levine, M.S. (1977). *Canonical analysis and factor comparison.* Beverly Hills, CA: Sage.

Levine, N.R. (1971). Validation of the Quick Test for intelligence screening of the elderly. *Psychological Reports, 29,* 167–172.

Levinson, E.M., & Folino, L. (1994). Correlations of scores on the Gifted Evaluation Scale with those on the WISC-III and the Kaufman Brief Intelligence Test with students referred for gifted education. *Psychological Reports, 74,* 419–424.

Levinson, E.M., & Folino, L. (1995). The relationship between the WISC-III and the Kaufman Brief Intelligence Test with students referred for gifted education. *Special Services in the Schools, 8,* 155–159.

Levitt, E.E., & Truumaa, A. (1972). *The Rorschach technique with children and adolescents: Application and norms.* New York: Grune & Stratton.

Levy, I.S. (1971). The Goodenough–Harris Drawing Test and educable mentally retarded adolescents. *Journal of Mental Deficiency, 75,* 760–761.

Lewinsohn, P.M. (1973). Psychological assessment of patients with brain injury. Unpublished manuscript, University of Oregon, Eugene.

Lewis, C.D., & Lorentz, S. (1994). Comparison of the Leiter International Performance Scales and the Wechsler Intelligence Scales. *Psychological Reports, 74,* 521–522.

Lewis, M., Jaskir, J., & Enright, M.K. (1986). The development of mental abilities in infancy. *Intelligence, 10,* 331–354.

Lewis, R.D., & Lorion, R.P. (1988). Discriminative effectiveness of the Luria–Nebraska Neuropsychological Battery for LD adolescents. *Learning Disability Quarterly, 11,* 62–70.

Lewis, S., Campbell, A., Takushi-Chinen, R., Brown, A., Dennis, G., Wood, D., & Weir, R. (1997). Visual organization test performance in an African-American population with unilateral cerebral lesions. *International Journal of Neuroscience, 91,* 295–302.

Lezak, M.D. (1979). Recovery of memory and learning functions following traumatic brain injury. *Cortex, 15,* 63–72.

Lezak, M.D. (1982). The test–retest stability and reliability of some tests commonly used in neuropsychological assessment. Presented at fifth European Conference of the International Neuropsychological Society, Deauville, France.

Lezak, M.D. (1983). *Neuropsychological assessment* (2nd ed.). New York: Oxford University Press.

Lezak, M.D. (1995). *Neuropsychological assessment* (3rd ed.). New York: Oxford University Press.

Lezak, M.D., & Glaudin, V. (1969). Differential effects of physical illness on MMPI profiles. *Newsletter for Research in Psychology, 11,* 27–28.

Libb, J.W., & Coleman, J.M. (1971). Correlations between the WAIS and Revised Beta, Wechsler Memory Scale, and Quick Test in a vocational rehabilitation center. *Psychological Reports, 29,* 863–865.

Liberman, J.N., Stewart, W., Seines, O., & Gordon, B. (1994). Rater agreement for the Rey–Osterrieth Complex Figure. *Journal of Clinical Psychology, 50,* 615–624.

Libon, D.J., Malamut, B.L., Swenson, R., Sands, L.P., & Cloud, B.S. (1996a). Further analysis of clock drawings among demented and nondemented older subjects. *Archives of Clinical Neuropsychology, 11,* 193–205.

Libon, D.J., Mattson, R.E., Glosser, G., Kaplan, E., Malamut, B.L., Sands, L.P., Swenson, R., & Cloud, B.S. (1996b). A nine-word dementia version of the California Verbal Learning Test. *The Clinical Neuropsychologist, 10,* 237–244.

Lichtenberg, P.A., & Christensen, B. (1992). Extended normative data for the Logical Memory Subtests of the

Wechsler Memory Scale-Revised: Responses from a sample of cognitively intact elderly medical patients. *Psychological Reports, 71,* 745–746.

Lichtenberg, P.A., Ross, T., & Christensen, B. (1994). Preliminary data on the Boston Naming Test for an older urban population. *The Clinical Neuropsychologist, 8,* 109–111.

Lichtenberg, P.A., Millis, S.R., & Nanna, M. (1995). Use of the Visual Form Discrimination Test with urban geriatric medical inpatients. *The Clinical Neuropsychologist, 8,* 462–465.

Lichtenberg, P.A., Vangel, S.J., Kimbarow, M.L., & Ross, T.P. (1996). The Boston Naming Test-Clinical utility. *Clinical Gerontologist, 16,* 69–72.

Lichtenberg, P.A., Ross, T.P., Youngblade, L., & Vangel, S.J., Jr. (1998). Normative studies research project test battery: Detection of dementia in African American and European American urban elderly patients. *The Clinical Neuropsychologist, 12,* 146–154.

Liebetrau, A.M. (1983). *Measures of association.* Beverly Hills, CA: Sage.

Likert, R., & Quasha, W.H. (1948). *The revised Minnesota Paper Form Board Test.* New York: The Psychological Corporation.

Lin, Y., & Rennick, P.M. (1973). WAIS correlates of the Minnesota Percepto-Diagnostic Test in a sample of epileptic patients: Differential patterns for men and women. *Perceptual and Motor Skills, 37,* 643–646.

Lindgren, S.D., & Benton, A.L. (1980). Developmental patterns of visuospatial judgement. *Journal of Pediatric Psychology, 5,* 217–225.

Lindsay, P.H., Shapiro, A., Musselman, C.R., & Wilson, A. (1988). Predicting language development in deaf children using the Leiter International Performance Scales. *Canadian Journal of Psychology, 42,* 144–162.

Lippold, S., & Claiborn, J.M. (1983). Comparison of the Wechsler Adult Intelligence Scale and the Wechsler Adult Intelligence Scale-Revised. *Journal of Consulting and Clinical Psychology, 51,* 315.

Livingston, R.B., Mears, G., Marshall, R., Gray, R., & Haak, R.A. (1996). Psychostimulant effects on neuro-psychological, intellectual, and achievement measures for children and adolescents with attention deficit hyperactivity disorder. *Applied Neuropsychology, 3,* 174–177.

Livingston, R.B., Gray, R.M., Haak, R.A., & Jennings, E. (1997a). Factor structure of the Halstead–Reitan Neuropsychological Test Battery for Older Children. *Child Neuropsychology, 3,* 176–191.

Livingston, R.B., Pritchard, D.A., Moses, J.A. Jr., Haak, R.A., Marshall, R., & Gray, R. (1997b). Modal profiles for the Halstead–Reitan Neuropsychological Battery for Children. *Archives of Clinical Neuropsychology, 12,* 459–476.

Livingston, R.B., Gray, R.M., & Haak, R.A. (1999). Internal consistency of three tests from the Halstead–Reitan Neuropsychological Battery for Older Children. *Assessment, 6,* 93–99.

LoBello, S.G. (1991a). A table for determining probability of obtaining verbal and performance scale discrepancies on the Wechsler Preschool and Primary Scale of Intelligence-Revised. *Psychology in the Schools, 28,* 93–94.

LoBello, S.G. (1991b). Significant differences between individual subtest scaled scores and average scaled scores on the Wechsler Preschool and Primary Scale of Intelligence-Revised. *Psychology in the Schools, 28,* 15–18.

LoBello, S.G. (1991c). A short form of the Wechsler Preschool and Primary Scale of Intelligence-Revised. *Journal of School Psychology, 29,* 229–236.

LoBello, S.G. (1991d). Subtest scatter as an indicator of the inaccuracy of short-form estimates of IQ. *Psychological Reports, 68,* 1115–1118.

LoBello, S.G., & Guelgoez, S. (1991). Factor analysis of the Wechsler Preschool and Primary Scale of Intelligence-Revised. *Psychological Assessment, 3,* 130–132.

LoBello, S.G., Thompson, A.P., & Evani, V. (1998). Supplementary WAIS-III tables for determining strengths and weaknesses. *Journal of Psychoeducational Assessment, 16,* 196–200.

Loewenstein, D.A., Amigo, D.A., Duara, R., Guterman, A., Hurwitz, D., Berkowitz, N., Wilkie, F., Weinberg, G., Black, B., Gittelman, B., & Eisdorfer, C. (1989). A new scale for the assessment of functional status in Alzheimer's disease and related disorders. *Journal of Gerontology: Psychological Sciences, 44,* 114–121.

Logue, P., & Wyrick, L. (1979). Initial validation of Russell's Revised Wechsler Memory Scale: A comparison of normal aging versus dementia. *Journal of Consulting and Clinical Psychology, 47,* 176–178.

Logue, P.E., Tupler, L.A., D'Amico, C., & Schmitt, F.A. (1993). The Neurobehavioral Cognitive Status Examination: Psychometric properties in use with psychiatric inpatients. *Journal of Clinical Psychology, 49,* 80–89.

Lowman, M.G., Schwanz, K.A., & Kamphaus, R.W. (1996). WISC-III third factor: Critical measurement issues. *Canadian Journal of School Psychology, 12,* 15–22.

Lord, F. (1952). A theory of test scores. *Psychometrika,* Monograph No. 7.

Lord, F.M. (1980). *Applications of item response theory to practical testing problems*. Hillsdale, NJ: Lawrence J. Erlbaum.

Lord, F.M., & Novick, M.R. (1968). *Statistical theories of mental test scores*. Reading, MA: Addison-Wesley.

Loring, D.W. (1989). The Wechsler Memory Scale-Revised or the Wechsler Memory Scale-Revisited? *Clinical Neuropsychologist, 3*, 59–69.

Loring, D.W., Lee, G.P., & Meador, K.J. (1988). Revising the Rey–Osterrieth: Rating right hemisphere recall. *Archives of Clinical Neuropsychology, 3*, 239–247.

Loring, D.W., Lee, G.P., Martin, R.C., & Meador, K.J. (1989). Verbal and Visual Memory Index discrepancies from the Wechsler Memory Scale-Revised: Cautions in interpretation. *Psychological Assessment, 1*, 198–202.

Loring, D.W., Martin, R.C., Meador, K.J., & Lee, G.P. (1990). Psychometric construction of the Rey–Osterrieth Complex Figure: Methodological considerations and interrater reliability. *Archives of Clinical Neuropsychology, 5*, 1–14.

Loring, D.W., Meador, K.J., & Lee, G.P. (1994). Effects of temporal lobectomy on generative fluency and other language functions. *Archives of Clinical Neuropsychology, 9*, 229–238.

Lorig, T.S., Gehring, W.J., & Hyrn, D.L. (1986). Period analysis of the EEG during performance of the Trail Making Test. *International Journal of Clinical Neuropsychology, 8*, 97–99.

LoSasso, G.L., Rapport, L.J., Axelrod, B.N., & Reeder, K.P. (1998). Intermanual and alternate-form equivalence on the Trail Making Tests. *Journal of Clinical and Experimental Neuropsychology, 20*, 107–110.

Love, H.G.I. (1970). Validation of the Hooper Visual Organization Test on a New Zealand psychiatric hospital population. *Psychological Reports, 27*, 915–917.

Loveland, N.T. (1961). Epileptic personality and cognitive functioning. *Journal of Projective Techniques, 25*, 54–68.

Lowe, J.D., Anderson, H.N., Williams, A., & Currie, B.B. (1987). Long-term predictive validity of the WPPSI and WISC-R with Black school children. *Personality and Individual Differences, 8*, 551–559.

Lowrance, D., & Anderson, H.N. (1979). A comparison of the Slosson Intelligence Test and the WISC-R with elementary school children. *Psychology in the Schools, 16*, 361–364.

Lubin, B., & Sands, E.W. (1992). Bibliography of the psychometric properties of the Bender Visuo-Motor Gestalt Test. *Perceptual and Motor Skills, 75*, 385–386.

Lucas, J.A., Ivnik, R.J., Smith, G.E., Bohac, D.L., Tangalos, E.G., Kokmen, E., Graff-Radford, N.R., & Petersen, R.C. (1998a). Mayo's Older Americans Normative Studies: Category fluency norms. *Journal of Clinical and Experimental Neuropsychology, 20*, 194–200.

Lucas, J.A., Ivnik, R.J., Smith, G.E., Bohac, D.L., Tangalos, E.G., Kokmen, E., Graff-Radford, N.R., & Petersen, R.C. (1998b). Normative data for the Matttis Dementia Rating Scale. *Journal of Clinical and Experimental Neuropsychology, 20*, 536–547.

Lucas, J.A., Ivnik, R.J., Smith, G.E., Bohac, D.L., Tangalos, E.G., Graff-Radford, N.R., & Petersen, R.C. (1998). Mayo's Older Americans Normative Study: Category fluency norms. *Journal of Clinical and Experimental Neuropsychology, 20*, 194–200.

Lukatela, K., Malloy, P., Jenkins, M., & Cohen, R. (1998). The naming deficit in early Alzheimer's and vascular dementia. *Neuropsychology, 12*, 565–572.

Lukens, J., & Hurrell, R.M. (1996). A comparison of the Stanford–Binet IV and the WISC-III with mildly retarded children. *Psychology in the Schools, 33*, 24–27.

Luo, C.R. (1999). Semantic competition as the basis for the Stroop interference: Evidence from color-word matching tasks. *Psychological Science, 10*, 35–40.

Luria, A.R. (1966). *Higher cortical functions in man* (1st ed.; B. Heigh, Trans.). New York: Basic Books and Plenum Press.

Lynn, R., Mylotte, A., Ford, F., & McHugh, M. (1997). The heritability of intelligence and social maturation in four to six year olds: A study of Irish twins. *Irish Journal of Psychology, 18*, 439–443.

Lysaker, P., Bell, M., & Beam-Goulet, J. (1995). Wisconsin Card Sorting Test performance in schizophrenia. *Psychiatry Research, 56*, 45–51.

Macciocchi, S.N., Fowler, P.C., & Ranseen, J.D. (1992). Trait analyses of the Luria–Nebraska Intellectual Processes, Motor Functions, and Memory Scales. *Archives of Clinical Neuropsychology, 7*, 541–551.

MacInnes, W.D., Golden, C.J., McFadden, J.E., & Wilkening, G.N. (1983). Relationship between the Booklet Category Test and the Wisconsin Card Sorting Test. *International Journal of Neuroscience, 21*, 257–264.

Mack, J.L. (1979). The MMPI and neurological dysfunction. In C.S. Newmark (Ed.), *MMPI: Current clinical and research trends*. New York: Praeger.

Mack, W.J., Freed, D.M., Williams, B.W., & Henderson, V.W. (1992). Boston Naming Test: Shortened version for use in Alzheimer's disease. *Journal of Gerontology, 47*, P154–P158.

Maddrey, A.M., Cullum, C.M., Weiner, M.F., & Filley, C.M. (1996). Premorbid intelligence estimation and level of dementia in Alzheimer's disease. *Journal of the International Neuropsychological Society, 2*, 551–555.

Maier, L.R., & Abidin, R. (1967). Validation attempt of Hovey's five-item MMPI index for central nervous system disorders. *Journal of Consulting Psychology, 31*, 542.

Majdan, A., Sziklas, V., & Jones-Gotman, M. (1996). Performance of healthy subjects and patients with resection from the anterior temporal lobe on matched tests of verbal learning and visuoperceptual learning. *Journal of Clinical and Experimental Neuropsychology, 18*, 416–430.

Malec, J. (1978). Neuropsychological assessment of schizophrenia versus brain damage: A review. *The Journal of Nervous and Mental Disease, 166*, 507–516.

Malina, A.C., Bowers, D.A., Millis, S.R., & Uekert, S. (1998). Internal consistency of the Warrington Recognition Memory Test. *Perceptual and Motor Skills, 86*, 1320–1322.

Maller, S.J., & Ferron, J. (1997). WISC-III factor invariance across deaf and standardization samples. *Educational and Psychological Measurement, 57*, 987–994.

Maller, S.J., Konold, T.R., & Glutting, J.J. (1998). WISC-III factor invariance across samples of children exhibiting appropriate and inappropriate test-session behaviors. *Educational and Psychological Measurement, 58*, 467–474.

Malloy, P.F., & Webster, J.S. (1981). Detecting mild brain impairment using the Luria–Nebraska Neuropsychological Battery. *Journal of Consulting and Clinical Psychology, 49*, 768–770.

Malmo, H.P. (1974). On frontal lobe functions: Psychiatric patient controls. *Cortex, 10*, 231–237.

Mandes, E., & Gessner, T. (1988). Differential effects on verbal-performance achievement levels on the WAIS-R as a function of progressive error rate on the Memory For Designs Test (MFD). *Journal of Clinical Psychology, 44*, 317–320.

Mandes, E., & Gessner, T. (1989). The principle of additivity and its relation to clinical decision making. *Journal of Psychology, 123*, 485–490.

Mandes, E., Massimino, C., & Mantis, C. (1991). A comparison of borderline and mild mental retardates assessed on the Memory For Designs and the WAIS-R. *Journal of Clinical Psychology, 47*, 562–567.

Mangiaracina, J., & Simon, M.J. (1986). Comparison of the PPVT-R and WAIS-R in state hospital psychiatric patients. *Journal of Clinical Psychology, 42*, 817–820.

Manly, J.J., Jacobs, D.M., Sano, M., Bell, K., Merchant, C.A., Small, S., & Stern, Y. (1998a). Cognitive test performance among nondemented elderly African American and Whites. *Neurology, 50*, 1238–1245.

Manly, J.J., Miller, S.W., Heaton, R.K., Byrd, D., Reilly, J., Velasquez, R.J., Sacuzzo, D.P., Grant, I., and the HIV Neurobehavioral Research Center (HRNC) Group. (1998b). The effect of African-American acculturaltion on neuropsychological test performance in normal and HIV-positive individuals. *Journal of the International Neuropsychological Society, 4*, 291–302.

Mann, U., Staedt, D., Kappos, L., Wense A.V., & Haubitz, I. (1989). Correlation of MRI findings and neuropsychological results in patients with multiple sclerosis. *Psychiatry Research, 29*, 293–294.

Marciso, D.S., & Wagner, E.E. (1990). A comparison of the Lacks and Pascal–Suttell Bender–Gestalt scoring methods for diagnosing brain damage in an outpatient sample. *Journal of Clinical Psychology, 46*, 868–877.

Marcopulos, B.A., McLain, C.A., & Giuliano, A.J. (1997). Cognitive impairment or inadequate norms: A study of healthy, rural, older adults with limited education. *Clinical Neuropsychologist, 11*, 111–131.

Marcotte, T.D., van Gorp, W., Hinkin, C.H., & Osato, S. (1997). Concurrent validity of the Neurobehavioral Cognitive Status Exam subtests. *Journal of Clinical and Experimental Neuropsychology, 19*, 386–395.

Margolin, D.I., Pate, D.S., Friedrich, F.J., & Elia, E. (1990). Dysnomia in dementia and stroke patients: Different underlying cognitive deficits. *Journal of Clinical and Experimental Neuropsychology, 12*, 597–612.

Margolis, R.B., Greenlief, C.L., & Taylor, J.M. (1985). Relationship between the WAIS-R and WRAT in a geriatric sample with suspected dementia. *Psychological Reports, 56*, 287–292.

Margolis, R.B., Taylor, J.M., & Greeenlief, C.L. (1986). A cross-validation of two short forms of the WAIS-R in a geriatric sample suspected of dementia. *Journal of Clinical Psychology, 42*, 145–146.

Marieen, P., Mampaey, E., Vervaet, A., Saerens, J., & DeDeyn, P.P. (1998). Normative data for the Boston Naming Test in native Dutch-speaking Belgian elderly. *Brain and Language, 65*, 447–467.

Marini, A.E. (1990). Concurrent, criterion-related validity of the Quick Test based on a sample of gifted students. *Psychological Reports, 67*, 1007–1010.

Mark, R., Beal, A.L., & Dumont, R. (1998). Validation of a WISC-III short form for the identification of Canadian gifted students. *Canadian Journal of School Psychology, 14*, 1–10.

Markowitz, H.J. (1973). The differential diagnosis of acute schizophrenia and organic brain damage. Doctoral dissertation, West Virginia University.

Marmorale, A.M., & Brown, F. (1977). Bender–Gestalt performance of Puerto Rican, white, and black children. *Journal of Clinical Psychology, 33,* 224–228.

Marsh, G.C., & Hirsch, S.H. (1982). Effectiveness of two tests of visual retention. *Journal of Clinical Psychology, 38,* 115–118.

Marson, D.C., Dymek, M.P., Duke, L.W., & Harrell, L.E. (1997). Subscale validity of the Mattis Dementia Rating Scale. *Archives of Clinical Neuropsychology, 12,* 269–275.

Martin, J.D., Blair, G.E., & Vickers, D.M. (1979). Correlation of the Slosson Intelligence Test with the California Short-Form Test of Mental Maturity and the Shipley Institute of Living Scale. *Educational and Psychological Measurement, 39,* 193–196.

Martin, J.D., Blair, G.E., & Bledsoe, J.R. (1990). Measures of concurrent validity and alternate-form reliability of the Test of Nonverbal Intelligence. *Psychological Reports, 66,* 503–508.

Martin, R.C., Franzen, M.D., & Orey, S. (1998). Magnitude of error as a strategy to detect feigned memory impairment. *The Clinical Neuropsychologist, 12,* 84–91.

Martino, A.A., Pizzamiglio, L., & Razzano, C. (1976). A new version of the "Token Test" for aphasics: A concrete objects form. *Journal of Communication Disorders, 9,* 1–5.

Maruish, M.E., Sawicki, R.F., Franzen, M.D., & Golden, C.J. (1985). Alpha coefficient reliabilities for the Luria–Nebraska summary and localization scales by diagnostic category. *International Journal of Clinical Neuropsychology, 7,* 10–12.

Mason, E.M. (1992). Percent agreement among raters and rater reliability of the Copying subtest of the Stanford–Binet Intelligence Scale: Fourth Edition. *Perceptual and Motor Skills, 74,* 347–353.

Massman, P.J., & Bigler, E.D. (1993). A quantitative review of the diagnostic utility of the WAIS-R Fuld profile. *Archives of Clinical Neuropsychology, 8,* 417–428.

Massoth, N.A. (1985). The McCarthy Scales of Children's Abilities as a predictor of achievement: A five-year follow-up. *Psychology in the Schools, 22,* 10–13.

Matarazzo, J.D., & Herman, D.O. (1984). Base rate information for the WAIS-R: Test–retest stability and VIQ-PIQ differences. *Journal of Clinical Neuropsychology, 6,* 351–366.

Matarazzo, J.D., Wiens, A.N., Matarazzo, R.G., & Goldstein, S. (1974). Psychometric and clinical test–retest reliability of the Halstead–Reitan Impairment Index in a sample of healthy, young, normal men. *The Journal of Nervous and Mental Disease, 158,* 37–49.

Matarazzo, J.D., Matarazzo, R.G., Wiens, A.N., Gallo, A.E., & Klonoff, H. (1976). Retest reliability of the Halstead Impairment Index in a normal, a schizophrenic, and two samples of organic patients. *Journal of Clinical Psychology, 32,* 338–349.

Matarazzo, J.D., Carmody, T.P., & Jacobs, L.D. (1980). Test–retest reliability and stability of the WAIS: A literature review with implications for clinical practice. *Journal of Clinical Neuropsychology, 2,* 89–105.

Matthews, C.G., & Booker, H.E. (1972). Pneumonecephalographic measurements and neuropsychological test performance in human adults. *Cortex, 8,* 69–92.

Matthews, C.G., & Haaland, K.Y. (1979). The effect of symptom duration on cognitive and motor performance in Parkinsonism. *Neurology, 29,* 951–956.

Matthews, C.G., Shaw, D.J., & Klove, H. (1966). Psychological test performance in neurologic and "pseudo-neurologic" subtests. *Cortex, 2,* 244–253.

Matthews, C.G., Dikmen, S., & Harley, J.P. (1977). Age of onset and psychometric correlates of MMPI profiles in major epilepsy. *Diseases of the Nervous System, 38,* 173–176.

Mattis, S. (1988). *Dementia Rating Scale.* Odessa, FL: Psychological Assessment Resources.

Mattis, P.J., Hannay, H.J., & Meyers, C.A. (1992). Efficacy of the Satz–Mogel short form WAIS-R for tumor patients with lateralized lesions. *Psychological Assessment, 4,* 357–362.

Matz, P.A., Altepeter, T.S., & Perlman, B. (1992). MMPI-2: Reliability with college students. *Journal of Clinical Psychology, 48,* 330–334.

McBurnett, K., Hynd, G.W., Lahey, B.B., & Town, P.A. (1988). Do neuropsychological measures contribute to the prediction of academic achievement? The predictive validity of the LNNB-CR Pathognomonic scale. *Journal of Psychoeducational Assessment, 6,* 162–167.

McCaffrey, R.J., Cousins, J.P., Westervelt, H.J., Martynowics, M., Remick, S.C., Szebenyi, A., Wagle, W.A., Bottomly, P.A., Hardy, C.J., & Haase, R.F. (1995). Practice effects withe NIMH AIDS abbreviated neuropsychological battery. *Archives of Clinical Neuropsychology, 14,* 241–250.

McCallum, R.S., & Bracken, B.A. (1981). Alternate forms reliability of the PPVT-R for black and white preschool children. *Psychology in the Schools, 18*, 422–425.

McCallum, R.S., Karnes, F., & Crowell, M. (1988). Factor structure of the Stanford–Binet Intelligence Scale (4th ed.) for gifted children. *Contemporary Educational Psychology, 13*, 331–338.

McCann, J.T. (1998). Defending the Rorschach in court: An analysis of admissibility using legal and professional standards. *Journal of Personality Assessment, 70*, 125–144.

McCara, E. (1953). The Wechsler Memory Scale with average and superior normal adults. *Bulletin of the Maritime Psychology Association*, pp. 30–33.

McCarthy, D. (1972). *McCarthy Scales of Children's Abilities manual*. New York: The Psychological Corporation.

McCarty, S.M., Logue, P.E., Power, D.G., Ziesat, H.A., & Rosenstiel, A.K. (1980). Alternate-form reliability and age related scores of Russell's Revised Wechsler Memory Scale. *Journal of Consulting and Clinical Psychology, 48*, 296–298.

McCracken, L.M., & Franzen, M.D. (1992). Principal-components analysis of the equivalence of alternate forms of the Trail Making Test. *Psychological Assessment, 4*, 235–238.

McCrowell, K.L., & Nagle, R.J. (1994). Comparability of the WPPSI-R and the S-B:IV among preschool children. *Journal of Psychoeducational Assessment, 12*, 126–134.

McCusker, P.J. (1994). Validation of Kaufman, Ishikuma, and Kaufman–Packard's Wechsler Adult Intelligence Scale-Revised short forms on a clinical sample. *Psychological Assessment, 6*, 246–248.

McDowell, C., & Acklin, M.W. (1996). Standardizing procedures for calculating Rorschach interrater reliability: Conceptual and empirical foundations. *Journal of Personality Assessment, 66*, 308–320.

McElwain, D.W., Kearney, G.E., & Ord, I.G. (n.d.). *The Queensland Test*. Brisbane, Australia: Craftsman Press.

McFie, J., & Piercy, M.F. (1952). The relation of lesion to performance on Weigl's sorting test. *Journal of Mental Science, 98*, 299–305.

McGhee, R.L., & Lieberman, L.R. (1991). Test–retest reliability of the Test of Nonverbal Intelligence (TONI). *Journal of School Psychology, 28*, 351–353.

McGilligan, R.P., Yater, A.C., & Hulsing, R. (1971). Goodenough–Harris Drawing Test reliabilities. *Psychology in the Schools, 8*, 359–362.

McGlone, J. (1977). Sex differences in the cerebral organization of verbal functions in patients with unilateral brain lesions. *Brain, 100*, 775–793.

McGlone, J. (1978). Sex differences in functional brain asymmetry. *Cortex, 14*, 122–128.

McGlynn, S.M., & Kazniak, A.W. (1991). When metacognition fails: Impaired awareness of deficits in Alzheimer's disease. *Journal of Cognitive Neuroscience, 3*, 183–189.

McGlynn, S.M., & Schacter, D.L. (1989). Unawareness of deficit in neuropsychological syndromes. *Journal of Clinical and Experimental Neuropsychology, 11*, 143–205.

McGrew, K.S. (1987). Exploratory factor analysis of the Woodcock–Johnson Tests of Cognitive Ability. *Journal of Psychoeducational Assessment, 5*, 200–216.

McGrew, K., & Murphy, S. (1995). Uniqueness and general factor characteristics of the Woodcock–Johnson Tests of Cognitive Ability-Revised. *Journal of School Psychology, 33*, 421–428.

McGrew, K.S., & Wrightson, W. (1997). The calculation of new and improved WISC-III subtest reliability, uniqueness and general factor characteristic information through the use of data smoothing procedures. *Psychology in the Schools, 34*, 181–195.

McIntosh, D.E., Dunham, M.D., Dean, R.S., & Kundert, D.K. (1995). Neuropsychological characteristics of learning disabled/gifted children. *International Journal of Neurosciences, 83*, 123–130.

McIntosh, D.E., Waldo, S.L., & Koller, J.R. (1997). Exploration of the underlying dimension and overlap between the Kaufman Adolescent and Adult Intelligence Test and the Wechsler Memory Test-Revised. *Journal of Psychoeducational Assessment, 15*, 15–26.

McKay, S.E., & Golden, C.J. (1981a). The assessment of specific neuropsychological skills using scales derived from factor analysis of the Luria–Nebraska Neuropsychological Battery. *International Journal of Neuroscience, 14*, 189–204.

McKay, S.E., & Golden, C.J. (1981b). Re-examination of the factor structure of the Receptive Language scale of the Luria–Nebraska Neuropsychological Battery. *International Journal of Neuroscience, 14*, 183–188.

McKay, S., & Ramsey, R. (1984). Neuropsychological correlates of sociometric status in alcoholics. *International Journal of Clinical Neuropsychology, 6*, 191–195.

McKinley, J.C., & Hathaway, S.R. (1942). A multiphasic personality schedule (Minnesota): 4. Psychasthenia. *Journal of Applied Psychology, 26*, 614–624.

McKinley, J.C., & Hathaway, S.R. (1944). The MMPI: 5. Hysteria, hypomania, and psychopathic deviate. *Journal of Applied Psychology, 28,* 153–174.

McKinzey, R.K., & Russell, E.W. (1997a). Detection of malingering on the Halstead–Reitan Battery: A cross-validation. *Archives of Clinical Neuropsychology, 12,* 584–589.

McKinzey, R.K., & Russell, E.W. (1997b). A partial cross-validation of a Halstead–Reitan Battery malingering formula. *Journal of Clinical and Experimental Neuropsychology, 19,* 484–488.

McKinzey, R.K., Podd, M.H., Krehbiel, M.A., Mensch, A.J., & Trombka, L. (1997). Detection of malingering on the Luria–Nebraska Neuropsychological Battery: An initial and cross-validation. *Archives of Clinical Neuropsychology, 12,* 505–512.

McKinzey, R.K., Roecker, C.E., Puente, A.E., & Rogers, E.B. (1998). Performance of normal adults on the Luria–Nebraska Neuropsychological Battery, Form I. *Archives of Clinical Neuropsychology, 13,* 397–413.

McNeil, M.R., & Prescott, T.E. (1978). *Revised Token Test.* Baltimore: University Park Press.

McNulty, J.L., Graham, J.R., Ben-Porath, Y.S., & Stein, L.A.R. (1997). Comparative validity of MMPI-2 scores of African American and Caucasian mental health center clients. *Psychological Assessment, 9,* 404–470.

McSweeny, A.J., Grant, I., Heaton, R.K., Prigatano, G.P., & Adams, K.M. (1985). Relationship of neuropsychological status to everyday functioning in healthy and chronically ill persons. *Journal of Clinical and Experimental Neuropsychology, 7,* 281–291.

McSweeny, A.J., Naugle, R.I., Chelune, G.J., & Lueders, H. (1993). "T Scores for Change": An illustration of a regression approach to depicting change in clinical neuropsychology. *The Clinical Neuropsychologist, 7,* 300–312.

Meador, K.J., Moore, E.E., Nichols, M.E., Abney, O.L., Taylor, H.S., Zamrini, E.Y., & Loring, D.W. (1993). The role of the cholinergic systems in visuospatial processing. *Journal of Clinical and Experimental Neuropsychology, 15,* 832–842.

Meek, P.S., Clark, W., & Solana, V.L. (1989). Neurocognitive impairment: The unrecognized component of dual diagnosis in substance abuse treatment. *Journal of Psychoactive Drugs, 21,* 153–160.

Megaree, E.I. (1997). Using the Megaree MMPI-based classification system with the MMPI-2s of female prison inmates. *Psychological Assessment, 9,* 75–82.

Megaree, E.I., & Dorhut, B. (1977). A new classification system for criminal offenders, III: Revision and refinement of the classificatory rules. *Criminal Justice and Behavior, 4,* 125–148.

Megaree, E.I., & Bohn, M.J., Jr. (with Meyer, J. & Sink, F.). (1979). *Classifying criminal offenders: A new system based on the MMPI.* Beverly Hills, CA: Sage.

Mehlman, B., & Rand, M.E. (1960). Face validity on the MMPI. *Journal of General Psychology, 63,* 171–178.

Mehryar, A.H., Tashakkori, A., Yousefi, F., & Khajavi, F. (1987). The application of the Goodenough–Harris Draw-A-Man test to a group of Iranian children in the city of Shiraz. *British Journal of Educational Psychology, 57,* 401–406.

Meier, M.J. (1969). The regional localization hypothesis and personality changes associated with focal cerebral lesions and ablations. In J.N. Butcher (Ed.), *MMPI: Research developments and clinical applications.* New York: McGraw-Hill.

Meier, M.J., & French, L.A. (1965). Some personality correlates of unilateral and bilateral EEG abnormalities in psychomotor epileptics. *Journal of Clinical Psychology, 21,* 3–9.

Meier, M.J., & Story, J.L. (1967). Selective impairment of Porteus Maze performance after right subthalamotomy. *Neuropsychologia, 5,* 181–189.

Mekarski, J.E., Cutmore, T.R.H., & Suborski, W. (1996). Gender differences during processing of the Stroop task. *Perceptual and Motor Skills, 83,* 563–568.

Meloy, R.J., Hansen, T.L., & Weiner, I.B. (1997). Authority of the Rorschach: Legal citations during the past 50 years. *Journal of Personality Assessment, 69,* 53–62.

Mendez, M.F., Cherrier, M., Perryman, K.M., Pachana, N., Miller, B.L., & Cummings, J.L. (1996). Fronto-temporal dementia versus Alzheimer's disease: Different cognitive features. *Neurology, 47,* 1189–1193.

Mensch, A.J., & Woods, D.J. (1986). Patterns of feigning brain damage on the LNNB. *International Journal of Clinical Neuropsychology, 8,* 59–63.

Mentzel, H.J., Gaser, C., Volz, H.P., Rzanny, R., Hager, F., Sauer, H., & Kaiser, W.A. (1998). Cognitive stimulation with the Wisconsin Sorting Test: Functional MR imaging at 1.5 T. *Radiology, 207,* 399–404.

Mercer, W.N., Harrell, E.H., Miller, D.C., Childs, H.W., & Rockers, D.M. (1997). Performance of brain-injured versus healthy adults on three versions of the Category Test. *The Clinical Neuropsychologist, 11,* 174–179.

Meyer, G.J. (1993). The impact of response frequency on the Rorschach constellation indices and on their validity with diagnostic and MMPI-2 criteria. *Journal of Personality Assessment, 60,* 153–180.

Meyer, G.J. (1997a). Assessing reliability: Critical corrections for a critical examination of the Rorschach Comprehensive System. *Psychological Assessment, 9,* 480–489.

Meyer, G.J. (1997b). Thinking clearly about reliability: More critical corrections regarding the Rorschach Comprehensive System. *Psychological Assessment, 9,* 495–498.

Meyer, J., Jr., & Megaree, E.I. (1972). Development of an MMPI-based typology of youthful offenders. *FCI Research Reports, 2,* 1–24. Tallahassee, FL: Federal Correction Institute.

Meyers, J.E, Bayless, J., & Meyers, K. (1996). The Rey Complex Figure, Memory error patterns and functional abilities. *The Clinical Neuropsychologist, 8,* 153–166.

Meyers, J.E., & Lange, D. (1994). Recognition subtests for the Complex Figure. *The Clinical Neuropsychologist, 8,* 153–166.

Meyers, J.E., & Meyers, K.R. (1995a). Rey Complex Figure Test under four different administration procedures. *The Clinical Neuropsychologist, 9,* 63–67.

Meyers, J., & Meyers, K. (1995b). *Rey Complex Figure and Recognition Trial: Professional manual.* Odessa, FL: Psychological Assessment Resources.

Meyers, J.E., & Volbrecht, M. (1998a). Validation of memory error patterns on the Rey Complex Figure and Recognition Trial. *Applied Neuropsychology, 5,* 120–131.

Meyers, J.E., & Volbrecht, M. (1998b). Validation of reliable digits for detection of malingering. *Assessment, 5,* 303–307.

Miceli, G., Caltagirone, C., Gainotti, G., Masullo, C., & Silveri, M.C. (1981). Neuropsychological correlates of localized cerebral lesions in non-aphasic brain damaged patients. *Journal of Clinical Neuropsychology, 3,* 53–63.

Michell, J. (1986). Measurement scales and statistics: A clock of paradigms. *Psychological Bulletin, 100,* 398–407.

Miller, E. (1971). On the nature of the memory disorder in presenile dementia. *Neuropsychologia, 9,* 75–81.

Miller, E. (1973). Short and long term memory in patients with presenile dementia (Alzheimer's disease). *Psychological Medicine, 3,* 221–224.

Miller, H.B., & Paniak, C.E. (1995). MMPI and MMPI-2 profile and code type congruence in a brain-injured sample. *Journal of Clinical and Experimental Neuropsychology, 17,* 58–64.

Miller, L.T., & Lee, C.J. (1993). Construct validation of the Peabody Picture Vocabulary test-Revised: A structural equation model of the acquisition order of words. *Psychological Assessment, 5,* 438–441.

Millis, S.R. (1992). The recognition memory test in the detection of malingered and exaggerated memory deficits. *The Clinical Neuropsychologist, 6,* 406–414.

Millis, S.R. (1995). Factor structure of the California Verbal Learning Test in moderate and severe closed head injury. *Perceptual and Motor Skills, 80,* 219–224.

Millis, S.R., & Putnam, S. (1994). The recognition memory test in the assessment of memory impairment after financially compensable mild head injury: A replication. *Archives of Clinical Neuropsychology, 9,* 163.

Millis, S.R., & Ricker, J.H. (1994). Verbal learning patterns in moderate and severe traumatic brain injury. *Journal of Clinical and Experimental Neuropsychology, 16,* 498–507.

Millis, S.R., Rosenthal, M., & Lourie, I.F. (1994). Predicting community integration after traumatic brain injury with neuropsychological measures. *International Journal of Neuroscience, 79,* 165–167.

Millis, S.R., Putnam, S.H., Adams, K.M., & Ricker, J.H. (1995). The California Verbal Learning Test in the detection of incomplete effort in neuropsychological evaluation. *Psychological Assessment, 7,* 463–471.

Millis, S.R., Ross, S.R., & Ricker, J.H. (1998). Detection of incomplete effort on the Wechsler Adult Intelligence Scale-Revised: A cross-validation. *Journal of Clinical and Experimental Neuropsychology, 20,* 167–173.

Milner, B. (1963). Effects of different brain lesions on card sorting. *Archives of Neurology, 9,* 90–100.

Milner, B. (1971). Interhemispheric differences in the localization of psychological processes in man. *British Medical Bulletin, 27,* 272–277.

Milner, B. (1972). Disorders of learning and memory after temporal lobe lesions in man. *Clinical Neurosurgery, 19,* 421–446.

Milrod, R.J., & Rescorla, L. (1991). A comparison of the WPPSI-R and WPPSI with high-IQ children. *Journal of Psychoeducational Assessment, 9,* 255–262.

Mishra, S.P. (1982). The WISC-R and evidence of item bias for Native-American Navajos. *Psychology in the Schools, 19,* 458–464.

Mishra, S.P. (1983). Validity of WISC-R IQ's and factor scores in predicting achievement for Mexican-American children. *Psychology in the Schools, 20,* 442–444.

Mitrushina, M., Satz, P., & Chervinsky, A.B. (1990). Efficiency of recall on the Rey–Osterrieth Complex Figure in normal aging. *Brain Dysfunction, 3,* 148–150.

Mitrushina, M., Satz, P., Chervinsky, A., & D'Elia, L. (1991). Performance of four age groups of normal elderly on the Rey Auditory–Verbal Learning Test. *Journal of Clinical Psychology, 47,* 351–357.

Mitrushina, M., Abara, J., & Blumenfeld, A. (1996). A comparison of cognitive profiles in schizophrenia and other psychiatric disorders. *Journal of Clinical Psychology, 52,* 177–190.

Mitrushina, M.N., Boone, K.B., & D'Elia, L.F. (1999). *Handbook of normative data for neuropsychological assessment.* New York: Oxford University Press.

Mittenberg, W., Thompson, G.B., & Schwartz, J.A. (1991). Abnormal and reliable differences among Wechsler Memory Scale-Revised subtests. *Psychological Assessment, 3,* 492–495.

Mittenberg, W., Burton, D.B., Darrow, E., & Thompson, G.B. (1992). Normative data for the Wechsler Memory Scale-Revised: 24–34-year-olds. *Psychological Assessment, 4,* 363–368.

Mittenberg, W., Azrin, R., Millsaps, C. & Heilbronner, R. (1993). Identification of malingered head injury on the Wechsler Memory Scale-Revised. *Psychological Assessment, 5,* 34–40.

Mittenberg, W., Theroux-Fichera, S., Zielincki, R.E., Fichera, K., & Heilbronner, R. (1995). Identification of malingered head injury on the Wechsler Adult Intelligence Scale-Revised. *Professional Psychology: Research and Practice, 26,* 491–498.

Mittenberg, W., Rotholc, A., Russell, E., & Heilbronner, R. (1996a). Identification of malingered head injury on the Halstead–Reitan Battery. *Archives of Clinical Neuropsychology, 11,* 271–281.

Mittenberg, W., Tremont, G., & Rayls, K.R. (1996b). Impact of cognitive function on MMPI-2 validity in neurologically impaired patients. *Assessment, 3,* 157–163.

Moore, A.D., Stambrook, M., Hawryluk, G.A., Peters, L.C., Gill, D.D., & Hyman, M.M. (1990). Test retest stability of the Wechsler Adult Intelligence Scale-Revised in the assessment of head–injured patients. *Psychological Assessment, 2,* 98–100.

Moore, C., O'Keefe, S.L., & Laehorn, D. (1998). Concurrent validity of the Snijders–Oomen Nonverbal Intelligence Test 2½–7 with the Wechsler Preschool and Primary Scale of Intelligence-Revised. *Psychological Reports, 82,* 619–625.

Moore, P.M., & Baker, G.A. (1997). Psychometric properties and factor structure of the Wechsler Memory Scale-Revised in a sample of persons with intractable epilepsy. *Journal of Clinical Neuropsychology, 19,* 897–905.

Moose, D., & Brannigan, G.G. (1997). Comparison of preschool children's scores on the modified version of the Bender–Gestalt Test and the Developmental Test of Visual–Motor Integration. *Perceptual and Motor Skills, 85,* 766.

Morey, L.C. (1991). *Personality Assessment Inventory.* Odessa, FL: Psychological Assessment Resources.

Morey, L.C. (1994). Critical issues in construct validation: Comment on Boyle and Lennon (1994). *Journal of Psychopathology and Behavioral Assessment, 17,* 393–401.

Morey, L.C. (1995). Critical issues in construct validation: Comment on Boyle and Lennon (1994). *Journal of Psychopathology and Behavioral Assessment, 17,* 393–401.

Morey, L.C., & Lanier, V.W. (1998). Operating characteristics of six response distortion features for the Personality Assessment Inventory. *Assessment, 5,* 203–214.

Morgan, D.W., Weitzel, W.D., Guyden, T.E., Robinson, J.A., & Hedlund, J.L. (1972). Comparing MMPI statements and mental status items. *American Journal of Psychiatry, 129,* 693–697.

Morgan, S.B., & Brown, T.L. (1988). Luria–Nebraska Neuropsychological Battery-Children's revision with three learning disability subtypes. *Journal of Consulting and Clinical Psychology, 56,* 463–466.

Morgan, S.F. (1991). Effect of true memory impairment on a test of memory complaint validity. *Archives of Clinical Neuropsychology, 6,* 327–334.

Morgan, S.F., & Hatsukami, D.K. (1987). Use of the Shipley Institute of Living Scale for neuropsychological screening of the elderly: Is it an appropriate measure for this population? *Journal of Clinical Psychology, 42,* 796–798.

Morgan, S.F., Tidwell, L.C., & Takarae, Y. (1996). Examining the relationship between educational attainment and performance on the WRAT-R among a group of injured workers. *Vocational Evaluation and Work Adjustment Bulletin, 29,* 40–46.

Morris, J., Kunka, J.M., & Rosini, E.D. (1997). Development of alternate paragraphs for the Logical Memory subtest of the Wechsler Memory Scale-Revised. *The Clinical Neuropsychologist, 11,* 370–374.

Morris, R.G., Abrahams, S., & Polkey, C.E. (1995). Recognition memory for words and faces following unilateral temporal lobectomy. *British Journal of Clinical Psychology, 34,* 571–576.

Morrison, M.W. (1994). The use of psychological tests to detect malingered intellectual impairment. *American Journal of Forensic Psychology, 12,* 47–64.

Moscovitch, M. (1994). Cognitive resources and the dual-task interference effects at retrieval in normal people: The role of the frontal lobes and medial temporal cortex. *Neuropsychology, 8,* 524–534.

Moses, J.A., Jr. (1983). An orthogonal factor solution of the Luria–Nebraska Neuropsychological Battery items: I. Motor, Rhythm, Tactile, and Visual·Scales. *International Journal of Clinical Neuropsychology, 5,* 181–185.

Moses, J.A., Jr. (1984a). The effect of presence or absence of neuroleptic medication treatment on Luria–Nebraska Neuropsychological Battery performance in a schizophrenic population. *International Journal of Clinical Neuropsychology, 6,* 249–251.

Moses, J.A., Jr. (1984b). An orthogonal factor solution of the Luria–Nebraska Neuropsychological Battery items: II. Receptive Speech, Expressive Speech, Writing, and Reading scales. *International Journal of Clinical Neuropsychology, 6,* 24–28.

Moses, J.A., Jr. (1984c). An orthogonal factor solution of the Luria–Nebraska Neuropsychological Battery items: III. Arithmetic, Memory, and Intelligence scales. *International Journal of Clinical Neuropsychology, 6,* 103–106.

Moses, J.A., Jr. (1984d). An orthogonal factor solution of the Luria–Nebraska Neuropsychological Battery items: IV. Pathognomonic, Right Hemisphere, and Left Hemisphere scales. *International Journal of Clinical Neuropsychology, 6,* 161–165.

Moses, J.A., Jr. (1984e). Performance as a function of sensorimotor impairment in a brain damaged sample. *International Journal of Clinical Neuropsychology, 6,* 123–126.

Moses, J.A., Jr. (1984f). The relative effects of cognitive and sensorimotor deficits in Luria–Nebraska Neuropsychological Battery performance in a brain damaged population. *International Journal of Clinical Neuropsychology, 6,* 8–12.

Moses, J.A., Jr. (1985a). Internal consistency of standard and short forms of three itemized Halstead–Reitan Neuropsychological Battery Tests. *International Journal of Clinical Neuropsychology, 7,* 164–166.

Moses, J.A., Jr. (1985b). Relationship of the profile elevation and impairment scales of the Luria–Nebraska Neuropsychological Battery in neurological examination. *International Journal of Clinical Neuropsychology, 7,* 183–190.

Moses, J.A., Jr. (1985c). The relative contribution of Luria–Nebraska Neuropsychological Battery and WAIS subtest variables to cognitive performance level. *International Journal of Clinical Neuropsychology, 7,* 125–130.

Moses, J.A., Jr. (1986a). Factor analysis of the Luria–Nebraska Neuropsychological Battery by sensorimotor, speech, and conceptual item bands. *International Journal of Clinical Neuropsychology, 8,* 26–35.

Moses, J.A., Jr. (1986b). Factor structure of Benton's tests of Visual Retention, Visual Construction, and Visual Form Discrimination. *Archives of Clinical Neuropsychology, 1,* 147–156.

Moses, J.A., Jr. (1989). Replicated factor structure of Benton's tests for visual retention, visual construction, and visual form discrimination. *International Journal of Clinical Neuropsychology, 11,* 30–37.

Moses, J.A., Jr. (1997). The Luria–Nebraska Neuropsychological Battery: Advances in interpretation. In A. MacN. Horton, D. Wedding, & J. Webster (Eds.), *The Neuropsychology Handbook: Vol. 1, Foundations and assessment* (pp. 255–289). New York: Springer Publishing Company.

Moses, J.A., Jr., & Maruish, M.E. (1987). A critical review of the Luria–Nebraska Neuropsychological Battery literature: I. Reliability. *International Journal of Clinical Neuropsychology, 9,* 149–157.

Moses, J.A., Jr., & Maruish, M.E. (1988a). A critical review of the Luria–Nebraska Neuropsychological Battery literature: II. Construct validity. *International Journal of Clinical Neuropsychology, 10,* 5–11.

Moses, J.A., Jr., & Maruish, M.E. (1988b). A critical review of the Luria–Nebraska Neuropsychological Battery: III. Concurrent validity. *International Journal of Clinical Neuropsychology, 10,* 12–19.

Moses, J.A., Jr. & Maruish, M.E. (1988c). A critical review of the Luria–Nebraska Neuropsychological Battery literature: IV. Cognitive deficit in schizophrenia and related disorders. *International Journal of Clinical Neuropsychology, 10,* 51–62.

Moses, J.A., Jr., & Maruish, M.E. (1988d). A critical review of the Luria–Nebraska Neuropsychological Battery: V. Cognitive deficit in miscellaneous psychiatric disorders. *International Journal of Clinical Neuropsychology, 10,* 63–73.

Moses, J.A., Jr., & Maruish, M.E. (1988e). A critical review of the Luria–Nebraska Neuropsychological Battery literature: VI. Neurologic cognitive deficit parameters. *International Journal of Clinical Neuropsychology,* *10*, 130–140.

Moses, J.A., Jr., & Maruish, M.E. (1988f). A critical review of the Luria–Nebraska Neuropsychological Battery: VII. Specific neurologic syndromes. *International Journal of Clinical Neuropsychology, 10*, 178–188.

Moses, J.A., Jr., & Maruish, M.E. (1989a). A critical review of the Luria–Nebraska Neuropsychological Battery literature: VIII. New summary indices. *International Journal of Clinical Neuropsychology, 11*, 9–20.

Moses, J.A., Jr., & Maruish, M.E. (1989b). A critical review of the Luria–Nebraska Neuropsychological Battery: IX. Alternate forms. *International Journal of Clinical Neuropsychology, 11*, 97–110.

Moses, J.A., Jr., & Maruish, M.E. (1989c). A critical review of the Luria–Nebraska Neuropsychological Battery: X. Critiques and rebuttals. *International Journal of Clinical Neuropsychology, 11*, 145–162.

Moses, J.A., Jr., & Chiu, M.L. (1993). Nonequivalence of Forms I and II of the Luria–Nebraska Neuropsychological Battery for adults. Paper presented at the meeting of the National Academy of Neuropsychology, October, Phoenix, AZ.

Moses, J.A., Jr., & Pritchard, D.A. (1999). Performance scales for the Luria–Nebraska Neuropsychological Battery-Form I. *Archives of Clinical Neuropsychology, 14*, 285–302.

Moses, J.A., Jr., & Schefft, B.K. (1985). Interrater reliability analyses of the Luria–Nebraska Neuropsychological Battery. *International Journal of Clinical Neuropsychology, 7*, 31–38.

Moses, J.A., Jr., Golden, C.J., Ariel, R.N., & Gustavson, J.L. (1983a). *Interpretation of the Luria–Nebraska Neuropsychological Battery* (Vol. 1). New York: Grune & Stratton.

Moses, J.A., Jr., Johnson, G.L., & Lewis, G.P. (1983b). Reliability analyses of the Luria–Nebraska Neuropsychological Battery summary, localization and factor scales. *International Journal of Neuroscience, 20*, 149–154.

Moses, J.A., Csernansky, J.G., & Leiderman, D.B. (1988). Neuropsychological criteria for identification of cognitive deficit in limbic epilepsy. *International Journal of Clinical Neuropsychology, 10*, 106–112.

Moses, J.A., Jr., Schefft, B.K., Wong, J.L., & Berg, R.A., (1992). Revised norms and decision rules for the Luria–Nebraska Neuropsychological Battery, Form II. *Archives of Clinical Neuropsychology, 7*, 251–269.

Moses, J.A., Pritchard, D.A., & Faustman, W.O. (1994). Modal profiles for the Luria–Nebraska Neuropsychological Battery. *Archives of Clinical Neuropsychology, 9*, 15–30.

Moses, J.A., Jr., Pritchard, D.A., & Adams, R.L. (1996). Modal profiles for the Halstead–Reitan Neuropsychological Battery. *Archives of Clinical Neuropsychology, 11*, 469–480.

Moses, J.A., Jr., Pritchard, D.A., & Adams, R.L. (1997). Neuropsychological Information in the Wechsler Adult Intelligence Scale-Revised. *Archives of Clinical Neuropsychology, 12*, 97–109.

Moses, J.A., Jr., Pritchard, D.A., & Adams, R.L. (1999). Normative corrections for the Halstead–Reitan Neuropsychological Battery. *Archives of Clinical Neuropsychology, 14*, 445–454.

Mueller, H., Hasse-Sander, I., Horn, R., Helmstaedter, C., & Elger, C.E. (1997). Rey Auditory–Verbal Learning Test: Structure of a modified German version. *Journal of Clinical Psychology, 53*, 663–671.

Munford, P.R., Meyerowitz, B.E., & Munford, A.M. (1980). A Comparison of black and white children's WISC/WISC-R differences. *Journal of Clinical Psychology, 36*, 471–475.

Mungas, D. (1983). Differential clinical sensitivity of specific parameters of the Rey Auditory Verbal Learning Test. *Journal of Consulting and Clinical Psychology, 51*, 848–855.

Myers, D., Sweet, J.J., Deysach, R., & Myers, F.C. (1989). Utility of the Luria–Nebraska Neuropsychological Battery-Children's Revision in the evaluation of reading disabled children. *Archives of Clinical Neuropsychology, 4*, 201–215.

Mysiw, W.J., Beegan, J.G., & Gatens, P.F. (1989). Prospective cognitive assessment of stroke patients before inpatient rehabilitation. *American Journal of Physical Medicine and Rehabilitation, 68*, 168–171.

Nabors, N.A., Vangel, S.J., & Lichtenberg, P.A. (1996). Visual Form Discrimination Test with elderly medical inpatients. *Clinical Gerontologist, 17*, 43–53.

Nabors, N.A., Millis, S.R., & Rosenthal, M. (1997a). Use of the Neurobehavioral Cognitive Status Examination (Cognistat) in traumatic brain injury. *Journal of Head Trauma Rehabilitation, 12*, 79–84.

Nabors, N.A., Vangel, S.J., Lichtenberg, P., & Walsh, P. (1997b). Normative and clinical utility of the Hooper Visual Organization Test with geriatric medical inpatients. *Journal of Clinical Geropsychology, 3*, 191–198.

Nadler, J.D., Grace, J., White, D.A., Butters, M.A., & Malloy, P.F. (1996). Laterality differences in quantitative and qualitative Hooper performance. *Archives of Clinical Neuropsychology, 11*, 223–229.

Nagahama, Y., Fukuyama, H., Yamauchi, H., Matsuzaki, S., Konishi, J., Shibaski, H., & Kimura, J. (1996). Cerebral activation during performance of a card sorting test. *Brain, 119*, 1667–1675.

Nagel, J.A., Harrell, E., & Gray, S.G. (1997). Prediction of achievement scores using the Luria–Nebraska Neuropsychological Battery Form II. *Psychology—A Quarterly Journal of Human Behavior, 34*, 41–47.

Nagle, R.J. (1993). The relationship between WAIS-R and academic achievement among EMR adolescents. *Psychology in the Schools, 30*, 37–39.

Nagle, R.J., & Bell, N.L. (1993). Validation of Stanford–Binet Intelligence Scale: Fourth Edition abbreviated batteries with college students. *Psychology in the Schools, 30*, 227–231.

Nagle, R.J., & Bell, N.L. (1995a). Clinical utility of Kaufman's "amazingly" short forms of the WAIS-R with educable mentally retarded adolescents. *Journal of Clinical Psychology, 51*, 396–400.

Nagle, R.J., & Bell, N.L. (1995b) Validation of an item-reduction short form of the Stanford–Binet Intelligence Scale: Fourth Edition with college students. *Journal of Clinical Psychology, 51*, 63–70.

Naglieri, J.A. (1982). Two types of tables for use with the WAIS-R. *Journal of Consulting and Clinical Psychology, 50*, 319–321.

Naglieri, J.A. (1984). Predictive validity of the PPVT-R for Navajo children. *Psychological Reports, 55*, 297–298.

Naglieri, J.A. (1985). Normal children's performance on the McCarthy Scales, Kaufman Assessment Battery, and Peabody Individual Achievement Test. *Journal of Psychoeducational Assessment, 3*, 123–129.

Naglieri, J.A., & Maxwell, S. (1981). Inter-rater reliability and concurrent validity of the Goodenough–Harris and McCarthy Draw-A-Child scoring systems. *Perceptual and Motor Skills, 53*, 343–348.

Naglieri, J.A., & Parks, J.C. (1980). Wide Range Achievement Test: A one year stability study. *Psychological Reports, 47*, 1028–1030.

Naglieri, J.A., & Pfeiffer, S.I. (1983). Stability and concurrent validity of the Peabody Individual Achievement Test. *Psychological Reports, 52*, 672–674.

Nash, M.M., & Schwaller, R.L. (1985). A multiple-choice format for the Quick Test. *Psychological Reports, 57*, 1297–1298.

Naugle, R.J. (1993). The relationship between the WAIS-R and academic achievement among EMR adolescents. *Psychology in the Schools, 30*, 37–39.

Naugle, R.I., Chelune, G.J., Cheek, R., & Luders, H. (1993a). Detection of changes in material-specific memory following temporal lobectomy using the Wechsler memory Scale-Revised. *Archives of Clinical Neuropsychology, 8*, 381–395.

Naugle, R.I., Chelune, G.J., & Tucker, G.D. (1993b). Validity of the Kaufman Brief Intelligence Test. *Psychological Assessment, 5*, 182–186.

Nebes, R.D., Martin, D.C., & Horn, L.C. (1984). Sparing of semantic memory in Alzheimer's disease. *Journal of Abnormal Psychology, 93*, 321–330.

Nehil, J., Agathon, M., Greif, J.L., Delagrange, G., & Rondepierre, J.P. (1965). Contribution a 'etude comparative des tests psychometriques de deterioration et des traces EEG. *Review of Neurology, 112*, 293–296.

Nelson, H.E. (1976). A modified card sorting test sensitive to frontal lobe defects. *Cortex, 12*, 313–324.

Nelson, H.E. (1982). *National Adult Reading Test Manual*. Windsor, UK: NFER-Nelson.

Nelson, H.E., & McKenna, P. (1975). The use of current reading ability in the assessment of dementia. *British Journal of Social and Clinical Psychology, 14*, 259–267.

Nelson, H.E., & O'Connell, D. (1978). Dementia: The estimate of premorbid intelligence levels using the New Adult Reading Test. *Cortex, 14*, 234–244.

Nesselroade, J.R., Stigler, S.M., & Baltes, P.B. (1980). Regression toward the mean and the study of change. *Psychological Bulletin, 88*, 622–637.

Nester, M.J., Sakati, N., & Greer, W. (1992). Unknown dysmorphic syndromes and developmental delay in Saudi Arabia. *Journal of Child Neurology, 7*(suppl.), S64–S68.

Nestor, P.G., Shenton, M.E., McCarley, R.W., Haimson, J., Smith, R.S., O'Donnell, B., Kimble, M., Kikinis, R., & Jolesz, F.A. (1993). Neuropsychological correlates of MRI temporal lobe abnormalities. *American Journal of Psychiatry, 150*, 1849–1855.

Neuringer, C., Dombrowski, P.S., & Goldstein, G. (1975). Cross-validation of an MMPI scale of differential diagnosis of brain damage from schizophrenia. *Journal of Clinical Psychology, 31*, 268–271.

Newby, R.F., Hallenback, C.E., & Embretson, S. (1983). Confirmatory factor analysis of four general models with a modified Halstead–Reitan Battery. *Journal of Clinical Neuropsychology, 5*, 115–133.

Newcombe, F., Oldfield, R.C., Ratcliffe, G.G., & Wingfield, A. (1971). Recognition and naming of object drawings by men with focal brain wounds. *Journal of Neurology, Neurosurgery, and Psychiatry, 34*, 329–340.

Newman, P.J., & Sweet, J.J. (1986) The effects of clinical depression on the Luria–Nebraska Neuropsychological Battery. *International Journal of Clinical Neuropsychology, 8,* 109–114.

Neyens, L.G.J., & Aldenkemp, A.P. (1997). Stability of cognitive measures in children of average ability. *Child Neuropsychology, 3,* 161–170.

Nicholson, C.L. (1977). Correlations between the Quick Test and the Wechsler Intelligence Scale for Children-Revised. *Psychological Reports, 40,* 523–526.

Nicholson, R.A., Mouton, G.J., Bagby, R.M., Buis, T., Peterson, S.A., & Buigas, R.A. (1997). Utility of MMPI-2 indicators of response distortion: Receiver operating characteristic analysis. *Psychological Assessment, 9,* 471–479.

Nielsen, H., Lolk, A., & Kragh-Sorensen, P. (1995). Normative data for eight neuropsychological tests, gathered from a random sample of Danes aged 64–83. *Nordisk Psykologi, 47,* 241–255.

Nies K.J., & Sweet, J.J. (1994). Neuropsychological assessment and malingering: A critical review of the past and present strategies. *Archives of Clinical Neuropsychology, 9,* 501–552.

Nijenhuis, J., & van der Flier, H. (1997). Comparability of GATB scores for immigrants and majority group members: Some Dutch findings. *Journal of Applied Psychology, 82,* 675–687.

Northern California Neurobehavioral Group (1988). *Manual for the Neurobehavioral Cognitive Status Examination.* Fairfax, CA: Author.

Norton, J.C. (1975). Patterns of neuropsychological test performance in Huntington's disease. *Journal of Nervous and Mental Disease, 161,* 276–279.

Norton, J.C. (1978). The Trail Making Test and Bender Gestalt background interference procedure as screening devices. *Journal of Clinical Psychology, 34,* 916–922.

Norton, J.C. (1979). Wechsler variables as a function of age and neurologic status. *Journal of Clinical Psychiatry, 219,* 21–23.

Norton, J.C., & Romano, P.O. (1977). Validation of the Watson–Thomas rules for MMPI diagnosis. *Diseases of the Nervous System, 38,* 773–775.

Novack, T.A., Kofoed, B.A., & Crosson, B. (1995). Sequential performance on the California Verbal Learning Test following traumatic brain injury. *The Clinical Neuropsychologist, 9,* 38–43.

Novick, M., & Lewis, M. (1967). Coefficient alpha and the reliability of composite measurements. *Psychometrika, 32,* 1–13.

Nunnally, J.C. (1978). *Psychometric theory.* New York: McGraw-Hill.

Oakland, T., & Feigenbaum, D. (1979). Multiple sources of test bias on the WISC-R and Bender Gestalt test. *Journal of Consulting and Clinical Psychology, 47,* 968–974.

O'Carroll, R.E. (1987). The inter-rater reliability of the National Adult Reading Test (NART): A pilot study. *British Journal of Clinical Psychology, 26,* 229–230.

O'Carroll, R.E., & Badenoch, L.D. (1994). The inter-rater reliability of the Wechsler Memory Scale-Revised Visual Memory test. *British Journal of Clinical Psychology, 33,* 208–210.

O'Carroll, R.E., & Gilleard, C.J. (1986). Estimation of premorbid intelligence in dementia. *British Journal of Clinical Psychology, 25,* 157–158.

O'Carroll, R.E., Baikie, E.M., & Whittick, J.E. (1987). Does the National Adult Reading Test hold in dementia? *British Journal of Clinical Psychology, 26,* 315–316.

O'Donnell, W.E., & Reynolds, D. McQ. (1983). *Neuropsychological Impairment Scale manual.* Annapolis, MD: Annapolis Neuropsychological Services.

O'Donnell, W.E., Reynolds, D. McQ., & De Soto, C.B. (1983). Neuropsychological Impairment Scale (NIS): Initial validation study using Trailmaking Test (A&B) and WAIS Digit Symbol (Scaled Score) in a mixed grouping of psychiatric, neuropsychological, and normal patients. *Journal of Clinical Psychology, 39,* 746–748.

O'Donnell, W.E., Reynolds, D. McQ., & De Soto, C.B. (1984a). Validity and reliability of the Neuropsychological Impairment Scale (NIS). *Journal of Clinical Psychology, 40,* 549–553.

O'Donnell, W.E., De Soto, C.B., & Reynolds, D. McQ. (1984b). Sensitivity and specificity of the Neuropsychological Impairment Scale (NIS). *Journal of Clinical Psychology, 40,* 553–555.

O'Donnell, W.E., De Soto, C.B., & De Soto, J.L. (1993). Validity and reliability of the revised Neuropsychological Impairment Scale (NIS). *Journal of Clinical Psychology, 49,* 372–382.

O'Donnell, W.E., De Soto, C.B., & De Soto, J.L. (1994a). Neuropsychological symptoms in a cross-sectional sample of abstinent alcoholics. *Psychological Reports, 75,* 1475–1484.

O'Donnell, W.E., De Soto, C.B., De Soto, J.L., & Reynolds, D.McQ. (1994b). *The Neuropsychological Impairment Scale (NIS) Manual.* Los Angeles, CA: Western Psychological Services.

O'Grady, K.E. (1983). A confirmatory maximum likelihood factor analysis of the WAIS-R. *Journal of Consulting and Clinical Psychology, 51,* 826–831.

Okubu, Y., Suhara, T., Suzuki, K., Kobayashi, K., Inoue, O., Terasaki, O., Someya, Y., Sassa, T., Sudo, Y., Matsushima, E., Iyo, M., Tateno, Y., & Toru, M. (1997). Decreased prefrontal dopamine D1 receptors in schizophrenia revealed by PET. *Nature, 385,* 634–636.

Oldfield, R.C., & Wingfield, A. (1965). Response latencies in naming objects. *The Quarterly Journal of Experimental Psychology, 17,* 273–281.

Ollo, C., Lindquist, T., Alim, T.N., & Deutsch, S.I. (1995). Predicting premorbid functioning in crack-cocaine abusers. *Drug and Alcohol Dependence, 40,* 173–175.

Oltmanns, T. (1978). Selective attention in schizophrenia and manic psychoses: The effect of distraction on information processing. *Journal of Abnormal Psychology, 87,* 212–225.

O'Mahony, J.F., & Doherty, B. (1993). Patterns of intellectual performance among recently abstinent alcohol abusers on the WAIS-R and WMS-R subtests. *Archives of Clinical Neuropsychology, 8,* 373–380.

O'Maille, P.S., & Fine, M.A. (1995). Personality disorder scales for the MMPI-2: An assessment of psychometric properties in a correctional population. *Journal of Personality Disorders, 9,* 235–246.

O'Malley, P.M., & Bachman, J.G. (1976). Longitudinal evidence for the validity of the Quick Test. *Psychological Reports, 38,* 1247–1252.

Orgass, B., & Poeck, K. (1966). Clinical validation of a new test for aphasia: An experimental study on the Token Test. *Cortex, 2,* 222–243.

Orpen, C. (1974). The susceptibility of the Quick Test to instructional sets. *Journal of Clinical Psychology, 30,* 507–509.

Orsini, A., Schiappa, O., & Grossi, D. (1981). Sex and cultural differences in children's spatial and verbal memory span. *Perceptual and Motor Skills, 53,* 39–42.

Osato, S.S., Van Gorp, W.G., Kern, R.S., Satz, P., & Steinman, L. (1989). The Satz–Mogel short form of the WAIS-R in an elderly, demented population. *Psychological Assessment, 1,* 339–341.

Osato, S.S., Yang, J., & LaRue, A. (1993). The Neurobehavioral Cognitive Status Examination in an older psychiatric population: An exploratory study of validity. *Neuropsychiatry, Neuropsychology, and Behavioral Neurology, 6,* 98–102.

Osborne, D., & Davis, L.J. (1978). Standard scores for Wechsler Memory Scale subtests. *Journal of Clinical Psychology, 34,* 115–116.

Osmon, D.C. (1992). Modified Wisconsin Card Sorting Test with scores to fractionate executive processes. Paper presented at the Annual meeting of the National Academy of Neuropsychology, Pittsburgh, PA.

Osmon, D.C., & Golden, C.J. (1978). Minnesota Multiphasic Personality Inventory correlates of neuropsychological deficits. *International Journal of Neurosciences, 3,* 113–122.

Osmon, D.C., & Suchy, Y. (1996). Fractionating frontal lobe functions: Factors of the Milwaukee Card Sorting Test. *Archives of Clinical Neuropsychology, 11,* 541–552.

Osmon, D.C., Smet, I.C., Winegarden, B., & Gandhavadi, B. (1992). Neurobehavioral Cognitive Status Examination: Its use with unilateral stroke patients in a rehabilitation setting. *Archives of Physical Medicine and Rehabilitation, 73,* 414–418.

Osterlind, S.J. (1983). *Test item bias.* Beverly Hills, CA: Sage.

Ostreicher, J.M., & O'Donnell, J.P. (1995). Validation of the General Neuropsychological Deficit Scale with nondisabled, learning-disabled, and head-injured young adults. *Archives of Clinical Neuropsychology, 10,* 185–191.

Ostrosky, F., Jaime, R.M., & Ardila, A. (1998). Memory abilities during normal aging. *International Journal of Neuroscience, 93,* 151–162.

Otto, M.W., Bruder, G.E., Fava, M., Delis, D.C., Quitkin, F.M., & Rosenbaum, J.F. (1994). Norms for depressed patients for the California Verbal Learning Test: Associations with depression severity and self-report of cognitive difficulties. *Archives of Clinical Neuropsychology, 9,* 81–88.

Ottosson, J. (1960). Experimental studies of memory impairment after electroconvulsive therapy. *Acta Psychiatrica et Neurologica, 145*(suppl. 35), 103–132.

Pachana, N.A., Boone, K.B., Miller, B.L., Cummings, J.L., & Berman, N. (1996). Comparison of neuropsychological functioning in Alzheimer's disease and frontotemporal dementia. *Journal of the International Neuropsychological Society, 2,* 505–510.

Paletz, M.D., & Hirshoren, A. (1972). A comparison of two tests of visual–sequential memory ability. *Journal of Learning Disabilities, 5,* 46–47.

Palmer, B.W., Boone, K.B., Allman, L., & Castro, D.B. (1995). Co-occurrence of brain lesions and cognitive deficit exaggeration. *The Clinical Neuropsychologist, 9*, 68–73.

Palmer, B.W., Boone, K.B., Lesser, I.M., & Wohl, M.A. (1998). Base rates of "impaired" neuropsychological test performance among healthy older adults. *Archives of Clinical Neuropsychology, 13*, 503–511.

Paniak, C., Miller, H.B., Murphy, D., Andrews, A., & Flynn, J. (1997). Consonant Trigrams Test for Children: Development and norms. *The Clinical Neuropsychologist, 11*, 198–200.

Paniak, C., Murphy, D., Miller, H., & Lee, M. (1998). Wechsler Memory Scale-Revised Logical Memory and Visual Reproduction norms for 9- to 15-year olds. *Developmental Neuropsychology, 14*, 555–562.

Pantano, L.T., & Schwartz, M. (1978). Differentiation of neurologic and pseudo-neurologic patients with combined MMPI mini-mull and pseudo-neurologic scale. *Journal of Clinical Psychology, 34*, 55–60.

Paolo, A.M., & Ryan, J.J. (1991). Application of WAIS-R short forms to persons 75 years of age and older. *Journal of Psychoeducational Assessment, 9*, 345–352.

Paolo, A.M., & Ryan, J.J. (1992). Generalizability of two methods of estimating premorbid intelligence in the elderly. *Archives of Clinical Neuropsychology, 7*, 135–143.

Paolo, A.M., & Ryan, J.J. (1993). Test–retest stability of the Satz–Mogel WAIS-R Short Form in a sample of normal persons 75–87 years of age. *Archives of Clinical Neuropsychology, 8*, 397–404.

Paolo, A.M., & Ryan, J.J. (1996). Stability of WAIS-R scatter indices in the elderly. *Archives of Clinical Neuropsychology, 11*, 503–511.

Paolo, A.M., Troster, A.I., Axelrod, B.N., & Koller, W.C. (1995). Construct validity of the WCST in normal elderly and persons with Parkinson's disease. *Archives of Clinical Neuropsychology, 10*, 463–473.

Paolo, A.M., Axelrod, B.N., Troster, A.I., Blackwell, K.T., & Koller, W.C. (1996a). Utility of a Wisconsin Card Sorting Test short form in persons with Alzheimer's and Parkinson's disease. *Journal of Clinical and Experimental Neuropsychology, 18*, 892–897.

Paolo, A.M., Cluff, R.B., & Ryan, J.J. (1996b). Influence of perceptual organization and naming abilities on the Hooper Visual Organization Test: A replication and extension. *Neuropsychiatry, Neuropsychology, and Behavioral Neurology, 9*, 254–257.

Paolo, A.M., Ryan, J.J., Troster, A.I., & Hilmer, C.D. (1996c). Demographically based regression equations to estimate WAIS-R subtest scaled scores. *The Clinical Neuropsychologist, 10*, 130–140.

Paolo, A.M., Troster, A.I., & Ryan, J.J. (1997a). California Verbal Learning Test normative data for the elderly. *Journal of Clinical and Experimental Neuropsychology, 19*, 220–234.

Paolo, A.M., Troster, A.I., & Ryan, J.J. (1997b). Test–retest stability of the California Verbal Learning Test in older persons. *Neuropsychology, 11*, 613–616.

Paolo, A.M., Troster, A.I., & Ryan, J.J. (1998a). Continuous Visual Memory Test performance in healthy persons 60–94 years of age. *Archives of Clinical Neuropsychology, 13*, 333–337.

Paolo, A.M., Troster, A.I., & Ryan, J.J. (1998b). Test–retest stability of the Continuous Visual Memory Test in elderly persons. *Archives of Clinical Neuropsychology, 13*, 617–621.

Paradiso, S., Andreason, N.C., O'Leary, D.S., Arndt, S., & Robinson, R.G. (1997). Cerebellar size and cognition: Correlations with IQ, verbal memory, and motor dexterity. *Neuropsychiatry, Neuropsychology, and Behavioral Neurology, 10*, 1–8.

Paramesh, C.R. (1982). Relationship between the Quick Test and WISC-R and reading ability as used in a juvenile setting. *Perceptual and Motor Skills, 55*, 881–882.

Parker, J.W. (1957). The validity of some current tests for organicity. *Journal of Consulting Psychology, 21*, 425–428.

Parker, K. (1983). Factor analysis of the WAIS-R at nine age levels between 16 and 74 years. *Journal of Consulting and Clinical Psychology, 51*, 302–308.

Parker, K.C., & Atkinson, L. (1995). Computation of Wechsler Adult Intelligence Scale-Revised factor scores: Equal and differential weights. *Psychological Assessment, 7*, 456–462.

Parker, K.C., Hanson, R.K., & Hunsley, J. (1988). MMPI, Rorschach, and WAIS: A meta-analytic comparison of reliability, stability, and validity. *Psychological Bulletin, 103*, 367–373.

Parker, L.D. (1993). The Kaufman Brief Intelligence Test: An introduction and review. *Measurement and Evaluation in Counseling and Development, 26*, 152–156.

Parkin, A.J., & Leng, N.R.C. (Eds.) (1993). *Neuropsychology of the Amnesic Syndrome.* Hove, UK: Lawrence J. Erlbaum.

Parkinson, S.R. (1980). Aging and amnesia: A running span analysis. *Bulletin of the Psychonomic Society, 15*, 215–217.

Parmar, R.S. (1989). Cross-cultural transfer of non-verbal intelligence tests: An (in)validity study. *British Journal of Educational Psychology, 59,* 378–388.

Parsons, O.A. (1970). Clinical neuropsychology. In C.D. Spielberger (Ed.), *Current topics in clinical and community psychology* (Vol. 2). New York: Academic Press.

Parsons, O.A. (1977). Neuropsychological deficits in alcoholics: Facts and fancies. *Alcoholism: Clinical and Experimental Research, 1,* 51–56.

Parsons, O.A., & Prigatano, G.P. (1978). Methodological consideration in clinical neuropsychological research. *Journal of Consulting and Clinical Psychology, 46,* 608–619.

Pauker, J.D. (1977). Adult norms for the Halstead–Reitan Neuropsychological Test Battery: Preliminary data. Paper presented at the fifth annual meeting of the International Neuropsychological Society, Santa Fe.

Paul, D.S., Franzen, M.D., Cohen, S.H., & Fremouw, W. (1992). An investigation into the reliability and validity of two tests used in the detection of dissimulation. *International Journal of Clinical Neuropsychology, 14,* 1–9.

Peavy, G., Jacobs, D., Salmon, D.P., Butters, N., Delis, D.C., Taylor, M., Massman, P., Stout, J., Heindel, W.C., Kirson, D., Atkinson, J.H., Chndler, J.L., & Grant, I. (1994). Verbal memory performance of patients with human immunodeficiency virus infection: Evidence of subcortical dysfunction. *Journal of Clinical and Experimental Neuropsychology, 16,* 508–523.

Peck, D.F. (1970). The conversion of Progressive Matrices and Mill Hill Vocabulary raw scores into deviation IQs. *Journal of Clinical Psychology, 26,* 67–70.

Peebles, J., & Moore, R.J. (1998). Detecting socially desirable responding with the Personality Assessment Inventory: The Positive Impression Management Scale and the Defensiveness Index. *Journal of Clinical Psychology, 54,* 621–628.

Peirson, A.R., & Jansen, P. (1997). Comparability of the Rey–Osterrieth and Taylor forms if the Complex Figure Test. *The Clinical Neuropsychologist, 11,* 244–248.

Pendleton, M.G., & Heaton, R.K. (1982). A comparison of the Wisconsin Card Sorting Test and the Category Test. *Journal of Clinical Psychology, 38,* 392–396.

Perez, E., Slate, J.R., Neeley, R., & McDaniel, M. (1995). Validity of the CELF-R, TONI, and SIT for children referred for auditory processing problems. *Journal of Clinical Psychology, 51,* 540–543.

Perez, S.A., Schlottmann, R.S., Holloway, J.A., & Ozolins, M.S. (1996). Measurement of premorbid intellectual ability following brain injury. *Archives of Clinical Neuropsychology, 11,* 491–501.

Peritti, P. (1969). Cross sex and cross educational performance in a color word interference test. *Psychonomic Science, 16,* 321–323.

Peritti, P. (1971). Effects of non-competitive, competitive instructions and sex on performance in color word interference test. *Journal of Psychology, 79,* 67–70.

Perlstein, W.M., Carter, C.S., Barch, D.M., & Baird, J.W. (1998). The Stroop task and attention deficits in schizophrenia: A critical review of card and single trial Stroop methodology. *Neuropsychology, 12,* 414–425.

Perry, W., McDougall, A., & Viglione, D. (1995). A five-year follow-up on the stability of the Ego Impairment Index. *Journal of Personality Assessment, 63,* 112–118.

Pershad, D., & Lubey, B.L. (1974). Some experience with a memory test in the aged cases. *Indian Journal of Psychology, 49,* 305–312.

Pershad, D., & Verma, S.K. (1980). Clinical utility of Hooper's Visual Organization test (VOT): A preliminary investigation. *Indian Journal of Clinical Psychology, 7,* 67–70.

Peters, B.A., Lewis, E.G., Dustman, R.E., Straight, R.C., & Beck, E.C. (1976). Sensory, perceptual, motor, and cognitive functioning following oral administration of tetrahydrocannabinol. *Psychopharmacology, 47,* 141–148.

Peterson, L.R., & Peterson, M.J. (1959). Short term retention of individual verbal items. *Journal of Experimental Psychology, 58,* 193–198.

Pheley, A.M., & Klesges, R.C. (1986). The relationship between experimental and neuropsychological measures of memory. *Archives of Clinical Neuropsychology, 1,* 231–241.

Phelps, L. (1995). Exploratory factor analysis of the WRAML with academically at-risk students. *Journal of Psychoeducational Assessment, 13,* 384–390.

Phelps, L., Rosso, M., & Falasco, S.L. (1984). Correlations between the Woodcock–Johnson and the WISC-R for a behavior disordered population. *Psychology in the Schools, 21,* 442–446.

Phelps, L., Rosso, M., & Falasco, S.L. (1985). Multiple regression data using the WISC-R and the Woodcock–Johnson Tests of Cognitive Ability. *Psychology in the Schools, 22,* 46–49.

Piedmont, R.L., Sokolove, R.L., & Fleming, M.Z. (1989). On WAIS-R difference scores in a psychiatric sample. *Psychological Assessment, 1,* 155–159.

Piercy, M., & Smith, V.O.G. (1962). Right hemisphere dominance for certain non-verbal intellectual skills. *Brain, 85,* 775–790.

Piguet, O., Saling, M.M., O'Shea, M.F., Berkovic, S.F., & Bladin, P.F. (1994). Rey figure distortions reflect nonverbal differences between right and left foci in unilateral temporal lobe epilepsy. *Archives of Clinical Neuropsychology, 9,* 451–460.

Pihl, R.O., & Nimrod, G. (1976). The reliability and validity of the Draw-A-Person test in IQ and personality assessment. *Journal of Clinical Psychology, 32,* 470–472.

Pinkerman, J.E., Haynes, J.P., & Keiser, T. (1993) Characteristics of practice in juvenile court clinics. *American Journal of Forensic Psychology, 11,* 3–12.

Piotrowski, Z. (1937). The Rorschach inkblot method in organic disturbances of the central nervous system. *Journal of Nervous and Mental Disease, 86,* 525–537.

Piotrowski, Z. (1940). Positive and negative Rorschach organic reactions. *Rorschach Research Exchange, 4,* 147–151.

Pisoneault, T.B. (1996). Equivalency of computer-assisted and paper-and-pencil administered versions of the Minnesota Multiphasic Personality-2. *Computers in Human Behavior, 12,* 291–300.

Plaisted, J.R., & Golden, C.J. (1982). Test–retest reliability of the clinical, factor, and localization scales of the Luria–Nebraska Neuropsychological Battery. *International Journal of Neuroscience, 17,* 163–167.

Plante, L.G., Plante, T.G., Rahm, P., Brentar, J.T., & Couchman, C. (1997). Administering the Digit Span subtest of the WISC-III to children with attentional, emotional, and learning difficulties: Should the examiner make eye contact or not? *Assessment, 4,* 351–357.

Pogge, D.L., Stokes, J.M., Frank, J., Wong, H., & Harvey, P.D. (1997). Association of MMPI validity scales and therapist ratings of psychopathology in adolescent psychiatric inpatients. *Assessment, 4,* 17–27.

Poitrenaud, J., & Barrere, H. (1972). Etude sur la signification diagnostique des certaines erreurs de reproduction au V.R.T. de Benton. *Review of Applied Psychology, 22,* 43–56.

Pollock, B. (1942). The validity of the Shipley–Hartford Retreat Test for "deterioration." *Psychiatric Quarterly, 16,* 119–131.

Porch, A.M., Ross, T.P., & Whitman, R.D. (1995). Reexamination of executive function in psychosis-prone college students. *Personality and Individual Differences, 18,* 535–539.

Porteus, S.D. (1959). *The Maze Test and clinical psychology.* Palo Alto, CA: Pacific Books.

Porteus, S. (1965). *Porteus maze test: Fifty years' application.* Palo Alto, CA: Pacific Books.

Poteat, G.M., Wuensch, K.L., & Gregg, N.B. (1988). An investigation of differential prediction with the WISC-R. *Journal of School Psychology, 26,* 59–68.

Powell, J.B., Cripe, L.I., & Dodrill, C.B. (1991). Assessment of brain impairment with the Rey Auditory Verbal Learning Test: A comparison with other neuropsychological measures. *Archives of Clinical Neuropsychology, 6,* 241–249.

Prado, W.M., & Taub, D.V. (1966). Accurate prediction of individual intellectual functioning by the Shipley–Hartford. *Journal of Clinical Psychology, 22,* 294–296.

Prakash, I.J., & Bhogle, S. (1992). Benton's Visual Retention Test: Norms for different age groups. *Journal of the Indian Academy of Applied Psychology, 18,* 33–36.

Prewett, P.N. (1992a). The relationship between the Kaufman Brief Intelligence Test (K-BIT) and the WISC-R with incarcerated juvenile delinquents. *Educational and Psychological Measurement, 52,* 977–982.

Prewett, P.N. (1992b). The relationship between the Kaufman Brief Intelligence Test (K-BIT) and the WISC-R with referred students. *Psychology in the Schools, 29,* 25–27.

Prewett, P.N. (1992c). Short forms of the Stanford–Binet Intelligence Scale: Fourth Edition. *Journal of Psychoeducational Assessment, 10,* 257–264.

Prewett, P.N. (1995). A comparison of two screening tests (the Matrix Analogies Test-Short Form and the Kaufman Brief Intelligence Test) with the WISC-III. *Psychological Assessment, 7,* 69–72.

Prewett, P.N., & Fowler, D.B. (1992). Predictive validity of the Slosson Intelligence Test with the WISC-R and the WRAT-R Level 1. *Psychology in the Schools, 29,* 17–21.

Prewett, P.N., & MacCaffrey, L.K. (1993). A comparison of the Kaufman Brief Intelligence Test (K-BIT) with the Stanford–Binet, a two-subtest short form, and the Kaufman Test of Educational Achievement (K-TEA) Brief Form. *Psychology in the Schools, 30,* 299–304.

Price, L.J., Fein, G., & Feinberg, I. (1979). Cognitive and neuropsychological variables in the normal elderly. Paper presented at the American Psychological Association convention, New York City.

Price, D.R., Herbert, D.A., Walsh, M.L., & Law, J.G. (1990). Study of WAIS-R, Quick Test, and PPVT IQs for neuropsychiatric patients. *Perceptual and Motor Skills, 70,* 1320–1322.

Prifitera, A., & Ledbetter, M. (1992, November). Normative delayed recall rates based on the Wechsler Memory Scale-Revised standardization sample. Paper presented at the 12th annual meeting of the National Academy of Neuropsychology, Pittsburgh, PA.

Prifitera, A., & Ryan, J.J. (1981). Validity of the Luria–Nebraska Neuropsychological Battery Intellectual Processes scale as a measure of adult intelligence. *Journal of Consulting and Clinical Psychology, 49,* 755–756.

Prifitera, A., & Ryan, J.J. (1982). Concurrent validity of the Luria–Nebraska Neuropsychological Battery Memory scale. *Journal of Clinical Psychology, 38,* 378–379.

Prigatano, G.F. (1978). Wechsler Memory Scale: A selective review of the literature (monograph). *Journal of Clinical Psychology, 34,* 816–832.

Prigatano, G.P., & Amin, K. (1993). Digit Memory Test: Unequivocal cerebral dysfunction and suspected malingering. *Journal of Clinical and Experimental Neuropsychology, 15,* 537–546.

Prigatano, G.P., & Parsons, O.A. (1976). Relationship of age and education to Halstead Test performance in different patient populations. *Journal of Consulting and Clinical Psychology, 44,* 527–533.

Prigatano, G.P., Parsons, D., Wright, E., Levin, D.C., & Hawryluk, G. (1983). Neuropsychological test performance in mildly hypoxic patients with chronic obstructive pulmonary disease. *Journal of Consulting and Clinical Psychology, 51,* 108–116.

Prigatano, G.P., Smason, I., Lamb, D.G., & Bortz, J.J. (1997). Suspected malingering and the Digit Memory test: A replication and extension. *Archives of Clinical Neuropsychology, 12,* 609–619.

Prout, H.T., & Schwartz, J.F. (1984). Validity of the Peabody Picture Vocabulary Test-Revised. *Journal of Clinical Psychology, 40,* 584–587.

Psychological Corporation (1997). WAIS-III/WMS-III technical manual. San Antonio: The Psychological Corporation-Harcourt Brace & Company.

Puente, A.E., Heidelberg-Sanders, C., & Lund, N.L. (1982). Discrimination of schizophrenia with and without nervous system damage using the Luria–Nebraska Neuropsychological Battery. *International Journal of Neuroscience, 16,* 59–62.

Pugh, G.M., & Boer, D.P. (1991). Normative data on the validity of Canadian substitute items for the WAIS-R Information subtest. *Canadian Journal of Behavioural Science, 23,* 149–158.

Putman, L.R. (1981). Minnesota Percepto-Diagnostic Test and reading achievement. *Perceptual and Motor Skills, 53,* 235–238.

Putnam, S.H., Kurtz, J.E., & Houts, D.C. (1996). Four-month test–retest reliability of the MMPI-2 with normal male clergy. *Journal of Personality Assessment, 67,* 341–353.

Putzke, J.D., Williams, M.A., Adams, W., & Boll, T.J. (1999a). Does memory performance in children become more consistent with age?: Cross-sectional comparison using the WRAML. *Journal of Clinical and Experimental Neuropsychology, 20,* 835–845.

Putzke, J.D., Williams, M.A., Daniel, F.J., & Boll, T.J. (1999b). The utility of K-correction to adjust for a defensive response set on the MMPI. *Assessment, 6,* 61–70.

Qataee, A. (1993). Factorial similarity and accuracy of measurement of the Saudi version of the WISC-R across sex at six age groups. *Journal of Social Sciences, 21,* 253–264.

Quattrochi, M.M., & Golden, C.J. (1983). Peabody Picture Vocabulary Test-Revised and Luria–Nebraska Neuropsychological Battery for Children: Intercorrelations for normal youngsters. *Perceptual and Motor Skills, 56,* 632–634.

Quereshi, M.Y., & Seitz, R. (1994a). Non-equivalence of WPPSI, WPPSI-R, and WISC-R scores. *Current Psychology: Development, Learning, Personality, Social, 13,* 210–225.

Quereshi, M.Y., & Seitz, R. (1994b). Gender differences on the WPPSI, the WISC-R, and the WPPSI-R. *Current Psychology: Developmental, Learning, Personality, Social, 13,* 117–123.

Quereshi, M.Y., Treis, K.M., & Riebe, A.L. (1989). The equivalence of the WAIS-R and the WISC-R at age 16. *Journal of Clinical Psychology, 45,* 633–641.

Query, W.T., & Berger, R.A. (1980). AVLT memory scores as a function of age among general, medical, neurologic, and alcoholic patients. *Journal of Clinical Psychology, 36,* 1009–1012.

Query, W.T., & Megran, J. (1983). Age related norms for a AVLT in a male patient population. *Journal of Clinical Psychology, 39,* 136–138.

Raggio, D.J. (1993). Correlations of the Kahn Intelligence Test and the WAIS-R IQS among mentally retarded adults. *Perceptual and Motor Skills, 76,* 252–254.

Raglund, J.D., Glahn, D.C., Gur, R.C., Censits, D.M., Smith, R.J., Mozley, P.D., Alavi, A., & Gur, R.E. (1997). PET retional cerebral blood flow during working and declarative memory: Relationship with task performance. *Neuropsychology, 11*, 222–231.

Raguet, M.L., Campbell, D.A., Berry, D.T.R., Schmitt, F.A., & Smith, G.T. (1996). Stability of intelligence and intellectual predictors in older persons. *Psychological Assessment, 8*, 154–160.

Randolph, C., Mohr, E., & Chase, T.N. (1993). Assessment of intellectual functioning in dementing disorders: Validity of WAIS-R short forms for patients with Alzheimer's, Huntington's, and Parkinson's disease. *Journal of Clinical and Experimental Neuropsychology, 15*, 743–753.

Randolph, C., Gold, J.M., Kozora, E., & Cullum, C.M. (1994). Estimating memory function: Disparity of Wechsler memory Scale-Revised and California Verbal Learning Test indices in clinical and normal samples. *Clinical Neuropsychologist, 8*, 99–108.

Rapcsak, S.Z., Polster, M.R., Comer, J.F., & Rubens, A.B. (1994). False identification and misidentification of faces following right hemisphere damage. *Cortex, 30*, 565–583.

Rapport, L.J., Dutra, R.L., Webster, J.S., Charter, R., & Morrill, B. (1995). Hemispatial deficits on the Rey–Osterrieth Complex Figure Drawing. *The Clinical Neuropsychologist, 9*, 169–179.

Rapport, L.J., Axelrod, B.N., Theisen, M.E., Brines, D.B., Kalechstein, A.D., & Ricker, J.H. (1997a). Relationship of IQ to verbal learning and memory: Test and retest. *Journal of Clinical and Experimental Neuropsychology, 19*, 655–666.

Rapport, L.J., Charter, R.A., Dutra, R.L., Farchione, T.J., & Kingsley, J.J. (1997b). Psychometric properties of the Rey–Osterrieth Complex Figure: Lezak–Osterrieth vs. Denman scoring systems. *The Clinical Neuropsychologist, 11*, 46–63.

Rapport, L.J., Farchione, T.J., Coleman, R.D., & Axelrod, B.N. (1998). Effects of coaching on malingered motor function profiles. *Journal of Clinical and Experimental Neuropsychology, 20*, 89–97.

Raskin, S.A., & Rearick, E. (1996). Verbal fluency in individuals with mild traumatic brain injury. *Neuropsychology, 10*, 416–422.

Rasmusson, D.X., Bylsma, F.W., & Brandt, J. (1995). Stability of performance on the Hopkins Verbal Learning Test. *Archives of Clinical Neuropsychology, 10*, 21–26.

Rasmusson, D.X., Carson, K.A., Brookmeyer, R., Kawas, C., & Brandt, J. (1996). Predicting rate of cognitive decline in probable Alzheimer's disease. *Brain and Cognition, 31*, 133–147.

Rasmusson, D.X., Zonderman, A.B., Kawas, C., & Resnick, S.M. (1998). Effects of age and dementia on the Trail Making Test. *The Clinical Neuropsychologist, 12*, 169–178.

Ratcliffe, K.J., & Ratcliffe, M.W. (1979). The Leiter Scales: A review of validity findings. *American Annals of the Deaf, 124*, 38–44.

Rathbun, J., & Smith, A. (1982). Comment on the validity of Boyd's validation study of the Hooper Visual Organization Test. *Journal of Consulting and Clinical Psychology, 50*, 281–283.

Ravindran, A. (1995). Bender Gestalt test: A tool of neuropsychological impairment in epilepsy. *Journal of Personality and Clinical Studies, 11*, 11–15.

Rausch, R., Lieb, J.P., & Crandall, P.H. (1978). Neuropsychological correlates of depth spike activity in epileptics. *Archives of Neurology, 35*, 699–705.

Raven, J.C., Court, J.H., & Raven, J. (1977). *Manual for Raven's Progressive Matrices and Vocabulary Scales*. London: H.K. Lewis.

Rawlings, D.B., & Crewe, N.M. (1992). Test–retest practice effects and test score changes of the WAIS-R in recovering traumatically brain-injured survivors. *The Clinical Neuropsychologist, 6*, 415–430.

Ray, E.C., Engum, E.S., Lambert, E.W., Bane, G.F., Nash, M.R., & Bracy, O.L. (1997). Ability of the Cognitive Behavioral Driver's Inventory to distinguish malingerers from brain-damaged subjects. *Archives of Clinical Neuropsychology, 12*, 491–503.

Raz, S., Shah, F., & Sander, C.J. (1996). Differential effects of perinatal hypoxic risk on early developmental outcome: A twin study. *Neuropsychology, 10*, 429–436.

Records, N.L., Tomblin, J.B., & Buckwalter, P.R. (1995). Auditory verbal learning and memory in young adults with specific language impairment. *The Clinical Neuropsychologist, 9*, 187–193.

Reed, H.B.C., & Reitan, R.M. (1963). Changes in psychological test performance associated with the normal aging process. *Journal of Gerontology, 18*, 271–274.

Reeder, K.P., & Boll, T.J. (1992). A shortened intermediate version of the Halstead Category Test. *Archives of Clinical Neuropsychology, 7*, 53–62.

Rees, L.M., Tombaugh, T.N., Gansler, D.A., & Moczynski, N.P. (1998). Five validation experiments of the Test of Memory Malingering. *Psychological Assessment, 10,* 10–20.

Reeve, R.R., French, J.L., & Hunter, M. (1983). A validation of the Leiter International Performance Scale with kindergarten children. *Journal of Consulting and Clinical Psychology, 51,* 458–459.

Reid, D.B., & Kelly, M.P. (1993). Wechsler Memory Scale-Revised in closed head injury. *Journal of Clinical Psychology, 49,* 245–254.

Reitan, R.M. (1955a). Affective disturbances in brain-damaged patients. *Archives of Neurology and Psychiatry, 73,* 530–532.

Reitan, R.M. (1955b). Certain differential effects of left and right cerebral lesions in human adults. *Journal of Comparative and Physiological Psychology, 48,* 474–477.

Reitan, R.M. (1955c). An investigation of the validity of Halstead's measures of biological intelligence. *Archives of Neurology and Psychiatry, 73,* 28–35.

Reitan, R.M. (1959). The comparative effects of brain damage on the Halstead Impairment Index and the Wechsler–Bellevue Scale. *Journal of Clinical Psychology, 15,* 281–285.

Reitan, R.M. (1966). A research program on the psychological effects of brain lesions in human beings. In N.R. Ellis (Ed.), *International review of research in mental retardation* (Vol. 1). New York: Academic Press.

Reitan, R.M. (1967). Psychological assessment of deficits associated with brain lesions in subjects with normal and subnormal intelligence. In J.L. Khanna (Ed.), *Brain damage and mental retardation: A psychological evaluation.* Springfield, IL: Charles C. Thomas.

Reitan, R.M. (1969). *Manual for administration of neuropsychological batteries for adults and children.* Indianapolis, IN: Author.

Reitan, R.M. (1976). Neurological and physiological bases of psychopathology. *Annual Review of Psychology, 27,* 189–216.

Reitan, R.M., & Davison, L.A. (1974). *Clinical neuropsychology: Current status and applications.* Washington, DC: Winston.

Reitan, R.M., & Wolfson, D. (1992). *Neuropsychological evaluation of older children.* Tucson, AZ: Neuropsychology Press.

Reitan, R.M., & Wolfson, D. (1993). *The Halstead–Reitan Neuropsychological Battery: Theory and clinical interpretation.* Tucson, AZ: Neuropsychology Press.

Reitan, R.A., & Wolfson, D. (1995a). Influence of age and education on neuropsychological test results. *The Clinical Neuropsychologist, 9,* 151–158.

Reitan, R.A., & Wolfson, D. (1995b). Cross-validation of the General Neuropsychological Deficit Scale (GNDS). *Archives of Clinical Neuropsychology, 10,* 125–131.

Reitan, R.M., & Wolfson, D. (1995c). Consistency of responses on retesting among head-injured subjects in litigation versus head-injured subjects not in litigation. *Applied Neuropsychology, 2,* 67–71.

Reitan, R.M., & Wolfson, D. (1995d). Category Test and Trail Making Test as measures of frontal lobe functions. *The Clinical Neuropsychologist, 9,* 50–56.

Reitan, R.M., & Wolfson, D. (1996a). The question of validity of neuropsychological test scores among head-injured litigants: Development of a dissimulation index. *Archives of Clinical Neuropsychology, 11,* 573–580.

Reitan, R.M., & Wolfson, D. (1996b). Relationships between specific and general tests of cerebral functioning. *The Clinical Neuropsychologist, 10,* 37–42.

Reitan, R.M., & Wolfson, D. (1997). Consistency of neuropsychological test scores of head-injured subjects involved in litigation compared with head-injured subjects not involved in litigation: Development of the retest consistency index. *The Clinical Neuropsychologist, 11,* 69–76.

Resnick, S.M., Trotman, K.M., Kawas, C., & Zonderman, A.B. (1995). Age-associated changes in specific errors on the Benton Visual Retention Test. *Journals of Gerontology Series B- Psychological Sciences and Social Sciences, 50B,* P171–P178.

Retzlaff, P.D., & Morris, G.L. (1996). Event-related potentials during the Continuous Visual Memory Test. *Journal of Clinical Psychology, 52,* 43–47.

Retzlaff, P., Slicner, N., & Gibertini, M. (1986). Predicting WAIS-R scores from the Shipley Institute of Living Scale in a homogeneous sample. *Journal of Clinical Psychology, 42,* 357–359.

Rey, A. (1964). *L'examen clinique en psychologie.* Paris: Presses Universitaires de France.

Reynolds, C.R. (1997). Forward and backward memory span should not be combined for clinical analysis. *Archives of Clinical Neuropsychology, 12,* 29–40.

Reynolds, C.R. (1998). Reliability of performance on the Test of Memory and Learning (TOMAL) by an adolescent learning disability sample. *Educational and Psychological Measurement, 58,* 832–835.

Reynolds, C.R., & Bigler, E.D. (1994). *Test of memory and learning.* Austin, TX: PRO-ED.

Reynolds, C.R., & Bigler, E.D. (1996). Factor structure, factor indexes, and other useful statistics for interpretation of the Test of Memory and Learning (TOMAL). *Archives of Clinical Neuropsychology, 11,* 29–43.

Reynolds, C.R., & Gutkin, T.B. (1979). Predicting the premorbid intellectual status of children using demographic data. *Clinical Neuropsychology, 1,* 36–38.

Reynolds, C.R., & Gutkin, T.B. (1980). Statistics related to profile interpretation of the Peabody Individual Achievement Test. *Psychology in the Schools, 17,* 316–319.

Reynolds, C.R., & Ford, L. (1994). Comparative three-factor structure solutions of the WISC-III and WISC-R at 11 age levels between 6½ and 16½ years. *Archives of Clinical Neuropsychology, 9,* 553–570.

Reynolds, C.R., Sanchez, S., & Willson, V.L. (1996). Normative tables for calculating the WISC-III Performance and Full Scale IQS when Symbol Search is substituted for Coding. *Psychological Assessment, 8,* 378–382.

Riccio, C.A., & Hynd, G.W. (1993). Validity of Benton's Judgment of Line Orientation Test. *Journal of Psychoeducational Assessment, 10,* 210–218.

Riccio, C.A., Cohen, M.J., Hall, J., & Ross, C.M. (1997). The third and fourth factors of the WISC-III: What they don't measure. *Journal of Psychoeducational Assessment, 15,* 27–39.

Richards, H.C., Fowler, P.C., Berent, S., & Boll, T.J. (1980). Comparison of WISC-R factor patterns for younger and older epileptic children. *Journal of Clinical Neuropsychology, 2,* 333–341.

Ricker, J.H., & Axelrod, B.N. (1994). Analysis of an oral paradigm for the Trail Making Test. *Assessment, 1,* 47–51.

Ricker, J.H., & Axelrod, B.N. (1995). Hooper Visual Organization Test: Effects of naming ability. *The Clinical Neuropsychologist, 9,* 57–62.

Riddle, M., & Roberts, A.H. (1977). Delinquency, delay of gratification, recidivism, and the Porteus Maze Tests. *Psychological Bulletin, 84,* 417–425.

Riddle, M., & Roberts, A.H. (1978). Psychosurgery and the Porteus Maze Tests. *Archives of General Psychiatry, 35,* 493–497.

Riege, W.H., Kelly, K., & Klane, L.T. (1981). Age and error differences on Memory for Designs. *Perceptual and Motor Skills, 52,* 507–513.

Rippich, D.N., Carpenter, B., & Ziol, E. (1997). Comparison of African-American and white persons with Alzheimer's disease on language measures. *Neurology, 48,* 781–783.

Rissmiller, D.J., Wayslow, A., Madison, H., Hogate, P., Rissmiller, F.R., & Steer, R.A. (1998). Prevalence of malingering in inpatient suicide ideators and attempters. *Crisis, 19,* 62–66.

Ritter, D.R. (1974). Concurrence of psychiatric diagnosis and psychological diagnosis based on the MMPI. *Journal of Personality Assessment, 38,* 52–54.

Rixecker, H., & Hartje, W. (1980). Kimura's Recurring-Figures-Test: A normative study. *Journal of Clinical Psychology, 36,* 465–467.

Robin, R.W., & Shea, J.D.C. (1983). The Bender Gestalt Visual Motor Test in Papua New Guinea. *International Journal of Psychology, 18,* 263–270.

Robiner, W.N., Dossa, D., & O'Dowd, W. (1988). Abbreviated WAIS-R procedures: Use and limitations with head-injured patients. *The Clinical Neuropsychologist, 2,* 365–374.

Robinson, A.L., Heaton, R.K., Lehman, R.A.W., & Stilson, D.W. (1980). The utility of the Wisconsin Card Sorting Test in detecting and localizing frontal lobe lesions. *Journal of Consulting and Clinical Psychology, 48,* 605–614.

Robinson, A.L., Kester, D.B., Saykin, A.J., Kaplan, E.G., & Gur, R.C. (1991). Comparison of two short forms of the Wisconsin Card Sorting Test. *Archives of Clinical Neuropsychology, 6,* 27–33.

Robinson, N.M., Dale, P.S., & Landesman, S. (1990). Validity of Stanford–Binet IV with linguistically precocious toddlers. *Intelligence, 14,* 173–186.

Robinson-Whelan, S. (1992). Benton Visual Retention Test performance among normal and demented older adults. *Neuropsychology, 6,* 261–269.

Rodriguez, C.M., Treacy, L.A., Sowerby, P.J., & Murphy, L.E. (1998). Applicability of Australian adaptations of intelligence tests in new Zealand with a Dunedin sample of children. *New Zealand Journal of Psychology, 27,* 4–12.

Rogers, D.A. (1972). Review of the MMPI. In Oscar Burros (Ed.), *The seventh mental measurements yearbook.* Lincoln, NE: Burros Institute.

Rogers, R., Ornduff, S.R., & Sewell, K.W. (1993). Feigning specific disorders: A study of the Personality Assessment Inventory. *Journal of Personality Assessment, 60*, 554–560.

Rogers, R., Flores, J., Ustad, K., & Sewell, K.W. (1995). Initial validation of the Personality Assessment Inventory—Spanish version with clients from Mexican-American communities. *Journal of Personality Assessment, 64*, 340–348.

Rogers, R., Sewell, K.W., Morey, L.C., & Ustad, K.L. (1996). Detection of feigned mental disorders on the Personality Assessment Inventory: A discriminant analysis. *Journal of Personality Assessment, 67*, 629–640.

Rogers, R., Sewell, K.W., Cruise, K.R., Wang, E.W., & Ustad, K.L. (1998a). The PAI and feigning: A cautionary note on its use in forensic-correctional settings. *Assessment, 5*, 399–405.

Rogers, R., Ustad, K.L., & Salekin, R.T. (1998b). Convergent validity of the Personality Assessment Inventory: A study of emergency referrals in a correctional setting. *Assessment, 5*, 3–12.

Rohwer, W.D., & Lynch, S. (1968). Retardation, school strata, and learning efficiency. *American Journal of Mental Deficiency, 73*, 91–96.

Roid, G.H., & Worrall, W. (1997). Replication of the Wechsler Intelligence Scale for Children-Third Edition four factor model in the Canadian normative sample. *Psychological Assessment, 9*, 512–515.

Roid, G.H., Prifitera, A., & Ledbetter, M. (1988). Confirmatory analysis of the factor structure of the Wechsler Memory Scale-Revised. *The Clinical Neuropsychologist, 2*, 116–120.

Rojas, D.C., & Bennett, T.L. (1995). Single versus composite score discriminative validity with the Halstead–Reitan Battery and the Stroop test in mild brain injury. *Archives of Clinical Neuropsychology, 10*, 101–110.

Roman, D.D., Kubo, S.H., Ormaza, S., Francis, G.S., Bank, A.J., & Shumway, S.J. (1997). Memory improvement following cardiac transplantation. *Journal of Clinical and Experimental Neuropsychology, 19*, 692–697.

Roman, M.J., Delis, D.C., Willerman, L., Magulac, M., Demadura, T.L., de la Pena, J.L., Loftis, C., Walsh, J., & Kracun, M. (1998). Impact of pediatric traumatic brain injury on components of verbal memory. *Journal of Clinical and Experimental Neuropsychology, 20*, 245–258.

Roper, B.L., Ben-Porath, Y.S., & Butcher, J.N. (1995). Comparability and validity of computerized adaptive testing with the MMPI-2. *Journal of Personality Assessment, 65*, 358–371.

Roper, B.L., Bieliauskas, L.A., & Peterson, M.R. (1996). Validity of the Mini-Mental State Exam and the Neurobehavioral Cognitive Status Examination in cognitive screening. *Neuropsychiatry, Neuropsychology, and Behavioral Neurology, 9*, 54–57.

Rose, F.E., Hall, S., Szalda-Petree, A.D., & Bach, P. (1998). A comparison of four tests of malingering and the effects of coaching. *Archives of Clinical Neuropsychology, 13*, 349–363.

Rosenberg, S.J., Ryan, J.J., & Prifitera, A. (1984). Rey Auditory–Verbal Learning Test performance of patients with and without memory impairment. *Journal of Clinical Psychology, 40*, 785–787.

Rosenfeld, J.P., Sweet, J.J., Chuang, J., Ellwanger, J., & Song, L. (1996). Detection of simulated malingering using forced choice recognition enhanced with event-related potential recording. *The Clinical Neuropsychologist, 10*, 163–179.

Rosenthal, B.L., & Kamphaus, R.W. (1988). Interpretative tables for test scatter on the Stanford–Binet Intelligence Scale: Fourth Edition. *Journal of Psychoeducational Assessment, 6*, 359–370.

Rosenthal, R. (1984). *Meta-analytic procedures for social research.* Beverly Hills, CA: Sage.

Ross, S.R., Millis, S.R., & Rosenthal, M. (1997). Neuropsychological prediction of psychosocial outcome after traumatic brain injury. *Applied Neuropsychology, 4*, 165–170.

Ross, T.P., & Lichtenberg, P.A. (1997). Effects of age and education on neuropsychological test performance: A comparison of normal vs. cognitively impaired geriatric medical patients. *Aging Neuropsychology and Cognition, 4*, 74–79.

Ross, T.P., & Lichtenberg, P.A. (1998). Expanded norms for the Boston Naming Test for use with urban, elderly medical patients. *The Clinical Neuropsychologist, 12*, 475–481.

Ross, T.P., Lichtenberg, P.A., & Christensen, B.K. (1995). Normative data on the Boston Naming Test for elderly adults in a demographically diverse medical sample. *The Clinical Neuropsychologist, 9*, 321–325.

Ross, W.D., & Ross, S. (1944). Some Rorschach ratings of clinical value. *Rorschach Research Exchange, 8*, 1–9.

Rosselli, M., & Ardila, A. (1991). Effects of age, education, and gender on the Rey–Osterrieth Complex Figure. *The Clinical Neuropsychologist, 5*, 370–376.

Rossini, E.D., Kowalski, J.M., Dudish, S.A., & Telcher, S.L. (1991). Temporal consistency of the WAIS-R Memory/Freedom from Distractibility factor in a nonclinical sample. *Psychological Reports, 68*, 827–832.

Rosso, M., & Phelps, A. (1988). Factor analysis of the Woodcock–Johnson with conduct-disordered adolescents. *Psychology in the Schools, 25*, 105–110.

Rosso, M., Falasco, S.L., & Koller, J.R. (1984). Investigations into the relationship of the PPVT-R and the WISC-R with incarcerated delinquents. *Journal of Clinical Psychology, 40*, 588–591.

Rotatori, A.F. (1978). Test–retest reliability of the Quick Test for mentally retarded children. *Psychological Reports, 46*, 162.

Roth, D.L., Hughes, C.W., Monkowski, P.G., & Crosson, B. (1984). Investigation of validity of WAIS-R short-forms for patients suspected to have brain impairment. *Journal of Consulting and Clinical Psychology, 52*, 722–723.

Rothlisberg, B.A. (1987). Comparing the Stanford–Binet, Fourth Edition to the WISC-R: A concurrent validity study. *Journal of School Psychology, 25*, 193–196.

Rothstein, H.R., & McDaniel, M.A. (1992). Differential validity by sex in employment settings. *Journal of Business and Psychology, 7*, 45–62.

Rouse, S.V., Butcher, J.N., & Miller, K.B. (1999). Assessment of substance abuse in psychotherapy clients: The effectiveness of the MMPI-2 substance abuse scales. *Psychological Assessment, 11*, 101–107.

Royce, J.R., Yeudall, L.T., & Bock, C. (1976). Factor analytic studies of human brain damage: 1. 1st and 2nd order factors and their brain correlates. *Multivariate Behavioral Research, 11*, 381–418.

Rubin, H., Goldman, J.J., & Rosenfeld, J.G. (1990). A follow-up comparison of WISC-R and WAIS-R IQS in a residential mentally retarded population. *Psychology in the Schools, 27*, 309–310.

Ruddle, H.V., & Bradshaw, C.M. (1982). On the estimation of premorbid intelligence functioning: Validation of Nelson & McKenna's formula and some new normative data. *British Journal of Clinical Psychology, 21*, 159–165.

Ruff, C.F., Ayers, J.L., & Templer, D.I. (1977). The Watson and Hovey MMPI scales: Do they measure organicity or "functional" psychopathology? *Journal of Clinical Psychology, 33*, 732–734.

Ruff, R.M., Light, R.H., Parker, S.B., & Levin, H.S. (1996). Benton Controlled Oral Word Association Test: Reliability and updated norms. *Archives of Clinical Neuropsychology, 11*, 329–338.

Russell, E.W. (1975a). A multiple scoring system for the assessment of complex memory functions. *Journal of Consulting and Clinical Psychology, 43*, 800–809.

Russell, E.W. (1975b). Validation of a brain-damage vs. schizophrenia MMPI key. *Journal of Clinical Psychology, 31*, 659–661.

Russell, E.W. (1976). The Bender–Gestalt and the Halstead–Reitan battery: A case study. *Journal of Clinical Psychology, 32*, 355–361.

Russell, E.W. (1977). MMPI profiles of brain-damaged and schizophrenic subjects. *Journal of Clinical Psychology, 33*, 190–193.

Russell, E.W. (1980). Theoretical bases of Luria–Nebraska and Halstead–Reitan batteries. Paper presented at the American Psychological Association Convention, Montreal.

Russell, E.W. (1982). Factor analysis of the Revised Wechsler Memory Scale tests in a neuropsychological battery. *Perceptual and Motor Skills, 54*, 971–974.

Russell, E.W. (1984). Theory and development of pattern analysis methods related to the Halstead–Reitan battery. In P.E Logue & J.M. Schear (Eds.), *Clinical neuropsychology: A multidisciplinary approach* (pp. 50–98). Springfield, IL: Charles C Thomas.

Russell, E.W. (1986). The psychometric foundation of clinical neuropsychology. In S.B. Filskov & T.J. Boll (Eds.), *Handbook of clinical neuropsychology* (Vol. 2, pp. 45–80). New York: John Wiley & Sons.

Russell, E.W. (1987). Neuropsychological interpretation of the WAIS. *Neuropsychology, 1*, 2–6.

Russell, E.W. (1994). The cognitive-metric, fixed battery approach to neuropsychological assessment. In R.D. Vanderploeg (Ed.), *Clinician's guide to neuropsychological assessment* (pp. 211–258). Hillsdale, NJ: Lawrence J. Erlbaum.

Russell, E.W. (1997). Developments in the psychometric foundations of neuropsychological assessment. In G. Goldstein & T.M. Incagnoli (Eds.), *Contemporary approaches to neuropsychological assessment*. New York: Plenum.

Russell, E.W. (1998). In defense of the Halstead Reitan battery: A critique of Lezak's review. *Archives of Clinical Neuropsychology, 13*, 365–381.

Russell, E.W., & Levy, M. (1987). Revision of the Halstead Category Test. *Journal of Consulting and Clinical Psychology, 55*, 898–901.

Russell, E.W., Neuringer, C., & Goldstein, G. (1970). *Assessment of brain damage: A neuropsychological key approach*. New York: John Wiley & Sons.

Russo, M., & Vignolo, L.A. (1967). Visual figure-ground discrimination in patients with unilateral cerebral disease. *Cortex*, *3*, 118–127.

Rust, J.O., & Lindstrom, A. (1996). Concurrent validity of the WISC-III and Stanford–Binet IV. *Psychological Reports*, *79*, 618–620.

Rutter, M., Graham, P., & Yule W. (1970). *A neuropsychiatric study in childhood*. London: Spastics International Medical Publication.

Ryan, C.M., & Hendrickson, R. (1998). Evaluating the effects of treatment for medical disorders: Has the value of neuropsychological assessment been fully realized? *Applied Neuropsychology*, *5*, 209–219.

Ryan, J.J. (1984). Abnormality of subtest score and verbal–performance IQ differences on the WAIS-R. *International Journal of Clinical Neuropsychology*, *6*, 97–98.

Ryan, J.J. (1985). Application of a WAIS-R short form with neurological patients: Validity and correlational findings. *Journal of Psychoeducational Assessment*, *3*, 61–64.

Ryan, J.J., & Geisser, M.E. (1986). Validity and diagnostic accuracy of an alternate form of the Rey Auditory Verbal Learning Test. *Archives of Clinical Neuropsychology*, *1*, 209–217.

Ryan, J.J., & Lewis, C.V. (1988). Comparison of normal controls and recently detoxified alcoholics on the Wechsler Memory Scale-Revised. *The Clinical Neuropsychologist*, *2*, 173–180.

Ryan J.J., & Paolo, A.M. (1992). A screening procedure for estimating premorbid intelligence in the elderly. *The Clinical Neuropsychologist*, *6*, 53–62.

Ryan, J.J., & Prifitera, A. (1990). The WAIS-R Index for estimating premorbid intelligence: Accuracy of predicting short form IQ. *The International Journal of Clinical Neuropsychology*, *12*, 20–23.

Ryan, J.J., Morris, J., Yaffa, S., & Peterson, L. (1981). Test–retest reliability of the Wechsler Memory Scale, Form 1. *Journal of Clinical Psychology*, *37*, 847–848.

Ryan, J.J., Prifitera, A., & Powers, L. (1983). Scoring reliability of the WAIS-R. *Journal of Consulting and Clinical Psychology*, *51*, 149–150.

Ryan, J.J., Georgemiller, R.J., & McKinney, B.E. (1984a). Application of the four-subtest short form with an older clinical sample. *Journal of Clinical Psychology*, *40*, 1033–1036.

Ryan, J.J., Rosenberg, S.J., & DeWolfe, A.S. (1984b). Generalization of the WAIS-R factor structure with a vocational rehabilitation sample. *Journal of Consulting and Clinical Psychology*, *52*, 311–312.

Ryan, J.J., Rosenberg, S.J., & Mittenberg, W. (1984c). Factor analysis of the Rey Auditory–Verbal Learning Test. *International Journal of Clinical Neuropsychology*, *8*, 239–241.

Ryan, J.J., Georgemiller, R.J., Geisser, M.E., & Randall, D.M. (1985). Test–retest reliability of the WAIS-R in a clinical sample. *Journal of Clinical Psychology*, *41*, 552–556.

Ryan, J.J., Geisser, M.E., Randall, D.M., & Georgemiller, R.J. (1986). Alternate form reliability and equivalence of the Rey Auditory Verbal Learning Test. *Journal of Clinical and Experimental Neuropsychology*, *8*, 611–616.

Ryan, J.J., Nowak, T.J., & Geisser, M.E. (1987). On the comparability of the WAIS and WAIS-R: Review of the research and implications for clinical practice. *Journal of Psychoeducational Assessment*, *5*, 15–30.

Ryan, J.J., Utley, A.P., & Worthen, V.E. (1988). Comparison of two IQ conversion tables for the Vocabulary-Block Design short form. *Journal of Clinical Psychology*, *44*, 950–952.

Ryan, J.J., Paolo, A.M., & Brungardt, T.M. (1990). WAIS-R reliability and standard errors for persons 75 to 79, 80 to 84, and 85 and older. *Journal of Psychoeducational Assessment*, *8*, 9–14.

Ryan, J.J., Paolo, A.M., & Smith, A.J. (1992). Wechsler Adult Intelligence Scale-Revised intersubtest scatter on brain-damaged patients: A comparison with the standardization sample. *Psychological Assessment*, *4*, 63–66.

Ryan, J.J., Paolo, A.M., & Van Fleet, M. (1994). Comparative test–retest stability of four WAIS-R selected subtest short forms in persons 75–87 years old. *Assessment*, *1*, 401–405.

Ryan, J.J., Dunn, G.E., & Paolo, A.M. (1995a). Temporal stability of the MMPI-2 in a substance abuse sample. *Psychotherapy in Private Practice*, *14*, 33–41.

Ryan, J.J., Paolo, A.M., & Dunn, G.E. (1995b). Analysis of a WAIS-R old-age normative sample in terms of gender, years of education, and preretirement occupation. *Assessment*, *2*, 225–231.

Ryan, J.J., Weilage, M.E., Lopez, S.J., Paolo, A.M., Miller, D.A., & Morris, J. (1997). Application of the seven subtest short form of the WAIS-R in African Americans with brain damage. *Journal of Psychoeducational Assessment*, *15*, 314–321.

Ryan, J.J., Weilage, M.E., Paolo, A.M., Miller, D.A., & Morris, J. (1998). Utility of the seven subtest short form in a female sample with brain damage. *International Journal of Neuroscience*, *93*, 197–203.

Ryckman, D.B., Rentfrow, R., Fargo, G., & McCartin, R. (1972). Reliabilities of three tests of form copying. *Perceptual and Motor Skills, 34*, 917–918.

Sackett, P.R., & Wilk, S.L. (1994). Within-group norming and other forms of score adjustment in preemployment testing. *American Psychologist, 49*, 929–954.

Sacks, T.L., Clark, C.R., & Geffen, L.B. (1991). Comparability and stability of six alternate forms of the Dodrill–Stroop Colour–Word Test. *The Clinical Neuropsychologist, 5*, 220–225.

Sahgal, A., McKeith, I.G., Galloway, P.H., Tasker, N., & Steckler, T. (1995). Do differences in visuospatial ability between senile dementia of the Alzheimer's and Lewy body types reflect differences solely in mnemonic function? *Journal of Clinical and Experimental Neuropsychology, 17*, 35–43.

Saklofske, D.H., Schwean, V.L., Yakulic, R.A., & Quinn, D. (1994). WISC-III and S-B: FE performance of children with attention deficit hyperactivity disorder. *Canadian Journal of School Psychology, 10*, 167–171.

Salmon, D.P., Kow-on-Yuen, P.F., Henidel, W.C., Butters, N., & Thal, L.J. (1989). Differentiation of Alzheimer's disease and Huntington's disease with the Dementia Rating Scale. *Archives of Neurology, 46*, 1204–1208.

Salthouse, T.A. (1998). Independence of age-related influences on cognitive abilities across the life-span. *Developmental Psychology, 34*, 851–864.

Salvia, J. (1969). Four tests of color vision: A study of diagnostic accuracy with the mentally retarded. *American Journal of Mental Deficiency, 74*, 421–427.

Salvia, J., & Ysseldyke, J. (1972). Criterion validity of four tests for red–green color blindness. *American Journal of Mental Deficiency, 76*, 418–422.

Samuels, I., Butters, N., & Fedio, P. (1972). Short term memory disorders following temporal lobe removals in humans. *Cortex, 8*, 283–298.

Sand, P.L. (1973). Performance of medical patient groups with and without brain-damage on the Hovey (O) and Watson (SC-O) MMPI scales. *Journal of Clinical Psychology, 29*, 235–237.

Sanner, R., & McManis, D.L. (1978). Concurrent validity of the Peabody Individual Achievement Test and the Wide Range Achievement Test for middle-class elementary school children. *Psychological Reports, 42*, 19–24.

Sapp, G.L., Abbott, G., Hinckley, R., & Rowell, A. (1997). Examination of the validity of the WISC-III with urban exceptional students. *Psychological Reports, 81*, 1163–1168.

Satterfield, W.A., Martin, C.W., & Leiker, M. (1994). A comparison of four WAIS-R short forms in patients referred for psychological/neuropsychological assessments. *Journal of Psychoeducational Assessment, 12*, 364–371.

Sattler, J., & Atkinson, L. (1993). Item equivalence across scales: The WPPSI-R and WISC-III. *Psychological Assessment, 5*, 203–206.

Sattler, J.M., & Feldman, G.I. (1981). Comparisons of 1965, 1976, and 1978 norms for the Wide Range Achievement Test. *Psychological Reports, 49*, 115–118.

Sattler, J., & Gwynne, J. (1982a). Ethnicity and Bender Visual Motor Gestalt test performance. *Journal of School Psychology, 20*, 13–26.

Sattler, J.M., & Gwynne, J. (1982b). White examiners do not impede the intelligence test performance of black children: To debunk a myth. *Journal of Consulting and Clinical Psychology, 50*, 196–208.

Satz, P. (1966). A block rotation task: The application of multivariate and decision theory analysis for the prediction of organic brain damage. *Psychological Monographs: General and Applied, 80* (No. 269).

Satz, P., Fennell, E., & Reilly, C. (1970). Predictive validity of six neurodiagnostic tests: A decision theory analysis. *Journal of Consulting and Clinical Psychology, 34*, 375–381.

Savage, R.M., & Gouvier, W.D. (1992). Rey Auditory–Verbal Learning Test: The effects of age and gender, and norms for delayed recall and story recognition trials. *Archives of Clinical Neuropsychology, 7*, 407–414.

Sawicki, R.F., & Golden, C.J. (1984a). Multivariate techniques in neuropsychology: 1. Comparison of orthogonal rotation methods with the receptive scale of the Luria–Nebraska Neuropsychological Battery. *International Journal of Clinical Neuropsychology, 6*, 126–134.

Sawicki, R.F., & Golden, C.J. (1984b). The profile elevation scale and impairment scale: Two new summary scales for the Luria–Nebraska Neuropsychological Battery. *International Journal of Neuroscience, 23*, 81–90.

Sawrie, S.M., Chelune, G.J., Naugle, R.I., & Luders, H.O. (1996). Empirical methods for assessing meaningful neuropsychological change following epilepsy surgery. *Journal of the International Neuropsychological Society, 2*, 556–564.

Sawyer, R.N., Stanley, G.E., & Watson, T.E. (1979). A factor analytic study of the construct validity of the Pictorial Test of Intelligence. *Educational and Psychological Measurement, 39*, 613–622.

Sbordone, R.J., & Long, C.J. (1996). *Ecological validity of neuropsychological testing*. Del Ray Beach, FL: GR Press/St. Lucie Press.

Schagen, S., Schmand, B., de Sterke, S., & Lindeboom, J. (1997). Amsterdam short-term memory test: A new procedure for the detection of feigned memory deficits. *Journal of Clinical and Experimental Neuropsychology, 19*, 43–51.

Schear, J.M., & Croft, R.B. (1989). Examination of the concurrent validity of the California Verbal Learning Test. *The Clinical Neuropsychologist, 3*, 162–168.

Schear, J.M., Harrison, W.R., & Sherman, C.J. (1987). Estimating WAIS IQ of neuropsychiatric patients at three educational levels. *Psychological Reports, 58*, 947–950.

Schinka, J.A. (1995). Personality Assessment Inventory scale characteristics and factor structure in the assessment of alcohol dependency, *Journal of Personality Assessment, 64*, 101–111.

Schinka, J.A., & LaLone, L. (1997). MMPI-2 norms: Comparisons with a census-matched subsample. *Psychological Assessment, 9*, 307–311.

Schinka, J.A., Vanderploeg, R.D., & Greblo, P. (1998). Frequency of WISC-III and WAIS-R pairwise subtest differences. *Psychological Assessment, 10*, 171–175.

Schlosser, D., & Ivison, D. (1989). Assessing memory deterioration with the Wechsler Memory Scale, the National Adult Reading Test, and the Schonell Graded Reading Test. *Journal of Clinical and Experimental Neuropsychology, 11*, 785–792.

Schlottmann, R.S., & Johnsen, D.E. (1991). The Intellectual Correlates Scale and the prediction of premorbid intelligence in brain-damage adults. *Archives of Clinical Neuropsychology, 6*, 363–374.

Schludermann, E.H., Schludermann, S.M., Merryman, P.W., & Brown, B.W. (1983). Halstead's studies in the neuropsychology of aging. *Archives of Gerontology and Geriatrics, 2*, 49–172.

Schmand, B., Geerlings, M.I., Jonker, C., & Lindeboom, J. (1998). Reading ability as an estimator of premorbid intelligence: Does it remain stable in emergent dementia? *Journal of Clinical and Experimental Neuropsychology, 20*, 42–51.

Schmidt, I.W., Brouwer, W.H., Vanier, M., & Kemp, F. (1996). Flexible adaption to change task demands in severe closed head injury patients: A driving simulator study. *Applied Neuropsychology, 3*, 155–165.

Schmidt, M., Trueblood, W., Durham, L., & Merwon, M. (1994). How much do "Attention" tests tell us? *Archives of Clinical Neuropsychology, 9*, 383–394.

Schmidt, R., Freidl, W. Fazekas, F., Reinhart, P., Greishofer, P., Koch, M., Eber, B., Schumacher, M., Polmin, K., & Lechner, H. (1994). The Mattis Dementia Rating Scale: Normative data from 1,001 healthy volunteers. *Neurology, 44*, 964–966.

Schneider, M.A., & Spivack, G. (1979). An investigative study of the Bender–Gestalt: Clinical validation of its use in a reading disabled population. *Journal of Clinical Psychology, 35*, 346–351.

Schonell, F.J. (1942). *Backwardness in the basic subjects*. Edinburgh: Oliver & Boyd.

Schreiber, D.J., Goldman, H., Kleinman, K.M., Goldfader, P.R., & Snow, M.Y. (1976). The relationship between independent neuropsychological and neurological detection and localization of cerebral impairment. *Journal of Nervous and Mental Disease, 162*, 360–365.

Schretlen, D., & Ivnik, R.J. (1996). Prorating IQ scores for older adults: Validation of a seven-subtest WAIS-R with the Mayo Older Americans Normative Sample. *Assessment, 3*, 411–416.

Schretlen, D., Benedict, R.H.B., & Bobholz, J.H. (1994). Composite reliability and standard errors of measurement for a seven subtest short form of the Wechsler Adult Intelligence Scale-Revised. *Psychological Assessment, 6*, 188–190.

Schuerger, J.M., & Witt, A.C. (1989). The temporal stability of individually tested intelligence. *Journal of Clinical Psychology, 45*, 294–302.

Schultz, E.E., Keesler, T.Y., Friedenberg, L., & Sciara, A.D. (1984). Limitations in equivalence of alternate subtests for Russell's revision of the Wechsler Memory Scale: Causes and solutions. *Journal of Clinical Neuropsychology, 6*, 220–223.

Schultz, M.K. (1997). WISC-III and WJ-R Tests of Achievement: Concurrent validity and learning disability identification. *Journal of Special Education, 31*, 377–386.

Schultz, R.T., Carter, A.S., Gladstone, M., Scahill, L., Leckman, J.F., Peterson, B.S., Zhang, H., Cohen, D.J., & Pauls, D. (1998). Visual-motor integration functioning in children with Tourette's syndrome. *Neuropsychology, 12*, 134–145.

Schum, R.L., & Sivan, A.B. (1997). Verbal abilities in healthy elderly adults. *Applied Neuropsychology, 4*, 133–134.

Schutz, S.R., & Keisler, E.R. (1972). Young children's immediate memory of word classes in relation to social class. *Journal of Verbal Learning and Verbal Behavior, 11,* 13–17.

Schwamm, L.H., Van Dyke, C., Kiernan, R.J., Merrin, E.L., & Mueller, J. (1987). The Neurobehavioral Cognitive Status Examination: Comparison with the CCSE and MMSE in a neurosurgical population. *Archives of Internal Medicine, 107,* 486–491.

Schwarting, F.G., & Schwarting, K.R. (1977). The relationship of the WISC-R and WRAT: A study based upon a selected population. *Psychology in the Schools, 14,* 431–433.

Schwartz, M.S. (1969). "Organicity" and the MMPI 1-3-9 and 2-9 codes. Proceedings, 77th Annual Convention, American Psychological Association.

Schwartz, M.S., & Brown, J.R. (1973). MMPI differentiation on multiple sclerosis vs. pseudoneurologic patients. *Journal of Clinical Psychology, 29,* 471–474.

Schwartz, S., & Wiedel, T.C. (1981). Incremental validity of the MMPI in neurological decisionmaking. *Journal of Personality Assessment, 45,* 424–426.

Schwenn, E., & Postman, L. (1967). Studies of learning to learn. *Journal of Verbal Learning and Verbal Behavior, 6,* 566–573.

Scott, J.A., Krull, K.R., Williamson, D.J.G., Adams, R.L., & Iverson, G.L. (1997). Oklahoma Premorbid Intelligence Estimation (OPIE): Utilization in clinical samples. *The Clinical Neuropsychologist, 11,* 146–154.

Scott, L.H. (1981). Measuring intelligence with the Goodenough–Harris Drawing Test. *Psychological Bulletin, 89,* 483–505.

Scott, W.A. (1955). Reliability of content analysis: The case of nominal scale coding. *Public Opinion Quarterly, 19,* 321–325.

Scruggs, T.E., Mastropieri, M.A., & Argulewicz, E.D. (1983). Stability of performance on the PPVT-R for three ethnic groups attending a bilingual kindergarten. *Psychology in the Schools, 20,* 433–435.

Sechrest, L. (1963). Incremental validity: A recommendation. *Educational and Psychological Measurement, 23,* 153–158.

Seidel, W.T. (1994). Applicability of the Hooper Visual Organization Test to pediatric populations. *The Clinical Neuropsychologist, 8,* 59–68.

Seidenberg, M., Taylor, M.A., & Haltiner, A. (1994). Personality and self-report of cognitive functioning. *Archives of Clinical Neuropsychology, 9,* 353–361.

Seidman, L.J., Biederman, J., Faraone, S.V., Weber, W., & Ouelette, C. (1997). Toward defining a neuropsychology of attention deficit-hyperactivity disorder: Performance of children and adolescents from a large clinically referred sample. *Journal of Consulting and Clinical Psychology, 65,* 150–160.

Selby, M.J., Ling, N., Williams, J.M., & Dawson, A. (1998). Interferon beta 1-B in verbal memory functioning of patients with relapsing-remitting multiple sclerosis. *Perceptual and Motor Skills, 86,* 1099–1106.

Selnes, O.A., Jacobson, L., Machado, A.M., Becker, J.T. , Welsch, J., Miller, E.N., Viscsher, B., & McArthur, J.C. (1991). Normative data for a brief neuropsychological screening battery. *Perceptual and Motor Skills, 73,* 539–550.

Semrud-Clikeman, M., Hynd, G.W., Lorys, A.R., & Lahey, B.B. (1993). Differential diagnosis of children with ADHD and ADHD/co-occurring conduct disorder. *School Psychology International, 14,* 361–370.

Sewell, T.E. (1977). A comparison of the WPPSI and Stanford–Binet Intelligence Scale (1972) among lower SES black children. *Psychology in the Schools, 14,* 158–161.

Shah, A., & Holmes, N. (1985). The use of the Leiter International Performance Scale with autistic children. *Journal of Autism and Developmental Disorders, 15,* 195–203.

Shapiro, D.M., & Harrison, D.W. (1990). Alternate forms of the AVLT: A procedure and test for form equivalence. *Archives of Clinical Neuropsychology, 5,* 405–410.

Shapiro, D.M., & Simpson, R.G. (1994). Patterns and predictors of performance on the Bender–Gestalt and the Developmental Test of Visual Motor Integration in a sample of behaviorally and emotionally disturbed adolescents. *Journal of Psychoeducational Assessment, 12,* 254–263.

Sharp, H.C. (1958). A note on the reliability of the Leiter International Performance Scale 1948 Revision. *Journal of Consulting Psychology, 22,* 230.

Sharpe, K., & O'Carroll, (1991). Estimating premorbid intellectual level in dementia using the National Adult Reading Test: A Canadian study. *British Journal of Clinical Psychology, 30,* 381–384.

Shavelson, R.J., & Webb, N.M. (1991). *Generalizablity theory: A primer.* Newbury Park, CA: Sage.

Shaw, D.J. (1966). The reliability and validity of the Halstead Category Test. *Journal of Clinical Psychology, 20,* 176–180.

Shaw, F.J., & Matthews, C.G. (1965). Differential MMPI performance of brain-damaged versus pseudo-neurologic groups. *Journal of Clinical Psychology, 21*, 405–408.

Shay, K.A., Duke, L.W., Conboy, T., Harrell, L.E., Callaway, R., & Folks, D.G. (1991). The clinical validity of the Mattis Dementia Rating Scale in staging Alzheimer's disease. *Journal of Geriatric Psychiatry and Neurology, 4*, 18–25.

Shearn, C.R., Berry, D.F., & Fitzgibbons, D.J. (1974). Usefulness of the Memory For Designs Test in assessing mild organic complications in psychiatric patients. *Perceptual and Motor Skills, 38*, 1099–1104.

Shelley, C., & Goldstein, G. (1982). Psychometric relations between the Luria–Nebraska and Halstead–Reitan Neuropsychological Batteries in a neuropsychiatric setting. *Clinical Neuropsychology, 4*, 128–133.

Shelley, C., & Goldstein, G. (1983). Discrimination of chronic schizophrenia and brain damage with the Luria–Nebraska Neuropsychological Battery: A partially successful replication. *Clinical Neuropsychology, 5*, 82–85.

Shepard, L.A. (1982). Definitions of bias. In R.A. Berk (Ed.), *Handbook of methods for detecting test bias* (pp. 9–30). Baltimore, MD: Johns Hopkins University Press.

Sherer, M., & Adams, R.L. (1993). Cross-validation of Reitan and Wolfson's neuropsychological deficit scales. *Archives of Clinical Neuropsychology, 8*, 429–435.

Sherer, M., Scott, J.G., Parsons, O.A., & Adams, R.L. (1994). Relative sensitivity of the WAIS-R subtests and selected HRNB measures to the effects of brain damage. *Archives of Clinical Neuropsychology, 9*, 427–436.

Sherman, A.M., & Massman, P.J. (1999). Prevalence and correlates of category versus letter fluency discrepancies in Alzheimer's disease. *Archives of Clinical Neuropsychology, 14*, 411–418.

Sherman, M.S., Strauss, E., Spellacy, F., & Hunter, M. (1995). Construct validity of WAIS-R: Neuropsychological test correlates in adults referred for evaluation of possible head injury. *Psychological Assessment, 7*, 440–444.

Sherman, M.S., Strauss, E., & Spellacy, F. (1997). Validity of the Paced Auditory Serial Addition Test (PASAT) in adults referred for neuropsychological assessment after head injury. *The Clinical Neuropsychologist, 11*, 34–45.

Sheslow, D., & Adams, W. (1990). *Wide range assessment of memory and learning.* Wilmington, DE: Jastak.

Shichita, K., Hatano, S., Ohashi, Y., Shibata, H., & Matuzaki, T. (1986). Memory changes in the Benton Visual Retention Test between ages 70 and 75. *Journal of Gerontology, 41*, 385–386.

Shores, E.A., & Carstairs, J.R. (1998). Accuracy of the MMPI-2 computerized Minnesota Report in identifying fake-good and fake-bad response sets. *The Clinical Neuropsychologist, 12*, 101–106.

Short-DeGraff, M.A., & Holan, S. (1992). Self-drawing as a gauge of perceptual-motor skill. *Physical and Occupational Therapy in Pediatrics, 12*, 53–68.

Short-DeGraff, M.A., Slansky, L., & Diamond, K.E. (1989). Validity of pre-schoolers' self-drawings as an index of human figure drawing performance. *Journal of Clinical Psychology, 9*, 305–315.

Shukla, V., Tripathi, R.R., & Dhar, N.K. (1987). Validation of Pitrowski's Rorchach signs of "organicity" against Bender Visual Motor Gestalt test. *Indian Journal of Clinical Psychology, 14*, 84–86.

Shum, D.H.K., Murray, R.A., & Eadie, K. (1997). Effect of speed of presentation on administration of the Logical Memory subtest of the Wechsler Memory Scale-Revised. *The Clinical Neuropsychologist, 11*, 188–191.

Shuttleworth-Jordan, A.B. (1997). Age and education effects on brain-damaged subjects: "Negative" findings revisited. *The Clinical Neuropsychologist, 11*, 205–209.

Siegel, D.J., & Piotrowski, R.J. (1994). Reliability of WISC-III subtest composites. *Assessment, 1*, 249–253.

Sigmon, S.B. (1983). Performance of American school children on Raven's Progressive Matrices scale. *Perceptual and Motor Skills, 56*, 484–486.

Silberstein, R.B., Ciorciari, J., & Pipingas, A. (1995). Steady-state visually evoked potential topography during the Wisconsin Card Sorting Test. *Electroencephalography and Clinical Neurophysiology, 96*, 24–35.

Silverman, A.B. (1991). Reliability of score differences on Wechsler's intelligence scales. *Journal of Clinical Psychology, 47*, 264–266.

Silverstein, A.B. (1962). Perceptual, motor, and memory functions in the Visual Retention Test. *American Journal of Mental Deficiency, 66*, 613–617.

Silverstein, A.B. (1963). Qualitative aspects of performance on the Visual Retention Test. *American Journal of Mental Deficiency, 68*, 109–113.

Silverstein, A.B. (1980). A comparison of the 1976 and 1978 norms for the WRAT. *Psychology in the Schools, 17*, 313–315.

Silverstein, A.B. (1982a). Pattern analysis as simultaneous statistical inference. *Journal of Consulting and Clinical Psychology, 50*, 234–240.

Silverstein, A.B. (1982b). Factor structure of the Wechsler Adult Intelligence Scale-Revised. *Journal of Consulting and Clinical Psychology, 50,* 661–664.

Silverstein, A.B. (1985). Two- and four-subtest short forms of the WAIS-R: A closer look at validity and reliability. *Journal of Clinical Psychology, 41,* 95–97.

Silverstein, A.B. (1987). Equal weighting vs. differential weighting of subtest scores on short forms of Wechsler's intelligence scales. *Journal of Clinical Psychology, 43,* 714–720.

Silverstein, A.B. (1990a). Critique of a Doppelt-type short form of the WAIS-R. *Journal of Clinical Psychology, 46,* 333–339.

Silverstein, A.B. (1990b). Notes on the reliability of Wechsler short forms. *Journal of Clinical Psychology, 46,* 194–196.

Silverstein, A.B. (1991). Reliability of score differences on Wechsler's intelligence scales. *Journal of Clinical Psychology, 47,* 264–266.

Silverstein, M.L., McDonald, C., & Meltzer, H.Y. (1988). Differential patterns of neuropsychological deficit in psychiatric disorders. *Journal of Clinical Neuropsychology, 44,* 412–415.

Silverstein, S.M., Osborn, L.M., & Palumbo, D.R. (1998). Rey–Osterrieth Complex Figure Test performance in acute, chronic, and remitted schizophrenic patients. *Journal of Clinical Psychology, 54,* 985–994.

Simon, C.L., & Clopton, J.R. (1984). Comparison of WAIS- and WAIS-R scores of mildly and moderately retarded adults. *American Journal of Mental Deficiency, 89,* 301–303.

Simon, M.J. (1995). Relationship between the Quick Test and WAIS-R in low-functioning criminal defendants. *Psychological Reports, 77,* 1001–1002.

Simpson, R.G. (1982). Correlation between the General Information Subtest of the Peabody Individual Achievement Test and the Full Scale Intelligence Quotient of the WISC-R. *Educational and Psychological Measurement, 42,* 685–699.

Sinnett, E.R., Holen, M.C., & Davie, M.J. (1988). Quick Test scores among persons over sixty. *Psychological Reports, 62,* 397–398.

Siskind, G. (1976). Hovey's 5-item MMPI scale and psychiatric patients. *Journal of Clinical Psychology, 32,* 50.

Sivan, A.B. (1992). *Benton Visual Retention Test* (5th ed.). San Antonio, TX: The Psychological Corporation.

Ska, B., Poissant, A., & Joanette, Y. (1990). Line orientation judgment in normal elderly and subjects with dementia of the Alzheimer's type. *Journal of Clinical and Experimental Neuropsychology, 12,* 695–702.

Skillbeck, C.E., & Woods, R.T. (1980). The factorial structure of the Wechsler Memory Scale: Samples of neuropsychological and psychogeriatric patients. *Journal of Clinical Neuropsychology, 2,* 293–300.

Skillman, G., Dabbs, P., Mitchell, M., McGrath, M., Lewis, J. & Brems, C. (1992). Appropriateness of the Draw-A-Person test with Alaskan Native populations. *Journal of Clinical Psychology, 48,* 561–564.

Slate, J.R. (1995). Two investigations of the validity of the WISC-III. *Psychological Reports, 76,* 299–306.

Slate, J.R., & Jones, C.H. (1995). Preliminary evidence of the validity of the WISC-III for African American students undergoing special education evaluation. *Educational and Psychological Measurement, 55,* 1039–1046.

Slate, J.R., Jones, C.H., Graham, L.S., & Bower, J. (1994). Correlations of WISC-III, WRAT-R, KM-R, and PPVT-R scores in students with specific learning disabilities. *Learning Disabilities Research, and Practice, 9,* 104–107.

Slate, J.R., Graham, L.S., & Bower, J. (1996). Relationships of the WISC-R and K-BIT for an adolescent clinical sample. *Adolescence, 31,* 777–782.

Slater, E.J., & VanWagoner, S.L. (1988). Validity and utility of WAIS-R and WISC-R short forms with adolescents recovering from closed head injury. *Journal of Adolescent Research, 3,* 217–225.

Slick, D.J., Hopp, G., Strauss, E., & Spellacy, F.J. (1996). Victoria Symptom Validity Test: Efficiency for detecting feigned memory impairment and relationship to neuropsychological tests and MMPI-2 validity scales. *Journal of Clinical and Experimental Neuropsychology, 18,* 911–922.

Slick, D., Iverson, G.L., & Franzen, M. (1996, August). Evaluation of Wechsler Memory Scale-Revised savings scores in a sample of substance-abuse inpatients. Paper presented at the XXVI International Congress of Psychology, Montreal, Canada.

Sliwinski, M., Buschke, H., Stewart, W.F., Masur, D., & Lipton, R.B. (1997). The effect of dementia risk factors on comparative and diagnostic selective reminding norms. *Journal of the International Neuropsychological Society, 3,* 317–326.

Slosson, R.L. (1963). *Slosson Intelligence Test for Children and Adults.* East Aurora, NY: Slosson.

Small, J.G., Milstein, V., & Stevens, J.R. (1962). Are psychomotor epileptics different? A controlled study. *Archives of Neurology, 7,* 187–194.

Smirni, P., Villardita, C., & Zappala, G. (1983). Influence of different paths on spatial memory performance in the Block Tapping Test. *Journal of Clinical Neuropsychology, 5,* 355–359.

Smith, A. (1960). Changes in Porteus Maze scores of brain operated schizophrenics after an eight year interval. *The Journal of Mental Science, 106,* 967–978.

Smith, A., & Kinder, E.F. (1959). Changes in psychological test performances of brain-operated schizophrenics after eight years. *Science, 129,* 149–150.

Smith, G.E., Ivnik, R.J., Malec, J.F., & Tangalos, E.G. (1993). Factor structure of the Mayo Older Americans Normative Sample (MOANS) core battery: Replication in a clinical sample. *Psychological Assessment, 5,* 121–124.

Smith, G.E., Bohac, D.L., Ivnik, R.J., & Malec, J.F. (1997a). Using word recognition tests to estimate premorbid IQ in early dementia: Longitudinal data. *Journal of the International Neuropsychological Society, 3,* 528–533.

Smith, G.E., Wong, J.S., Ivnik, R.J., & Malec, J.F. (1997b). Mayo's Older American Normative Studies: Separate norms for WMS-R logical memory stories. *Assessment, 4,* 79–86.

Smith, R.S. (1983). A comparison of the Wechsler Adult Intelligence Scale and the Wechsler Adult Intelligence Scale-Revised in a college population. *Journal of Consulting and Clinical Psychology, 51,* 414–419.

Smith, S.T., Mann, V.A., & Shankweiler, D. (1986). Spoken sentence comprehension by good and poor readers: A study with the Token Test. *Cortex, 22,* 627–632.

Smith, T.C., Smith, B.L., & Dobbs, K. (1991). Relationship between the Peabody Picture Vocabulary Test-Revised, Wide Range Achievement Test-Revised, and the Wechsler Intelligence Scale for Children-Revised. *Journal of School Psychology, 29,* 53–56.

Smith-Seemiller, L., Franzen, M.D., & Bowers, D. (1997). Use of Wisconsin Card Sorting Test short forms in clinical samples. *The Clinical Neuropsychologist, 11,* 421–427.

Snitz, B.E., Roman, D.D., & Beniak, T.E. (1996). Efficacy of the Continuous Visual Memory Test in lateralizing temporal lobe dysfunction in chronic complex-partial epilepsy. *Journal of Clinical and Experimental Neuropsychology, 18,* 747–754.

Snow, J.H. (1998). Clinical use of the Benton Visual Retention Test for children and adolescents with learning disabilities. *Archives of Clinical Neuropsychology, 13,* 629–636.

Snow, J.H., Hynd, G.W., Hartlage, L.C., & Grant, D.H. (1983). The relationship between the Luria–Nebraska Neuropsychological Battery-Children's Revision and the Minnesota Percepto-Diagnostic Test with learning disabled students. *Psychology in the Schools, 20,* 415–419.

Snow, W.G., Freedman, L., & Ford, L. (1986). Lateralized brain damage, sex differences, and the Wechsler Scales: A reexamination of the literature. *Journal of Clinical and Experimental Neuropsychology, 8,* 179–189.

Snow, W.G., Tierney, M.C., Zorzitto, M.L., Fisher, R.H., & Reid, D.W. (1989). WAIS-R test–retest reliability in a normal elderly sample. *Journal of Clinical and Experimental Neuropsychology, 11,* 423–428.

Sobotka, K.R., & Black, F.W. (1978). A procedure for the rapid computation of WISC-R factor scores. *Journal of Clinical Psychology, 34,* 117–119.

Soethe, J.W. (1972). Concurrent validity of the Peabody Individual Achievement Test. *Journal of Learning Disabilities, 5,* 47–49.

Soukup, V.M., Ingram, F., Grady, J.J., & Scheiss, M.C. (1998). Trail Making Test: Issues in normative data selection. *Applied Neuropsychology, 5,* 65–73.

Spangler, R.S., & Sabatino, D.A. (1995). Temporal stability of gifted children's intelligence. *Roeper Review, 17,* 207–210.

Spellacy, F.J., & Spreen, O. (1969). A short form of the Token Test. *Cortex, 5,* 390–397.

Spiers, P.A. (1981). Have they come to praise Luria or to bury him? The Luria–Nebraska Neuropsychological Battery controversy. *Journal of Consulting and Clinical Psychology, 49,* 331–341.

Spiers, P.A. (1982). The Luria–Nebraska Neuropsychological Battery revisited: A theory in practice or just practicing? *Journal of Consulting and Clinical Psychology, 50,* 301–306.

Spiers, P.A. (1984). What more can I say? In reply to Hutchinson, one last comment from Spiers. *Journal of Consulting and Clinical Psychology, 52,* 546–552.

Spikman, J.M., van Zomeran, A.H., & Deelman, B.G. (1996). Deficits of attention after closed-head injury: Slowness only? *Journal of Clinical and Experimental Neuropsychology, 18,* 755–767.

Spillane, M.M., Ross, K.K., & Vasa, S.F. (1996). A comparison of eye-gaze and standard response mode on the PPVT-R. *Psychology in the Schools, 33*, 265–271.

Spitzform, M. (1982). Normative data in the elderly on Luria–Nebraska Neuropsychological Battery. *Clinical Neuropsychology, 4*, 103–105.

Spreen, O., & Benton, A.L. (1963). Sentence Repetition Test: Administration, scoring, and preliminary norms. Unpublished manuscript, University of Iowa.

Spreen, O., & Gaddes, W.H. (1969). Developmental norms for 15 neuropsychological tests, ages 6 to 15. *Cortex, 5*, 171–191.

Spreen, O., & Strauss, E. (1998). *A compendium of neuropsychological tests: Administration, norms, and commmentary*. New York: Oxford University Press.

Spruill, J. (1996). Composite SAS of the Stanford–Binet Intelligence Scale: Is it determined by only one area SAS? *Psychological Assessment, 8*, 328–330.

Spruill, J., & Beck, B. (1986). Relationship between the WAIS-R and Wide Range Achievement Test-Revised. *Educational and Psychological Measurement, 46*, 1037–1040.

Stallings, G., Boake, C., & Sherer, M. (1995). Comparison of the California Verbal Learning Test and the Rey Auditory Verbal Learning Test in head-injured patients. *Journal of Clinical and Experimental Neuropsychology, 17*, 706–712.

Stambrook, M.S. (1983). The Luria–Nebraska Neuropsychological Battery: A promise that may be only partly fulfilled. *Journal of Clinical Neuropsychology, 5*, 247–269.

Stanczak, D.E., Lynch, M.D., McNeil, C.K., & Brown, B. (1998). The expanded Trail Making Test: Rationale, development, and psychometric properties. *Archives of Clinical Neuropsychology, 13*, 473–487.

Starr, J.M., Whalley, L.J., Inch, S., & Shering, P.A. (1992). The quantification of the relative effects of age and BART-predicted IQ on cognitive function in healthy old people. *International Journal of Geriatric Psychiatry, 7*, 153–157.

Stebbins, G.T., Gilley, D.W., Wilson, R.S., Bernard, B.A., & Fox, J.H. (1990). Effects of language disturbance in permorbid estimates of IQ in mild dementia. *The Clinical Neuropsychologist, 4*, 18–24.

Stein, L.A.R., & Graham, J.R. (1999). Detecting fake-good MMPI-A profiles in a correctional facility. *Psychological Assessment, 11*, 386–395.

Stein, L.A.R., McClinton, B.K., & Graham, J.R. (1998). Long-term stability of MMPI-A scales. *Journal of Personality Assessment, 70*, 103–108.

Stein, L.A.R., Graham, J.R., Ben-Porath, Y.S., & McNulty, J.L. (1999). Using the MMPI-2 to detect substance abuse in an outpatient mental health setting. *Psychological Assessment, 11*, 94–100.

Stein, S. (1972). Psychometric test performance in relation to the psychopathology of epilepsy. *Archives of General Psychiatry, 26*, 532–538.

Steinmeyer, C.H. (1986). A meta-analysis of Halstead–Reitan test performance of non-brain damaged subjects. *Archives of Clinical Neuropsychology, 1*, 301–308.

Stern, R.A., Singer, E.A., Duke, L.M., Singer, N.G., Morey, C.E., Daughtrey, E.W., & Kaplan, E. (1994). The Boston Qualitative scoring system for the Rey–Osterrieth Complex Figure: Description and interrater reliability. *The Clinical Neuropsychologist, 8*, 309–322.

Sternberg, D.E., & Jarvik, M.E. (1976). Memory functions in depression: Improvement with antidepressant medication. *Archives of General Psychiatry, 33*, 219–224.

Sterne, D.M. (1966). The Knox Cube Test as a test of memory and intelligence with male adults. *Journal of Clinical Psychology, 22*, 191–193.

Sterne, D.M. (1973). The Hooper Visual Organization Test and the Trail Making Test as discriminants of brain injury. *Journal of Clinical Psychology, 29*, 212–213.

Stevenson, J.D. (1986). Alternate form reliability and concurrent validity of the PPVT-R for referred rehabilitation agency adults. *Journal of Clinical Psychology, 42*, 650–653.

Stewart, K.D., & Jones, E.C. (1976). Validity of the Slosson Intelligence Test: A ten year review. *Psychology in the Schools, 13*, 372–380.

Stinnett, J.L., & DiGiacomo, J.N. (1970). Daily administered unilateral ECT. *Biological Psychiatry, 3*, 303–306.

Stone, B.J., Gridely, B.E., & Gyurke, J.S. (1991). Confirmatory factor analysis of the WPPSI-R at the extreme ends of the age range. *Journal of Psychoeducational Assessment, 9*, 263–270.

Stone, M.H., & Wright, B.D. (1980). *Knox's Cube Test* (manual). Chicago: Stoelting.

Stoner, S.B. (1981). Alternate form reliability of the Revised Peabody Picture Vocabulary Test for Head Start children. *Psychological Reports, 49*, 628.

Tröester, A.I., Butters, N., Salmon, D.P., Cullum, C.M., Jacobs, D., Brandt, J., & White, R.F. (1993). The diagnostic utility of savings scores: Differentiating Alzheimer's and Huntington's diseases with the logical memory and visual reproduction tests. *Journal of Clinical and Experimental Neuropsychology, 15*, 773–788.

Trosset, M.W., & Kazniak, A.W. (1996) Measures of deficit unawareness for predicted performance experiments. *Journal of the International Neuropsychological Society, 2*, 315–322.

Troyer, A.K., Fisk, J.D., Archibald, C.J., Ritvo, P.G., & Murray, T.J. (1996). Conceptual reasoning as a mediator of verbal recall in patients with multiple sclerosis. *Journal of Clinical and Experimental Neuropsychology, 18*, 211–219.

Troyer, A.K., Moscovitch, M., & Winocur, G. (1997). Clustering and switching as two components of verbal fluency: Evidence from younger and older healthy adults. *Neuropsychology, 11*, 138–146.

Troyer, A.K., & Wishart, H.A. (1997). A comparison of qualitative scoring systems for the Rey–Osterrieth Complex Figure Test. *The Clinical Neuropsychologist, 11*, 381–390.

Trueblood, W., & Binder, L.M. (1997). Psychologists' accuracy in identifying neuropsychological test protocols of clinical malingerers. *Archives of Clinical Neuropsychology, 12*, 13–27.

Trueblood, W., & Schmidt, M. (1993). Malingering and other validity considerations in the neuropsychological evaluation of mild head injury. *Journal of Clinical and Experimental Neuropsychology, 15*, 578–590.

Trueman, M., Lynch, A., & Branthwaite, A. (1984). A factor analytic study of the McCarthy Scales of Children's Abilities. *British Journal of Educational Psychology, 54*, 331–335.

Tsushima, W.T. (1994). Short form of the WPPSI and WPPSI-R. *Journal of Clinical Psychology, 50*, 877–880.

Tsushima, W.T., & Newbill, W. (1996). Effects of headaches during neuropsychological testing of mild head injury patients. *Headache, 36*, 613–615.

Tsushima, W.T., & Wedding, D.A. (1979). A comparison of the Halstead–Reitan Neuropsychological Battery and computerized tomography in the identification of brain disorder. *Journal of Nervous and Mental Disease, 167*, 704–707.

Tulving, E. (1972). Episodic and semantic memory. In E. Tulving & W. Donaldson (Eds.), *Organization of memory* (pp. 381–403). New York: Academic Press.

Tuokko, H., & Crockett, D. (1987). Central cholinergic deficiency WAIS profiles in a nondemented sample. *Journal of Clinical and Experimental Neuropsychology, 9*, 224–227.

Tuokko, H., & Woodward, T.S. (1996). Development and validation of a demographic correction system for neuropsychological measures used in the Canadian Study of Health and Aging. *Journal of Clinical and Experimental Neuropsychology, 18*, 479–616.

Tupa, D.J., Wright, M.O'D., & Fristad, M.A. (1997). Confirmatory factor analysis of the WISC-III with child psychiatric inpatients. *Psychological Assessment, 9*, 302–306.

Tupper, D.E. (1990). Some observations on the use of the Woodcock–Johnson Tests of Cognitive Ability in adults with head injury. *Journal of Learning Disabilities, 23*, 306–310.

Tuppler, L.A., Coffey, C.E., Logue, P.E., Djang, W.T., & Fagan, S. (1992). Neuropsychological importance of subcortical white matter hyperintensity. *Archives of Neurology, 49*, 1248–1252.

Tuppler, L.A., Welsch, K.A., Asare-Aboagye, Y., & Dawson, D.V. (1995). Reliability of the Rey–Osterrieth Complex Figure in use with memory-impaired patients. *Journal of Clinical and Experimental Neuropsychology, 17*, 566–579.

Tymchuk, A.J. (1974). Comparison of Bender error and time scores for groups of epileptic, retarded, and behavior-problem children. *Perceptual and Motor Skills, 38*, 71–74.

Uchimaya, C.L., D'Elia, L.F., Dellinger, A.M., Becker, J.T., Selnes, O.A., Wesch, J.E., Chen, B.B., Satz, P., van Gorp, W., & Miller, E.N. (1995). Alternate forms of the Auditory Verbal Learning Test: Issue of test comparability, longitudinal reliability, and moderating variables. *Archives of Clinical Neuropsychology, 10*, 133–145.

Ullman, D.G., McKee, D.T., Campbell, K., Larrabee, G.J., & Trahan, D.E. (1997). Preliminary children's norms for the Continuous Visual Memory Test. *Child Neuropsychology, 3*, 171–175.

Upper, D., & Seeman, W. (1966). Brain-damage, schizophrenia, and five MMPI items. *Journal of Clinical Psychology, 24*, 444.

Urbina, S.P., & Clayton, J.P. (1991). WPPSI-R/WISC-R: A comparative study. *Journal of Psychoeducational Assessment, 9*, 247–254.

Urmer, A.H., Morris, A.B., & Wendland, L.V. (1960). The effect of brain damage on Raven's Progressive Matrices. *Journal of Clinical Psychology, 16*, 182–185.

U.S. Employment Service (1970). *Manual for the General Aptitude Test Battery*. Washington, DC: U.S. Department of Labor.

Uttl, B., & Graf, P. (1997). Color–Word Stroop Test performance across the adult life span. *Journal of Clinical and Experimental Neuropsychology, 19*, 405–420.

Vagrecha, Y.S., & Sen Mazumadar, D.P. (1974). Relevance of Piotrowski's signs in relation to intellectual deficit in organic (epileptic) and normal subjects. *Indian Journal of Clinical Psychology, 1*, 64–68.

Vakil, E., & Blachstein, H. (1993). Rey Auditory–Verbal Learning Test: Structure analysis. *Journal of Clinical Psychology, 49*, 883–890.

Vakil, E., & Blachstein, H. (1997). Rey AVLT: Developmental norms for adults and the sensitivity of different memory measures to age. *The Clinical Neuropsychologist, 11*, 356–369.

Vakil, E., Blachstein, H., Sheleff, P., & Grossman, S. (1989). BVRT: Scoring system and time delay in differentiation of lateralized hemispheric damage. *International Journal of Clinical Neuropsychology, 11*, 125–128.

Valencia-Flores, M., Bliwsie, D.L., Guilleminault, C., Cilveti, R., & Clerk, A. (1996). Cognitive function in patients with sleep apnea after acute nocturnal nasal continuous positive airflow pressure (CPAP) treatment: Sleepiness and hypoxemia effects. *Journal of Clinical and Experimental Neuropsychology, 18*, 197–210.

Valencia, R.R. (1984). The McCarthy scales and Kaufman's McCarthy short forms correlations with the Comprehensive Test of Basic Skills. *Psychology in the Schools, 21*, 141–147.

Valencia, R.R., & Rothwell, J.G. (1984). Concurrent validity of the WPPSI with Mexican-American preschool children. *Educational and Psychological Measurement, 44*, 955–961.

Vance, B. (1988). Concurrent validity of the Quick Test, the Test of Nonverbal Intelligence, and the WISC-R for a sample of special education students. *Psychological Reports, 62*, 443–446.

Vance, H.B., & Engin, A. (1978). Analysis of cognitive abilities of black children's performance on WISC-R. *Journal of Clinical Psychology, 34*, 452–456.

Vance, H., Blixt, S., & Ellis, C.R. (1980). Equivalence of Forms One and Three of the Quick Test. *Psychological Reports, 46*, 1184–1186.

Vance, H.B., Blixt, S., Ellis, R., & Bebell, S. (1981). Stability of the WISC-R for a sample of exceptional children. *Journal of Clinical Psychology, 37*, 397–399.

Vance, B., Lester, M.L., & Thatcher, R.W. (1983). Interscorer reliability of the Minnesota Percepto-Diagnostic Test-Revised. *Psychology in the Schools, 20*, 420–423.

Vance, H.B., Kitson, D., & Singer, M.G. (1985). Relationship between the standard scores of Peabody Picture Vocabulary Test-Revised and the Wide Range Achievement Test. *Journal of Clinical Psychology, 41*, 691–693.

Vance, B., Hankins, N., & Brown, W. (1988). Ethnic and sex differences on the Test of Nonverbal Intelligence, the Quick Test of Intelligence and the Wechsler Intelligence Scale for Children-Revised. *Journal of Clinical Psychology, 44*, 261–265.

Vance, H.B., Hankins, N., & Reynolds, F. (1988). Prediction of Wechsler Intelligence Scale for Children-Revised Full Scale IQ from the Quick Test of Intelligence and the Nonverbal Test of Intelligence for a referred sample of children and youth. *Journal of Clinical Psychology, 44*, 793–794.

Vance, B., West, R., & Kutsick, K. (1989). Prediction of Wechsler Preschool and Primary Scale of Intelligence IQ scores (WPPSI-R), Peabody Picture Vocabulary Test-R (PPVT-R), and the Expressive One-Word Picture Vocabulary test (EOWPVT). *Journal of Clinical Psychology, 45*, 642–644.

van den Broek, A., Golden, C.J., Loonstra, A., Ghinglia, K., & Goldstein, D. (1998). Short forms of the Wechsler memory Scale- Revised: Cross-validation and derivation of a two-subtest form. *Psychological Assessment, 10*, 38–40.

van den Burg, W., & Kingma, A. (1999). Performance of 225 Dutch children on Rey's Auditory Verbal Learning Test (AVLT): Parallel test–retest reliabilities with an interval of 3 months and normative data. *Archives of Clinical Neuropsychology, 14*, 545–599.

van der Hurk, P.R., & Hodges, J.R. (1995). Episodic and semantic memory in Alzheimer's disease and progressive supranuclear palsy: A comparative study. *Journal of Clinical and Experimental Neuropsychology, 17*, *59–471.

Vanderploeg, R.D. (1994). Estimating premorbid level of functioning. In R.D. Vanderploeg (Ed.), *Clinician's guide to neuropsychological assessment* (pp. 43–68). Hillsdale, NJ: Lawrence J. Erlbaum.

Vanderploeg, R.D., & Schinka, J.A. (1995). Predicting WAIS-R premorbid ability: Combining subtest performance and demographic variable predictors. *Archives of Clinical Neuropsychology, 10*, 225–239.

Vanderploeg, R.D., Schinka, J.A., & Retzlaff, P. (1994). Relationships between measures of auditory verbal learning and executive functioning. *Journal of Clinical and Experimental Neuropsychology, 16*, 243–252.

Vanderploeg, R.D., Schinka, J.A., & Axelrod, B.N. (1996). Estimation of WAIS-R premorbid intelligence: Current ability and demographic data used in a best performance fashion. *Psychological Assessment, 8*, 404–411.

Vanderploeg, R.D., Axelrod, B.N., Shere, M., Scott, J., & Adams, R.L. (1997a). The importance of demographic adjustments on neuropsychological test performance: A response to Reitan and Wolfson (1995). *The Clinical Neuropsychologist, 11*, 210–217.

Vanderploeg, R.D., LaLone, L.V., Greblo, P., & Schinka, J.A. (1997b). Odd–even short forms of the Judgment of Line Orientation Test. *Applied Neuropsychology, 4*, 244–246.

Van Dyke, C., Mueller, J., & Kiernan, R. (1987). The case for psychiatrists as authorities on cognition. *Psychosomatics, 28*, 87–89.

Vangel, S.J., & Lichtenberg, P.A. (1995). Mattis Dementia Rating Scale: Clinical utility and relationship with deomgraphic variables. *The Clinical Neuropsychologist, 9*, 209–213.

van Gorp, W.G., Satz, P., Kiersch, M.E., & Henry, R. (1986). Normative data on the Boston Naming Test for a group of normal older adults. *Journal of Clinical and Experimental Neuropsychology, 8*, 702–709.

van Gorp, W.G., Kalechstein, A.D., Moore, L.H., Hinkin, C.H., Mahler, M.E., Foti, D., & Mendez, M. (1997). A clinical comparison of two forms of the Card Sorting Test. *The Clinical Neuropsychologist, 11*, 155–160.

van Hagen, J., & Kaufman, A.S. (1975). Factor analysis of the WISC-R for a group of mentally retarded children and adolescents. *Journal of Consulting and Clinical Psychology, 43*, 661–667.

Varney, N.R. (1981). Letter recognition and visual form discrimination in aphasic alexia. *Neuropsychologia, 19*, 795–800.

Varney, N.R., & Benton, A.L. (1982). Qualitative aspects of pantomime recognition in aphasia. *Brain and Cognition, 1*, 132–139.

Vega, A., Jr., & Parsons, O.A. (1967). Cross-validation of the Halstead–Reitan tests for brain damage. *Journal of Consulting Psychology, 31*, 619–625.

Veiel, H.O.F. (1997a). A preliminary profile of neuropsychological deficits associated with major depression. *Journal of Clinical and Experimental Neuropsychology, 19*, 587–603.

Veiel, H.O.F. (1997b). CVLT recognition-recall discrepancies and retrieval deficits. A comment on Wilde et al. (1995). *Journal of Clinical and Experimental Neuropsychology, 19*, 141–143.

Velborsky, J. (1964). Der Benton-Test in der klinischen Praxis. *Diagnostica, 10*, 91–102.

Vendrell, P., Junque, C., Pujol, J., Jurado, M.A., Molet, J., & Grafman, J. (1995). The role of prefrontal regions in the Stroop task. *Neuropsychologia, 33*, 341–352.

Venkatesan, S. (1991). Bender Gestalt Visuo Motor Test as a measure of intelligence in mentally handicapped individuals. *Indian Journal of Clinical Psychology, 18*, 7–9.

Verma, S.K., Pershad, D., & Khanna, R. (1993). Hooper's Visual Organization Test: Item analysis on Indian subjects. *Indian Journal of Clinical Psychology, 20*, 5–10.

Viglione, D.J., Jr. (1997). Problems in Rorschach research and what to do about them. *Journal of Personality Research, 68*, 590–599.

Viglione, D., & Exner, J. (1983). Current research in the comprehensive Rorschach systems. In J. Butcher & C. Spielberger (Eds.), *Advances in personality assessment* (Vol. 1). Hillsdale, NJ: Lawrence J. Erlbaum.

Vincent, K.R. (1990). The fragile nature of MMPI code types. *Journal of Clinical Psychology, 46*, 800–802.

Vingerhoets, G., van Nooten, G., & Jannes, C. (1997). Neuropsychological impairment in candidates for cardiac surgery. *Journal of the International Neuropsychological Society, 3*, 480–484.

Vitaliano, P.P., Breen, A.R., Russo, J., Albert, M.S., Vitiello, M., & Prinz, P.N. (1984a). The clinical utility of the Dementia Rating Scale for assessing Alzheimer's patients. *Journal of Chronic Disability, 37*, 743–753.

Vitaliano, P.P., Breen, A.R., Russo, J., Albert, M.S., Vitiello, M., & Prinz, P.N. (1984b). Memory, attention, and functional status in community residing Alzheimer type dementia patients and optimally healthy aged individuals. *Journal of Gerontology, 39*, 58–64.

Vlachos, F.M., & Karapetsas, A.B. (1994). Visuomotor organization in the right-handed and the left-handed child: A comparative neuropsychological approach. *Applied Neuropsychology, 1*, 33–37.

Vogel, W. (1962). Some effects of brain lesions on MMPI profiles. *Journal of Consulting Psychology, 26*, 412.

Volkow, N.D., Gur, R.C., Wang, G.J., Fowler, J.S., Moberg, P.J., Ding, Y.S., Hitzeman, R., Smith, G., & Logan, J. (1998). Association between decline in brain dopamine activity with age and cognitive and motor impairment in healthy individuals. *American Journal of Psychiatry, 155*, 344–349.

Waber, B.P., & Bernstein, J.H. (1995). Performance of learning-disabled and non-learning-disabled children on the Rey–Osterrieth Complex Figure: Validation of the developmental scoring system. *Developmental Neuropsychology*, *11*, 237–252.

Waber, D.P., & Holmes, J.M. (1985). Assessing children's copy production of the Rey–Osterrieth Complex Figures. *Journal of Clinical and Experimental Neuropsychology*, *7*, 264–280.

Waber, D.P., & Holmes, J.M. (1986). Assessing children's memory production of the Rey–Osterrieth Complex Figures. *Journal of Clinical and Experimental Neuropsychology*, *8*, 563–580.

Wachter, K.W., & Straf, M.L. (1990). *The future of meta-analysis*. New York: Russell Sage Foundation.

Wagner, E.E., & Gianakos, I. (1985). Comparison of WAIS and WAIS-R scaled scores for an outpatient clinical sample retested over extended intervals. *Perceptual and Motor Skills*, *61*, 87–90.

Wahler, C. (1956). A comparison of reproductive errors made by brain-damaged and control patients on a memory-for-designs test. *Journal of Abnormal and Social Psychology*, *52*, 251–255.

Wake, F.R. (1956). Finger localization in Canadian school children. Presented at the Annual Meeting of the Canadian Psychological Association, June, Ottawa.

Wake, F.R. (1957). Finger localization scores in defective children. Presented at the Annual Meeting of the Canadian Psychological Association, June, Toronto.

Waldman, D.A., & Avolio, B.J. (1989). Homogeneity of test validity. *Journal of Applied Psychology*, *7*, 371–374.

Waldstein, S.R., Ryan, C.M., Jennings, J.R., Muldoon, M.F., & Manuck, S.B. (1997). Self-reported levels of anxiety do not predict neuropsychological performance in healthy men. *Archives of Clinical Neuropsychology*, *12*, 567–574.

Wallace, J.L. (1984). Wechsler Memory Scale. *International Journal of Clinical Neuropsychology*, *6*(suppl.), 216–226.

Wallbrown, F.H., & Fremont, T. (1980). The stability of Koppitz scores on the Bender Gestalt for reading disabled children. *Psychology in the Schools*, *17*, 181–184.

Wallbrown, F.H., & Fuller, G.B. (1984). A five step procedure for the clinical use of the MPD in neuropsychological assessment of children. *Journal of Clinical Psychology*, *40*, 220–229.

Wallbrown, F.H., Blaha, J., Wallbrown, J.D., & Engin, H. (1975). The hierarchical factor structure of the Wechsler Intelligence Scale for Children-Revised. *Journal of Psychology*, *77*, 223–235.

Wallbrown, F.H., Wallbrown, J.D., & Engin, A.W. (1976). Test–retest reliability of the Bender–Gestalt for first grade children. *Perceptual and Motor Skills*, *42*, 743–746.

Wallbrown, J.D., Wallbrown, F.H., & Engin, A.W. (1977). The validity of two clinical tests of visual-motor perception. *Journal of Clinical Psychology*, *33*, 491–495.

Walsh, P.F., Lichtenberg, P.A., & Rowe, R.J. (1997). Hooper Visual Organization Test performance in geriatric rehabilitation patients. *Clinical Gerontologist*, *17*, 3–11.

Walton, D. (1957). The validity of a psychological test of brain damage. *Bulletin of the British Psychological Society*, No. 34.

Walton, D., & Black, D.A. (1957). The validity of a psychological test of brain damage. *British Journal of Medical Psychology*, *30*, 270–279.

Walton, D., White, J.G., Black, D.A., & Young, A.J. (1959). The Modified New Word Learning Test: A cross-validation study. *The British Journal of Medical Psychology*, *32*, 213–220.

Wang, P.L. (1977). Visual organization ability in brain-damaged adults. *Perceptual and Motor Skills*, *45*, 723–728.

Wang, E.W., Rogers, R., Giles, C.L., Diamond, P.M., Herrington-Wang, L.E., & Taylor, E.R. (1997). A pilot study of the Personality Assessment Inventory (PAI) in corrections: Assessment of malingering, suicide risk, and aggression in male inmates. *Behavioral Sciences and the Law*, *15*, 469–482.

Ward, L.C. (1990). Prediction of Verbal Performance, and Full Scale IQS from seven subtests of the WAIS-R. *Journal of Clinical Psychology*, *46*, 436–440.

Ward, L.C., & Ryan, J.J. (1996). Validity and time savings in the selection of short forms of the Wechsler Adult Intelligence Scale-Revised. *Psychological Assessment*, *8*, 69–72.

Ward, C.L., & Ryan, J.J. (1997). Validity of quick short forms of the Wechsler Adult Intelligence Scale-Revised with brain damaged patients. *Archives of Clinical Neuropsychology*, *12*, 63–69.

Ward, L.O. (1982). Variables influencing children's formulation of criteria of classification as measured by a modification of the Weigl Sorting Test. *Journal of Psychology*, *111*, 211–216.

Warrington, E.K. (1984). *Recognition Memory Test*. Windsor, England: NFER-Nelson.

Warrington, E.K., & Weiskrantz, L. (1973) An analysis of short- and long-term memory defects in man. In J.A. Deutsch (Ed.), *The physiological basis of memory*. New York: Academic Press.

Warschausky, S., Kewman, D.G., & Selim, A. (1996). Attentional performance of children with traumatic brain injury: A quantitative and qualitative analysis of Digit Span. *Archives of Clinical Neuropsychology, 11*, 147–153.

Wasyliw, O.E., Benn, A.F., Grossman, L.S., & Haywood, T.W. (1998). Detection of minimization of psychopathology on the Rorschach in cleric and noncleric alleged sex offenders. *Assessment, 5*, 389–397.

Watkins, C.E., & Campbell, V.L. (1992). The test retest reliability and stability of the WAIS–R in a sample of mentally retarded adults. *Journal of Intellectual Disability Research, 36*, 265–268.

Watkins, C.E., Edinger, J.D., & Shipley, R.H. (1986). Validity of a WAIS-R screening instrument (Satz–Mogel) for medical inpatients. *Rehabilitation Psychology, 31*, 103–109.

Watkins, C.E., Himmell, C.D., Polk, N.E., & Reinberg, J.A. (1988). WAIS-R short forms with mentally retarded adults: A note of caution. *Journal of Mental Deficiency, 32*, 239–242.

Watkins, C.E., McKay, B.L., Parra, R.A., & Polk, N.E. (1987). Using WAIS-R short forms with clinical outpatients: A cautionary note. *Professional Psychology: Research and Practice, 18*, 397–398.

Watkins, K.E., Hewes, D.K., Connelly, A., Kendall, B.E., Kingsley, D.P., Evans, J.E., Gadian, D.G., Vargha-Khadem, F., & Kirkham, F.J. (1998). Cognitive deficits associated with frontal-lobe infarction in children with sickle cell disease. *Developmental Medicine and Child Neurology, 40*, 536–543.

Watkins, M.W., Marley, W., Kush, J.C., & Glutting, J.J. (1997). Discriminant and predictive validity of the WISC-III ACID profile among children with learning disabilities. *Psychology in the Schools, 34*, 309–319.

Watson, C.G. (1968). The separation of NP hospital organics from schizophrenics with three visual motor screening tests. *Journal of Clinical Psychology, 24*, 412–414.

Watson, C.G. (1971). An MMPI scale to separate brain-damaged patients from schizophrenics. *Journal of Consulting and Clinical Psychology, 36*, 121–125.

Watson, C.G. (1973). A simple bivariate screening technique to separate NP hospital organics from other psychiatric groups. *Journal of Clinical Psychology, 29*, 448–450.

Watson, C.G., & Plemel, D. (1978). An MMPI scale to separate brain-damaged from functional psychiatric patients in neuropsychiatric settings. *Journal of Consulting and Clinical Psychology, 46*, 1127–1132.

Watson, C.G., & Thomas, R.W. (1968). MMPI profiles of brain-damaged and schizophrenic patients. *Perceptual and Motor Skills, 27*, 567–573.

Watson, C.G., Felling, J., & Maceachern, D.G. (1967). Objective Draw-A-Person scales: An attempted cross-validation. *Journal of Clinical Psychology, 23*, 382–386.

Watson, C.G., Thomas, R.W., Felling, J., & Anderson, D. (1968). Differentiation of organics from schizophrenics with the Trail Making Dynamometer, Critical Flicker Fusion, and Light-Intensity Matching Tests. *Journal of Clinical Psychology, 25*, 130–133.

Watson, C.G., Gasser, B., Schaefer, A., Buranen, C., & Wold, J. (1981). Separation of brain damaged from psychiatric patients with ability and personality measures. *Journal of Clinical Psychology, 37*, 347–353.

Watson, C.G., Plemel, D., Schaefer, A., Raden, M., Alfano, A.M, Anderson, P.E.D., Thomas, D., & Anderson, D. (1992). The comparative concurrent validities of the Shipley Institute of Living Scale and the Henmon–Nelson Tests of Mental Ability. *Journal of Clinical Psychology, 48*, 233–239.

Watts, F.N., & Everitt, B.S. (1980). The factorial structure of the General Aptitude Test Battery. *Journal of Clinical Psychology, 36*, 763–767.

Wechsler, D. (1945). A standardized memory scale for clinical use. *Journal of Psychology, 19*, 87–95.

Wechsler, D. (1958). *The measurement and appraisal of adult intelligence* (4th ed.). Baltimore: Williams & Wilkins.

Wechsler, D. (1974). *Manual for the Wechsler Intelligence Scale for Children-Revised*. New York: The Psychological Corporation.

Wechsler, D. (1981). *WAIS-R manual*. New York: The Psychological Corporation.

Wechsler, D. (1987). *Wechsler Memory Scale-Revised manual*. San Antonio: The Psychological Corporation-Harcourt Brace Jovanovich.

Wechsler, D. (1991). *Wechsler Intelligence Scale for Children-Third Edition manual*. San Antonio, TX: The Psychological Corporation.

Wechsler, D. (1997a). *Wechsler Adult Intelligence Scale-Third Edition*. San Antonio TX: The Psychological Corporation.

Wechsler, D. (1997b). Wechsler Memory Scale-Third Edition. San Antonio, TX: The Psychological Corporation.

Wechsler, D., & Stone, C.P. (1973). *Wechsler Memory Scale Manual*. New York: The Psychological Corporation.

Wedding, D. (1983). Comparison of statistical and actuarial models for predicting lateralization of brain damage. *Clinical Neuropsychology, 5*, 15–20.

Weigl, E. (1941). On the psychology of so-called processes of abstraction. *Journal of Abnormal and Social Psychology, 36*, 3–33.

Weigner, S., & Donders, J. (1999). Performance on the Wisconsin Card Sorting Test after traumatic brain injury. *Assessment, 6*, 179–187.

Weinberg, J., Diller, L., Gerstman, L., & Schulman, P. (1972). Digit span in left and right hemiplegics. *Journal of Clinical Psychology, 28*, 361.

Weiner, I.B. (1996). Some observations on the validity of the Rorschach inkblot method. *Psychological Assessment, 8*, 206–213.

Weingarden, B.J., Yates, B.L., Moses, A.J., Jr., Benton, A.L., & Faustman, W.O. (1998). Development of an optimally reliable short form for the Judgment of Line Orientation. *The Clinical Neuropsychologist, 12*, 311–314.

Weingartner, H., & Silberman, E. (1982). Models of cognitive impairment: Cognitive changes in depression. *Psychopharmacology Bulletin, 18*(2), 27–42.

Weingold, H.P., Dawson, J.G., & Kael, H.C. (1965). Further examination of Hovey's "Index" for identification of brain lesions: Validation study. *Psychological Reports, 16*, 1098.

Weinman, J., & Cooper, R.L. (1981). Individual differences in perceptual problem solving ability: A response analysis approach. *Intelligence, 5*, 165–178.

Weinstein, S. (1964). Deficits concomitant with aphasia or lesions of either cerebral hemisphere. *Cortex, 1*, 154–169.

Weise, M.J., Struer, J.H., Piersel, W.C., & Schwarting, F.G. (1987). Stability of the WISC-R and WRAT factor scores for an intellectually retarded sample: A three year follow-up. *Journal of Psychoeducational Assessment, 5*, 364–369.

Weiss, D.J. (1985). Adaptive testing by computer. *Journal of Consulting and Clinical Psychology, 53*, 774–789.

Weiss, L.G., & Prifitera, A. (1995). An evaluation of differential prediction of WIAT achievement scores from WISC-III FSIQ across ethnic and gender groups. *Journal of School Psychology, 33*, 297–304.

Welch, L.W., Doineau, D., Johnson, S., & King, D. (1996). Educational and gender normative data for the Boston Naming Test in a group of older adults. *Brain and Language, 53*, 260–266.

Welsh, G.S. (1956). Factor dimensions A and R. In G.S. Welsh & W.G. Dahlstrom (Eds.), *Basic readings on the MMPI in psychology and medicine*. Minneapolis: University of Minnesota Press.

West, R., & Bell, M.A. (1997). Stroop color-word interference and electroencephalogram activation: Evidence for age-related decline of the anterior attention system. *Neuropsychology, 11*, 421–427.

Wetter, M.W., & Deitsch, S.E. (1996). Faking specific disorders and temporal response consistency on the MMPI-2. *Psychological Assessment, 8*, 39–47.

Wetzel, L., & Boll, T.J. (1987). *Short Category Test, Booklet Format*. Los Angeles: Western Psychological Services.

Wetzel, L., & Murphy, S.G. (1991). Validity of the use of a discontinue rule and evaluation of discriminability of the Hooper Visual Organization Test. *Neuropsychology, 5*, 119–122.

Wheeler, L., & Reitan, R.M. (1963). Discriminant functions applied to the problem of predicting cerebral damage from behavioral tests: A cross validation study. *Perceptual and Motor Skills, 16*, 681–701.

Wheeler, L., Burke, C.J., & Reitan, R.M. (1963). An application of discriminant functions to the problem of predicting brain damage using behavioral variables. *Perceptual and Motor Skills, 16*, 417–440.

White, F., Lynch, J.I., & Hayden, M.E. (1978). Use of the Leiter International Performance Scale with adult aphasics. *Journal of Clinical Psychology, 38*, 667–671.

White, J.G. (1959). Walton's Modified Word Learning Test with children. *British Journal of Medical Psychology, 32*, 221–225.

White, T.H. (1979). Correlations among the WISC-R, PIAT, and DAM. *Psychology in the Schools, 16*, 497–501.

Whitworth, R.H., & Gibbons, R.T. (1986). Cross-racial comparison of the WAIS and WAIS-R. *Educational and Psychological Measurement, 46*, 1041–1049.

Whorton, J.E., & Morgan, R.L. (1990). Comparison of the Test of Nonverbal Intelligence and Wechsler Intelligence Scale for Children-Revised in rural Native American and White children. *Perceptual and Motor Skills, 70*, 12–14.

Wickoff, R.L. (1978). Correlational and factor analysis of the Peabody Individual Achievement Test and the WISC-R. *Journal of Consulting and Clinical Psychology, 46*, 322–325.

Wickoff, R.L. (1979). The WISC-R as a predictor of achievement. *Psychology in the Schools, 16*, 364–366.

Widiger, T.A., Knudson, R.M., & Rorer, L.G. (1980). Convergent and discriminant validity of measures of cognitive styles and abilities. *Journal of Personality and Social Psychology, 39*, 116–129.

Wielkiewicz, R.M. (1990). Interpreting low scores on the WISC-R third factor: It's more than distractibility. *Psychological Assessment, 2*, 91–97.

Wiens, A.N., & Matarazzo, J.D. (1977). WAIS and MMPI correlates of the Halstead–Reitan Neuropsychological Battery in normal male subjects. *The Journal of Nervous and Mental Disease, 164*, 112–121.

Wiens, A.N., McMinn, M.R., & Crossen, J.R. (1988). Rey Auditory–Verbal Learning Test: Development of norms for healthy young adults. *The Clinical Neuropsychologist, 2*, 67–87.

Wiens, A.N., Bryan, J.E., & Crossen, J.R. (1993). Estimating WAIS-R FSIQ from the National Adult Reading Test-Revised in normal subjects. *The Clinical Neuropsychologist, 7*, 70–84.

Wiens, A.N., Tindall, A.G., & Crossen, J.R. (1994). California Verbal Learning Test: A normative study. *The Clinical Neuropsychologist, 8*, 75–90.

Wiens, A.N., Fuller, K.H., & Crossen, J.R. (1997). Paced Auditory Serial Attention Test: Adult norms and moderator variables. *Journal of Clinical and Experimental Neuropsychology, 19*, 473–483.

Wiese, M.J., Struer, J.H., Piersel, W.C., & Schwarting, F.G. (1987). Stability of the WISC-R and WRAT factor structure for an intellectually retarded sample: A 3-year follow-up. *Journal of Psychoeducational Assessment, 5*, 364–369.

Wiggins, E.C., & Brandt, J. (1988). The detection of simulated amnesia. *Law and Human Behavior, 12*, 57–78.

Wilde, M.C., & Boake, C. (1994). Factorial validity of the California Verbal Learning Test in head injury. *Archives of Clinical Neuropsychology, 9*, 202.

Wilde, M.C., Boake, C., & Scherer, M. (1995). Do recognition-free recall discrepancies detect retrieval deficits in closed head injury? An exploratory analysis with the California Verbal Learning Test. *Journal of Clinical and Experimental Neuropsychology, 17*, 849–855.

Wilde, M.C., Boake, C., & Scherer, M. (1997). Do recognition-free recall discrepancies detect retrieval deficits in closed head injury? A response to Veiel. *Journal of Clinical and Experimental Neuropsychology, 19*, 153–155.

Wilkinson, G.S. (1993). *The Wide Range Achievement Test-Third Edition Administration manual*. Wilmington, DE: Wide Range, Inc.

Williams, B.W., Mack, W., & Henderson, V.W. (1989). Boston Naming Test in Alzheimer's disease. *Neuropsychologia, 27*, 1073–1079.

Williams, H.L. (1952). The development of a caudality scale for the MMPI. *Journal of Clinical Psychology, 8*, 293–297.

Williams, J., & Dykman, R.A. (1994). Nonverbal factors derived from children's performances on neuropsychological test instruments. *Developmental Neuropsychology, 10*, 19–26.

Williams, J., & Haut, J. (1995). Differential performances on the WRAML in children and adolescents diagnosed with epilepsy, head injury, and substance abuse. *Developmental Neuropsychology, 11*, 201–213.

Williams, J., Rickert, V., Hogan, J., Zolten, A.J., Satz, P., D'Elia, L.F., Asarnow, R.F., Zaucha, K., & Light, R. (1995). Children's Color Trails. *Archives of Clinical Neuropsychology, 10*, 211–213.

Williams, J.M. (1987). *Cognitive behavior ratings scale manual*. Odessa, FL: Psychological Assessment Resources, Inc.

Williams, J.M. (1991). Memory assessment scales professional manual. Odessa, FL: Psychological Assessment Resources.

Williams, J.M. (1996). A practical model of everyday assessment. In R.J. Sbordone & C.J. Long (Eds.), *Ecological validity of neuropsychological testing*. Del Ray Beach, FL: GR Press/St. Lucie Press.

Williamson, D., Krull, K.R., & Scott, J.G. (1996). Revision and further validation of the Oklahoma Premorbid Intelligence Estimate. Paper presented at the Sixteenth Annual Meeting of the National Academy of Neuropsychology, Orlando, FL.

Willis, W.G. (1984). Reanalysis of an actuarial approach to neuropsychological diagnosis in consideration of base rates. *Journal of Consulting and Clinical Psychology, 52*, 567–569.

Wilson, J.D., & Spangler, P.F. (1974). The Peabody Individual Achievement Test as a clinical tool. *Journal of Learning Disabilities, 7*, 60–63.

Wilson, J.M., & Wolfensberger, W. (1963). Color–blindness testing as an aid in the etiological diagnosis of mental retardation. *American Journal of Mental Deficiency, 67*, 914–915.

Wilson, R.S., Rosenbaum, G., Brown, G., Rourke, D., Whitman, D., & Grisell, J. (1978). An index of premorbid intelligence. *Journal of Consulting and Clinical Psychology, 46*, 1554–1555.

Wilson, R.S., Rosenbaum, G., & Brown, G. (1979). The problem of premorbid intelligence in neuropsychological assessment. *Journal of Clinical Neuropsychology, 1,* 49–53.

Wilson, R.S., Bacon, L.D., Kaszniak, A.W., & Fox, J.H. (1982). The episodic-semantic distinction and paired associate learning. *Journal of Consulting and Clinical Psychology, 50,* 154–155.

Withers, E., & Hinton, J. (1971). Three forms of the Clinical Tests of the Sensorium and their reliability. *British Journal of Psychiatry, 119,* 1–8.

Witmer, L.R. (1935). The association value of three-place consonant syllables. *Journal of Genetic Psychology, 47,* 337–359.

Wolf, F.M. (1986). *Meta-analysis: Quantitative methods for research synthesis.* Beverly Hills, CA: Sage.

Woloszyn, D.B., Murphy, S.G., Wetzel, L., & Fisher, W. (1993) Interrater agreement on the Wechsler Memory Scale-Revised in a mixed clinical sample. *Clinical Neuropsychologist, 7,* 467–471.

Wong, J.L. (1993). Comparison of the Shipley vs. WAIS-R subtests and summary scores in predicting college grade point average. *Perceptual and Motor Skills, 76,* 1075–1078.

Wong, J.L., & Gilpin, A.R. (1993). Verbal vs. visual categories on the Wechsler Memory Scale-Revised: How meaningful a distinction? *Journal of Clinical Psychology, 49,* 175–179.

Wong, J.L., Schefft, B.K., & Moses, J.A., Jr. (1990). A normative study of the Luria–Nebraska Neuropsychological Battery, Form II. *International Journal of Clinical Neuropsychology, 12,* 175–179.

Wong, J.L., Regennitter, R.P., & Barrios, F. (1994). Base rate and simulated symptoms of mild head injury among normals. *Archives of Clinical Neuropsychology, 9,* 411–425.

Wood, J.M., Nezworski, M.T., & Stejskal, W.J. (1996). The Comprehensive System for the Rorschach: A critical examination. *Psychological Science, 7,* 3–10.

Wood, J.M., Nezworski, M.T., & Stejskal, W.J. (1997). The reliability of the Comprehensive System for the Rorschach: A comment on Wood (1997). *Psychological Assessment, 9,* 490–494.

Wood, J.M., Nezworski, M.T., Stejskal, W.J., Garvin, S., & West, S.G. (1999). Methodological issues in evaluating Rorschach validity: A comment on Burns (1996), Weiner (1996), and Ganellen (1996). *Assessment, 6,* 115–129.

Wood, W.D., & Strider, M.A. (1980). Comparison of two methods of administering the Halstead Category Test. *Journal of Clinical Psychology, 36,* 476–479.

Woodard, J.L. (1993). A prorating system for the Wechsler Memory Scale-Revised. *Clinical Neuropsychologist, 7,* 219–223.

Woodard, J.L., & Axelrod, B.N. (1995). Parsimonious prediction of Wechsler Memory Scale-Revised memory indices. *Psychological Assessment, 7,* 445–449.

Woodard, J.L., Benedict, R.H.B., Roberts, V.J., Goldstein, F.C., Kinner, K.M., Capruso, D.X., & Clark, A.N. (1996). Short-form alternatives to the Judgment of Line Orientation Test. *Journal of Clinical and Experimental Neuropsychology, 18,* 898–904.

Woodard, J.L., Benedict, R.H.B., Salthouse, T.A., Toth, J.P., Zgaljardic, D.J., & Hancock, H.E. (1998). Normative data for equivalent, parallel forms of the Judgment of Line Orientation Test. *Journal of Clinical and Experimental Neuropsychology, 20,* 457–462.

Woodcock, R.W., & Johnson, M.B. (1989,1990). *Woodcock–Johnson Psycho-Educational Battery-Revised.* Chicago: Riverside Publishing.

Woodcock, R.W., & Mather, N. (1989,1990). WJ-R Tests of Cognitive Ability-Standard and Supplementary Batteries: Examiner's Manual. In R.W. Woodcock & M.B. Johnson, *Woodcock & Johnson Psycho-Educational Battery-Revised.* Chicago: Riverside Publishing.

Woodward, C.A. (1982). The Hooper Visual Organization Test: A case against its use in neuropsychological assessment. *Journal of Consulting and Clinical Psychology, 50,* 286–288.

Woodward, C.A., Santa-Barbara, J., & Roberts, R. (1975). Test–retest reliability of the Wide Range Achievement Test. *Journal of Clinical Psychology, 31,* 81–84.

Woodward, H., & Donders, J. (1998). The performance of children with traumatic head injury on the Wide Range Assessment of Memory and Learning-Screening. *Applied Neuropsychology, 5,* 113–119.

Worrall, L.E., Yiu, E.M.-L., Hickson, L.M.H., & Barnett, H.M. (1995). Normative data for the Boston Naming Test for Australian elderly. *Aphasiology, 9,* 541–551.

Worthing, R.J., Phye, G.D., & Nunn, G.D. (1984). Equivalence and concurrent validity of PPVT-R forms L and M for school-age children with special needs. *Psychology in the Schools, 21,* 296–299.

Wright, B.D. (1977). Solving measurement problems with the Rasch model. *Journal of Educational Measurement, 14,* 97–114.

Wright, D., & DeMers, S.T. (1982). Comparison of the relationship between two measures of visual-motor coordination and academic achievement. *Psychology in the Schools, 19*, 473–477.

Wrobel, N.H., & Wrobel, T.A. (1996). The problem of assessing brain damage in psychiatric samples: Use of personality variables in prediction of WAIS-R scores. *Archives of Clinical Neuropsychology, 11*, 625–635.

Yater, A.C., Barclay, A.G., & McGilligan, R. (1969). Interrater reliability of scoring Goodenough–Harris drawings by disadvantaged preschool children. *Perceptual and Motor Skills, 28*, 281–282.

Yeates, K.O. (1994). Comparison of developmental norms for the Boston Naming Test. *The Clinical Neuropsychologist, 8*, 91–98.

Yeates, K.O., & Taylor, H.G. (1997). Predicting premorbid neuropsychological functioning following pediatric traumatic brain injury. *Journal of Clinical and Experimental Neuropsychology, 19*, 825–837.

Yeates, K.O., Blumenstein, E., Patterson, C.M., & Delis, D.C. (1995). Verbal learning and memory deficits following pediatric closed-head injury. *Journal of the International Neuropsychological Society, 1*, 78–87.

Yeudall, L.T., Fromm, D., Reddon, J.R., & Stefanyk, W.O. (1986). Normative information stratified by age and sex for 12 neuropsychological tests. *Journal of Clinical Psychology, 42*, 918–946.

York, C.D., & Cermak, S.A. (1995). Visual perception and praxis in adults after stroke. *American Journal of Occupational Therapy, 49*, 543–550.

Youngjohn, J.R., Larrabee, G.J., & Crook, T.H. (1993). New adult age- and education-correction norms for the Benton Visual Retention Test. *The Clinical Neuropsychologist, 7*, 155–160.

Youngjohn, J.R., Davis, D., & Wolf, I. (1997). Head injury and the MMPI-2 Paradoxical severity effects and the influence of litigation. *Psychological Assessment, 9*, 177–184.

Ysseldyke, J.E. (1990). Goodness of fit of the Woodcock–Johnson Psycho-Educational Battery-Revised to the Horn–Cattell Gf-Gc Theory. *Journal of Psychoeducational Assessment, 8*, 268–275.

Yun, X., Yao-Xian, G., & Matthews, J.R. (1987). The Luria–Nebraska Neuropsychological Battery Revised in China. *International Journal of Clinical Neuropsychology, 9*, 97–105.

Yuspeh, R.L., Vanderploeg, R.D., & Kershaw, D.A.J. (1998). Normative data on a measure of estimated premorbid abilities as part of a dementia evaluation. *Applied Neuropsychology, 5*, 149–153.

Zachary, R.A., Crumpton, E.M., & Spiegel, D.E. (1985). Estimating WAIS-R IQ from the Shipley Institute of Living Scale. *Journal of Clinical Psychology, 41*, 532–540.

Zaidel, D., & Sperry, R.W. (1973). Performance on the Raven's Colored Progressive Matrices Test by subjects with cerebral commissurotomy. *Cortex, 9*, 34–39.

Zaidel, E., Zaidel, D.W., & Sperry, R.W. (1981). Left and right intelligence: Case study of Raven's Progressive Matrices following brain bisection and hemidecortication. *Cortex, 17*, 167–186.

Zangwill, O.L. (1966). Psychological deficits associated with frontal lobe lesions. *International Journal of Neurology, 5*, 395–402.

Zappala, G., Measso, G., Cavareran, F., Grigoletto, F., Lebowitz, B., Pirozzolo, F., Amaducci, L., Massari, D., & Crook, T. (1995). Aging and memory: Corrections for age, sex, and education for three widely used memory tests. *Italian Journal of Neurological Sciences, 16*, 177–184.

Zielinski, J.J. (1993). A comparison of the Wechsler Memory Scale-Revised and the Memory Assessment Scales: Administrative, clinical, and interpretative issues. *Professional Psychology: Research and Practice, 24*, 353–359.

Zillmer, E.A., Waechtler, C., Harris, B., Khan, F., & Fowler, P.C. (1992). The effects of unilateral and multifocal lesions on the WAIS-R: A factor analytic study of stroke patients. *Archives of Clinical Neuropsychology, 7*, 29–40.

Zimmerman, I.L. (1965). Residual effects of brain-damage and five MMPI items. *Journal of Consulting Psychology, 29*, 394.

Zimmerman, I.L., & Woo-Sam, J.M. (1997). Review of the criterion-related validity of the WISC-III: The first five years. *Perceptual and Motor Skills, 85*, 531–546.

Zinn, S., McCumber, S., & Dahlstrom, W.G. (1999). Cross-validation and extension of the MMPI-A IMM scale. *Assessment, 6*, 1–6.

Zucker, S., & Copeland, E.P. (1988). K-ABC and McCarthy scale performance among "at-risk" and normal preschoolers. *Psychology in the Schools, 25*, 5–10.

Zucker, S., & Riordan, J. (1988). Concurrent validity of new and revised conceptual language measures. *Psychology in the Schools, 25*, 252–256.

Zwick, R. (1988). Another look at interrater agreement. *Psychological Bulletin, 103*, 374–378.

Index

ISBN 0-306-46344-X

90000